MW00581171

Tumors of the Eye and Ocular Adnexa

AFIP Atlas of Tumor Pathology

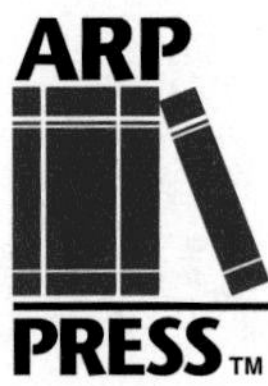

Editorial Director: Kelley S. Hahn
Production Editor: Dian S. Thomas
Editorial/Scanning Assistant: Mirlinda Q. Caton
Copy Editor: Audrey Kahn
Scanning Technician: Kenneth Stringfellow

Available from the American Registry of Pathology
Armed Forces Institute of Pathology
Washington, DC 20306-6000
www.afip.org
ISBN 1-881041-99-9

AFIP ATLAS OF TUMOR PATHOLOGY

Fourth Series
Fascicle 5

TUMORS OF THE EYE AND OCULAR ADNEXA

by

Ramon L. Font, MD
Director, Ophthalmic Pathology Laboratory
Professor of Pathology and Ophthalmology
Sarah Campbell Blaffer Professor of Ophthalmology
Cullen Institute, Baylor College of Medicine
Consultant in Pathology, University of Texas
M.D. Anderson Cancer Center, Houston, Texas

J. Oscar Croxatto, MD
Director of Laboratories and Research
Chairman, Department of Ophthalmic Pathology and Electron Microscopy
Fundación Oftalmológica Argentina Jorge Malbrán Azcuénaga
Buenos Aires, Argentina

Narsing A. Rao, MD
Professor of Pathology and Ophthalmology
University of Southern California School of Medicine
Los Angeles, California

Published by the
American Registry of Pathology
Washington, DC
in collaboration with the
Armed Forces Institute of Pathology
Washington, DC
2006

AFIP ATLAS OF TUMOR PATHOLOGY

EDITORS' NOTE

The Atlas of Tumor Pathology has a long and distinguished history. It was first conceived at a Cancer Research Meeting held in St. Louis in September 1947 as an attempt to standardize the nomenclature of neoplastic diseases. The first series was sponsored by the National Academy of Sciences-National Research Council. The organization of this Sisyphean effort was entrusted to the Subcommittee on Oncology of the Committee on Pathology, and Dr. Arthur Purdy Stout was the first editor-in-chief. Many of the illustrations were provided by the Medical Illustration Service of the Armed Forces Institute of Pathology (AFIP), the type was set by the Government Printing Office, and the final printing was done at the Armed Forces Institute of Pathology (hence the colloquial appellation "AFIP Fascicles"). The American Registry of Pathology (ARP) purchased the Fascicles from the Government Printing Office and sold them virtually at cost. Over a period of 20 years, approximately 15,000 copies each of nearly 40 Fascicles were produced. The worldwide impact of these publications over the years has largely surpassed the original goal. They quickly became among the most influential publications on tumor pathology, primarily because of their overall high quality but also because their low cost made them easily accessible the world over to pathologists and other students of oncology.

Upon completion of the first series, the National Academy of Sciences-National Research Council handed further pursuit of the project over to the newly created Universities Associated for Research and Education in Pathology (UAREP). A second series was started, generously supported by grants from the AFIP, the National Cancer Institute, and the American Cancer Society. Dr. Harlan I. Firminger became the editor-in-chief and was succeeded by Dr. William H. Hartmann. The second series' Fascicles were produced as bound volumes instead of loose leaflets. They featured a more comprehensive coverage of the subjects, to the extent that the Fascicles could no longer be regarded as "atlases" but rather as monographs describing and illustrating in detail the tumors and tumor-like conditions of the various organs and systems.

Once the second series was completed, with a success that matched that of the first, ARP, UAREP, and AFIP decided to embark on a third series. Dr. Juan Rosai was appointed as editor-in-chief, and Dr. Leslie H. Sobin became associate editor. A distinguished Editorial Advisory Board was also convened, and these outstanding pathologists and educators played a major role in the success of this series, the first publication of which appeared in 1991 and the last (number 32) in 2003.

The same organizational framework will apply to the current fourth series, but with UAREP no longer in existence, ARP will play the major role. New features will include a hardbound cover, illustrations almost exclusively in color, and an accompanying electronic version of each Fascicle. There will also be increased emphasis (wherever appropriate) on the cytopathologic (intraoperative, exfoliative, and/or fine needle aspiration) and molecular features that are important in diagnosis and prognosis. What will not change from the three previous series, however, is the goal of providing the practicing pathologist with thorough, concise, and up-to-date information on the nomenclature and classification; epidemiologic, clinical, and pathogenetic features; and, most importantly, guidance in the diagnosis of the tumors and tumorlike lesions of all major organ systems and body sites.

As in the third series, a continuous attempt will be made to correlate, whenever possible, the nomenclature used in the Fascicles with that proposed by the World Health Organization's Classification of Tumors, as well as to ensure a consistency of style throughout. Close cooperation between the various authors and their respective liaisons from the Editorial Board will continue to be emphasized in order to minimize unnecessary repetition and discrepancies in the text and illustrations.

Particular thanks are due to the members of the Editorial Advisory Board, the reviewers (at least two for each Fascicle), the editorial and production staff, and—first and foremost—the individual Fascicle authors for their ongoing efforts to ensure that this series is a worthy successor to the previous three.

Steven G. Silverberg, MD
Leslie H. Sobin, MD

PREFACE

In the Fourth Series, the tumors of the eye and ocular adnexa are organized to reflect an anatomic approach, with emphasis on ocular tumors followed by adnexal neoplasms. Chapters reflect various anatomic sites: conjunctiva, uvea, retina, optic nerve, eyelids, lacrimal gland, and orbit. In order to provide a structured approach, the chapters list salient anatomic and histologic features of the involved tissues followed by a section on general considerations. The latter includes the incidence of various tumors at an anatomic site, for example, the incidence of conjunctival tumors, in a referral ophthalmic pathology laboratory such as at the Armed Forces Institute of Pathology (AFIP) and at university hospitals such as the University of Southern California and Baylor College of Medicine. Where available, the etiology of the ocular tumor is discussed, followed by demographic features and common clinical presentations. Relevant microscopic grading of these tumors, and treatment and overall prognosis of the patients, are included. Our main objective is to emphasize the important features that are of special interest to general and surgical pathologists.

Following the general considerations, each chapter lists the benign and malignant tumors that appear at each anatomic site. Similar to the Third Series Fascicle, tumors are classified on the basis of histologic type and biologic behavior. For instance, conjunctival tumors are classified into epithelial tumors, melanocytic tumors, lymphoid tumors, and others. Since a large number of tumors develop at various ocular and adnexal sites, those that are unique to the eye and those that are encountered in related anatomic sites (eyelids, orbit) are included, provided such tumors are of clinical importance and biologic significance as a prototypic example of cancer biology (e.g., retinoblastoma). Although melanocytic lesions, like nevi, are covered in the Fascicle on skin tumors, conjunctival nevi exhibit distinct histologic features (e.g., cystic compound nevus) and the conjunctiva is the only site for the development of premalignant lesions such as primary acquired melanosis. Such entities are discussed in detail under the following subheadings: definition of the tumor; general features, which includes a brief history; pathogenesis and epidemiologic observations; clinical features; gross and microscopic findings; cytology (if applicable); differential diagnosis; and special studies. When applicable, the studies include immunohistochemistry and molecular approaches including ploidy, gene translocations, oncogenes, gene rearrangement for lymphomas, microdissection, and polymerase chain reaction–based amplification to detect genes of interest, as well as prognosis and treatment.

There are ocular and adnexal tumors that appear elsewhere in the body as well, for example, basal cell carcinoma and lymphomas (except primary intraocular large B-cell lymphoma of the retina and vitreous). These entities are briefly described along with appropriate references to other Fascicles for additional details. Moreover, we included relevant anatomic references relating to gross examination of ocular specimens and techniques for cutting the eye, as well as important anatomic landmarks. General guidelines on the processing of ocular specimens are also included.

Ramon L. Font, MD
J. Oscar Croxatto, MD
Narsing A. Rao, MD

ACKNOWLEDGEMENTS

This Fourth Series Fascicle, Tumors of the Eye and Ocular Adnexa, builds upon the work that appeared in the previous series, the contributions of ophthalmic pathologists that appeared in the ophthalmic pathology text and atlas edited by Spencer, and the 1978 World Health Organization monograph on ophthalmic neoplasms by Zimmerman. A vast majority of the illustrations used in the current Fascicle are from the files of the Ophthalmic Pathology Laboratory of the Armed Forces Institute of Pathology; the Cullen Eye Institute, Baylor College of Medicine; and the Doheny Eye Institute, Keck School of Medicine, University of Southern California.

For preparation of this Fascicle we had the assistance of several people whom it is a pleasure to acknowledge. Dr. Krishna Kumar compiled the data on the distribution of various ocular and adnexal tumors filed at the Doheny Eye Institute.

We greatly appreciate the photographic and computer expertise and support provided by Mrs. Jo Anne Johnson, Department of Ophthalmology, Baylor College of Medicine, Houston, Texas.

We are deeply grateful for the support and caring provided by our spouses, Hilda, Mirtha, and Sarojini, and for their patience in allowing our work to be a top priority.

Ramon L. Font, MD

J. Oscar Croxatto, MD

Narsing A. Rao, MD

Permission to use copyrighted illustrations has been granted by:

American Academy of Ophthalmology
Ophthalmic Anatomy: A Manual with Some Clinical Application, 1970. For Figure 7-1.

CONTENTS

1 TUMORS OF THE CONJUNCTIVA AND CARUNCLE

ANATOMY AND HISTOLOGY

The conjunctiva, a mucous membrane composed of epithelium and substantia propria, covers and connects the anterior surface of the eye and the inner surface of the eyelids. Although the conjunctiva is a continuous layer, for descriptive purposes it is divided into a palpebral portion (tarsal) lining the undersurface of the eyelid, a forniceal portion or intermediate part forming a conjunctival cul de sac where it reflects onto the surface of the globe, a bulbar portion covering the exposed part of the eyeball to the cornea (fig. 1-1), and associated elements, the plica semilunaris and the caruncle.

The epithelium of the conjunctiva is continuous with the corneal epithelium and with the epidermis of the eyelid margin through a transition zone of nonkeratinized stratified squamous epithelium. The conjunctival epithelium is composed of cuboidal and cylindrical cells arranged in two to five layers, with the addition of mucus-secreting goblet cells (fig. 1-2). The superficial epithelial cells may resemble apocrine cells due to the presence of eosinophilic cytoplasm and apical snouts. Goblet cells are abundant toward the fornix and at the nasal side of the bulbar conjunctiva. Other cells present in the conjunctival epithelium include melanocytes, Langerhans cells, and wandering intraepithelial lymphocytes. The limbal conjunctiva is the anular area that extends from the cornea to about 3 mm on the bulbar portion. The basal epithelial layers of the limbal conjunctiva contain the stem cells that repopulate the corneal epithelium. Branching dendritic melanocytes are abundant in this region and are often associated with melanin-containing basal epithelial cells.

The substantia propria of the bulbar conjunctiva is composed of loose connective tissue and a deeper dense collagenous layer. The connective tissue is composed of haphazardly arranged collagen fibers, loosely intermixed fibroblasts, blood vessels, lymphatic vessels, scattered mast cells, macrophages, lymphocytes, plasma cells, polymorphonuclear leukocytes, and eosinophils. The substantia propria of the palpebral conjunctiva is more uniform, and is closely

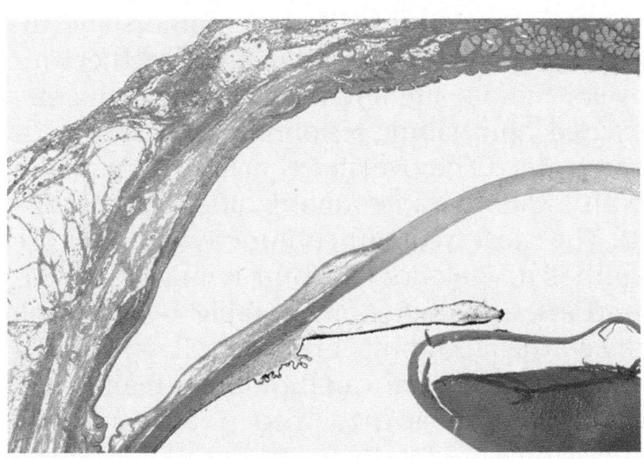

Figure 1-1

NORMAL CONJUNCTIVA

The different appearances of the bulbar, forniceal, and palpebral portions of the conjunctiva are illustrated.

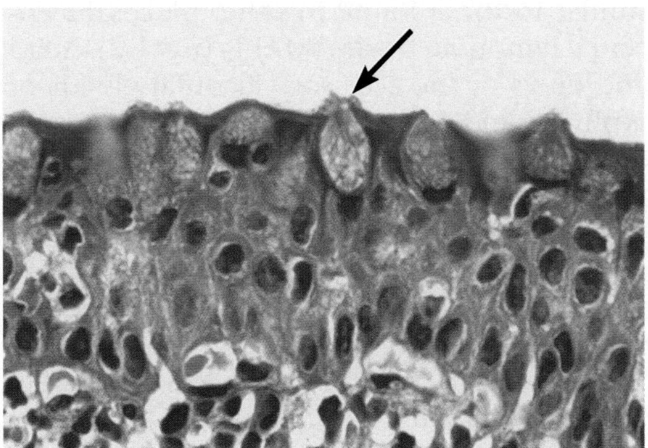

Figure 1-2

BULBAR CONJUNCTIVAL EPITHELIUM

The stratified cuboidal or cylindrical conjunctival epithelium shows prominent mucus-secreting goblet cells (arrow) in different stages of maturation, from the base to the surface layer.

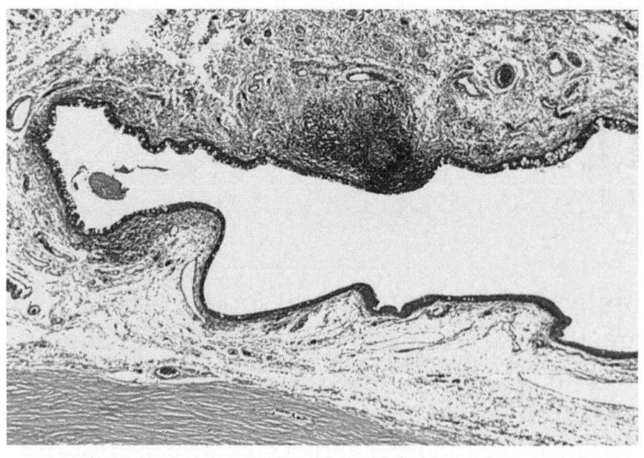

Figure 1-3

CONJUNCTIVAL CUL DE SAC

A collection of lymphocytes resembling a lymph follicle is seen in the loose substantia propria of the forniceal conjunctiva.

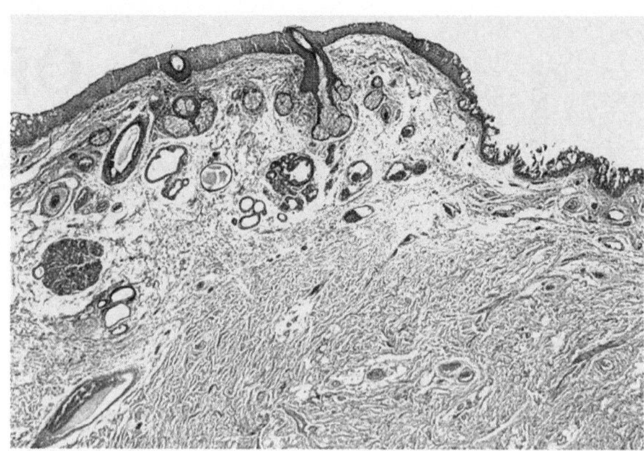

Figure 1-4

NORMAL CARUNCLE

The caruncle has a nodular configuration and is covered by stratified squamous epithelium. Goblet cells, pilosebaceous units, and adnexal glandular structures are seen.

attached to the tarsus. Inner buddings of the surface epithelium extend into the subepithelial connective tissue to form tubular and cystic structures, "pseudoglands of Henle," whose epithelium is made up of cuboidal cells and goblet cells. The blood vessels of the substantia propria (arterioles and venules) support and drain a complex capillary network. The connective tissue contains myelinated and unmyelinated branches of the trigeminal nerve. Close to the fornices are lymphocytic aggregates, with or without reactive follicles and plasma cells, similar to those found in other mucosal-associated lymphoid tissues (MALT) (fig. 1-3). Acini and ducts of the accessory lacrimal glands of Wolfring and Krause are observed in the subepithelial tissues of the palpebral conjunctiva, at the upper edge of the tarsus and close to the fornices, respectively. Nasally, a fold of loose conjunctiva forms the plica semilunaris, where smooth muscle cells and cartilage may occasionally be found.

The caruncle, which is a transition zone between the skin and the conjunctiva, is located at the inner canthus; it measures 5 x 3 mm (fig. 1-4). The surface of the caruncle is composed of columnar and nonkeratinized squamous epithelium. The subepithelial connective tissue may contain pilosebaceous units, accessory lacrimal gland tissue, smooth muscle fibers, and adipose tissue.

Lymphatic Drainage

Superficial, radial, and deep lymphatic vessels comprise the lymphatic channels that are located in the substantia propria. Large lymphatic vessels merge into major nasal and temporal trunks. The nasal trunk drains into the submandibular lymph nodes, and the temporal one drains into the preauricular and parotid lymph nodes. The submandibular lymph nodes receive the lymphatic drainage from the caruncle.

CLASSIFICATION AND FREQUENCY

Conjunctival tumors are classified as benign, premalignant, and malignant. Tumors and tumor-like lesions of the conjunctiva, together with eyelid tumors, are among the most frequently excised ophthalmic lesions that a pathologist encounters. The overall frequency of tumors in both locations varies among different series (1–4). The most frequent conjunctival tumors are epithelial, melanocytic, and lymphoid proliferations, and choristomas (Table 1-1). Among the epithelial tumors, intraepithelial neoplasia and squamous cell carcinoma are mainly encountered in adults, and papilloma and choristoma are mostly found in children. Forty-four percent of the excised pigmented lesions are nevi, and approximately 36 percent are melanomas (Table 1-2). A precursor of melanoma, primary acquired melanosis, is a distinctive melanocytic lesion of the conjunctiva that has characteristic clinical features and microscopic

Table 1-1

TUMORS OF THE CONJUNCTIVA[a]

Type of Tumor	Number of Cases (%) Doheny 1970-2000	AFIP 1984-1989
Epithelial	522 (48.3)	509 (40.5)
Melanocytic	327 (30.3)	542 (43.1)
Soft tissue	67 (6.0)	29 (2.3)
Lymphocytic and hematopoietic	113 (10.5)	117 (9.3)
Adnexal glands	22 (2.0)	24 (1.9)
Choristomatous	29 (2.7)	37 (2.9)
Total	1080	1258

[a]Frequency distribution of conjunctival tumors and tumor-like lesions from the pathology files of the Doheny Eye Institute and the Armed Forces Institute of Pathology (AFIP) Registry of Ophthalmic Pathology.

Table 1-2

CONJUNCTIVAL TUMORS OF MELANOCYTIC ORIGIN[a]

Type of Tumor	Number of Cases (%)
Nevus	145[b] (44.3)
Primary acquired melanosis without atypia	42 (12.8)
Primary acquired melanosis with atypia	18 (5.5)
Melanoma	120 (36.7)
Metastatic melanoma	2 (0.6)

[a]Frequency distribution of 327 melanocytic lesions from the pathology files of the Doheny Eye Institute collected between 1970 and 2000.
[b]Thirty-nine were associated with inflammation.

findings. Lymphoid proliferations are less frequent in the conjunctiva than in the orbit. A wide variety of soft tissue tumors may arise from the substantia propria of the conjunctiva; they are similar to their counterparts in other locations, and will be only briefly discussed.

EPITHELIAL NEOPLASMS

Papilloma

Definition. *Conjunctival papilloma* is a benign acquired papillary lesion. It is composed of branching fibrovascular cores covered by acanthotic, nonkeratinized squamous epithelium that contains a variable number of mucus-secreting cells (fig. 1-5). Synonyms include *squamous cell papilloma, conjunctival papilloma, infectious papilloma*, and *conjunctival wart*.

Clinical Features. Papillomas may develop at any age but are more frequent in children. They are solitary or multiple, unilateral or bilateral. They arise mainly from the region of the caruncle and the semilunar fold at the inner canthus or from the fornix. There may be secondary or multicentric involvement of the bulbar and palpebral conjunctivae. In adults they may originate from the limbus and adopt a sessile appearance (fig. 1-6). Human papillomavirus (HPV) serotypes 6, 11, and 16 have been demonstrated in 50 to 92 percent of the lesions (5–8).

Microscopic Findings. Squamous papillomas are exophytic lesions that are often covered by multilayered, nonkeratinized squamous cells; occasionally, oval or spindle-shaped cells confer a transitional appearance. Most papillomas in children have a variable number of mucus-secreting goblet cells. Acute inflammatory cells often permeate the exposed epithelium. Although HPV has been demonstrated in these lesions, the presence of koilocytosis is uncommon. Papillomas arising from the limbal region often are sessile and covered by acanthotic squamous epithelium (fig. 1-7). Some cells have larger and more hyperchromatic nuclei, suggesting a mild degree of dysplasia. Conjunctival papillomas with dysplasia have no risk of malignant transformation in children.

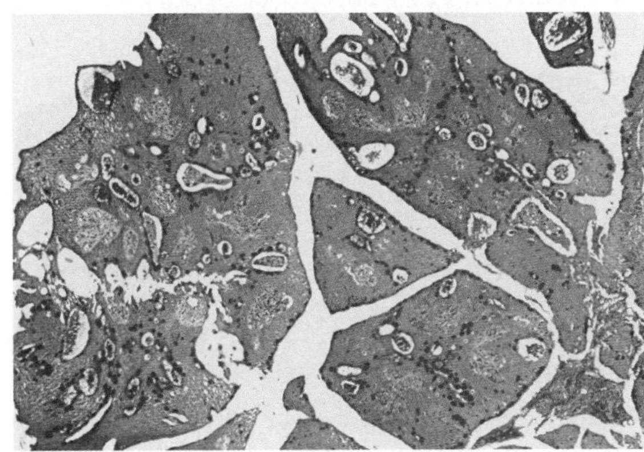

Figure 1-5

PAPILLOMA

Conjunctival papilloma contains fibrovascular cores covered by squamous or columnar epithelium.

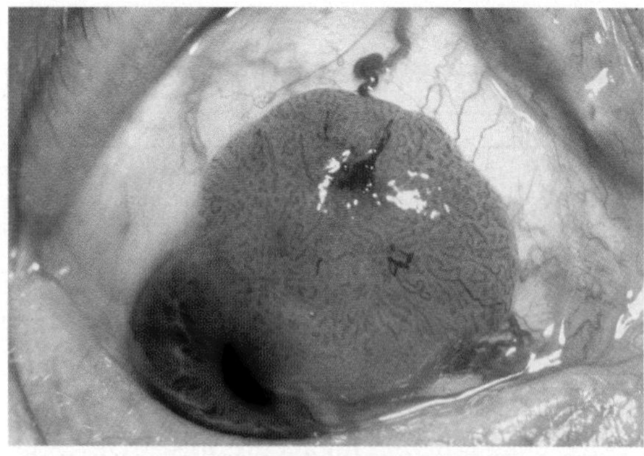

Figure 1-6

CLINICAL APPEARANCE OF A LIMBAL PAPILLOMA

The flat circumscribed lesion has multiple arborizing blood vessels, giving it a raspberry-like appearance.

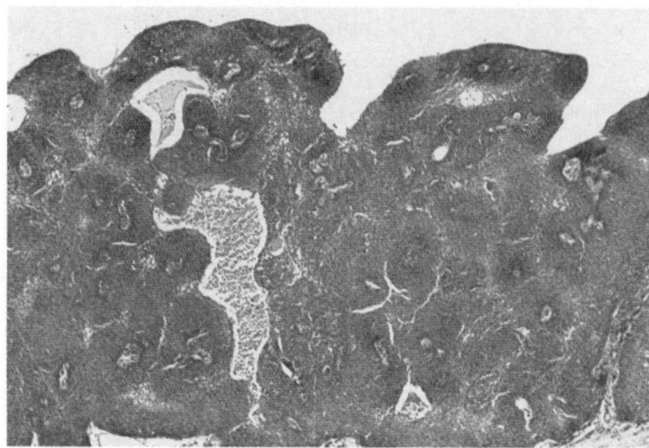

Figure 1-7

SESSILE PAPILLOMA

Arborizing fibrovascular cores are covered by acanthotic squamous epithelium.

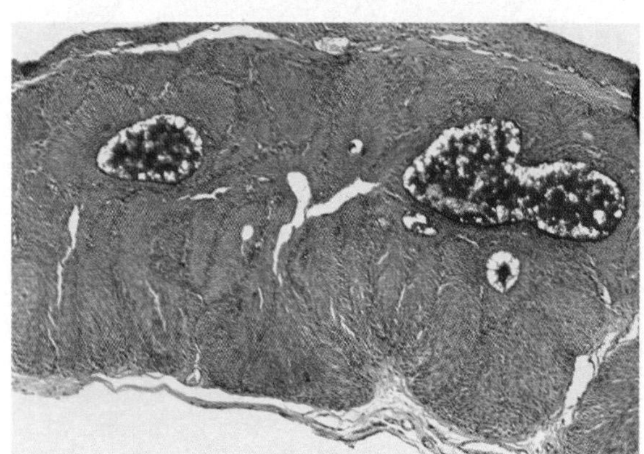

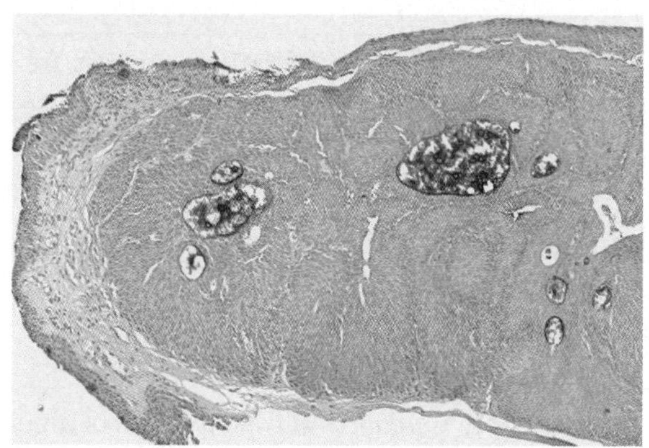

Figure 1-8

INVERTED PAPILLOMA

Left: The fibrovascular cores and acanthotic epithelium are growing within the substantia propria.
Right: The epithelium contains a number of mucus-secreting cells.

An endophytic variant of the papilloma, *inverted mucoepidermoid papilloma,* is characterized by invaginated lobules of proliferating, nonkeratinized squamous epithelial cells containing goblet cells (fig. 1-8) (9,10).

Differential Diagnosis. Exophytic papillomas in children are rarely confused with other conjunctival tumors. The differential diagnosis of a limbal papilloma in an adult may include carcinoma in situ and squamous cell carcinoma. The presence of frank atypia in a limbal papilloma is rare. Inverted papilloma of the conjunctiva must be differentiated from low-grade infiltrating mucoepidermoid carcinoma.

Treatment and Prognosis. Symptomatic conjunctival papillomas are surgically excised by the use of cryotherapy at the base and lateral surgical margins. The lesions tend to recur after excision. Extensive and recurrent papillomas may be treated with topical interferon (11), mitomycin C (12), or oral cimetidine (13).

Keratoacanthoma

Definition. *Keratoacanthoma* is an uncommon, rapidly growing, crater-like squamous cell proliferative tumor that mimics squamous cell carcinoma and pseudoepitheliomatous hyperplasia.

Clinical Features. The lesion tends to originate in the sun-exposed part of the bulbar conjunctiva (14–16). It grows rapidly in a period of few weeks, and then either regresses spontaneously or remains unchanged if untreated. The surrounding conjunctiva is usually inflamed.

Microscopic Findings. The lobules of proliferating squamous epithelium grow upward and inward, and may contain an increased number of mitotic figures, raising the suspicion of well-differentiated squamous cell carcinoma. The deep edges are well circumscribed and have a regular shape when seen on low-power magnification. The epithelial cells may have a glassy appearance, with vesicular nuclei and prominent eosinophilic nucleoli; true parakeratosis is rare. The acanthotic epithelium may be infiltrated by acute and chronic inflammatory cells, which may extend into the surrounding conjunctival connective tissue.

Differential Diagnosis. Keratoacanthoma may be confused with and difficult to differentiate from squamous cell carcinoma (17). In such cases, it is prudent to indicate in the pathology report that squamous cell carcinoma cannot be definitively excluded, and only the biologic behavior of the lesion will differentiate keratoacanthoma from a well-differentiated squamous cell carcinoma of the conjunctiva.

Treatment and Prognosis. The treatment of choice for a rapid-growing tumor with the clinical appearance of a keratoacanthoma is surgical removal. Since the diagnosis of squamous cell carcinoma cannot be ruled out, primary treatment may include cryotherapy of the surgical margins. Recurrences are rare.

Hereditary Benign Intraepithelial Dyskeratosis

Definition. *Hereditary benign intraepithelial dyskeratosis* (HBID) is a rare, autosomal dominant disease with incomplete penetrance. It is characterized by acanthotic and dyskeratotic epithelium involving the conjunctival and oral mucosa. This entity is also known as *Witkop-von Sallman syndrome* and *congenital benign hereditary dyskeratosis*.

General Features. HBID was originally described in Haliwa Indians, a triracial community whose ancestors include Africans, Europeans, and Native Americans of North Carolina, United States (18,19). Subsequently, cases have been described from other sites in the United States and Europe (20). Recent DNA analysis demonstrates a linkage to the telomeric region of 4q35, with duplication alleles that may be involved in causation (21).

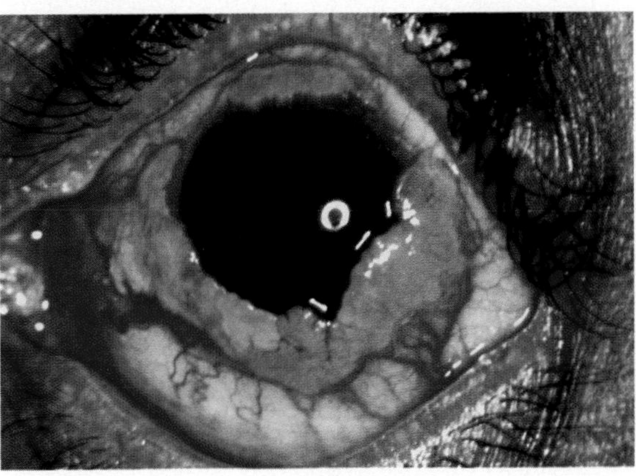

Figure 1-9

HEREDITARY BENIGN INTRAEPITHELIAL DYSKERATOSIS

Diffuse limbal and conjunctival involvement by a flat white lesion.

Clinical Features. In childhood, bilateral, grayish white, inflamed, horseshoe-shaped conjunctival lesions develop that often involve the interpalpebral region nasally and temporally (fig. 1-9). Similar lesions are also seen in the oral mucosa. The disease has a chronic relapsing course, and the lesions are usually resistant to medical and surgical intervention.

Microscopic Findings. The conjunctival epithelium is thickened and the middle and superficial cell layers are replaced by large squamous-like cells and dyskeratotic cells without nuclear atypia (fig. 1-10). Large dyskeratotic cells are usually observed at the surface. Malignant transformation has not been reported. There usually is a chronic inflammatory cell infiltrate in the subepithelial connective tissue.

Ultrastructural Findings. Ultrastructural findings reveal the presence of numerous vesicular bodies in immature dyskeratotic cells and densely packed tonofilaments filling the cytoplasm of mature dyskeratotic cells. Cellular interdigitations and desmosomes disappear in the latter cells (22).

Differential Diagnosis. Although the lesions resemble conjunctival epithelial dysplasia, individual cells in HBID do not have atypical

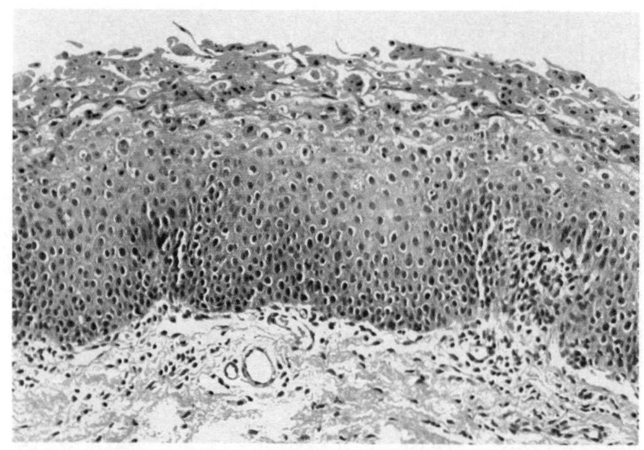

Figure 1-10

HEREDITARY BENIGN INTRAEPITHELIAL DYSKERATOSIS

The normal epithelium is replaced by acanthotic squamous epithelium with dyskeratotic cells.

changes. In addition, the presence of affected family members, bilaterality, and simultaneous involvement of the oral mucosa help distinguish these two lesions.

Treatment and Prognosis. The conjunctival lesions are managed by surgical excision, but recurrences are common. Malignant change has not been observed.

OTHER BENIGN EPITHELIAL LESIONS

Epithelial Cysts

The majority of *conjunctival epithelial cysts* are acquired, although some are congenital. Cysts are acquired secondary to surgical or accidental trauma, foreign body, and chronic inflammation (23). They are more frequently located on the nasal conjunctiva and lower fornix. The cysts have a translucent appearance, although light scattering may give them a bluish discoloration (24). They are lined by nonkeratinized squamous epithelium that contains a variable number of mucus-secreting goblet cells (25). Sometimes, one or two layers of cuboidal epithelium that have the peculiar apical snouts of the superficial layer (resembling apocrine glands) line the cysts. Simple excision is usually curative.

Nonspecific Keratotic (Leukoplakic) Lesions

Nonspecific keratotic lesions include a variety of isolated, grayish white epithelial lesions of the bulbar conjunctiva that have no malignant potential. The name *Bitot spot* describes a white focus of keratinization. These lesions are areas of squamous metaplasia and hyperkeratosis that originate spontaneously or are associated with vitamin A deficiency. The epithelium shows epidermalization and exhibits loss of goblet cells. Acanthosis, rete ridge formation, and focal surface keratinization are frequently noted. Cellular atypia is usually not seen. Conjunctival epithelial changes characterized by acanthosis, loss of mucus-secreting cells, and keratinization may be similarly observed in primary or secondary diseases of the ocular surface associated with drying of the conjunctiva (xerosis) such as keratoconjunctivitis sicca, Sjögren's syndrome, and radiotherapy.

Pseudoepitheliomatous (Pseudocarcinomatous) Hyperplasia

Pseudoepitheliomatous hyperplasia is a reactive proliferation of the surface epithelium secondary to an inflammatory or infectious process. The lesion develops rapidly and may become ulcerated. The proliferative squamous epithelium forms irregular lobules with variable degrees of acanthosis and keratinization. The epithelial cells may exhibit reactive changes and increased mitotic activity. The border between the proliferating epithelial lobules and the subepithelial connective tissue may be ill-defined by the inflammatory infiltrate, which often extends into the epithelium. In lesions with features of a mixed acute and chronic granulomatous inflammatory cell infiltrate, including multinucleated giant cells, a fungal infection should be considered. Special stains for fungi and bacteria may disclose the causative microorganism (26). *Pseudoadenomatous hyperplasia* refers to a gland-like proliferation that may mimic mucoepidermoid carcinoma. Pseudoepitheliomatous hyperplasia often resolves after elimination of the causative process (27).

Leukoplakic Lesions (Ultraviolet Light Related)

This group of *leukoplakic lesions* of the limbal conjunctiva features acanthosis and dysplasia of the epithelium overlying elastotic degeneration of the substantia propria from ultraviolet (UV) light damage. The World Health Organization (WHO) classifies these lesions as *actinic keratosis* (28,29). They involve the interpalpebral

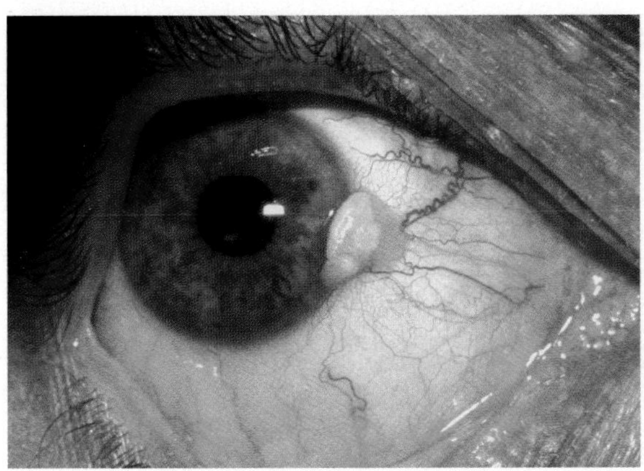

Figure 1-11

LEUKOPLAKIC LESION OF THE CONJUNCTIVA

The white lesion in the interpalpebral region of the conjunctiva is most likely related to exposure to ultraviolet (UV) light.

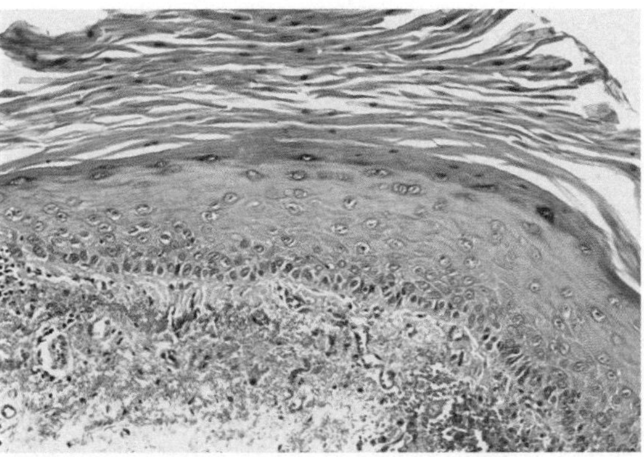

Figure 1-12

UV-RELATED LEUKOPLAKIC LESION

Acanthosis and parakeratosis are seen in a circumscribed area of transformed conjunctival epithelium. The substantia propria shows fibrillar degeneration of collagen fibers.

bulbar conjunctiva and are frequently found at the advancing head of the pterygium (fig. 1-11). The presence of parakeratosis and keratinization give them a "leukoplakic" grayish white appearance (29). In general, the lesions consist of a circumscribed area of transformed epithelium, with acanthosis, parakeratosis, and hyperkeratosis, that may exhibit dysplasia (figs. 1-12, 1-13). The subepithelial connective tissue shows elastotic degeneration and a lymphocytic inflammatory infiltrate.

Pterygia are fleshy lesions arising from the interpalpebral region of the bulbar conjunctiva and involve the cornea. The surface epithelium may be atrophic and thickened, or show dysplastic changes and keratosis. There is basophilic fibrillar degeneration of collagen fibers, increased vascularization, and scarring in the subepithelial connective tissue. A recurrent pterygium is characterized by abnormal hyperplastic scarring associated with increased vascularization.

CONJUNCTIVAL INTRAEPITHELIAL NEOPLASIA

Definition. *Conjunctival intraepithelial neoplasia* (CIN) includes a wide range of neoplastic intraepithelial changes ranging from dysplasia to full-thickness epithelial neoplasia or carcinoma in situ. Synonyms include *mild, moderate,* and *severe dysplasia, carcinoma in situ, ocular surface squamous neoplasia, intraepithelial epithelioma,* and *bowenoid type of dyskeratosis* (30).

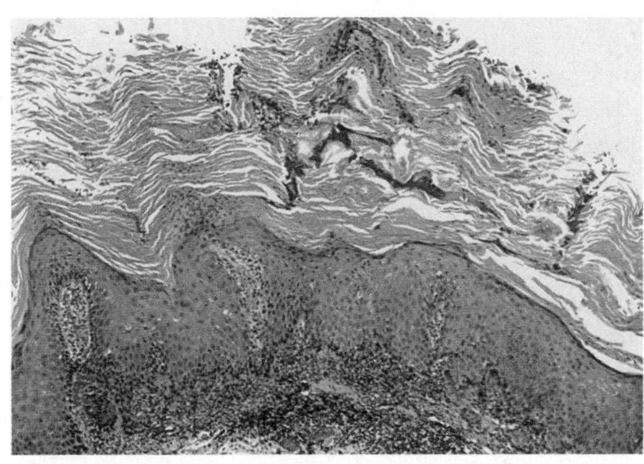

Figure 1-13

UV-RELATED LEUKOPLAKIC LESION

The hyperkeratosis and lymphocytic infiltrate within the substantia propria are more marked than in figure 1-12.

General Features. The incidence of dysplasia, carcinoma in situ, and invasive carcinoma of conjunctiva and cornea is estimated to be 1.9 cases/100,000 population/year, as averaged for 10 years in the Brisbane metropolitan area of Australia (31). The development of CIN is associated with ocular pigmentation, nonoffice and nonprofessional workers, and exposure to petroleum products and cigarette smoking (32). CIN has been reported after long-term use of systemic cyclosporine therapy in organ transplant recipients. HPV types 6 and 11 are found in 38 percent and HPV type 16 in 30 to 58 percent of

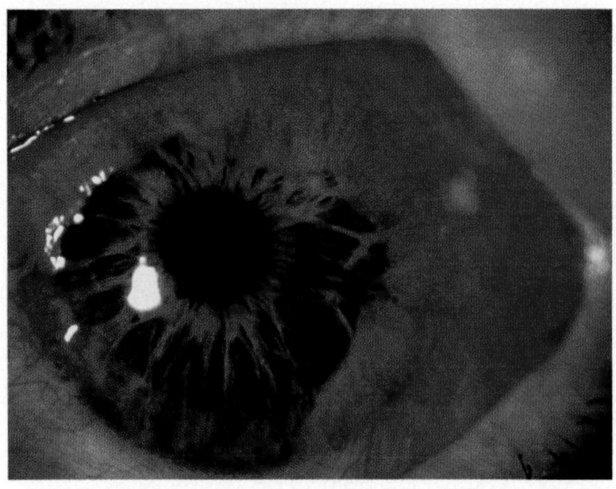

Figure 1-14

CONJUNCTIVAL INTRAEPITHELIAL NEOPLASIA

An annular, proliferative, gelatinous lesion of the limbal conjunctiva.

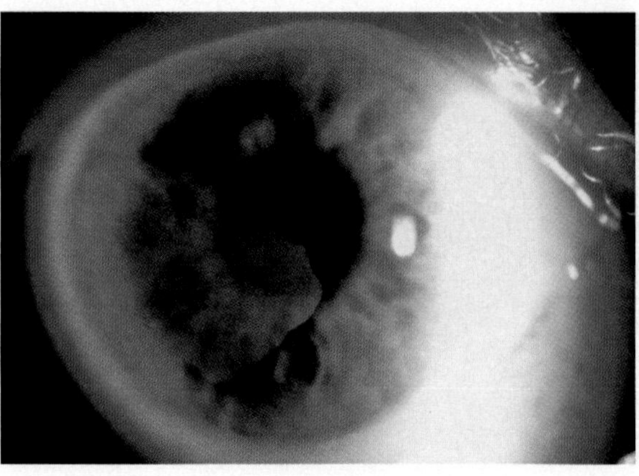

Figure 1-15

CORNEAL INTRAEPITHELIAL NEOPLASIA

Indirect illumination illustrates a delicate opaque epithelial proliferation of the cornea.

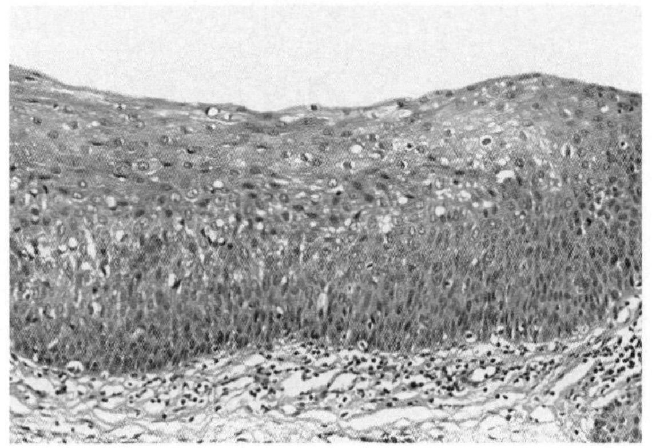

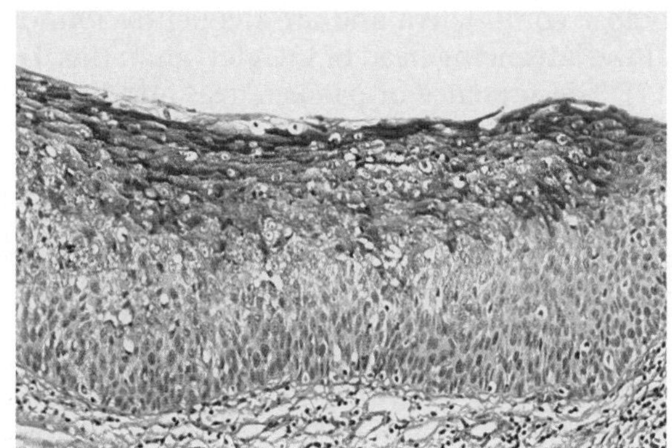

Figure 1-16

DYSPLASIA

Left: The middle third of the conjunctival epithelium is transformed. The upper layer shows large squamous cells with maturation towards the surface.

Right: Periodic acid–Schiff (PAS) stain discloses the presence of glycogen in non-neoplastic superficial squamous cells.

patients with conjunctival dysplasia; HPV type 18 is found in 50 to 57 percent of those with CIN (33–35). The demonstration of HPV 16 and 18 mRNA (E6 region) suggests an etiologic role in some cases of CIN (36).

Clinical Features. Clinically, the lesions are sharply demarcated from the surrounding normal epithelium and arise at the limbus, where corneal stem cells are located, with either or both conjunctival (fig. 1-14) and corneal (fig. 1-15) involvement (37,38). Most lesions are nonkeratinized, well-vascularized, and pink, and have a raspberry-like configuration. Rarely, the epithelial changes spontaneously regress (39).

Microscopic Findings. Intraepithelial dysplastic changes originate in the basal layers and extend towards the surface (fig. 1-16). The epithelial cells may transform to large squamous cells, small epithelial cells, and spindle-shaped epithelial cells, among others. Keratinization and dyskeratosis are not a common feature of CIN. Atypical mitoses are frequent and may be

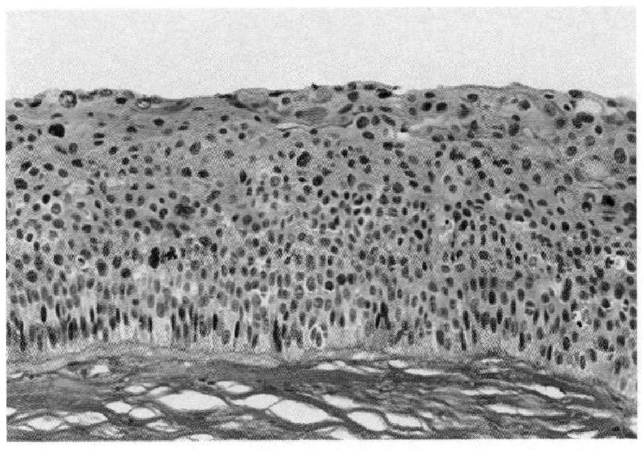

Figure 1-17

SEVERE DYSPLASIA

The cellular proliferation with squamous transformation failed to stain with PAS. This is indicative of severe dysplasia.

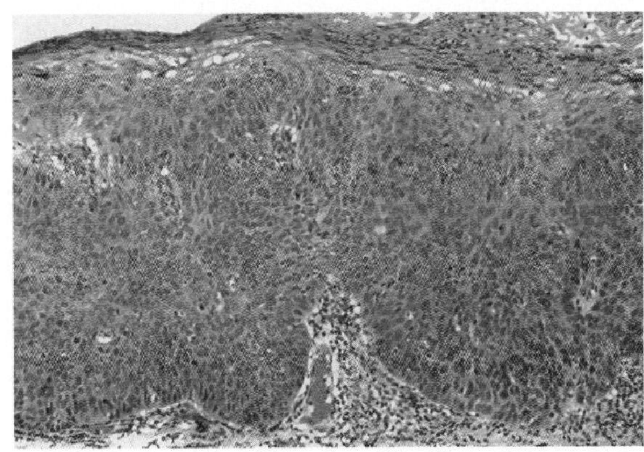

Figure 1-18

CARCINOMA IN SITU

The full thickness of the epithelium is replaced by atypical cells.

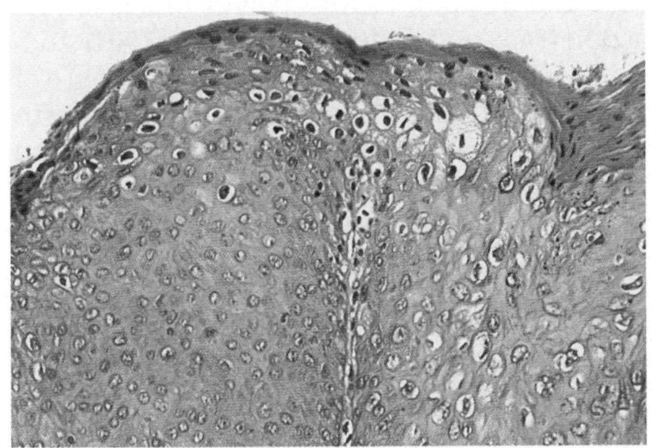

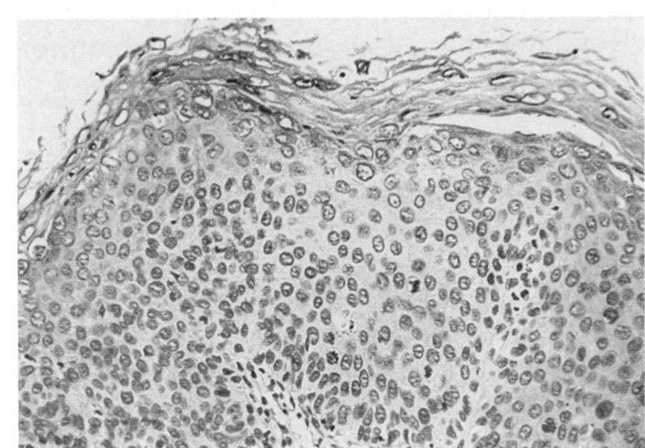

Figure 1-19

HUMAN PAPILLOMA VIRUS (HPV)-RELATED CONJUNCTIVAL INTRAEPITHELIAL NEOPLASIA

Left: Koilocytes are present within the transformed squamous epithelium.
Right: Immunohistochemistry demonstrates the presence of HPV proteins within the koilocytotic cells.

located at all levels of the epithelium. There is a sharp demarcation between the normal and diseased epithelium. The epithelial basal membrane remains intact. Fronds of proliferating blood vessels and connective tissue extend along the area involved by the transformed hyperplastic epithelium, giving rise to a configuration simulating sessile papilloma. The intraepithelial dysplastic changes are graded as mild, moderate, or severe (figs. 1-17, 1-18), based on the thickness of intraepithelial involvement. Rarely, koilocytes are identified, suggesting HPV infection (fig. 1-19).

Proliferating cell nuclear antigen (PCNA), p53 immunostaining, and argyrophilic nucleolar organizer region (AgNOR) staining may be useful for grading the dysplastic lesions and for correlation with clinical morphologic findings (40).

Differential Diagnosis. The differential diagnosis includes UV-related epithelial hyperplasias, intraepithelial sebaceous gland carcinoma, and rarely, intraepithelial invasion by an adenocarcinoma originating from the apocrine glands of Moll. Immunohistochemical analysis for HMB45, Melan-1, and S-100 protein is often helpful in distinguishing the lesions of primary acquired melanosis from CIN.

Treatment and Prognosis. CIN is treated by complete surgical excision. Recurrences are seen in 10 to 70 percent of cases. The main predictors of recurrence are histologic grade of the lesion and degree of differentiation (well, moderate, or poorly differentiated), corneal location, and size of the lesion (over 2 mm). Recurrences after excision depend on completeness of the surgical procedure and the use of adjunctive treatments such as cryotherapy to eradicate the diseased epithelium. Although exceptions do occur, most lesions remain intraepithelial in successive recurrences. In cases with diffuse involvement and recurrence, adjunctive chemotherapy with topical application of mitomycin-C (41), 5-fluorouracil (42), and interferon alpha-2b (43) have been used successfully with minor drug-related complications.

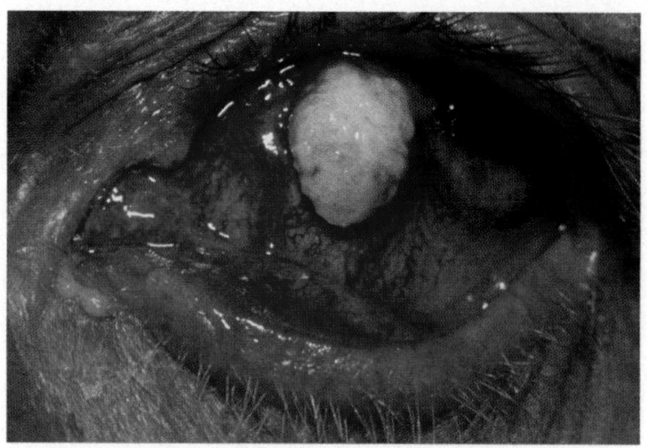

Figure 1-20

SQUAMOUS CELL CARCINOMA

Exophytic squamous cell carcinoma of the bulbar and limbal conjunctivae with extensive keratinization.

SQUAMOUS CELL CARCINOMA

Definition. *Squamous cell carcinomas* (SCC) of the conjunctiva are invasive keratinizing tumors arising from the epithelial conjunctival surface. They tend to recur but rarely metastasize except in advanced neglected cases.

General Features. The incidence of SCC varies from 0.03/100,000 population in the United States to 3.5/100,000 in Uganda (44,45). In the United States the rate is 5-fold higher among males and whites (44). Exposure to solar UV light is highly associated with the development of SCC (44,45). Usually, patients present during their early sixties, with a male predominance (ratio 2.3 to 1). Asian, African, and Latin American patients may be younger (less than 40 years) (46,47). An increased incidence of this malignancy has been observed in African countries in patients who are human immunodeficiency virus (HIV) seropositive (48). In patients with acquired immunodeficiency syndrome (AIDS), SCC and CIN may show aggressive histologic features.

Although most SCCs originate from actinic-related keratotic lesions, there are other predisposing conditions, including xeroderma pigmentosum, albinism, toxic exposure to chemicals, and physical factors. Polymerase chain reaction (PCR) and in situ hybridization (ISH) studies on tumor tissue have revealed the presence of HPV 16 and 18 in 55 percent of patients with SCC (47). HPV 16 has been detected in bilateral SCC, and in conjunctival dysplasia, suggesting a probable role for this virus in the progression of diffuse, multicentric, and bilateral precancerous and cancerous epithelial lesions (49).

Clinical Features. Usually the tumors are located in the bulbar conjunctiva, reaching the limbus at the interpalpebral region (fig. 1-20). They have a grayish white, exophytic, crater-like appearance, and are surrounded by an inflamed conjunctiva (50,51). Rarely, the tumors grow diffusely, disclosing multiple papillary fronds and variable degrees of keratinization.

Microscopic Findings. Well-differentiated SCC is characterized by infiltrating lobules, nests, and cords of variable size, extending from the surface neoplastic epithelium into the subepithelial connective tissue (fig. 1-21). The dense collagenous scleral tissue usually limits the deepest infiltrating margins. The epithelial lobules display keratinization with either the presence of cells arranged concentrically around a central focus of acellular keratin or multiple foci of cellular keratinization. The large squamous cells have eosinophilic or clear cytoplasm and intercellular bridges, and many show individual cell dyskeratosis. At the edge of the infiltrating

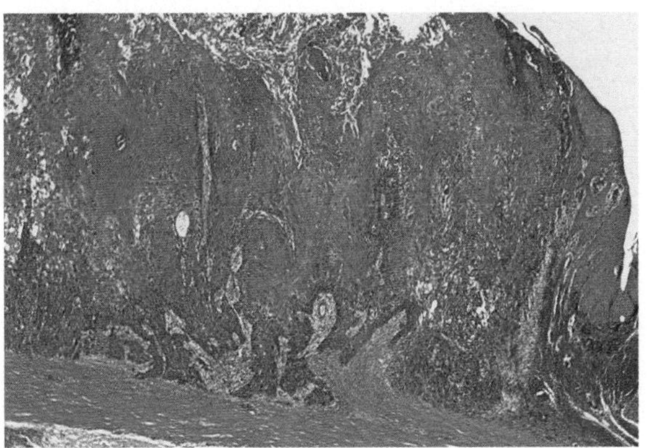

Figure 1-21

SQUAMOUS CELL CARCINOMA

Because of the endurance of the sclera, this well-differentiated squamous cell carcinoma demonstrates typical exophytic growth.

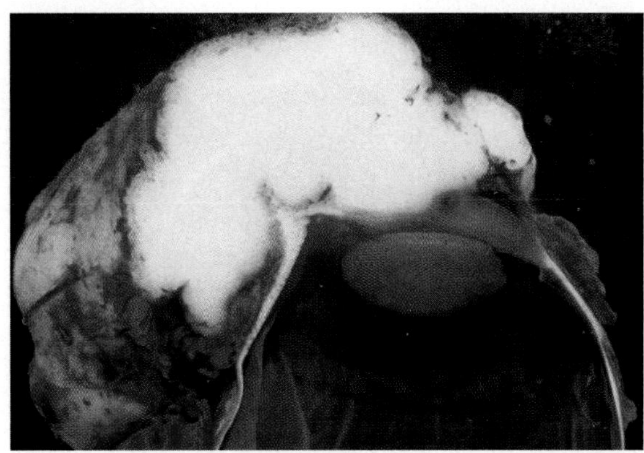

Figure 1-22

SQUAMOUS CELL CARCINOMA

A young patient with xeroderma pigmentosum developed a well-differentiated squamous cell carcinoma of the conjunctiva that invaded intraocularly.

lobules, the cells have a more atypical appearance, with darker cytoplasm and pleomorphic nuclei. The latter have coarse chromatin and prominent nucleoli. Mitotic activity is usually low, with abnormal mitotic figures haphazardly distributed within the lobules. In heavily pigmented patients, melanin pigment may be found within the benign and malignant epithelial cells, simulating melanoma.

Immunohistochemical Findings. The neoplastic squamous cells express high molecular weight cytokeratin, epithelial membrane antigen, and other epithelial markers. The main use of these antibodies is to differentiate SCC from other undifferentiated neoplasms.

Special Studies. DNA and cytomorphometric analyses show that the SCC cells are most frequently aneuploid, with a high mean DNA index and multiploid peaks, while hyperplastic epithelial lesions are nonaneuploid (52). Several emerging molecular markers, such as epidermal growth factor receptor, transforming growth factor-alpha, cyclin D1, and p53, may provide valuable prognostic information. At present, however, none of the these are used routinely as prognostic markers.

Cytologic Findings. Cytologic studies can help diagnose cases with diffuse involvement, identify recurrences, and evaluate the efficacy of topical chemotherapy (53). The specimens are obtained with a platinum spatula, cytobrush, or impression cytology for evaluation of cells attached to a nitrocellulose membrane. Some studies have shown a high sensitivity for the detection of atypical cells in dysplasia, carcinoma in situ, and SCC cytologic studies (54).

Differential Diagnosis. Since most SCCs of the conjunctiva are well differentiated, the main distinction is with keratoacanthoma and pseudoepitheliomatous hyperplasia. Rarely, pigmented SCC can be confused with melanoma, and in such cases immunohistochemical studies for keratin readily establish the diagnosis.

Treatment and Prognosis. Complete surgical excision, with a 3 to 5 mm surgical margin, is the treatment of choice. Intraoperative control of the surgical margins and adjunctive cryotherapy at the surgical margins may result in better tumor control (55,56). Recurrences, which occur in approximately 6 percent of the cases, have a slow growth rate and are usually observed 6 months to a year after the original excision (57). Topical 5-fluorouracil has been used to treat cases with diffuse involvement, incompletely excised lesions, and recurrences. Deeper structures are locally invaded with varying frequency, including sclera (37 percent), intraocular contents (13 percent), and orbital tissues (11 percent). Invasion of the intraocular structures is usually a late event after several recurrences (fig. 1-22) (58). Orbital involvement by conjunctival SCC is the most commonly encountered cause of secondary orbital tumors in older patients in some high-risk geographic areas (fig. 1-23) (59).

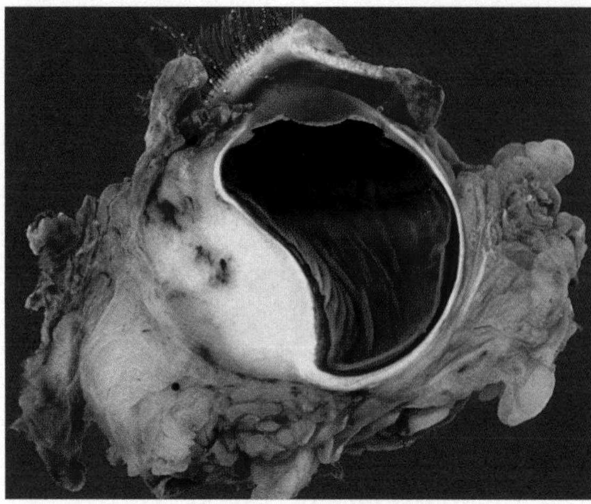

Figure 1-23

SQUAMOUS CELL CARCINOMA INVADING THE ORBIT

This exenteration specimen shows an extensive squamous cell carcinoma of the conjunctiva that invaded the orbital tissues.

Risk factors for metastasis are large size, neglected tumors, and multiple recurrences (60). The initial sites of metastasis include the parotid, submandibular, preauricular, and cervical lymph nodes; other sites include lung and bone. In recent years, because of early clinical diagnosis and adequate excision, metastatic SCC is rarely seen (61).

Pathologic Staging. See Table 1-3.

Table 1-3

PATHOLOGIC STAGING OF SQUAMOUS CELL CARCINOMA OF CONJUNCTIVA[a]

Primary Tumor (T)	
TX	Primary tumor cannot be assessed
T0	No evidence of primary tumor
Tis	Carcinoma in situ
T1	Tumor 5 mm or less in greatest dimension
T2	Tumor more than 5 mm in greatest dimension, without invasion of adjacent structures
T3	Tumor invades adjacent structures, excluding the orbit
T4	Tumor invades the orbit
Regional Lymph Nodes	
NX	Regional lymph nodes cannot be assessed
N0	No regional lymph node metastasis
N1	Regional lymph node metastasis
Distant Metastasis (M)	
MX	Distant metastasis cannot be assessed
M0	No distant metastasis
M1	Distant metastasis
Histopathologic Grade (G)	
GX	Grade cannot be assessed
G1	Well differentiated
G2	Moderately differentiated
G3	Poorly differentiated
G4	Undifferentiated

[a]Data from reference 62.

VARIANTS OF SQUAMOUS CELL CARCINOMA

Mucoepidermoid Carcinoma

Mucoepidermoid carcinoma of the conjunctiva is a rare neoplasm that clinically resembles SCC (63). The age at the time of clinical presentation varies from 36 to 81 years, with an average age of 67.3 years. Usually, it develops from the limbus and bulbar conjunctiva and characteristically shows local aggressiveness in the form of orbital and intraocular invasion (63–65). Histologically, there is an admixture of epidermoid cells, intermediate cells, and mucus-producing cells. The different cellular components may vary within the same tumor. Sheets or cords of large squamous epithelial cells displaying eosinophilic cytoplasm and mucin-containing cells may predominate (fig. 1-24). In infiltrating areas, the neoplastic cells may surround pools of mucin that stain brightly with Alcian blue, colloidal iron, and the mucicarmine method (fig. 1-25). The presence of squamous pearls is the exception rather than the rule.

Rapid recurrence is usually observed following simple excision. Recurrences are seen in about 85 percent of the cases. The recommended treatment is wide local excision with free surgical margins. Plaque radiotherapy with I^{125} has been used for recurrent lesions (66). Mucoepidermoid carcinoma is more aggressive than conventional SCC, tends to invade the intraocular structures and orbit, and can metastasize to regional lymph nodes, lungs, and bone.

Spindle Cell Carcinoma

Spindle cell carcinoma of the conjunctiva, also referred as *polypoid carcinoma of the conjunctiva,* resembles a spindle cell fibroblastic-like tumor

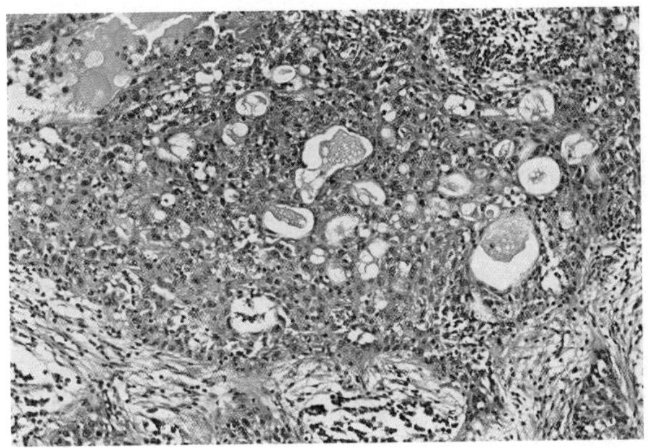

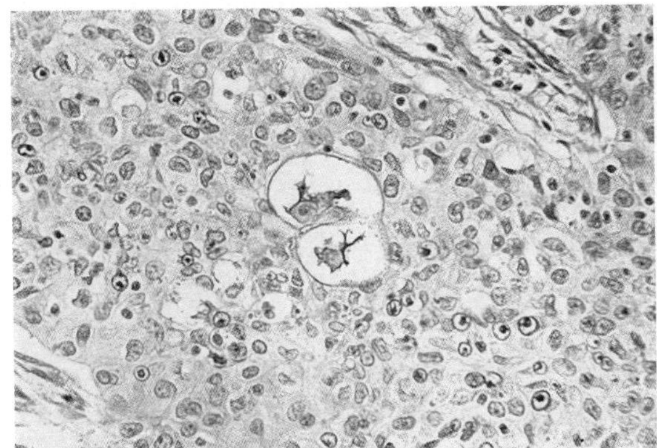

Figure 1-24

MUCOEPIDERMOID CARCINOMA

Left: Solid sheets of infiltrating squamous cells.
Right: Alcian blue stain discloses the presence of mucin within the tumor cells.

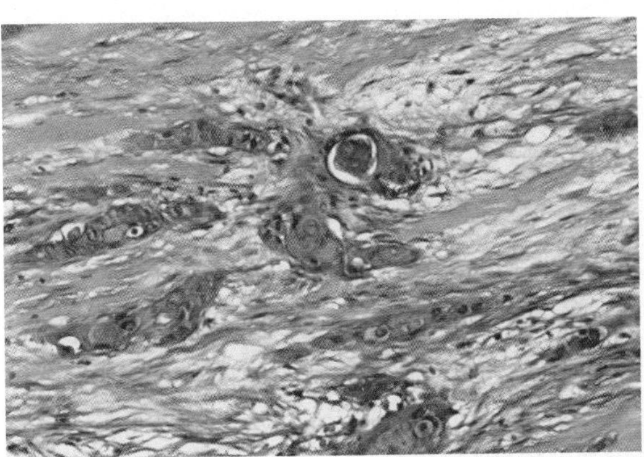

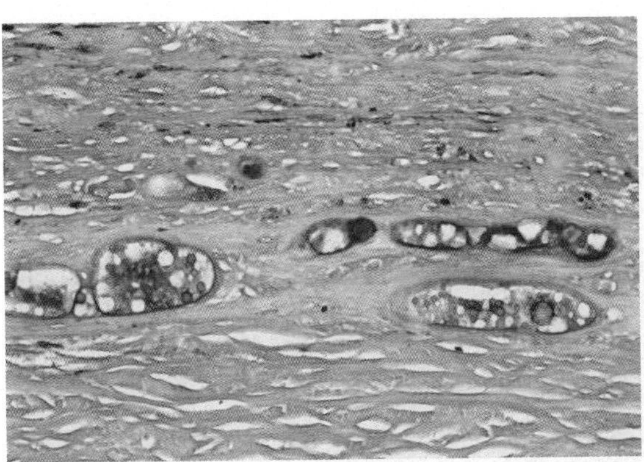

Figure 1-25

MUCOEPIDERMOID CARCINOMA

Left: Intraocular invasion by infiltrating cords of atypical squamous cells with empty spaces and occasional vacuolated cytoplasm.

Right: Alcian blue stain discloses the presence of extracellular and intracellular mucin.

with subtle continuity with the surface epithelium. It presents clinically as a localized, elevated, smooth-surfaced, reddish lesion arising from the limbus or bulbar conjunctiva in elderly patients (figs. 1-26, 1-27) (67–69).

Histologic examination shows an acanthotic epithelium with a varying degree of dysplasia; infiltrating cells have a spindle-shaped configuration, oval vesicular nuclei, and large basophilic or eosinophilic nucleoli (fig. 1-28). The most superficial infiltrating cells resemble those of the basal layer, with foci of dysplasia and even carcinoma in situ. Mitotic figures are variable but may be prominent in some tumors. The cells may be arranged in fascicles and associated with desmoplasia. A chronic inflammatory response associated with endothelial cell hyperplasia may obscure the neoplastic epithelial cells. Immunohistochemistry demonstrates the presence of keratin (fig. 1-29), vimentin, actin filaments, and epithelial membrane antigen (EMA) (70, 71). Electron microscopy may help demonstrate the true epithelial nature of the lesion (desmosomes and tonofilaments), although features of epithelial cells may not be evident in the most deeply located spindle-shaped cells.

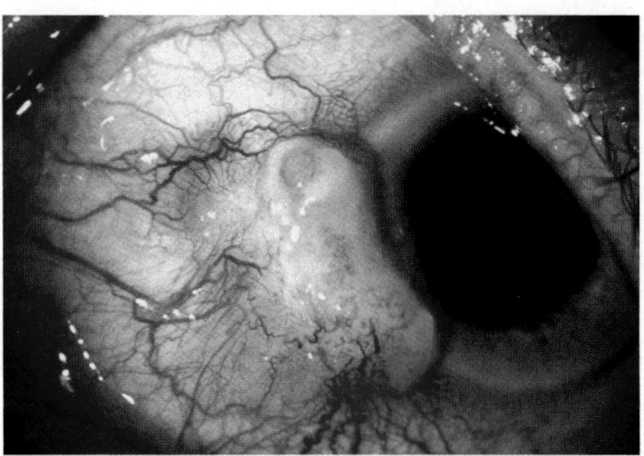

Figure 1-26

SPINDLE CELL CARCINOMA

An elevated nodular lesion at the limbus.

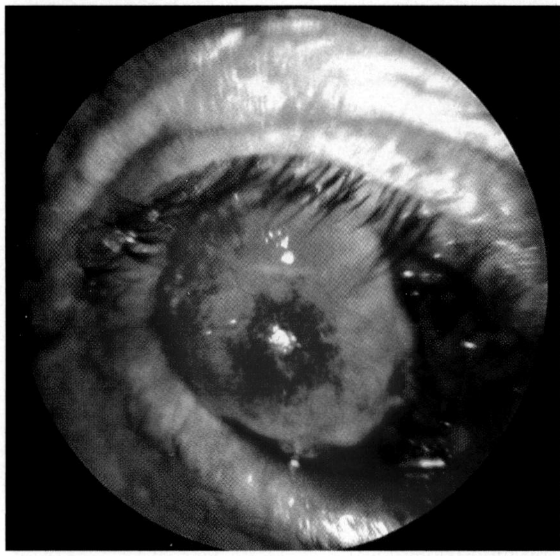

Figure 1-27

SPINDLE CELL CARCINOMA

A polypoidal reddish mass arises from the bulbar conjunctiva.

Most spindle cell carcinomas of the conjunctiva are initially misdiagnosed clinically and histologically as atypical fibroxanthoma, malignant fibrous histiocytoma, amelanotic spindle cell melanoma, and exuberant granulation tissue. Treatment is complete surgical excision. Recurrence, invasion of sclera, and intraocular spread have been reported (69).

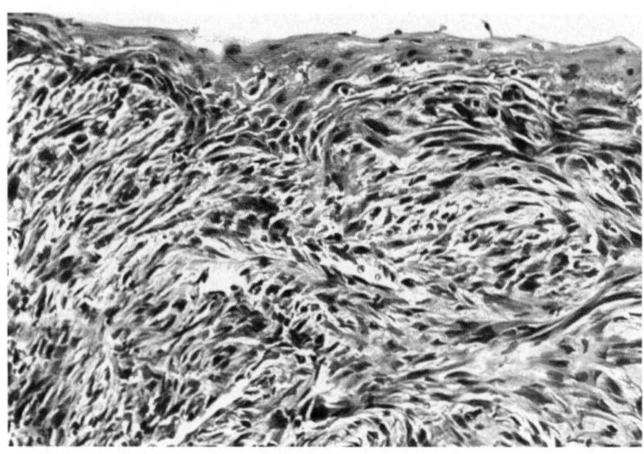

Figure 1-28

SPINDLE CELL CARCINOMA

The substantia propria is infiltrated by spindle-shaped cells that are clearly continuous with the surface epithelium. Intraepithelial atypia is seen in the surface epithelium.

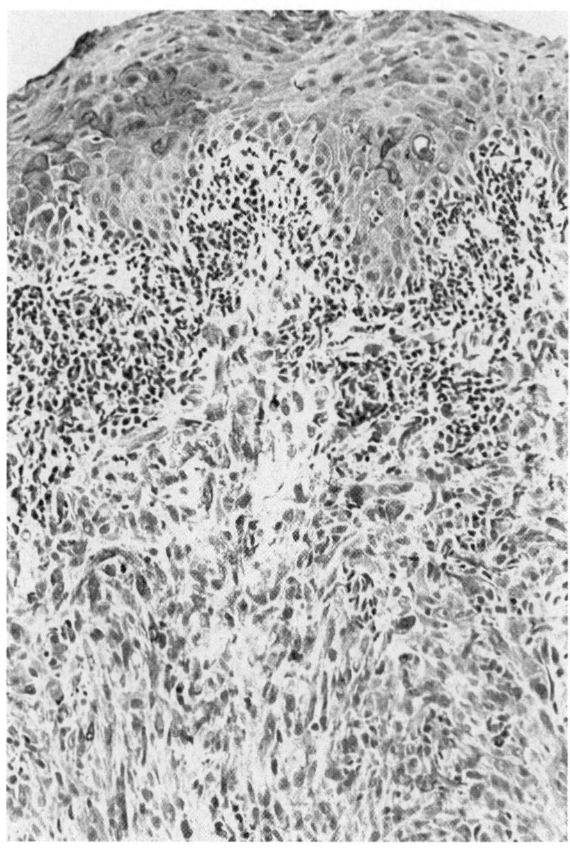

Figure 1-29

SPINDLE CELL CARCINOMA

Demonstration of epithelial differentiation in the spindle cell proliferation with anticytokeratin antibody.

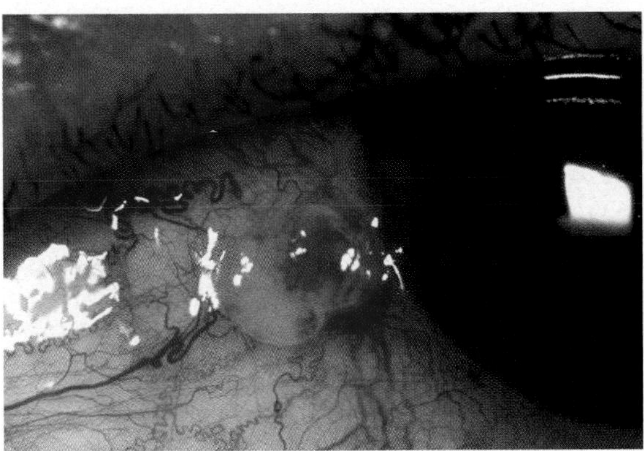

Figure 1-30

BASAL CELL CARCINOMA

Circumscribed nodular tumor at the temporal limbus.

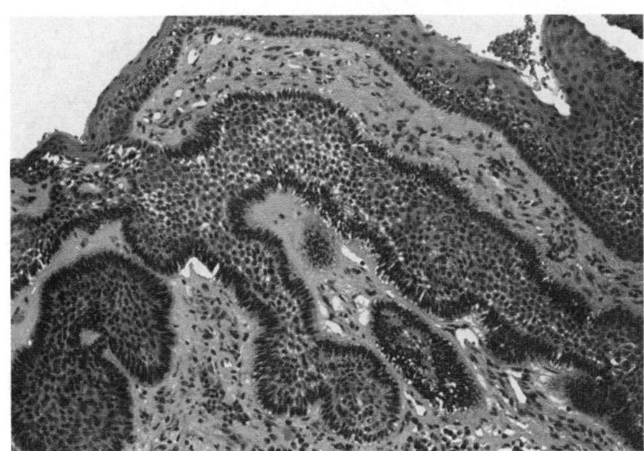

Figure 1-31

BASAL CELL CARCINOMA

Infiltrating lobules of atypical basal cells arise from the surface epithelium of the conjunctiva.

Adenoid Squamous Cell Carcinoma

Adenoid squamous cell carcinoma is characterized by islands of atypical squamous cells with foci of acantholysis and pseudoglandular spaces. Synonyms include *acantholytic squamous cell carcinoma, adenoacanthoma,* and *pseudoglandular squamous cell carcinoma.* Patients may present with a mass at the limbus or bulbar conjunctiva that is associated with signs of severe inflammation (72). These tumors have an aggressive biologic behavior: they may recur or infiltrate the deep orbital tissues. Surgical excision with frozen section control of the margins is the treatment of choice.

OTHER CARCINOMAS OF THE CONJUNCTIVA

Basal Cell Carcinoma

Rarely, *basal cell carcinoma* arises from the conjunctiva and caruncle without any adjacent lesion in the skin of the eyelid (73). The tumor is reported to occur in men aged 24 to 66 years (74,75). The tumor presents as a white nodular growth of the conjunctiva (fig. 1-30) (74,75). Microscopic examination reveals a nodular and cystic tumor composed of atypical basaloid cells, indistinguishable from tumors originating in the skin (fig. 1-31).

Sebaceous Carcinoma

Occurrence of *intraepithelial sebaceous neoplasia of the conjunctiva* without any evidence of a sebaceous gland tumor of the ocular adnexa is rare (76,77). The neoplasia may be caused by intraepithelial transformation of conjunctival cells or the result of spontaneous regression of an underlying meibomian gland carcinoma. In most cases, there is an occult sebaceous carcinoma with secondary pagetoid spread into the conjunctival epithelium.

Clinically, the conjunctival involvement masquerades as inflammatory disease (chronic keratoconjunctivitis) resulting in delayed diagnosis (78). Infiltration of the conjunctival epithelium varies from isolated neoplastic cells, with foamy or vacuolated cytoplasm, permeating the epithelial layers (pagetoid spread), to replacement of the entire thickness of the epithelium by contiguous neoplastic cells (bowenoid spread) (fig. 1-32). The differential diagnosis is facilitated by immunohistochemical demonstration of milk fat globule, breast carcinoma-1 antibody, OM-1 (ovarian cystadenocarcinoma antigen), and EMA. Oil red-O staining of frozen sections helps in the differential diagnosis (fig. 1-33). Map biopsies are required to determine the severity and extension of the tumor. Analysis of isolated reported cases indicates that this lesion may remain in situ for prolonged periods without evolving to an invasive carcinoma. Cryotherapy has been used to treat intraepithelial extension of sebaceous carcinoma of the eyelid (79).

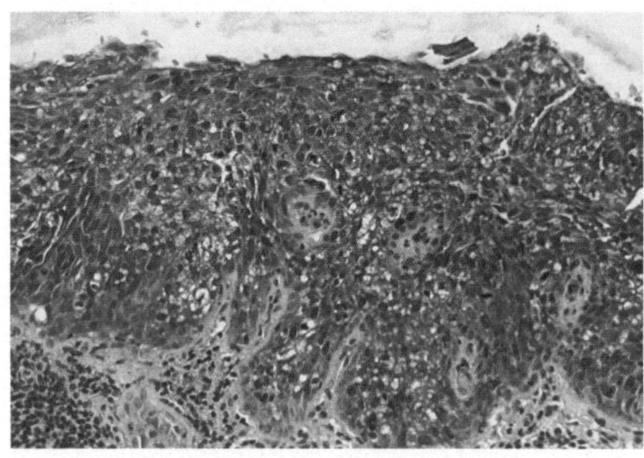

Figure 1-32

SEBACEOUS GLAND CARCINOMA

The conjunctival epithelium is replaced by confluent atypical epithelial cells with finely vacuolated cytoplasm.

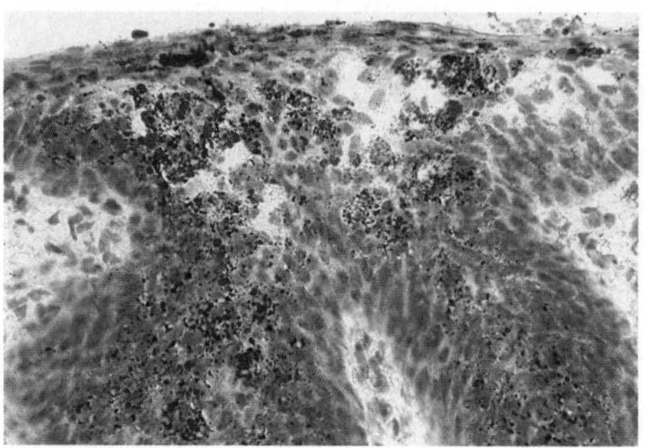

Figure 1-33

SEBACEOUS GLAND CARCINOMA

By the demonstration of lipid within the cytoplasm of the atypical cells, oil red-O stain reveals the sebaceous origin of the neoplastic intraepithelial cells.

Lymphoepithelioma-Like Carcinoma

Lymphoepithelioma-like carcinoma is a rare tumor in the conjunctiva. It is seen most commonly in the nasopharynx of individuals from south China and Taiwan, and is strongly associated with the Epstein-Barr virus. It is characterized histologically by nonkeratinizing, undifferentiated SCC with lymphocytic infiltration. Clinically, the lesions are white-yellow and behave as aggressive tumors that invade the cornea, eyelid, and orbit (80).

MELANOCYTIC TUMORS

Melanocytic lesions (classified in Table 1-4) are the second most common conjunctival lesions submitted to ophthalmic pathology laboratories (see Table 1-1). Although benign lesions outnumber malignant tumors, a correct interpretation of the histopathologic findings is important to guide clinical and surgical management, and preclude unnecessary systemic metastatic workups. Secondary pigmentation by migration of melanocytes, epithelial cells, or macrophages containing melanin may occur after chronic inflammation or trauma and may be associated with benign or malignant epithelial tumors. Pigment resembling melanin may be observed clinically in patients on topical and systemic medications such as epinephrine, tetracycline, or silver-containing products; with metabolic diseases such as ochronosis; and in cases of foreign bodies containing iron.

Nevi

General Features. *Conjunctival nevi* first appear in childhood as small, circumscribed, flat lesions which may or may not be pigmented (81). Their incidence is 0.012/100,000 population/year (82). The most frequent locations of conjunctival nevi are the bulbar conjunctiva and limbus in the interpalpebral region (fig. 1-34), the caruncle, the semilunar fold, and, rarely, the tarsal conjunctiva at the lid margin. Pigmentation may vary from amelanotic lesions to heavily pigmented tumors; however, most are pink to yellow-tan or brown (fig. 1-35). Growth of a nevus may be the result of factors other than melanocytic proliferation, such as inflammatory cell infiltration; nevi are capable of growth especially during puberty and pregnancy.

Microscopic Findings. Conjunctival nevi are classified as junctional, compound, and subepithelial. A *junctional nevus* is composed of contiguous nests of round to spindle-shaped melanocytes that have oval nuclei and small nucleoli, aligned along the basal cell region. The cells may show loss of cohesion and have larger vesicular nuclei with prominent basophilic nucleoli, but there is no atypia.

Cells of the more common *compound nevus* are present in both the epithelium and the subepithelial connective tissue. Because of the thin conjunctival epithelium, nests of nevus cells may seem to replace the full thickness of the

Table 1-4

CLASSIFICATION OF MELANOCYTIC LESIONS OF THE CONJUNCTIVA

- I. **Congenital**
  - Epithelial
    - Racial pigmentation
    - Benign epithelial melanosis
    - Ephelis
  - Subepithelial
    - Ocular melanocytosis
    - Oculodermal melanocytosis
- II. **Nevi**
  - Congenital
  - Acquired
    - Junctional
    - Subepithelial
    - Compound
    - Variants
      - Spindle/epithelioid
      - Blue nevus
      - Combined nevus
      - Melanocytoma
- III. **Acquired Melanosis**
  - Bilateral
    - Racial
    - Metabolic
    - Toxic
  - Unilateral
    - Secondary melanosis
    - Primary acquired melanosis
- IV. **Melanoma**
  - In primary acquired melanosis
  - De novo
  - In nevi
  - Secondary from uveal melanoma
  - Metastatic

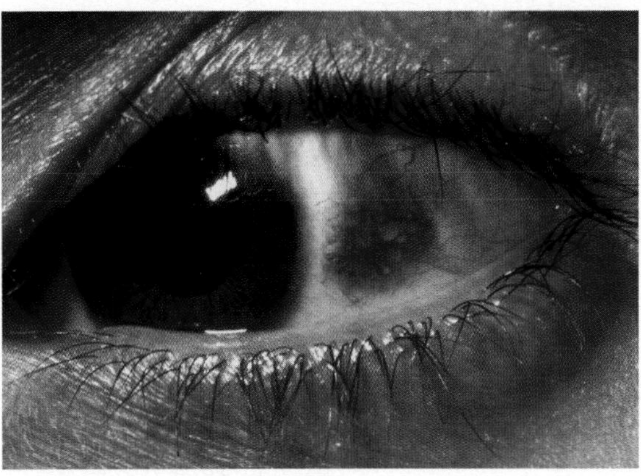

Figure 1-34

CONJUNCTIVAL NEVUS

Young patient with a circumscribed pigmented lesion of the conjunctiva. Round whitish areas correspond to cystic structures.

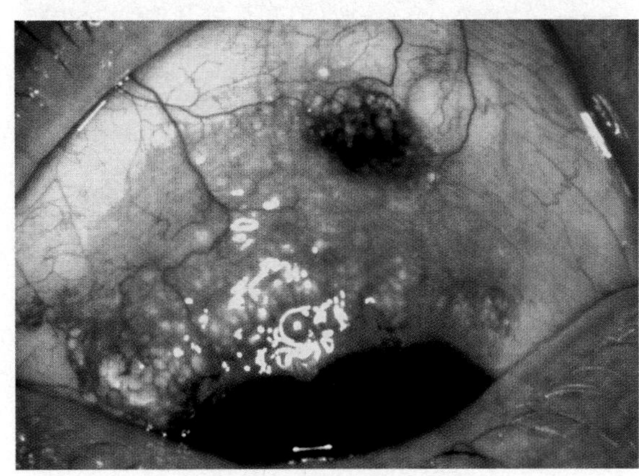

Figure 1-35

CONJUNCTIVAL NEVUS

Large conjunctival nevus of the superior limbus.

conjunctival epithelium. These nevi characteristically have cells with intranuclear inclusions and cysts of variable size lined by cuboidal cells and goblet cells. The cysts may be large and obscure the lightly pigmented nevus cells (figs. 1-36, 1-37). Compound nevi may have pigmented cells that are large and have prominent basophilic nucleoli. These cells are located at the basal layers of the epithelium and extend into the superficial stroma; they are regarded as manifesting junctional activity. The same nevi in deeper regions may disclose smaller cells with round nuclei (fig. 1-38). Mitotic figures are usually absent. Inflammation is a common finding, and it is seen in 86 percent of the cases (fig. 1-39). The inflammatory cells are represented by lymphocytes, plasma cells, monocytes, polymorphonuclear leukocytes, and, especially in children, eosinophils.

The last stage of conjunctival nevus ontogeny is represented by nevus cells with bland nuclei entirely located in the subepithelial connective tissue. These *subepithelial nevi* are usually nonpigmented. Occasionally, most of the nevus cells have clear cytoplasm due to the presence of lipid (lipidized nevus cells) and this type of nevus has been termed *balloon cell nevus* (fig. 1-40) (83).

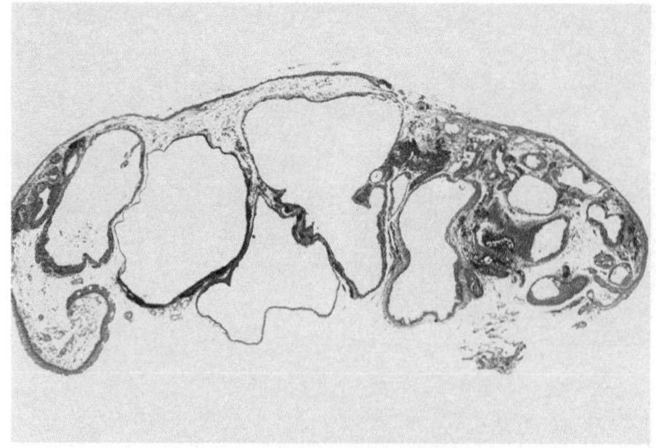

Figure 1-36

CONJUNCTIVAL NEVUS

Low-power magnification of a conjunctival nevus shows a well-circumscribed symmetrical lesion with cysts.

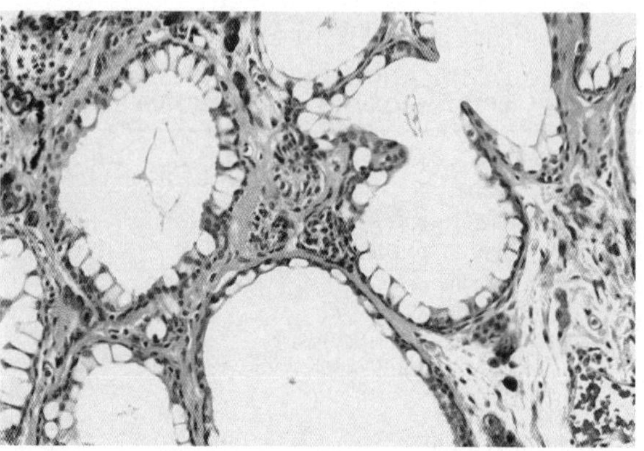

Figure 1-37

CONJUNCTIVAL NEVUS

Pigmented nevus cells surround large cystic spaces lined by cuboidal epithelium. The epithelium contains mucus-secreting goblet cells.

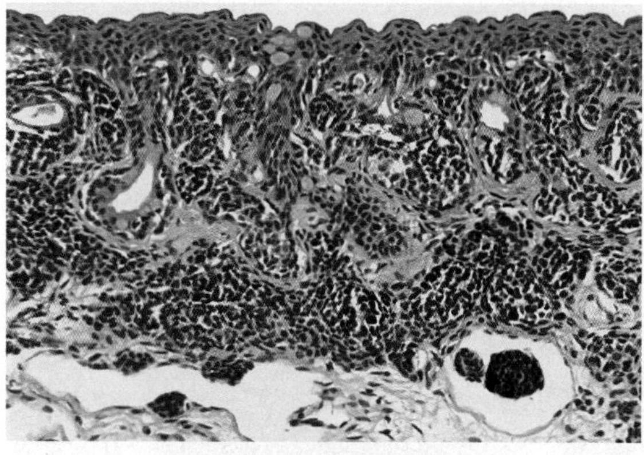

Figure 1-38

CONJUNCTIVAL NEVUS

Small nevus cells are within the lumen of lymphatic channels in the deepest part of the lesion.

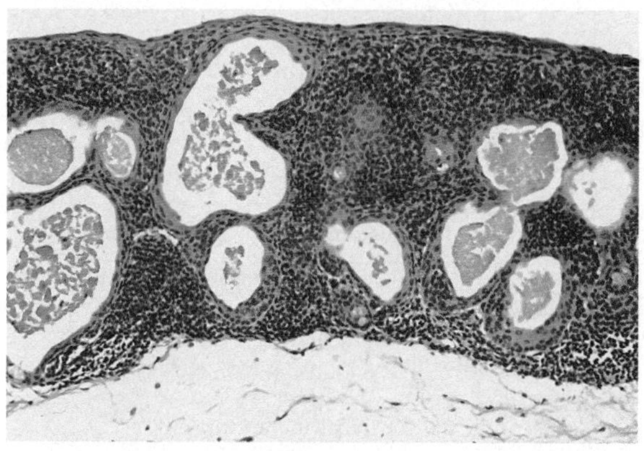

Figure 1-39

INFLAMMED CONJUNCTIVAL NEVUS

Lightly pigmented nevus cells are infiltrated by small lymphocytes.

Differential Diagnosis. Common nevi of the conjunctiva may change color, become elevated, and grow large, particularly during puberty and adolescence. A growing nevus may show atypical cellular features and occasional mitotic figures. The absence of an atypical intraepithelial component, atypical mitotic figures, and necrosis, however, is helpful for the differentiation from melanoma. Malignant transformation of a nevus occurs in 1 of 150,000 lesions (84). Despite careful histopathologic examination, a group of indeterminate melanocytic lesions exists that cannot be classified by pathologists as benign or malignant (85).

Treatment and Prognosis. In children, because conjunctival nevi rarely progress to malignant melanoma, excision of all pigmented lesions is not indicated. Indications for surgical treatment include newly acquired pigmented lesions in adults, clinical evidence of growth, change in pigmentation associated with increased vascularization, and cosmetic reasons. Complete excision is the treatment of choice. Biopsy is only indicated in very large lesions at the time of presentation for histopathologic study and accurate diagnosis before definitive therapy is instituted. The rate of recurrence is 2.7 percent following local excision (86).

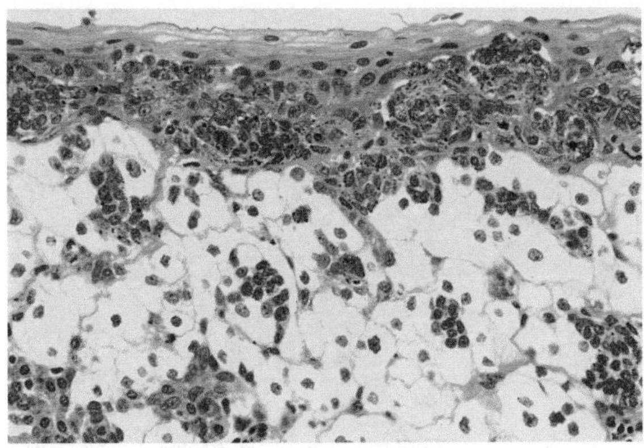

Figure 1-40

BALLOON CELL NEVUS

Most of the cells have clear cytoplasm and a hyperchromatic, centrally located nucleus.

Nevus Variants

Spindle and Epithelioid Cell Nevus. This is the conjunctival counterpart of the Spitz epithelioid nevus of the skin (87,88). The lesion is seen mainly in childhood as a nonpigmented lesion with a pink-yellow nodular appearance that may or may not be associated with rapid growth. The cellular component has an admixture of uniform, large, epithelioid-like cells with lightly pigmented spindle cells that often exhibit a "wind-blown" pattern. The cells are located mainly in the subepithelial connective tissue (87,88). The *pigmented spindle cell nevus* described by Reed (89) is best regarded as a pigmented variant of a Spitz nevus. Histologically, the pigmented nevus cells are arranged in nests in the basal cell layer and "rain down" into the subepithelial connective tissue (89).

Blue Nevus and Cellular Blue Nevus. These lesions are bluish brown because of the superficial location and lack of dermis-like collagenous tissue between the pigmented cells and the surface (90,91). Pigmented spindle and dendritic melanocytic nevus cells extend within the collagenous stroma.

Combined Nevus. Combined nevus of the conjunctiva has been recognized recently (92). It combines the histologic features of a compound or subepithelial acquired melanocytic nevus and a pigmented blue nevus. The importance of its recognition is not to misinterpret the spindle-shaped melanocytic nevus cells as malignant transformation.

Melanocytoma (Magnocellular Nevus). Melanocytoma is a rare, benign, deeply pigmented melanocytic nevus of the optic nerve and uveal tissue that rarely may arise in the conjunctiva (93). The lesion is heavily pigmented, disclosing a uniform brown to jet-black color. It is composed of large, polygonal melanocytic cells heavily loaded with pigment that obscures the nuclei. After bleaching, the cells disclose round nuclei with evenly distributed chromatin and small nucleoli. Melanocytic spindle cells may be present among the polygonal nevus cells.

OTHER BENIGN MELANOCYTIC LESIONS

Racial Pigmentation and Benign Epithelial Melanosis

Conjunctival pigmentation seen in pigmented individuals is termed *racial pigmentation, racial melanosis, complexion-associated conjunctival pigmentation*, and *benign epithelial melanosis*. The incidence of conjunctival pigmentation varies: 92.5 percent in blacks, 36 percent in Asians, 28 percent in Hispanics, and 4.9 percent in whites (94). This bilateral pigmentation is denser at the junction between the peripheral cornea and limbus and fades towards the bulbar conjunctiva. The melanocytes are not increased in number. Microscopically, the basal layer of the epithelium is pigmented and melanin typically accumulates in a supranuclear location. The pigmented cells should not be confused with early stages of benign primary acquired melanosis without atypia, where melanin is located in the epithelial cells and is associated with variable, benign melanocytic proliferation.

Ephelides

Ephelides, or *freckles,* are congenital focal lesions found in the interpalpebral conjunctiva that become pigmented in childhood and adolescence. The localized pigmented foci are not elevated, and the surrounding conjunctiva is normal. Histologically, the conjunctival epithelium has a normal appearance except for the presence of a well-circumscribed area of hyperpigmented basal cells. The pigmentation remains stable over time.

Congenital Pigmentation (Ocular Melanocytosis, Oculodermal Melanocytosis)

Abnormal migration of melanocytes during development may result in unusual sectorial or diffuse pigmentation of the ocular and periocular tissues. *Ocular melanocytosis* refers to the pigmentation of ocular structures while *oculodermal melanocytosis,* or *nevus of Ota*, includes, in addition, ipsilateral pigmentation of the periocular skin in the region innervated by the trigeminal nerve. Although these conditions may predispose to the development of uveal and orbital melanoma, there are no reported cases of conjunctiva melanoma arising in patients with congenital ocular melanocytosis. Microscopically, the pigmentation is localized to the episclera, and consists of pigmented dendritic or spindle melanocytes distributed among collagen fibers. The epithelium and subepithelial connective tissue are not involved.

PRIMARY ACQUIRED MELANOSIS

Definition. *Primary acquired melanosis* (PAM) is a clinicopathologic term used to describe a unilateral intraepithelial proliferation of abnormal melanocytes of the conjunctiva that possess variable biologic behavior, from benign to locally spreading to malignant (95). Several names have been used to designate this entity in the past, including precancerous and cancerous melanosis of Reese, epithelial melanosis, primary idiopathic acquired melanosis, conjunctival hypermelanosis, benign acquired melanosis, intraepithelial atypical melanocytic hyperplasia, premalignant melanosis, malignant acquired melanosis, melanoma in situ, and melanoma radial growth phase. The World Health Organization adopted the term primary acquired melanosis as a unifying concept to describe the varied clinicopathologic manifestations (96,28).

General Features. Epidemiologic studies suggest that PAM is a frequent lesion of the conjunctiva, seen in about 36 percent of adult Caucasians (97). Similar lesions are also noted in Asians, but in this racial group PAM has a benign biologic behavior without malignant potential (98). Approximately one third of cases of PAM confirmed histologically develop into melanoma (99). The average time from a confirmed diagnosis of PAM with atypia to melanoma is 2.5 years (100).

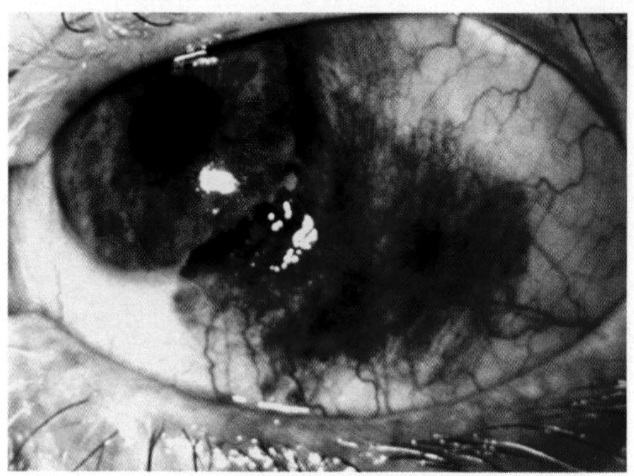

Figure 1-41

PRIMARY ACQUIRED MELANOSIS

Extensive pigmentation of the bulbar and limbal conjunctivae as well as pigmentation of the margin of the eyelid.

Clinical Features. The first clinical manifestation is the slowly progressive appearance of a golden-brown, flat pigmentation of the conjunctiva in middle-aged white patients. The predominant location is the bulbar conjunctiva (in any of its quadrants), but also the forniceal and palpebral conjunctivae are involved (fig. 1-41). The pigmented lesions begin insidiously and progress relentlessly, involving other areas of the conjunctiva. The corneal epithelium has a fine, dusty, golden-brown pigmentation due to the extension of the melanocytic intraepithelial proliferation. In some patients, the palpebral pigmentation is contiguous with lentigo maligna (Hutchinson's melanotic freckle) of the adjacent skin of the eyelid.

Microscopic Findings. Usually, there is a spectrum of epithelial involvement by abnormal melanocytes (fig. 1-42). The early stage is represented by pigmentation of the basilar epithelial layer, either as the only finding or associated with minimal melanocytic hyperplasia. Abnormal melanocytes produce pigment that is transferred to, or phagocytized by, the adjacent epithelial cells. Discharged melanin may also be phagocytized by macrophages in the substantia propria. Lesions composed of melanocytes without pigment are called *acquired melanosis "sine pigmento"* (101,102).

With progression, melanocytes proliferate as a layer of transformed isolated cells in the basal location, termed *basilar melanocytic hyperplasia,*

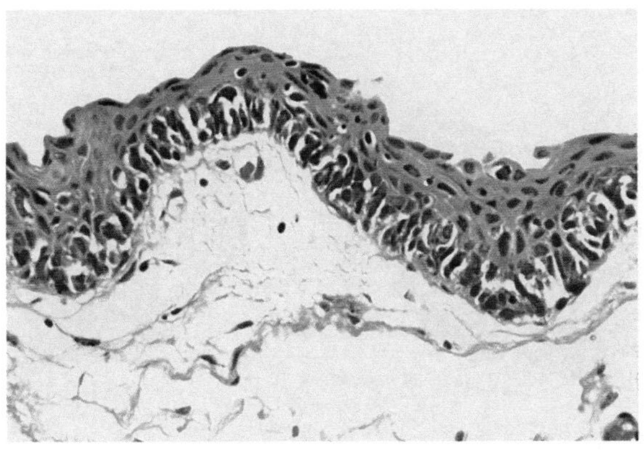

Figure 1-42

PRIMARY ACQUIRED MELANOSIS

Diffuse involvement of the basal epithelial layer by pigmented atypical melanocytes.

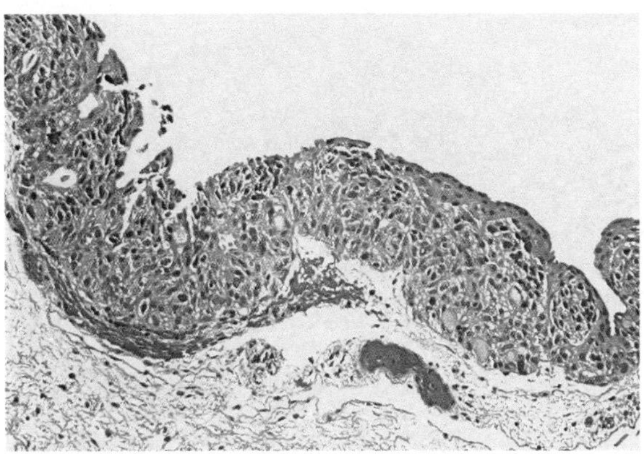

Figure 1-43

PRIMARY ACQUIRED MELANOSIS

Atypical melanocytes are arranged in nests within the conjunctival epithelium.

while basilar nests push the overlying epithelium without extending into the superficial epithelium. The proliferating melanocytes may detach from the basal location and form intraepithelial nests (fig. 1-43). Round, epithelioid, atypical melanocytes move upward into the superficial epithelial layers, adopting a pagetoid growth pattern that resembles extramammary Paget's disease. Individual atypical melanocytes have retracted cytoplasm; nuclei are usually larger than those of the surrounding epithelial cells, with clumping of the chromatin and prominent basophilic nucleoli. Four types of atypical melanocytes may be found: small polyhedral cells with small round nuclei and scanty cytoplasm, epithelioid cells with abundant cytoplasm, spindle cells, and large dendritic melanocytes. Occasional mitotic figures may be identified.

In more advanced stages, melanophages and a patchy inflammatory infiltrate composed of lymphocytes and mononuclear cells are seen in the substantia propria. Microinvasive melanoma develops in areas of marked confluent intraepithelial melanocytic atypia. Most commonly, the infiltrating neoplastic cells have the same configuration as the intraepithelial melanocytic cells. In other cases, the early subepithelial invasive component is composed of variably pigmented spindled melanocytes that appear mildly atypical and are oriented parallel to the basal epithelial layer. Actinic damage of the collagen and foci of benign nevus cells are observed in 20 percent of cases. These findings are unrelated to the development of PAM and do not have any prognostic significance (103).

PAM is currently classified as without atypia and with atypia. PAM without atypia includes those lesions with hyperpigmented basal epithelial cells and basilar melanocytic hyperplasia without cytologic atypia. The identification of atypical melanocytes with nuclear atypia and epithelioid features establishes the diagnosis of PAM with atypia, independent of the degree of intraepithelial involvement. PAM with atypia is divided into low risk and high risk for the development of malignant melanoma, based on either the absence or presence of atypical melanocytes with an epithelioid cell configuration or an intraepithelial growth pattern resembling intraepithelial melanoma in situ other than basilar melanocytic hyperplasia (104).

Immunohistochemical Findings. Immunohistochemistry is useful for differentiating PAM from nonmelanocytic lesions. The melanocytic cells stain consistently with HMB45 (fig. 1-44), S-100 protein, vimentin, and Melan-A, and are negative for cytokeratin and EMA.

Ultrastructural Findings. Although electron microscopy is not routinely used for the diagnosis of PAM, certain ultrastructural features help assess the progress to malignancy (104). PAM without atypia shows melanocytes with dendritic processes and transferred melanin in the epithelial cells. This change is regarded as grade 1. Grade 2 PAM consists of melanocytic cells

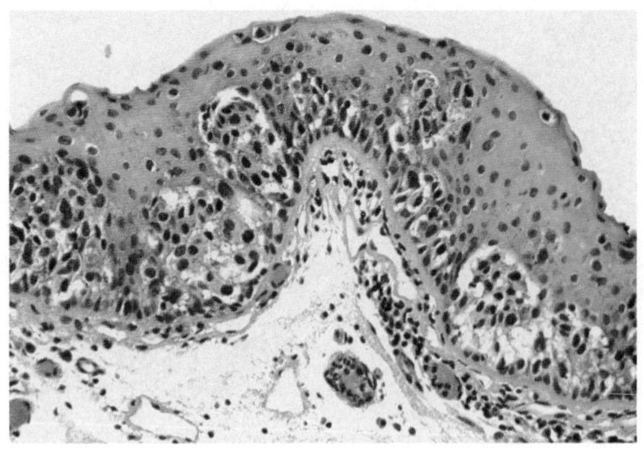

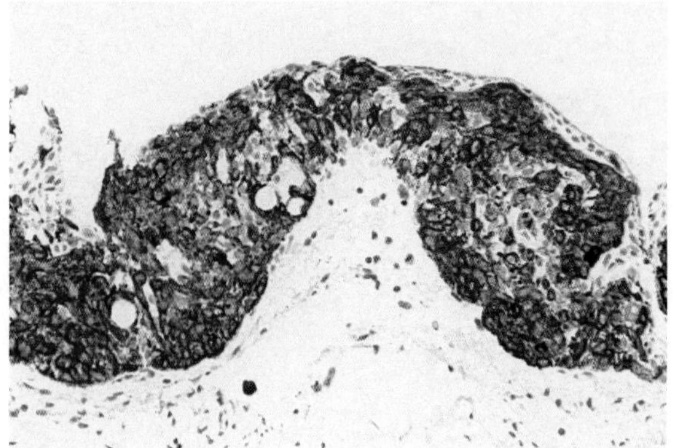

Figure 1-44

PRIMARY ACQUIRED MELANOSIS

Left: The conjunctival epithelium is almost completely replaced by atypical melanocytes resembling melanoma in situ. Right: The atypical melanocytes are positive for HMB45 antibody.

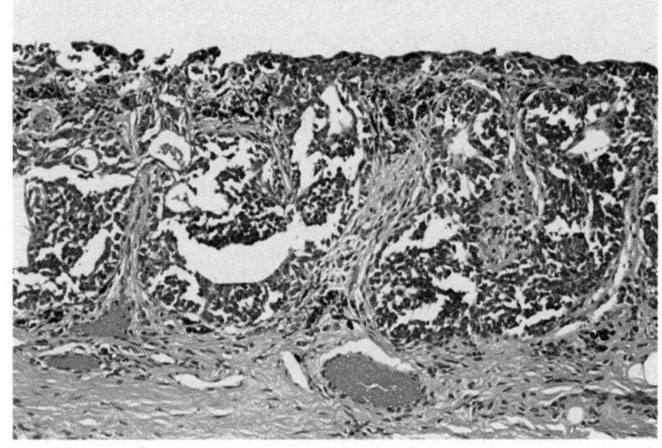

Figure 1-45

PRIMARY ACQUIRED MELANOSIS

Atypical melanocytes infiltrate the epithelium of the pseudoglands of Henle.

having shorter dendritic processes, with incomplete melanization and immature melanosomes, more irregular nuclei with clumped heterochromatin, and large nucleoli. The presence of epithelioid cells corresponds to grade 3. These cells do not have cytoplasmic processes; they have large irregular nuclei with large prominent nucleoli and abnormal melanogenesis.

Cytologic Findings. Examination of cytologic samples as a screening method for diagnosis discloses the presence of atypical melanocytes in 73 percent of the cases (105).

Differential Diagnosis. Differentiation of a junctional nevus from PAM in the absence of clinical data may be difficult. Junctional nevi occur primarily in children, whereas PAM is seen in adults. Microscopic features that help distinguish PAM are the presence of polygonal cells, nuclear atypia, a mixture of isolated melanocytic cells and nests, and irregular involvement of the epithelium.

In the palpebral conjunctiva, PAM may involve the pseudoglands of Henle, and such lesions are occasionally misinterpreted as invasive melanoma (fig. 1-45). Other pitfalls are misinterpretation of melanophages as invasive pigmented cells and not recognizing spindle-shaped melanocytic cells with bland nuclei as malignant.

Treatment and Prognosis. Any nodular lesion, enlarging flat lesion, pigmented lesion of the cul de sac and palpebral conjunctiva, or clinically suspicious pigmentation should be either completely excised or biopsied based on lesion size. Some authors have suggested that any flat speckled lesion greater than 2 to 3 mm in diameter should be excised. Based on the diagnosis, the presence and degree of cytologic atypia, and the completeness of excision, patients may receive additional treatment and should be followed at regular intervals. Because of the diffuse involvement of PAM, the use of topical mitomycin C and 5-fluorouracil has theoretical advantages and has shown promising results (106,107). Biopsies of PAM after topical chemotherapy with mitomycin may show epithelial atrophy, dyskeratosis, pyknotic nuclei,

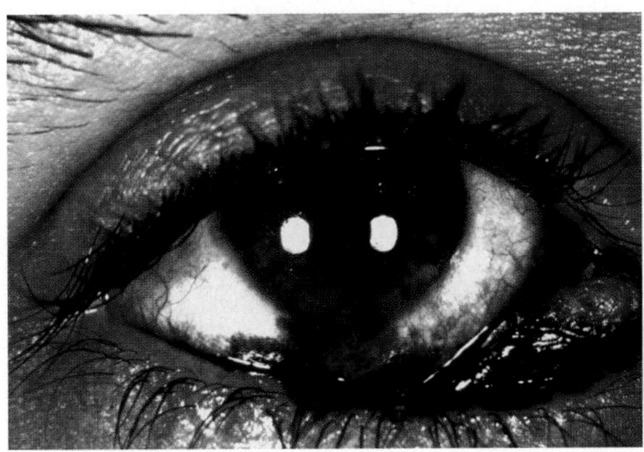

Figure 1-46

MALIGNANT MELANOMA ARISING FROM PRIMARY ACQUIRED MELANOSIS

There is involvement of the bulbar conjunctiva nasally and the inner canthal area.

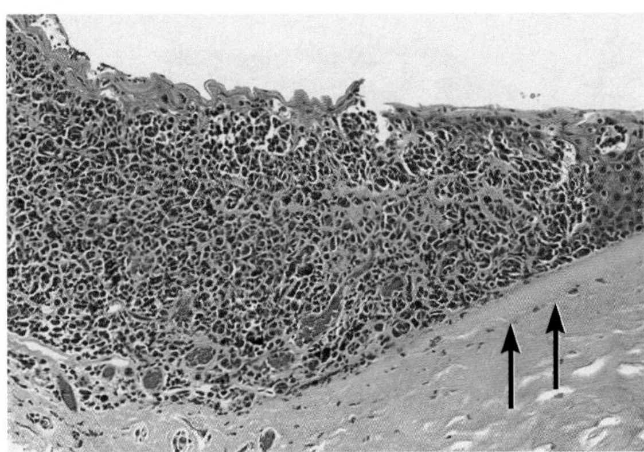

Figure 1-47

MALIGNANT MELANOMA ARISING FROM PRIMARY ACQUIRED MELANOSIS

Melanoma of the conjunctiva at the limbus involves the corneal epithelium. Note the presence of the Bowman layer at the corneal edge (arrows).

and focal keratinization associated with subepithelial inflammation. Recurrences or the development of new foci is the rule rather than the exception in cases of PAM with atypia. If progression of PAM to melanoma is not observed after the first 10 years after diagnosis, the patient is at low risk for the development of malignant melanoma (108).

MELANOMA

General Features. *Melanoma of the conjunctiva* accounts for approximately 2 percent of ocular malignancies and 5 percent of ocular melanomas (109,110). It is the second most frequent malignant neoplasm of the conjunctiva after SCC. The annual age-adjusted incidence of conjunctival melanoma in the United States is approximately 0.012 cases/100,000 population, 0.024/100,000 in Sweden, and 0.052/100,000 in Denmark (111–113). The development of melanoma in black patients is rare (114). Melanomas may originate from preexisting PAM, from nevi, or de novo. The former preexisting condition is noted in 25 to 75 percent of cases (fig. 1-46) (115,116). About 20 to 30 percent of patients with conjunctival melanoma, with or without PAM, have histologic evidence of a preexisting nevus or give a history of a conjunctival pigmented lesion from childhood (116). In about 18 to 25 percent of the cases there is no preexisting PAM or nevus (116,117). Most melanomas of the conjunctiva are heavily vascularized, pigmented, nodular or elevated tumors that usually arise in areas of preexisting conjunctival pigmentation. The average mean age at the time of diagnosis from several studies is in the fifth decade (116), with an age range of 11 to 89 years (118,119). Melanomas are extremely rare in children and adolescents (120). Although they are most frequent in the interpalpebral region of the bulbar conjunctiva (fig. 1-47), they may be observed arising from the fornix, palpebral conjunctiva, and inner canthus.

Microscopic Findings. By definition, the invasion of atypical melanocytes into the subepithelial connective tissue, no matter how superficial, qualifies the lesion as melanoma. Typical malignant melanoma of the conjunctiva is not difficult to diagnose histopathologically. The surface epithelium is usually very thin and contains atypical melanocytes. Most commonly, the tumor is composed of bizarre, polygonal, epithelioid cells with eosinophilic cytoplasm; atypical large vesicular nuclei; and prominent eosinophilic nucleoli. Mitotic activity and lacunar round cells undergoing apoptosis may be present. A mixture of other cell types, including small polyhedral cells, smaller spindle cells with oval nuclei, and balloon cells with clear multivacuolated cytoplasm containing lipid and nuclear indentation, may be present. Other melanomas are composed entirely of small epithelioid cells with irregular nuclei,

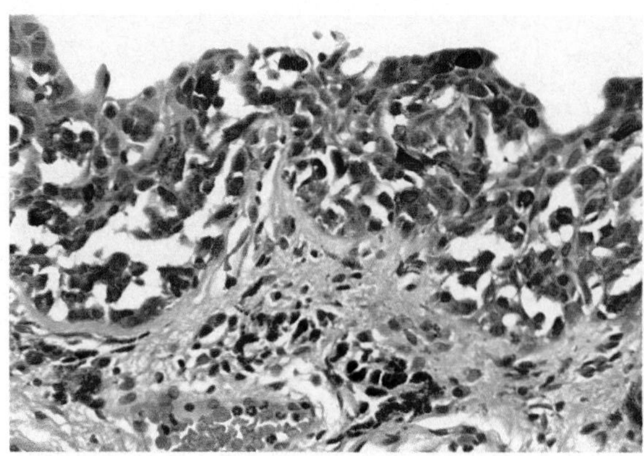

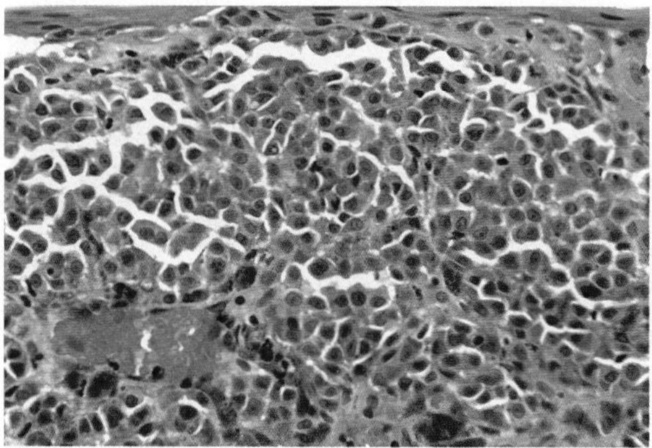

Figure 1-48

MALIGNANT MELANOMA ARISING FROM PRIMARY ACQUIRED MELANOSIS

Left: The epithelium of the bulbar conjunctiva is infiltrated by atypical melanocytes.
Right: Section of the melanoma in the same patient is composed of atypical epithelioid melanocytes.

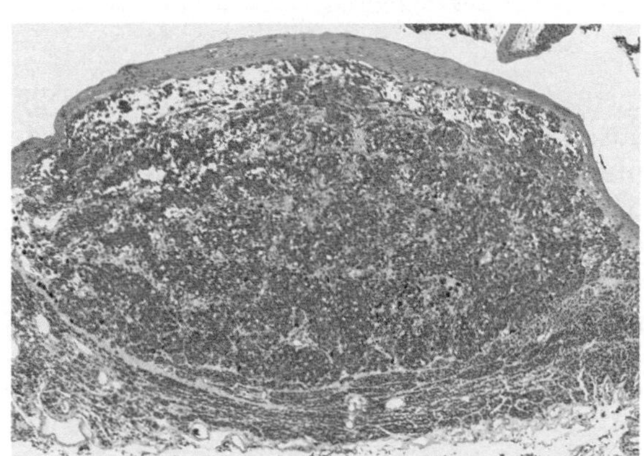

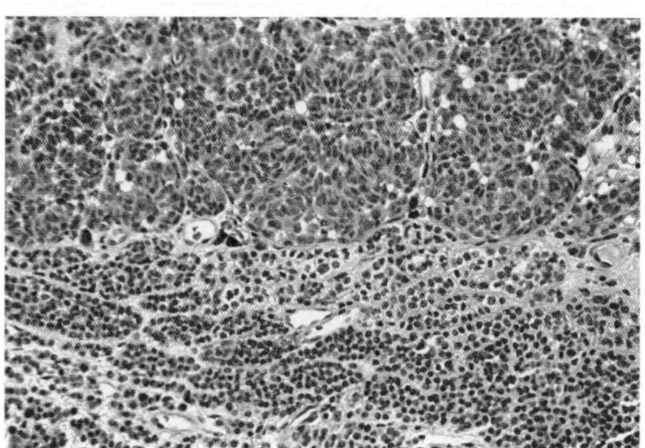

Figure 1-49

MALIGNANT MELANOMA ARISING FROM NEVUS

Left: Low-power magnification shows a malignant melanoma with a nevus in the deep part of the lesion.
Right: Higher magnification reveals small nonpigmented nevus cells (bottom) underneath malignant melanoma cells (top).

clumped granular chromatin disclosing basophilic nucleoli, or spindle-shaped cells. Lymphocytes are often observed among the neoplastic cells and at the base and infiltrating edges of the lesion. The degree of pigmentation and necrosis is variable.

An important histologic feature is whether or not PAM is present (fig. 1-48). Because large melanomas at the time of excision show an ulcerated surface, examination of the epithelium at the edge of the excision may reveal findings of PAM such as pagetoid spread and atypical intraepithelial epithelioid melanocytes. There may be histologic evidence of a subjacent nevus (fig. 1-49).

One clinicopathologic criterion for melanomas arising de novo is a definite statement from the patient, relatives, and the ophthalmologist that there was no evidence of abnormality or pigmentation of the conjunctiva before the development of the melanoma. In these cases, careful ophthalmologic examination shows no evidence of pigmentation on the remaining conjunctival epithelium. Adequate sampling and histopathologic examination of the surrounding conjunctiva show neither evidence of hyperpigmentation nor proliferation of melanocytes throughout the epithelium.

Immunohistochemical Findings and Special Studies. Immunohistochemical studies are valuable for confirming the diagnosis of a nonpigmented melanoma and for differentiating melanoma from other primary or secondary undifferentiated malignant neoplasms of the conjunctiva. Conjunctival melanoma cells are consistently positive for HMB45, vimentin, S-100 protein, and Melan-A. Aggressive melanomas composed of epithelioid cells may show focal positivity for cytokeratin. Proliferative nuclear and cytoplasmic antigens such as PCNA and Ki-67 (MIB-1) may be used as a proliferative index in addition to the mitotic rate (121,122). Studies of nucleolar organizer regions have suggested a cutoff value of 4.0 (mean silver staining of nucleolar organizer regions per cell) to differentiate melanoma and PAM with atypia from nevi and PAM without atypia (123).

Ultrastructural Findings. In rare cases that cannot be resolved with immunohistochemical stains, ultrastructural studies may provide valuable diagnostic information (124).

Differential Diagnosis. Primary melanoma of the conjunctiva should be differentiated from metastatic melanoma and "in transit" metastasis, and extraocular extension from a primary uveal melanoma. Metastatic melanoma has a circumscribed appearance when observed under low-power magnification. The tumor is not connected to the epithelium, which is uninvolved and often separated by a more compact collagen layer. Melanomas of the ciliary body and iris may present with a subconjunctival mass. Careful ophthalmologic examination readily rules out an anterior uveal melanoma. Nonpigmented spindle cell melanoma of the conjunctiva also may resemble the spindle variant of SCC and other soft tissue spindle cell and fibrous histiocytic tumors.

During the first two decades of life melanoma of the conjunctiva is rare. The pathologist should be cautious in making the diagnosis of melanoma in children; however, because of the difficulty in making a definite diagnosis, clear recommendations for management and follow-up should be provided to a child with a pigmented lesion.

Treatment and Prognosis. Primary treatment of malignant melanoma of the conjunctiva consists of complete surgical excision of the tumor and application of cryotherapy to the surgical edges and base of the lesion. Postoperative topical chemotherapy and radiotherapy are additional treatments for patients in whom the tumor cannot be excised completely or in whom there were previous recurrences or melanomas associated with PAM with atypia. Exenteration of the orbit does not preclude the development of metastasis and death and is used as a palliative procedure for advanced local disease (fig. 1-50) (125). Local tumor recurrences vary from 23 to 56 percent (117,126). Recurrences are primarily related to the initial method of treatment and should be expected in incompletely excised tumors (119). In one study, the time interval from excision to recurrence varied from 3 months to 14 years, with a mean interval of 2.5 years (117). The presence of one or more recurrences is associated with an increased incidence of distant metastasis (117). The development of new primary melanomas of the conjunctiva should be expected in patients with PAM with atypia.

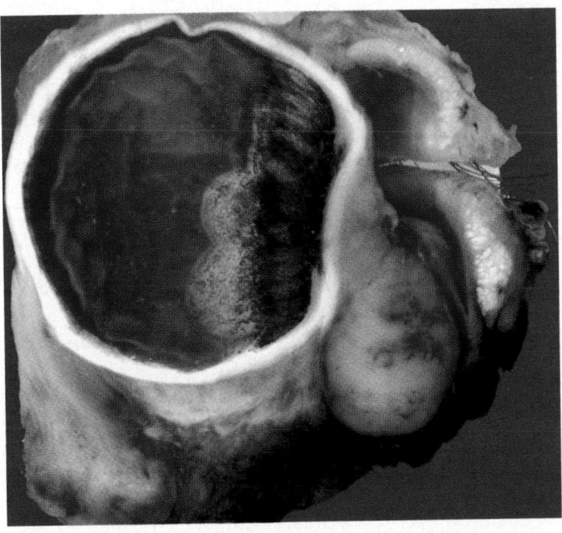

Figure 1-50

MALIGNANT MELANOMA ARISING FROM PRIMARY ACQUIRED MELANOSIS "SINE PIGMENTO"

Exenteration specimen shows nodular tumors infiltrating the orbital tissue.

Since the conjunctival layers differ totally from their cutaneous counterpart, the classifications of skin melanomas according to Clark's grading and Breslow's thickness measurements

Table 1-5

STAGING OF MELANOMA OF CONJUNCTIVA[a]

Clinical Classification (cTNM)	
Primary Tumor (T)	
TX	Primary tumor cannot be assessed
T0	No evidence of primary tumor
T1	Tumor(s) of bulbar conjunctiva occupying one quadrant or less
T2	Tumor(s) of bulbar conjunctiva occupying more than one quadrant
T3	Tumor(s) of conjunctival fornix and/or palpebral conjunctiva and/or caruncle
T4	Tumor invades eyelid, cornea, and/or orbit
Regional Lymph Nodes (N)	
NX	Regional lymph nodes cannot be assessed
N0	No regional lymph node metastasis
N1	Regional lymph node metastasis
Distant Metastasis (M)	
MX	Distant metastasis cannot be assessed
M0	No distant metastasis
M1	Distant metastasis
Pathologic Classification (pTNM)	
Primary Tumor (pT)	
pTX	Primary tumor cannot be assessed
pT0	No evidence of primary tumor
pT1	Tumor(s) of bulbar conjunctiva occupying one quadrant or less and 2 mm or less in thickness
pT2	Tumor(s) of bulbar conjunctiva occupying more than one quadrant and 2 mm or less in thickness
pT3	Tumor(s) of conjunctival fornix and/or palpebral conjunctiva and/or caruncle or tumor(s) of the bulbar conjunctiva, more than 2 mm in thickness
pT4	Tumor invades eyelid, cornea, and/or orbit
Regional Lymph Nodes (pN)	
pNX	Regional lymph nodes cannot be assessed
pN0	No regional lymph node metastasis
pN1	Regional lymph node metastasis
Distant Metastasis (pM)	
MX	Distant metastasis cannot be assessed
pM0	No distant metastasis
pM1	Distant metastasis
Histopathologic Grade (G)	
GX	Origin cannot be assessed
G0	Primary acquired melanosis
G1	Malignant melanoma arises from a nevus
G2	Malignant melanoma arises from primary acquired melanosis
G3	Malignant melanoma arises de novo

[a]Data from reference 62.

cannot be applied to conjunctival melanoma. Tumor thickness is measured from the surface of the lesion to the deepest margin of tumor invasion by using a calibrated micrometer grid. Some studies have shown that 1.8 mm of thickness separates lethal from nonlethal cases (127). Recent studies, however, have reduced the thickness threshold to 0.8 mm (8). The death rate is two times higher with tumor thickness of 1 to 4 mm and four times higher in tumors greater than 4 mm thick. Histologic factors suggesting a poor prognosis include origin from PAM with pagetoid intraepithelial spread; tumors composed of epithelioid cells rather than spindle cells; greater than 5 mitotic figures per 10 high-power fields; lack of lymphocytic host response; the presence of lymphatic, vascular, or perineural invasion; and invasion of the episcleral tissue, sclera, cornea, and orbit (115,116,125–131). Patients with tumors in anatomic locations other than the limbus, as well as those with multifocal nodules, have a guarded prognosis (119).

Conjunctival melanomas disseminate first to the preauricular and intraparotid lymph nodes, followed by submandibular and cervical lymph nodes, followed by lung, brain, skin, liver, and bone metastases. Regional lymph node dissection (sentinel node) is performed only in high-risk patients and in those with positive clinical or image studies. The presence of positive lymph nodes is not always followed by dissemination to other sites. On the other hand, lymph node dissection does not preclude the development of systemic metastasis. The overall mortality rate from metastatic spread of conjunctival melanoma is 25 percent and varies from 14 to 32 percent (113,116,117,119,125). The 5-year and 10-year survival rates in different series are 77 to 86 percent and 64 to 73 percent, respectively (115, 126,132). Survival rates appear to be lower in Asians: 53 percent after 5 years (131). The average time from diagnosis to metastasis is 3.6 years, and from diagnosis to death, 4.4 years (117).

Staging. Staging is based on complete resection of the primary site and histologic study of the margins and deep tissues (Table 1-5). Resection or needle biopsy of enlarged regional lymph nodes or orbital masses is desirable.

SOFT TISSUE TUMORS

The nonepithelial tissues of the conjunctiva include vascular and lymphatic structures, peripheral nerves, adipose tissue in the caruncle, and mesenchymal elements, all of which give

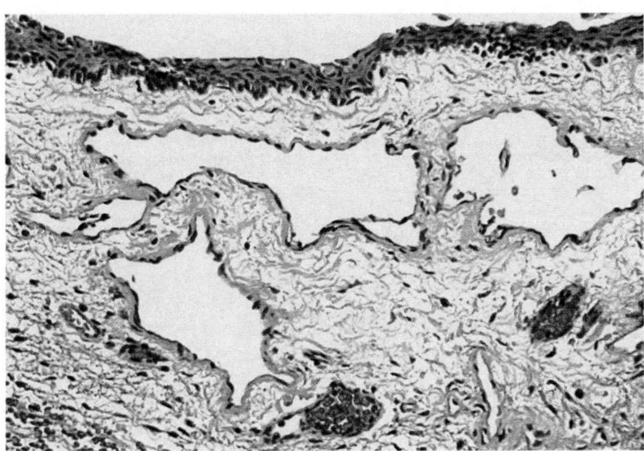

Figure 1-51

LYMPHANGIECTASIA

There are three dilated lymphatic channels in the bulbar conjunctiva.

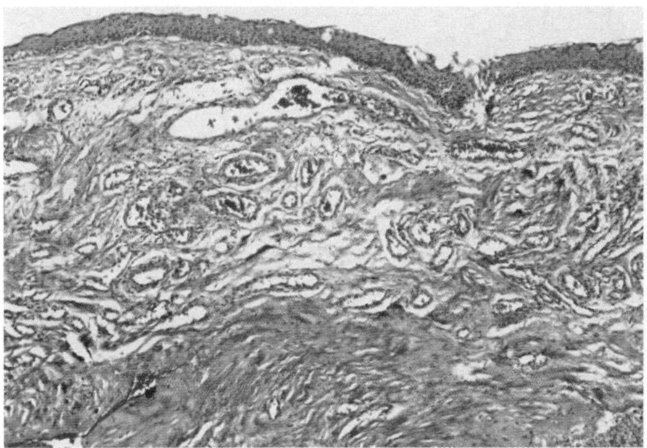

Figure 1-52

CAPILLARY HEMANGIOMA

This vascular tumor of the conjunctiva is composed of small capillary vessels.

rise to several types of soft tissue tumors (133–142). Most of these tumors do not differ from those originating in other locations in regards to gross features, microscopic findings, and behavior, and most are benign. Exceptions are the botryoid variant of embryonal rhabdomyosarcoma, malignant fibrous histiocytoma, and Kaposi's sarcoma involving the conjunctiva and eyelid in patients with AIDS. Following is a discussion and presentation of some characteristic features of conjunctival soft tissue lesions. A more detailed description is found in the chapter on tumors of the orbit.

Vascular Tumors

Vascular lesions of the conjunctiva are frequently seen clinically and include *capillary telangiectasias, vascular tortuosities* and *varix*, and *lymphangiectases* (fig. 1-51). Vascular tortuosity and lymphangiectases of the conjunctiva are seen as part of congenital systemic malformation syndromes termed phakomatoses, including Sturge-Weber syndrome and ataxia telangiectasia (Louis-Bar syndrome).

Hemangiomas of the capillary type may be isolated or associated with a large capillary hemangioma affecting the eyelid and periocular skin. They do not differ from capillary hemangiomas arising elsewhere (fig. 1-52). The differential diagnosis of acquired capillary hemangioma includes pyogenic granuloma and Kaposi's sarcoma. *Cavernous hemangiomas* are composed of enlarged, round, blood-filled vessels that are lined by endothelial cells and are surrounded by pericytes and scattered smooth muscle cells, arranged in a loose collagenous stroma.

Lymphangiomas of the conjunctiva should be considered as part of a larger lesion that already has or may progress to affect the orbit and the eyelids. Microscopically, the lesion shows a sinusoidal pattern of vascular empty spaces lined by flat endothelial cells without pericytes. Scattered lymphoid follicles and secondary foci of hemorrhage may be observed. The malformed lymph vessels of lymphangioma should be differentiated from excised local lymphangiectases, which resembles small cysts clinically, and the normal vascular conjunctival bed.

Pyogenic granulomas are hyperplastic vascular lesions that usually occur following surgery, as a foreign body reaction, or from an inflammatory disease associated with a chalazion. Typically, the lesions are fleshy, polypoid, and red or yellow, and have a rapid growth phase followed by regression or stabilization. They show a lobulated appearance of anastomosing capillary vessels within a variable edematous collagenous stroma; the stroma contains acute and chronic inflammatory cells. The surface is often ulcerated and covered by a fibrinous exudate. There may be local recurrences after simple excision.

Myxoma

Myxomas are rare benign mesenchymal tumors that may originate anywhere, including the eyelid and conjunctiva (143,144). In the

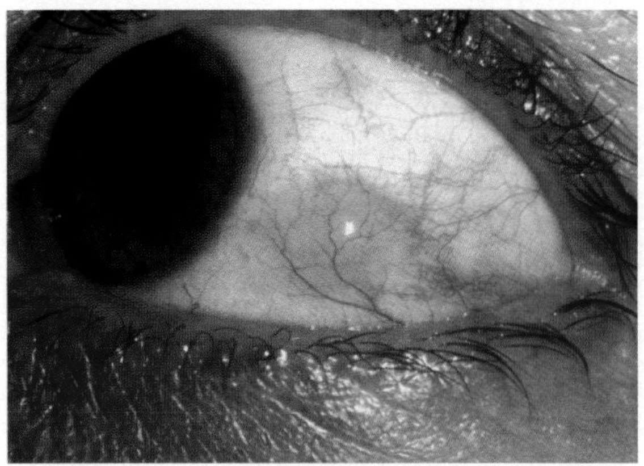

Figure 1-53

MYXOMA

A pale yellow nodule arises from the bulbar conjunctiva temporally.

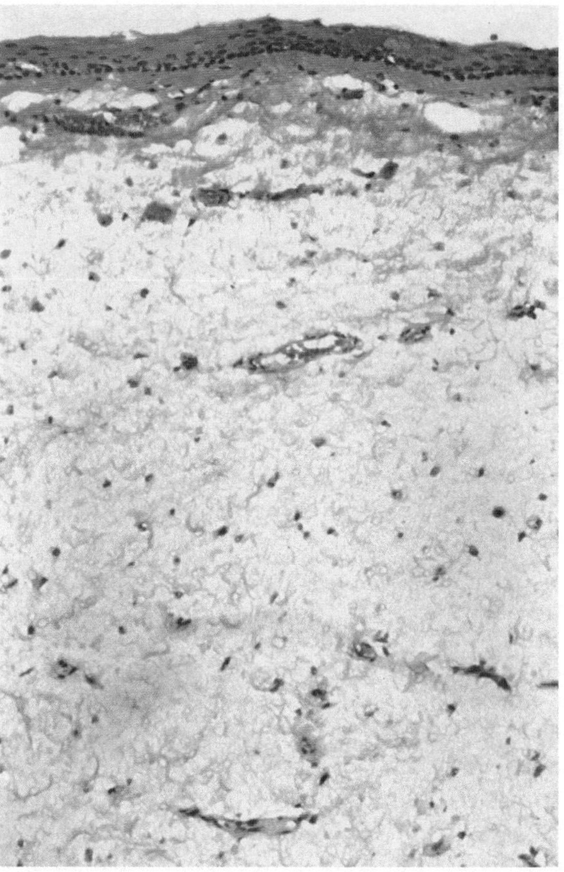

Figure 1-54

MYXOMA

Histopathologic examination of the lesion illustrated in figure 1-53 shows a proliferation of stellate cells in a myxoid matrix.

periocular location, myxomas are either isolated and usually located in the conjunctiva, or part of the Carney complex (145). They are painless, circumscribed, smooth, gelatinous lesions of the bulbar (temporal) conjunctiva (fig. 1-53) (146). Light microscopy shows a hypocellular lesion composed of stellate- and spindle-shaped cells with delicate cytoplasmic processes and small intranuclear vacuoles (fig. 1-54). Between the cells the stroma contains large amounts of Alcian blue–positive, hyaluronidase-sensitive acid mucopolysaccharides and chondroitin sulfate; vascularization is minimal.

Conjunctival myxomas should be differentiated from other benign and malignant tumors with myxomatous stroma including myxoid neurofibroma, nerve sheath myxoma, spindle cell lipoma, and lymphangioma. Surgical excision is required to rule out childhood rhabdomyosarcoma, which may have a similar clinical appearance. Simple local excision is curative. No recurrences have been reported after excision of isolated myxomas of the conjunctiva (146).

Fibrous Histiocytoma

Fibrous histiocytoma is a common mesenchymal neoplasm of the ocular adnexa that occasionally arises from the soft tissues of the conjunctiva. Benign and malignant variants of fibrous histiocytoma of the conjunctiva have been reported (147,148). Fibrous histiocytomas of the conjunctiva more frequently arise from the limbus or epibulbar conjunctiva and have a fleshy, yellowish, nodular appearance. Histologically, they resemble fibrous histiocytomas from other sites of the body. Treatment is complete surgical excision. Recurrence and metastasis are related to the completeness of the initial excision, depth and size of the lesion, and histologic grade.

EMBRYONAL RHABDOMYOSARCOMA, BOTRYOID SUBTYPE

The *botryoid type of rhabdomyosarcoma* is an embryonal rhabdomyosarcoma that affects mucosal surfaces including the conjunctiva (149,150). Children usually present with a fleshy, gelatinous mass that may be clinically

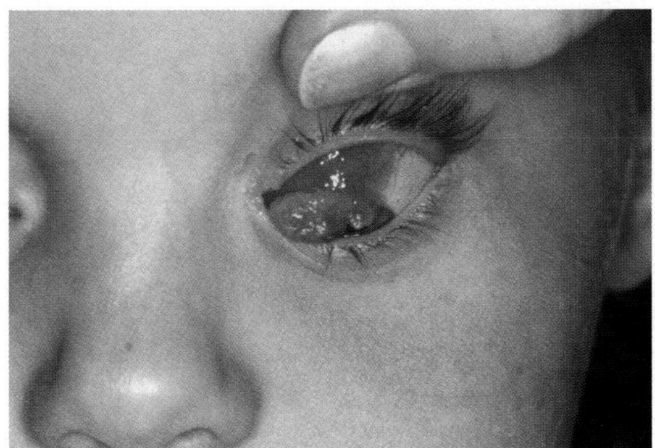

Figure 1-55

EMBRYONAL RHABDOMYOSARCOMA (SARCOMA BOTRYOIDES)

A fleshy mass arises from the superior fornix and inner canthus.

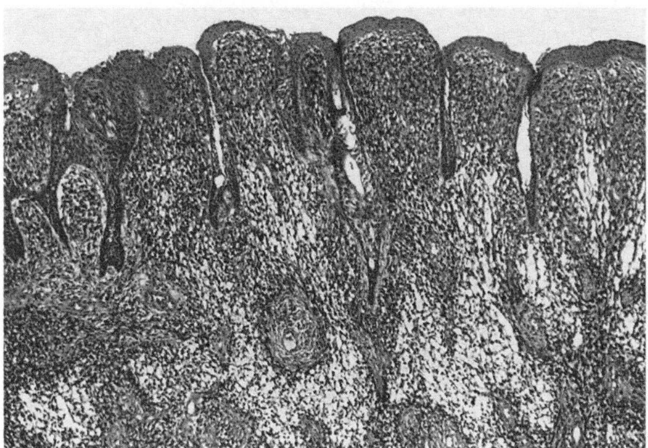

Figure 1-56

EMBRYONAL RHABDOMYOSARCOMA (SARCOMA BOTRYOIDES)

Low-power magnification shows an attenuated epithelium and an underlying cambium layer characterized by a band-like distribution of spindle-shaped cells.

mistaken for an epithelial or lymphatic cyst (fig. 1-55). Characteristically, in the early stages the lesion enlarges rapidly, without associated inflammation, conjunctival redness, or lid edema.

The myxoid hypercellular tumor is separated from the surface epithelium by multiple layers of neoplastic spindle cells, termed the cambium layer (fig. 1-56). Spindle cells and round rhabdomyoblasts showing an eosinophilic cytoplasm and enlarged, hyperchromatic and pleomorphic nuclei are observed. Small spindle-shaped cells with little cytoplasm and small homogeneous nuclei are present in the tumor matrix; the matrix is composed of pools of extracellular mucopolysaccharides and edema resembling cystic spaces. Cross-striations are seen in less than 10 percent of the cases. The cells are positive for desmin, muscle-specific actin, vimentin, and, rarely, myosin.

Rhabdomyosarcoma should always be suspected in children with a rapidly growing orbital or subconjunctival tumor, and a biopsy should be performed promptly. If the diagnosis is embryonal rhabdomyosarcoma, primary chemotherapy and adjunctive radiotherapy are prescribed (151).

Kaposi's Sarcoma

Kaposi's sarcoma (KS) *of the conjunctiva and eyelid* occurs in about 20 percent of patients with AIDS, and in 4 to 14 percent of these patients it may be the first manifestation of the disease

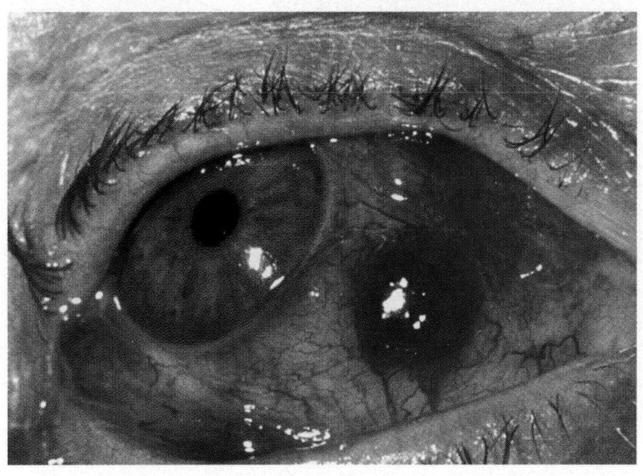

Figure 1-57

KAPOSI'S SARCOMA

A young patient with two reddish nodules on the nasal and inferior bulbar conjunctivae.

(fig. 1-57). A diagnosis of KS of the periocular tissues in an asymptomatic HIV-seropositive individual reclassifies the patient as having AIDS (153). The incidence of KS in AIDS patients has declined with the use of hyperactive antiretroviral therapy (HAART) (152).

The clinicopathologic classification of ocular adnexal KS proposed by Dugel et al. (154) is useful for diagnosis and management, and for predicting clinical behavior after excision. These authors proposed three types of KS: type I

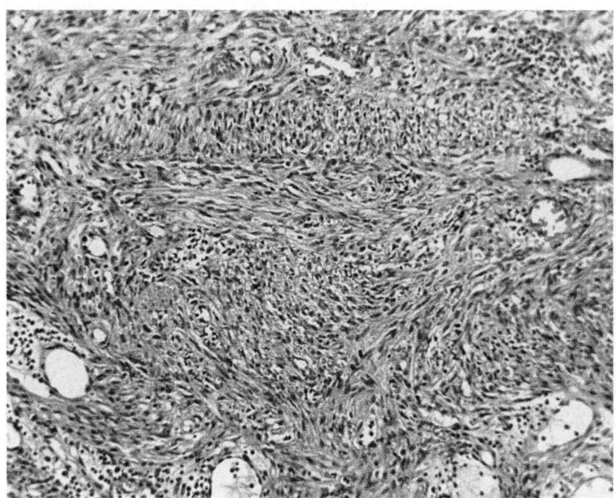

Figure 1-58

KAPOSI'S SARCOMA

A conjunctival tumor is composed of a spindle cell proliferation with slit-like spaces containing red blood cells.

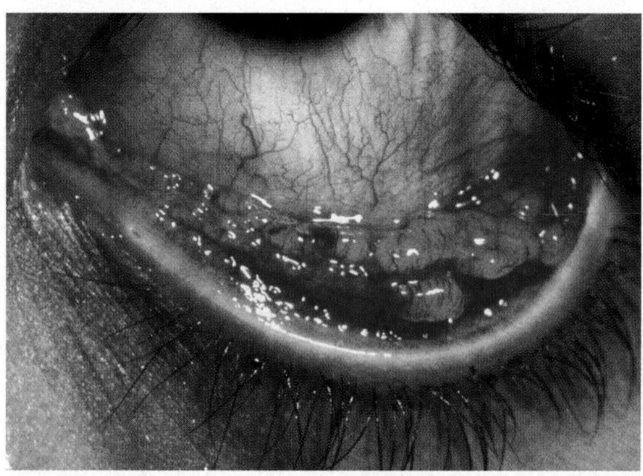

Figure 1-59

REACTIVE FOLLICULAR LYMPHOID HYPERPLASIA

Reddish thickening of the inferior fornix, with nodularity of the surface.

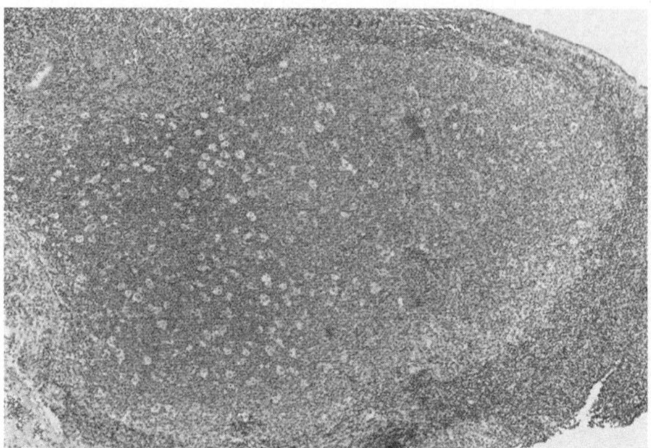

Figure 1-60

REACTIVE FOLLICULAR LYMPHOID HYPERPLASIA

Large, well-circumscribed follicular center cells are surrounded by a mantle of small lymphocytes.

lesions are patchy and flat and less than 3 mm in thickness, composed of thin and dilated vascular channels filled with erythrocytes, and lined by endothelial cells, without spindle cells or mitotic activity; type II lesions consist of flat tumors less than 3 mm thickness, empty vascular channels lined by plump, fusiform endothelial cells with hyperchromatic nuclei but no mitoses and only few spindle cells; and type III lesions are nodular, measure more than 3 mm in thickness, and usually have a duration of 4 months or longer. Histologically, they are composed of packed spindle cells with hyperchromatic nuclei and mitotic figures, and slit-like spaces containing erythrocytes (fig. 1-58).

KS may resemble other conjunctival vascular tumors clinically and histologically. Lesions to be considered in the differential diagnosis include angiosarcoma, angiolymphoid hyperplasia with eosinophilia, bacillary angiomatosis, and other spindle cell tumors. Local excision is indicated for isolated conjunctival lesions or large lesions that compromise vision. Local therapy should include excision with 1 to 2 mm of normal tissue followed by cryotherapy. Recurrences are expected with type III nodular tumors. Alternative treatments include cryotherapy, radiotherapy, local injection of chemotherapeutic agents, and intralesional interferon alpha (155).

LYMPHOID TUMORS

Lymphoid tumors of the conjunctiva are noninflammatory, slow-growing lesions that originate either as primary tumors without any evidence of systemic lymphoma or as secondary infiltrates, as part of a systemic disease (156, 157). They include a spectrum of benign (figs. 1-59, 1-60), malignant, and atypical or indeterminate lymphoid proliferations. Conjunctival lymphoid lesions account for approximately 20 percent of ocular adnexal tumors. Patients present either with a nonpainful mass associated with photophobia, redness, and irritation, or with

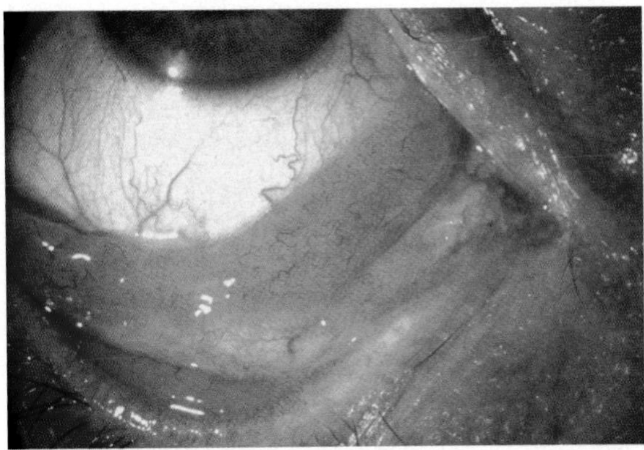

Figure 1-61

MALIGNANT LYMPHOMA

The diffuse salmon-colored mass has a smooth surface.

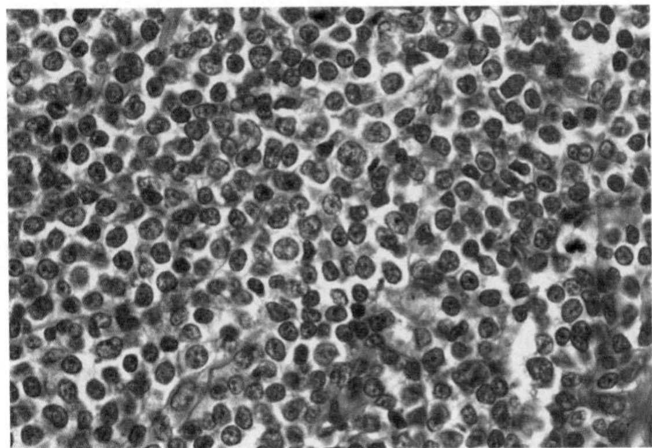

Figure 1-62

MALIGNANT LYMPHOMA

High-power magnification shows a diffuse proliferation of atypical lymphocytes.

an incidentally found conjunctival lesion. Most frequently, the tumors are located in the fornix, inner canthal area, and bulbar conjunctiva, and typically are a salmon red, pink, or orange (fig. 1-61). Bilateral lesions occur in more than 25 percent of cases, independent of whether the tumor is benign or malignant.

Most conjunctival lymphomas are classified as *extranodal marginal zone lymphomas* (EMZL) *of mucosa-associated lymphoid tissues* (MALT). EMZL should be differentiated from other, less frequent types of conjunctival lymphoma including mantle cell lymphoma, follicular lymphoma, lymphoplasmacytic lymphoma, and B-cell chronic lymphocytic leukemia and small lymphocytic lymphoma (fig. 1-62). Despite the occasional presence of germinal centers in normal lymphoid tissue of the conjunctiva, follicular lymphoma is rare. The workup of patients with lymphoma of the conjunctiva includes computerized tomography (CT) or magnetic resonance imaging (MRI) of the head and neck, thorax, and abdomen, and lymph node examination. A precise classification of the type of lymphoma is important mainly to determine whether the patient requires special studies (158). The incidence of nonocular lymphoma in patients with conjunctival lymphoma is less than 40 percent (159). EMZL has an indolent course without extraocular involvement in about 70 percent of the patients. Patients with mantle cell lymphoma, on the other hand, have a more ominous prognosis because of its aggressive clinical behavior, with a median survival period of 3 to 5 years. A detailed description of various types of lymphoid tumors appears in the chapter on tumors of the orbit.

PLASMACYTOMA

The conjunctiva may be affected by multiple myeloma or may rarely be the site of localized plasmacytic proliferations (160). Localized disease has been termed *solitary plasmacytoma* or *primary extramedullary solitary plasmacytoma*. The tumors are circumscribed, reddish lesions usually arising from the fornix, bulbar, or tarsal conjunctiva, and rarely, the caruncle. Clinically, they resemble an inflammatory or vascular lesion. Unusual cases may be associated with monoclonal serum immunoglobulin spikes. The differential diagnosis includes unusual cases of plasmacytic conjunctivitis with immunoglobulin crystals (161). The majority of the reported cases of solitary plasmacytoma of the conjunctiva have an indolent clinical course and are managed conservatively (160).

METASTATIC TUMORS OF THE CONJUNCTIVA

Metastasis to the conjunctiva in patients with advanced systemic malignancy is rare. The most frequent primary sites are breast, lung, and skin (cutaneous melanoma) (162). Conjunctival metastatic lesions are solitary, with either bulbar or palpebral involvement. Most metastatic melanomas to the conjunctiva develop from a primary of the skin of a lower extremity or

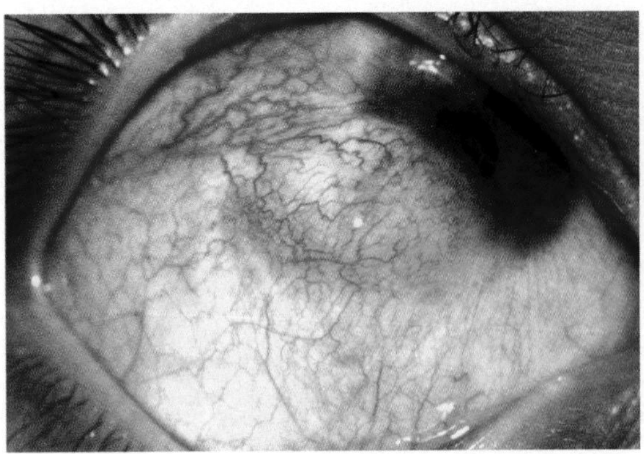

Figure 1-63

LIMBAL DERMOID

A well-circumscribed white mass is located at the inferior temporal limbus.

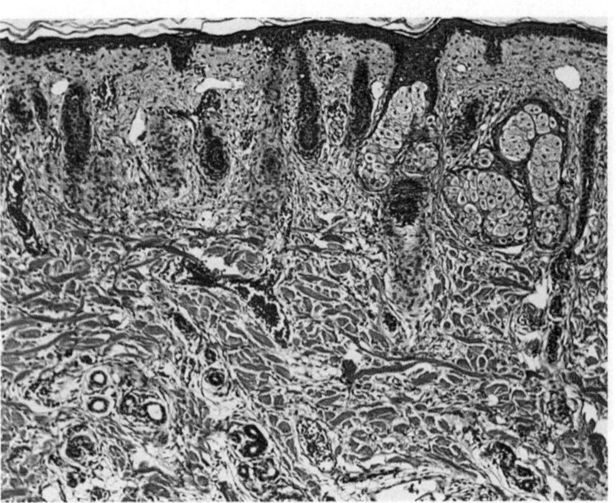

Figure 1-64

LIMBAL DERMOID

Squamous epithelium, dense collagenous stroma, and pilosebaceous units are seen.

trunk. Satellite foci of a metastatic melanoma should not be confused with primary acquired melanosis. Survival after diagnosis is poor.

TUMOR-LIKE CONGENITAL LESIONS

Choristomas are congenital non-neoplastic tumor growths formed by tissue elements that although cytologically normal in appearance, are not normally found in that location. Choristomas constitute 22 to 33 percent of epibulbar tumors in children (163,164). They may be confused with other clinical lesions or associated with other ocular abnormalities (165). Although conjunctival choristomas may grow after birth, none possess malignant potential. Several abnormal tissues may be identified in conjunctival choristomas (e.g., hairs, sebaceous glands, adipose tissue, lacrimal and serous glands, smooth muscle, cartilage, bone, and brain). Simple and complex choristomas can be part of several syndromes including Goldenhar-Gorlin oculo-auriculovertebral syndrome, nevus sebaceous of Jadassohn, Proteus syndrome, and Schimmelpenning-Feuerstein-Mims syndrome (166–170).

Dermoid

Solid dermoids are circumscribed lesions composed of epidermal and dermal components (171). They are most frequently located at the inferotemporal limbus (fig. 1-63). Clinical examination discloses a solid, yellowish white, round lesion with a variable number of thin hairs on its surface.

Microscopic examination shows nonkeratinized or keratinized stratified squamous epithelium resembling epidermis without rete ridges, and dense paucicellular collagenous stroma that often contains pilosebaceous units and sweat glands (fig. 1-64). Lobules of adipose tissue may be found in the center or base of the lesion. Occasionally, the lesions are composed of dense fibrovascular tissue covered by thickened conjunctival epithelium without mucus-secreting cells. These lesions have been called *dermis-like dermoids*. Treatment includes deep surgical excision, with or without lamellar keratectomy.

Dermolipoma

Dermolipomas are fibrofatty conjunctival lesions that are usually located supertemporally and extend posteriorly between the lateral and superior rectus. A similar clinical appearance is observed in older patients with a defect in the anterior orbital septum resulting in subepithelial prolapse of orbital adipose tissue. The dermolipoma is composed of dense collagenous bundles resembling the reticular dermis and lobules of adipose tissue. The surface epithelium is smooth and mildly acanthotic. Due to the attachment to the rectus muscles and fascial tissues of the anterior orbit, only the anterior superficial part of the lesion is excised.

Table 1-6

FREQUENCY OF TUMORS OF THE CARUNCLE[a]

Type of Tumor	Luthra et al. (178)	Shields et al. (179)	Santos and Gomez-Leal (180)	Fernandez-Meijide et al. (192)
Cysts	7	7	19	7
Squamous papillomas	13	32	26	26
Sebaceous	9	4	7	9
Nevus	43	24	34	43
Melanoma	2	–	4	2
Soft tissue	6	11	8	12
Lymphoid and hematopoietic	5	2	4	1
Other	17	20	1	4
(Number of Cases)	(112 cases)	(57 cases)	(113 cases)	(58 cases)

[a]Frequency in percentage (total is more than 100% because of rounding).

Ectopic Lacrimal Gland

Occasionally, lobules of lacrimal gland tissue are found outside their normal locations and are called *ectopic lacrimal gland tissue* (172,173). They may either be isolated or found as a component of other choristomas. Many become apparent late in life. The acini and ducts often resemble normal lacrimal gland tissue.

Complex Choristoma

Complex choristoma is a conjunctival choristoma in which a mixture of tissues, including lacrimal gland, smooth muscle, cartilage, bone, and ectopic brain, are identified (174).

Smooth Muscle Hamartoma

A congenital tumor composed of spindle-shaped smooth muscle cells has been reported arising from the inferior fornix and tarsal conjunctival region (175). *Smooth muscle hamartoma* has a gray, cyst-like appearance. Histopathologic examination reveals large bundles of smooth muscle intermixed with a fibrous stroma and lobules of adipose tissue.

Osseous Choristoma

Osseous choristoma is a solid, movable, small, circumscribed, reddish white, epibulbar, bony lesion typically located supertemporally between the superior and lateral rectus and 4 to 10 mm behind the limbus (176,177). The clinical diagnosis is often supported by imaging studies. Light microscopy shows a subconjunctival solid nodule or plaque of compact lamellar bone surrounded by dense collagenous tissue. Bone marrow may occasionally be found within the bone. Rarely, ectopic islands of meningothelial cells are observed.

TUMORS OF THE CARUNCLE

The caruncle is the site of a large variety of tumors and tumor-like lesions (178–182). Tumors of the caruncle, however, are rare and comprise about 4 percent of conjunctival tumors. They occur in patients of a wide age range, from childhood to adulthood. The preoperative clinical diagnosis is correctly made in only half of the cases; the most frequent clinical diagnosis, papilloma and nevus, constitute about 70 percent of tumors of the caruncle (Table 1-6).

The caruncle contains sebaceous glands and therefore is prone to the development of sebaceous hyperplasia, sebaceous adenoma, and sebaceous carcinoma. Oncocytoma or oncocytic adenoma may arise from accessory lacrimal gland tissue located in the caruncle, conjunctiva, and inner canthus, as well as the ductal lacrimal system (183–186). Malignant tumors of the caruncle are rare and clinically unsuspected in half of the patients. Among different series, the frequency of malignant tumors is about 5 percent (178,180). Melanoma, squamous cell carcinoma, sebaceous gland carcinoma, and malignant lymphoma have been described. Rarely, the caruncle may be involved by contiguous primary tumors of the eyelid, conjunctiva, and lacrimal drainage system.

REFERENCES

Classification and Frequency

1. Grossniklaus HE, Green WR, Luckenbach M, Chan CC. Conjunctival lesions in adults. A clinical and histopathologic review. Cornea 1987;6:78–116.
2. McLean IW, Burnier MN, Zimmerman LE, Jakobiec FA. Tumors of the eye and ocular adnexa. Atlas of Tumor Pathology, 3rd Series, Fascicle 12. Washington DC: Armed Forces Institute of Pathology; 1994.
3. Seitz B, Fisher M, Holbach LM, Naumann GO. Differential diagnosis and prognosis of 112 excised epibulbar epithelial tumors. Klin Monatsbl Augenheilkd 1995;207:239–46.
4. Feng G, Yi Y, Li Y. [777 cases of the primary conjunctival neoplasms.] Yan Ke Xue Bao 1995; 11:211–5. (Chinese.)

Papilloma

5. Mantyjarvi M, Syrjanen S, Kaipiainen S, Mantyjarvi R, Kahlos T, Syrjanen K. Detection of human papillomavirus type 11 DNA in a conjunctival squamous cell papilloma by in situ hybridization with biotinylated probes. Acta Ophthalmol (Copenh) 1989;67:425–9.
6. Saegusa M, Takano Y, Hashimura M, Okayasu I, Shiga J. HPV type 16 in conjunctival and junctional papilloma, dysplasia, and squamous cell carcinoma. J Clin Pathol 1995;48:1106–10.
7. Egbert JE, Kersten RC. Female genital tract papillomavirus in conjunctival papillomas of infancy. Am J Ophthalmol 1997;123:551–2.
8. Sjo NC, Heegaard S, Prause JU, von Buchwald C, Lindeberg H. Human papillomavirus in conjunctival papilloma. Br J Ophthalmol 2001;85: 785–7.
9. Jakobiec FA, Harrison W, Aronian D. Inverted mucoepidermoid papillomas of the epibulbar conjunctiva. Ophthalmology 1987;94:283–7.
10. Chang T, Chapman B, Heathcote JG. Inverted mucoepidermoid papilloma of the conjunctiva. Can J Ophthalmol 1993;28:184–6.
11. Lass JH, Foster CS, Grove AS, et al. Interferon-alpha therapy of recurrent conjunctival papillomas. Am J Ophthalmol 1987;103:294–301.
12. Hawkins AS, Yu J, Hamming NA, Rubenstein JB. Treatment of recurrent conjunctival papillomatosis with mitomycin C. Am J Ophthalmol 1999;128:638–40.
13. Shields CL, Lally MR, Singh AD, Shields JA, Nowinski T. Oral cimetidine (Tagamet) for recalcitrant, diffuse conjunctival papillomatosis. Am J Ophthalmol 1999;128:362–4.

Keratoacanthoma

14. Roth AM. Solitary keratoacanthoma of the conjunctiva. Am J Ophthalmol 1978;85:647–50.
15. Schellini SA, Marques ME, Milanezi MF, Bacchi CE. Conjunctival keratoacanthoma. Acta Ophthalmol Scand 1997;75:335–7.
16. Coupland SE, Heimann H, Kellner U, Bornfeld N, Foerster MH, Lee WR. Keratoacanthoma of the bulbar conjunctiva. Br J Ophthalmol 1998;82:586.
17. Grossniklaus HE, Martin DF, Salomon AR. Invasive conjunctival tumor with keratoacanthoma features. Am J Ophthalmol 1990;109: 736–8.

Hereditary Benign Intraepithelial Dyskeratosis

18. Yanoff M. Hereditary benign intraepithelial dyskeratosis. Arch Ophthalmol 1968;79:291–3.
19. Reed JW, Cashwell F, Klintworth GK. Corneal manifestations of hereditary benign intraepithelial dyskeratosis. Arch Ophthalmol 1979; 297–300.
20. McLean IW, Riddle PJ, Schruggs JH, Jones DB. Hereditary benign intraepithelial dyskeratosis. A report of two cases from Texas. Ophthalmology 1981;82:164–8.
21. Allingham RR, Seo B, Ramperdaud E, et al. A duplication in chromosome 4q35 is associated with hereditary benign intraepithelial dyskeratosis. Am J Hum Genet 2001;68:491–4.
22. Sadeghi EM, Witkop CJ. Ultrastructural study of hereditary benign intraepithelial dyskeratosis. Oral Surg Oral Med Oral Pathol 1977;44:567–77.

Conjunctival Cysts

23. Goldstein JH. Conjunctival cysts following strabismus surgery. J Pediatr Ophthalmol Strabismus 1968;5:204–6.
24. Gloor P, Horio B, Klassen M, Eagle RC Jr. Conjunctival cyst. Arch Ophthalmol 1996;114:1020–1.
25. Srinivasan BD, Jakobiec FA, Iwamoto T, De Voe AG. Epibulbar mucogenic subconjunctival cysts. Arch Ophthalmol 1978;96:857–9.

Pseudoepitheliomatous Hyperplasia

26. Slack JW, Hyndiuk RA, Harris GJ, Simons KB. Blastomycosis of the eyelid and conjunctiva. Ophthal Plast Reconstr Surg 1992;8:143–9.
27. Margo CE, Grossnicklaus HE. Pseudoadenomatous hyperplasia of the conjunctiva. Ophthalmology 2001;108:135–8.

Leukoplakic Lesions

28. Campbell RJ, Sobin LH. Histological typing of tumours of the eye and its adnexa. World Health Organization, 2nd ed. Berlin: Springer Verlag; 1998.
29. Mauriello JA Jr, Napolitano J, McLean I. Actinic keratosis and dysplasia of the conjunctiva: a clinicopathological study of 45 cases. Can J Ophthalmol 1995;30:312–6.

Intraepithelial Neoplasia and Dysplasia

30. Pizzarello LD, Jakobiec FA. Bowen's disease of the conjunctiva: a misnomer. In: Jakobiec FA, ed. Ocular and adnexal tumors. Birmingham: Aesculapius Pub; 1978:553–71.
31. Lee GA, Hirst LW. Incidence of ocular surface epithelial dysplasia in metropolitan Brisbane. A 10-year survey. Arch Ophthalmol 1992;110: 525–7.
32. Napora C, Cohen EJ, Genvert GI, et al. Factors associated with conjunctival intraepithelial neoplasia: a case control study. Ophthalmic Surg 1990;21:27–30.
33. Saegusa M, Takano Y, Hashimura M, Okayasu I, Shiga J. HPV type 16 in conjunctival and junctional papilloma, dysplasia, and squamous cell carcinoma. J Clin Pathol 1995;48:1106–10.
34. Nakamura Y, Mashima Y, Kameyama K, Mukai M, Oguchi Y. Detection of human papillomavirus infection in squamous tumours of the conjunctiva and lacrimal sac by immunohistochemistry, in situ hybridisation, and polymerase chain reaction. Br J Ophthalmol 1997; 81:308–13.
35. Karcioglu ZA, Issa TM. Human papilloma virus in neoplastic and non-neoplastic conditions of the external eye. Br J Ophthalmol 1997;81:595–8.
36. Scott IU, Karp CL, Nuovo GJ. Human papillomavirus 16 and 18 expression in conjunctival intraepithelial neoplasia. Ophthalmology 2002;109:542–7.
37. Waring GO 3rd, Roth AM, Ekins MB. Clinical and pathologic description of 17 cases of corneal intraepithelial neoplasia. Am J Ophthalmol 1984;97:547–59.
38. Erie JC, Campbell RJ, Liesegang TJ. Conjunctival and corneal intraepithelial and invasive neoplasia. Ophthalmology 1986;93:176–83.
39. Morsman CD. Spontaneous regression of a conjunctival intraepithelial neoplastic tumor. Arch Ophthalmol 1989;107:1490–1.
40. Aoki S, Kubo E, Nakamura S, et al. Possible prognostic markers in conjunctival dysplasia and squamous cell carcinoma. Jpn J Ophthalmol 1998;42:256–61.
41. Rozenman Y, Frucht-Pery J. Treatment of conjunctival intraepithelial neoplasia with topical drops of mitomycin C. Cornea 2000;19:1–6.
42. Yeatts RP, Engelbrecht NE, Curry CD, Ford JG, Walter KA. 5-Fluorouracil for the treatment of intraepithelial neoplasia of the conjunctiva and cornea. Ophthalmology 2000;107:2190–5.
43. Karp CL, Moore JK, Rosa RH Jr. Treatment of conjunctival and corneal intraepithelial neoplasia with topical interferon alpha-2b. Ophthalmology 2001;108:1093–8.

Squamous Cell Carcinoma

44. Sun EC, Fears TR, Goedert JJ. Epidemiology of squamous cell conjunctival cancer. Cancer Epidemiol Biomarkers Prev 1997;6:73–7.
45. Waddell KM, Lewallen S, Lucas SB, Atenyi-Agaba C, Herrington CS, Liomba G. Carcinoma of the conjunctiva and HIV infection in Uganda and Malawi. Br J Ophthalmol 1996;80:503–8.
46. Muccioli C, Belfort R Jr, Burnier M, Rao N. Squamous cell carcinoma of the conjunctiva in a patient with the acquired immunodeficiency syndrome. Am J Ophthalmol 1996;121:94–6.
47. Poole TR. Conjunctival squamous cell carcinoma in Tanzania. Br J Ophthalmol 1999;83:177–9.
48. Kaimbo Wa Kaimbo D, Parys-Van Ginderdeuren R, Missotten L. Conjunctival squamous cell carcinoma and intraepithelial neoplasia in AIDS patients in Congo Kinshasa. Bull Soc Belge Ophtalmol 1998;268:135–41.
49. Odrich MG, Jakobiec FA, Lancaster WD, et al. A spectrum of bilateral squamous conjunctival tumors associated with human papillomavirus type 16. Ophthalmology 1991;98:68–35.
50. Zimmerman LE. Squamous cell carcinoma and related lesions of the bulbar conjunctiva. In: Boniuk M, ed. Ocular and adnexal tumors. New and controversial aspects. Saint Louis: The CV Mosby Company; 1964:49–74.
51. Tunc M, Char DH, Crawford B, Miller T. Intraepithelial and invasive squamous cell carcinoma of the conjunctiva: analysis of 60 cases. Br J Ophthalmol 1999;83:98–103.
52. Nadjari B, Kersten A, Ross B, et al. Cytologic and DNA cytometric diagnosis and therapy monitoring of squamous cell carcinoma in situ and malignant melanoma of the cornea and conjunctiva. Anal Quant Cytol Histol 1999;21:387–96.
53. Midena E, Angeli CD, Valenti M, de Belvis V, Boccato P. Treatment of conjunctival squamous cell carcinoma with topical 5-fluorouracil. Br J Ophthalmol 2000;84:268–72.

54. Cartsburg O, Kersten A, Sundmacher R, Nadjari B, Pomjanski N, Bocking A. [Treatment of 9 squamous epithelial carcinoma in situ lesions of the conjunctiva (CIN) with mitomycin C eyedrops in cytological and DNA image cytometric control.] Klin Monatsbl Augenheilkd 2001;218:429–34. (German.)
55. Buus DR, Tse DT, Folberg R, Buuns DR. Microscopically controlled excision of conjunctival squamous cell carcinoma. Am J Ophthalmol 1994;117:97–102.
56. Shields JA, Shields CL, De Potter P. Surgical management of conjunctival tumors. The 1994 Lynn B. McMahan Lecture. Arch Ophthalmol 1997;115:808–15.
57. Tabin G, Levin S, Snibson G, Loughnan M, Taylor H. Late recurrences and the necessity for long-term follow-up in corneal and conjunctival intraepithelial neoplasia. Ophthalmology 1997;104:485–92.
58. Iliff WJ, Marback R, Green WR. Invasive squamous cell carcinoma of the conjunctiva. Arch Ophthalmol 1975;93:119–22.
59. Johnson TE, Tabbara KF, Weatherhead RG, Kersten RC, Rice C, Nasr AM. Secondary squamous cell carcinoma of the orbit. Arch Ophthalmol 1997;115:75–8.
60. Tabbara KF, Kersten R, Daouk N, Blodi FC. Metastatic squamous cell carcinoma of the conjunctiva. Ophthalmology 1988;95:318–21.
61. Bhattacharyya N, Wenokur RK, Rubin PA. Metastasis of squamous cell carcinoma of the conjunctiva: case report and review of the literature. Am J Otolaryngol 1997;18:217–9.
62. AJCC cancer staging manual, 5th ed. American Joint Committee on Cancer. Philadelphia: Lippincott Williams & Wilkins; 1997.

Mucoepidermoid Carcinoma

63. Rao NA, Font RL. Mucoepidermoid carcinoma of the conjunctiva: a clinicopathologic study of five cases. Cancer 1976;38:1699–709.
64. Brownstein S. Mucoepidermoid carcinoma of the conjunctiva with intraocular invasion. Ophthalmology 1981;88:1226–30.
65. Hwang IP, Jordan DR, Brownstein S, Gilberg SM, McEachren TM, Prokopetz R. Mucoepidermoid carcinoma of the conjunctiva: a series of three cases. Ophthalmology 2000;107:801–5.
66. Ullman S, Augsburger JJ, Brady LW. Fractionated epibulbar I-125 plaque radiotherapy for recurrent mucoepidermoid carcinoma of the conjunctiva. Am J Ophthalmol 1995;119:102–3.

Spindle Cell Carcinoma

67. Cohen BH, Green WR, Iliff NT, Taxy JB, Schwab LT, de la Cruz Z. Spindle cell carcinoma of the conjunctiva. Arch Ophthalmol 1980;98:1809–13.
68. Schubert HD, Farris RL, Green WR. Spindle cell carcinoma of the conjunctiva. Graefes Arch Clin Exp Ophthalmol 1995;233:52–3.
69. Slusker-Shternfeld I, Syed NA, Sires BA. Invasive spindle cell carcinoma of the conjunctiva. Arch Ophthalmol 1997;115:288–9.
70. Huntington AC, Langloss J, Hidayat AA. Spindle cell carcinoma of the conjunctiva. An immunohistochemical and ultrastructural study of six cases. Ophthalmology 1990;97:711–7.
71. Ni C, Guo BK. Histological types of spindle cell carcinoma of the cornea and conjunctiva. A clinicopathologic report of 8 patients with ultrastructural and immunohistochemical findings in three tumors. Chin Med J (Engl) 1990;103:915–20.

Adenoid Squamous Carcinoma

72. Mauriello JA Jr, Abdelsalam A, McLean IW. Adenoid squamous carcinoma of the conjunctiva—a clinicopathological study of 14 cases. Br J Ophthalmol 1997;81:1001–5.

Basal Cell Carcinoma

73. Husain SE, Patrinely JR, Zimmerman LE, Font RL. Primary basal cell carcinoma of the limbal conjunctiva. Ophthalmology 1993;100:1720–2.
74. Quillen DA, Goldberg SH, Rosenwasser GO, Sassani JW. Basal cell carcinoma of the conjunctiva. Am J Ophthalmol 1993;116:244–5.
75. Cable MM, Lyon DB, Rupani M, Matta CS, Hidayat AA. Case reports and small case series: primary basal cell carcinoma of the conjunctiva with intraocular invasion. Arch Ophthalmol 2000;118:1296–8.

Sebaceous Gland Carcinoma

76. Margo CE, Lessner A, Stern GA. Intraepithelial sebaceous cell carcinoma of the conjunctiva and the skin of the eyelid. Ophthalmology 1992;99:227–31.
77. Margo CE, Grossniklaus HE. Intraepithelial sebaceous neoplasia without underlying invasive carcinoma. Surv Ophthalmol 1995;39:293–301.
78. Condon GP, Brownstein S, Codere F. Sebaceous carcinoma of the eyelid masquerading as superior limbic keratoconjunctivitis. Arch Ophthalmol 1985;103:1525–9.
79. Lisman RD, Jakobiec FA, Small P. Sebaceous carcinoma of the eyelids. The role of adjunctive cryotherapy in the management of conjunctival pagetoid spread. Ophthalmology 1989;96:1021–6.

Lymphoepithelioma-Like Carcinoma

80. Cervantes G, Rodriguez AA Jr, Leal AG. Squamous cell carcinoma of the conjunctiva: clinicopathological features in 287 cases. Can J Ophthalmol 2002;37:14–9.

Melanocytic Lesions: Nevus

81. Folberg R, Jakobiec FA, Bernardino VB, Iwamoto T. Benign conjunctival melanocytic lesions. Clinicopathologic features. Ophthalmology 1989;96:436–61.
82. Gerner N, Norregaard JC, Jensen OA, Prause JU. Conjunctival naevi in Denmark 1960-1980. A 21-year follow-up study. Acta Ophthalmol Scand 1996;74:334–7.
83. Pfaffenbach DD, Green WR, Maumenee AE. Balloon cell nevus of the conjunctiva. Arch Ophthalmol 1972;87:192–5.
84. Kabukcuoglu S, McNutt NS. Conjunctival melanocytic nevi of childhood. J Cutan Pathol 1999;26:248–52.
85. Grossniklaus HE, Margo CE, Solomon AR. Indeterminate melanocytic proliferations of the conjunctiva. Trans Am Ophthalmol Soc 1999;97:157–68.
86. McDonnell JM, Carpenter JD, Jacobs P, Wan WL, Gilmore JE. Conjunctival melanocytic lesions in children. Ophthalmology 1989;96:986–93.
87. Jakobiec FA, Zuckerman BD, Berlin AJ, Odell P, McRae DW, Tuthill RJ. Unusual melanocytic nevi of the conjunctiva. Am J Ophthalmol 1985; 100:100–13.
88. Kantelip B, Boccard R, Nores JM, Bacin F. A case of conjunctival Spitz nevus: review of literature and comparison with cutaneous locations. Ann Ophthalmol 1989;21:176–9.
89. Seregard S. Pigmented spindle cell naevus of Reed presenting in the conjunctiva. Acta Ophthalmol Scand 2000;78:104–6.
90. Holbach L, Nagel G, Naumann GO. [Blue nevi of the conjunctiva.] Klin Monatsbl Augenheilkd 1994;205:242–3. (German.)
91. Blicker JA, Rootman J, White VA. Cellular blue nevus of the conjunctiva. Ophthalmology 1992;99:1714–7.
92. Crawford JB, Howes EL Jr, Char DH. Combined nevi of the conjunctiva. Arch Ophthalmol 1999;117:1121–7.
93. Verdaguer J, Valenzuela H, Strozzi L. Melanocytoma of the conjunctiva. Arch Ophthalmol 1974;91:363–6.
94. Henkind P. Conjunctival melanocytic lesions: natural history. In: Jakobiec FA, ed. Ocular and adnexal tumors. Birmingham, Ala: Aesculapius Pub Co; 1978:572–82.

Primary Acquired Melanosis

95. Zimmerman LE. Criteria for management of melanosis. Arch Ophthalmol 1966;76:307.
96. Zimmerman LE, Sobin LH. World Health Organization. Histological typing of tumours of the eye and its adnexa. Geneva: World Health Organization; 1980.
97. Gloor P, Alexandrakis G. Clinical characterization of primary acquired melanosis. Invest Ophthalmol Vis Sci 1995;36:1721–9.
98. Chau KY, Hui SP, Cheng GP. Conjunctival melanotic lesions in Chinese: comparison with Caucasian series. Pathology 1999;31:199–201.
99. Folberg R, McLean IW, Zimmerman LE. Conjunctival melanosis and melanoma. Ophthalmology 1984;91:673–8.
100. Folberg R, McLean IW. Primary acquired melanosis and melanoma of the conjunctiva: terminology, classification, and biologic behavior. Hum Pathol 1986;17:652–4.
101. Paridaens AD, McCartney AC, Hungerford JL. Multifocal amelanotic conjunctival melanoma and acquired melanosis sine pigmento. Br J Ophthalmol 1992;76:163–5.
102. Jay V, Font RL. Conjunctival amelanotic malignant melanoma arising in primary acquired melanosis sine pigmento. Ophthalmology 1998;105:191–4.
103. Crawford JB. Conjunctival melanomas: prognostic factors a review and analysis of a series. Trans Am Ophthalmol Soc 1980;78:467–502.
104. Jakobiec FA, Folberg R, Iwamoto T. Clinicopathologic characteristics of premalignant and malignant melanocytic lesions of the conjunctiva. Ophthalmology 1989;96:147–66.
105. Paridaens AD, McCartney AC, Curling OM, Lyons CJ, Hungerford JL. Impression cytology of conjunctival melanosis and melanoma. Br J Ophthalmol 1992;76:198–201.
106. Finger PT, Czechonska G, Liarikos S. Topical mitomycin C chemotherapy for conjunctival melanoma and PAM with atypia. Br J Ophthalmol 1998;82:476–9.
107. Demirci H, McCormick SA, Finger PT. Topical mitomycin chemotherapy for conjunctival malignant melanoma and primary acquired melanosis with atypia: clinical experience with histopathologic observations. Arch Ophthalmol 2000;118:885–91.
108. Folberg R, McLean IW, Zimmerman LE. Primary acquired melanosis of the conjunctiva. Hum Pathol 1985;16:136–43.

Malignant Melanoma

109. Char DH. The management of lid and conjunctival malignancies. Surv Ophthalmol 1980;24: 679–89.

110. Osterlind A.Trends in incidence of ocular malignant melanoma in Denmark 1943-1982. Int J Cancer 1987;40:161–4.
111. Scotto J, Fraumeni JF Jr, Lee JA. Melanomas of the eye and other noncutaneous sites: epidemiologic aspect. J Natl Cancer Inst 1976;56: 489–91.
112. Seregard S, Kock E. Conjunctival malignant melanoma in Sweden 1969-91. Acta Ophthalmol (Copenh) 1992;70:289–96.
113. Norregaard JC, Gerner N, Jensen OA, Prause JU. Malignant melanoma of the conjunctiva: occurrence and survival following surgery and radiotherapy in a Danish population. Graefes Arch Clin Exp Ophthalmol 1996;234:569–72.
114. Singh AD, Campos OE, Rhatigan RM, Schulman JA, Misra RP. Conjunctival melanoma in the black population. Surv Ophthalmol 1998;43:127–33.
115. Desjardins L, Poncet P, Levy C, Schlienger P, Asselain B, Validire P. [Prognostic factors in malignant melanoma of the conjunctiva. An anatomo-clinical study of 56 patients.] J Fr Ophtalmol 1999;22:315–21. (French.)
116. Folberg R, McLean IW, Zimmerman LE. Malignant melanoma of the conjunctiva. Hum Pathol 1985;16:136–43.
117. De Potter P, Shields CL, Shields JA, Menduke H. Clinical predictive factors for the development of recurrence and metastasis in conjunctival melanoma: a review of 68 cases. Br J Ophthalmol 1993;77:624–30.
118. Croxatto JO, Iribarren G, Ugrin C, Ebner R, Zarate JO, Sampaolesi R. Malignant melanoma of the conjunctiva. Report of a case. Ophthalmology 1987;94:1281–5.
119. Shields CL, Shields JA, Gunduz K, et al. Conjunctival melanoma: risk factors for recurrence, exenteration, metastasis, and death in 150 consecutive patients. Arch Ophthalmol 2000;118: 1497–507.
120. McDonnell JM, Carpenter JD, Jacobs P, Wan WL, Gilmore JE. Conjunctival melanocytic lesions in children. Ophthalmology 1989;96:986–93.
121. Seregard S. Cell proliferation as a prognostic indicator in conjunctival malignant melanoma. Am J Ophthalmol 1993;116:93–7.
122. Stefani FH. A prognostic index for patients with malignant melanoma of the conjunctiva. Graefes Arch Clin Exp Ophthalmol 1986;224:580–2.
123. Saornil MA, Marcus DM, Doepner D, Apolone G, Torre V, Albert DM. Nucleolar organizer regions in determining malignancy of pigmented conjunctival lesions. Am J Ophthalmol 1993; 115:800–5.
124. Jakobiec FA. The ultrastructure of conjunctival melanocytic tumors. Trans Am Ophthalmol Soc 1984;82:599–752.
125. Paridaens AD, McCartney AC, Minassian DC, Hungerford JL. Orbital exenteration in 95 cases of primary conjunctival malignant melanoma. Br J Ophthalmol 1994;78:520–8.
126. Lommatzsch PK, Lommatzsch RE, Kirsch I, Fuhrmann P. Therapeutic outcome of patients suffering from malignant melanomas of the conjunctiva. Br J Ophthalmol 1990;74:615–9.
127. Silvers DN, Jakobiec FA, Freeman TR, et al. Melanoma of the conjunctiva: a clinicopathologic study. In: Jakobiec FA, ed. Ocular and adnexal tumors. Birmingham, Ala: Aesculapius Publishing Co; 1978:583–99.
128. Jakobiec FA, Folberg R, Iwamoto T. Clinicopathologic characteristics of premalignant and malignant melanocytic lesions of the conjunctiva. Ophthalmology 1989;96:147–66.
129. Fuchs U, Kivel T, Liesto K, Tarkkanen A. Prognosis of conjunctival melanomas in relation to histopathologic features. Br J Cancer 1989;59:261–7.
130. Paridaens AD, McCartney AC, Hungerford JL. Multifocal amelanotic conjunctival melanoma and acquired melanosis sine pigmento. Br J Ophthalmol 1992;76:163–5.
131. Matsumoto A, Inatomi T, Kinoshita S, et al. [Analysis of the long-term prognosis for conjunctival malignant melanomas in Japan.] Nippon Ganka Gakkai Zasshi 1999;103:449–55. (Japanese.)
132. Werschnik C, Lommatzsch PK. Long-term follow-up of patients with conjunctival melanoma. Am J Clin Oncol 2002;25:248–55.

Miscellaneous Soft Tissue Tumors

133. Jakobiec FA, Sacks E, Lisman RL, Krebs W. Epibulbar fibroma of the conjunctival substantia propria. Arch Ophthalmol 1988;106:661–4.
134. Lahoud S, Brownstein S, Laflamme MY. Fibrous histiocytoma of the corneoscleral limbus and conjunctiva. Am J Ophthalmol 1988;106:579–83.
135. Clinch TJ, Kostick DA, Menke DM. Tarsal fibroma. Am J Ophthalmol 2000;129:691–3.
136. Allaire GS, Corriveau C, Teboul N. Malignant fibrous histiocytoma of the conjunctiva. Arch Ophthalmol 1999;117:685–7.
137. White VA, Damji KF, Richards JS, Rootman J. Leiomyosarcoma of the conjunctiva. Ophthalmology 1991;98:1560–4.
138. Albert DL, Brownstein S, Codere F. Subconjunctival angiomyxoma. Can J Ophthalmol 1996; 31:315–8.

139. Sujatha S, Sampath R, Bonshek RE, Tullo AB. Conjunctival haemangiopericytoma. Br J Ophthalmol 1994;78:497–9.
140. Perry HD. Isolated neurofibromas of the conjunctiva. Am J Ophthalmol 1992;113:112–3.
141. Le Marc'hadour F, Romanet JP, Fdili A, Peoc'h M, Pinel N. Schwannoma of the bulbar conjunctiva. Arch Ophthalmol 1996;114:1258–60.
142. Charles NC, Fox DM, Avendano JA, Marroquin LS, Appleman W. Conjunctival neurilemoma. Report of 3 cases. Arch Ophthalmol 1997;115:547–9.

Myxoma

143. Stafford WR. Conjunctival myxoma. Arch Ophthalmol 1971;85:443–4.
144. Patrinely JR, Green WR. Conjunctival myxoma. A clinicopathologic study of four cases and a review of the literature. Arch Ophthalmol 1983;101:1416–20.
145. Kennedy RH, Waller RR, Carney JA. Ocular pigmented spots and eyelid myxomas. Am J Ophthalmol 1987;104:533–8.
146. Pe'er J, Hidayat AA. Myxomas of the conjunctiva. Am J Ophthalmol 1986;102:80–6.

Fibrous Histiocytoma

147. Iwamoto T, Jakobiec FA, Darrell RW. Fibrous histiocytoma of the corneoscleral limbus. The ultrastructure of a distinctive inclusion. Ophthalmology 1981;88:1260–8.
148. Margo CE, Horton MB. Malignant fibrous histiocytoma of the conjunctiva with metastasis. Am J Ophthalmol 1989;107:433–4.

Embryonal Rhabdomyosarcoma

149. Joffe L, Shields JA, Pearah D. Epibulbar rhabdomyosarcoma without proptosis. J Pediatr Ophthalmol 1977;14:364–7.
150. Cameron JD, Wick MR. Embryonal rhabdomyosarcoma of the conjunctiva. A clinicopathologic and immunohistochemical study. Arch Ophthalmol 1986;104:1203–4.
151. Sekundo W, Roggenkamper P, Fischer HP, Fleischhack G, Fluhs D, Sauerwein W. Primary conjunctival rhabdomyosarcoma: 2.5 years' follow-up after combined chemotherapy and brachytherapy. Graefes Arch Clin Exp Ophthalmol 1998;236:873–5.

Kaposi's Sarcoma

152. Chokunonga E, Levy LM, Bassett MT, et al. AIDS and cancer in Africa: the evolving epidemic in Zimbabwe. AIDS 1999;13:2583–8.
153. Dugel PU, Gill PS, Frangieh GT, Rao NA. Ocular adnexal Kaposi's sarcoma in acquired immunodeficiency syndrome. Am J Ophthalmol 1990;110:500–3.
154. Dugel PU, Gill PS, Frangieh GT, Rao NA. Treatment of ocular adnexal Kaposi's sarcoma in acquired immune deficiency syndrome. Ophthalmology 1992;99:1127–32.
155. Brun SC, Jakobiec FA. Kaposi's sarcoma of the ocular adnexa. Int Ophthalmol Clin 1997;37: 25–38.

Lymphoid and Hematopoietic Lesions

156. Hardman-Lea S, Kerr-Muir M, Wotherspoon AC, Green WT, Morell A, Isaacson PG. Mucosal-associated lymphoid tissue lymphoma of the conjunctiva. Arch Ophthalmol 1994;112:1207–12.
157. Wotherspoon AC, Hardman-Lea S, Isaacson PG. Mucosa-associated lymphoid tissue (MALT) in the human conjunctiva. J Pathol 1994;174:33–7.
158. Harris NL, Jaffe ES, Stein H, et al. A revised European-American classification of lymphoid neoplasms: a proposal from the International Lymphoma Study Group. Blood 1994;84:1361–92.
159. Shields CL, Shields JA, Carvalho C, Rundle P, Smith AF. Conjunctival lymphoid tumors. Clinical analysis of 177 cases and relationship to systemic lymphoma. Ophthalmology 2001; 108:979–84.

Plasmacytoma

160. Lugassy G, Rozenbaum D, Lifshitz L, Aviel E. Primary lymphoplasmacytoma of the conjunctiva. Eye 1992;6(Pt 3):326–7.
161. Rao NA, Font RL. Plasmacytic conjunctivitis with crystalline inclusions. Immunohistochemical and ultrastructural studies. Arch Ophthalmol 1980;98:836–41.

Metastatic Tumors of the Conjunctiva

162. Kiratli H, Shields CL, Shields JA, DePotter P. Metastatic tumours to the conjunctiva: report of 10 cases. Br J Ophthalmol 1996;80:1.

Choristomas

163. Elsas FJ, Green WR. Epibulbar tumors in childhood. Am J Ophthalmol 1975;79:1001–7.
164. Cunha RP, Cunha MC, Shields JA. Epibulbar tumors in children: a survey of 282 biopsies. J Pediatr Ophthalmol Strabismus 1987;24:249–54.
165. Mansour AM, Barber JC, Reinecke RD, Wang FM. Ocular choristomas. Surv Ophthalmol 1989;33:339–58.
166. Goldenhar M. Associations malformatives de l'oeil et de l'oreille: en particulier, le syndrome: dermoide epibulbaire-appendices auriculaires-fistula auris congenita et ses relations avec la dysostose mandibulo-faciale. J Genet Hum 1952;1:243–82.

167. Gorlin RJ, Jue KL, Jakobsen V, Goldschmidt E. Oculoauriculovertebral dysplasia. J Pediatr 1963;63:991–9.
168. Diven DG, Solomon AR, McNeely MC, Font RL. Nevus sebaceous associated with major ophthalmologic abnormalities. Arch Dermatol 1987;123:383–6.
169. De Becker I, Gajda DJ, Gilbert-Barness E, Cohen MM Jr. Ocular manifestations in Proteus syndrome. Am J Med Genet 2000;92:350–2.
170. Mayer UM, Meythaler FH, Naumann GO. [Eye symptoms in Schimmelpenning-Feuerstein-Mims syndrome, a rare phacomatosis.] Klin Monatsbl Augenheilkd 1997;210:370–5. (German.)
171. Dailey EG, Lubowitx RM. Dermoids of the limbus and cornea. Am J Ophthalmol 1962;53: 661–5.
172. Pfaffenbach DD, Green WR. Ectopic lacrimal gland. Int Ophthalmol Clin 1971;11:149–59.
173. Pokorny KS, Hyman BM, Jakobiec FA, Perry HD, Caputo AR, Iwamoto T. Epibulbar choristomas containing lacrimal tissue. Clinical distinction from dermoids and histologic evidence of an origin from the palpebral lobe. Ophthalmology 1987;94:1249–57.
174. Emamy H, Ahmadian H. Limbal dermoid with ectopic brain tissue. Report of a case and review of the literature. Arch Ophthalmol 1977; 95:2201–2.
175. Roper GJ, Smith MS, Lueder GT. Conjunctival smooth muscle hamartoma of the conjunctiva fornix. Am J Ophthalmol 1999;128:643–4.
176. Ferry AP, Hein HF. Epibulbar osseous choristoma within an epibulbar dermoid. Am J Ophthalmol 1970;70:764–6.
177. Ortiz JM, Yanoff M. Epipalpebral conjunctival osseous choristoma. Br J Ophthalmol 1979;63: 173–6.

Caruncle Tumors

178. Luthra CL, Doxanas MT, Green WR. Lesions of the caruncle: a clinicopathologic study. Surv Ophthalmol 1978;23:183–95.
179. Shield CL, Shields JA, White D, Augsburger JJ. Types and frequency of lesions of the caruncle. Am J Ophthalmol 1986;102:771–8.
180. Santos A, Gomez-Leal A. Lesions of the lacrimal caruncle. Clinicopathologic features. Ophthalmology 1994;101:943–9.
181. Hirsch C, Holz FG, Tetz M, Volcker HE. [Clinical aspects and histopathology of caruncular tumors.] Klin Monatsbl Augenheilkd 1997;210: 153–7. (German.)
182. Fernandez-Meijide N, Gonzalez-Virgili S, Croxatto JO. Frequencia de lesiones de caruncula. Estudio restrospectivo clinico-patologico. Arch Oftalmol B Aires 2000;75:12–6.
183. Greer CH. Oxyphil cell adenoma of the lacrimal caruncle. Report of two cases. Br J Ophthalmol 1969;53:198–202.
184. Biggs SL, Font RL. Oncocytic lesions of the caruncle and other ocular adnexa. Arch Ophthalmol 1977;95:474–8.
185. Riedel K, Stefani FH, Kampik A. [Oncocytoma of the ocular adnexa.] Klin Monatsbl Augenheilkd 1983;182:544–8. (German.)
186. Chang WJ, Nowinski TS, Eagle RC Jr. A large oncocytoma of the caruncle. Arch Ophthalmol 1995;113:382.

2 TUMORS OF THE UVEAL TRACT

ANATOMY AND HISTOLOGY

The uveal tract is the pigmented layer of the ocular coats that lies between the sclera externally and the retina internally. It is mainly composed of blood vessels, pigmented melanocytes, nerves, and supportive connective tissue. The uvea comprises the iris, the ciliary body, and the choroid. The iris is continuous with the ciliary body at the iris root, and the ciliary body blends into the choroid at the ora serrata. The iris and ciliary body have three components: the stroma arising from the neural crest, the inner epithelial layers and the iris dilator and sphincter muscles from the neuroectoderm, and the vascular endothelium from the mesoderm. The neuroectodermal layers of the iris are the most anterior part of the embryonic optic cup. The choroid is derived mainly from the neural crest, with the mesoderm providing the endothelium lining the blood vessels.

The Iris

The most anterior part of the uvea is the iris, a pigmented muscular-vascular diaphragm-like structure that regulates the amount of light entering the eye. It measures 12 mm in diameter and 0.5 mm in thickness. The color of the iris is dependent upon the amount of pigmentation from the dendritic melanocytes within the stroma. *Heterochromia iridis* refers to the iris being brown in one eye and lightly pigmented in the opposite eye.

Grossly, the iris consists of a circular zone bordering the pupil in which the sphincter muscle is located, an intermediate zone containing the dilator muscle, and the peripheral iris root. The surface of the iris contains pigmented furrows and excavated clear crypts of Fuchs. The anterior border layer is a condensation of stromal cells and melanocytes (fig. 2-1). Clusters of melanocytes on the anterior border layer are seen clinically as iris freckles. The stroma contains characteristic thick-walled blood vessels, dendritic melanocytes, and supportive connective tissue elements. Groups of heavily pigmented cells are observed next to the pupillary margin; these cells are most easily recognized in lightly pigmented irides. The cells are pigment-laden macrophages (type I, cells of Koganei) and polygonal, fully pigmented, neuroectodermal-derived cells (type II, neuroepithelial cells) that have large, uniform, pigmented melanosomes. The sphincter muscle is located next to the pupillary margin, has a circular arrangement, and is composed of smooth muscle cells. A double layer of pigment epithelium covers the posterior surface of the iris.

The cells of the anterior layer have basal cytoplasm containing fully melanized melanosomes, and facing the stroma, plate-like smooth muscle differentiation of the cytoplasm that forms the dilator muscle. The posterior layer of the iris pigment epithelium is composed of columnar, pigmented cells. Large, spherical or ovoid melanin granules of the pigment epithelium of neuroectodermal origin (iris, ciliary body, and retina) contrast with the smaller, uniform, ovoid granules of the uveal melanocytes derived from the neural crest cells. Such differentiation in

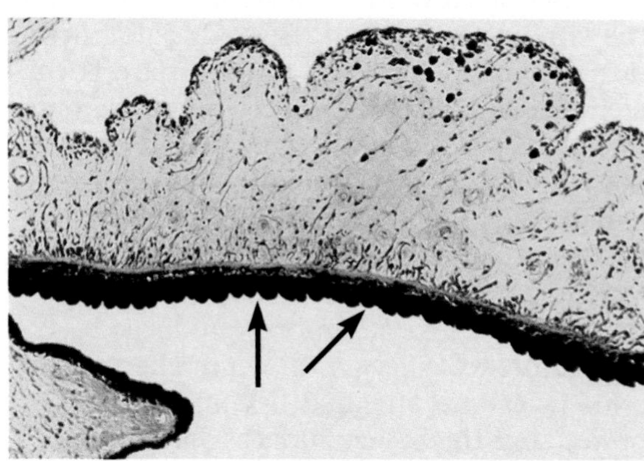

Figure 2-1

NORMAL IRIS

Layers of the middle third of the iris, between the pupillary area and the iris root. Arrows indicate the pigment epithelium.

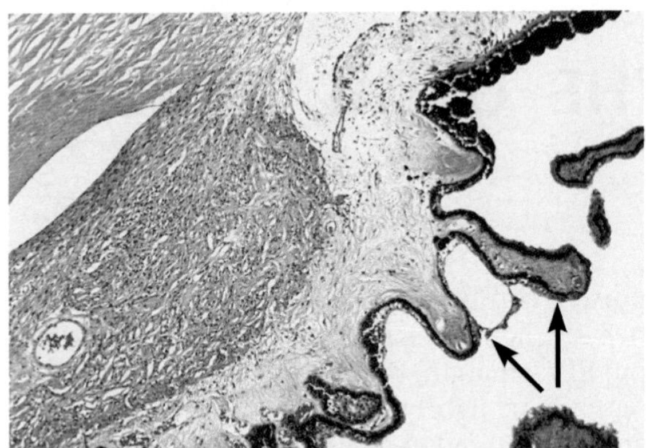

Figure 2-2

NORMAL CILIARY BODY

Pars plicata with ciliary processes (arrows), stroma, and the ciliary muscle.

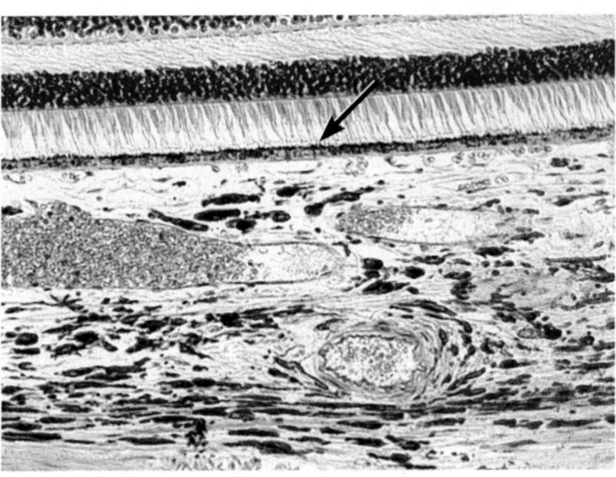

Figure 2-3

NORMAL CHOROID

The vascularized and pigmented choroid is located between the retina above and the collagenous sclera below. Arrow indicates the retinal pigment epithelium.

size, shape, and degree of melanization is sometimes useful for assessing the origin of a heavily pigmented intraocular tumor.

The Ciliary Body

The ciliary body measures 6 mm in length and extends from the anterior chamber angle and iris root to the ora serrata. The anterior part, or corona ciliaris, contains approximately 70 ciliary processes, radial ridges about 2-mm long (fig. 2-2). The posterior part is termed the pars plana ciliaris (orbicularis ciliaris). On cross section, the ciliary body has a triangular shape, with its base toward the anterior chamber angle, the inner side toward the posterior chamber and the vitreous cavity, and the outer side in contact with the sclera. The inner surface is covered by a double epithelial cell layer: the outer pigmented ciliary epithelium that is continuous with the iris pigment epithelium anteriorly and the retinal pigment epithelium posteriorly, and the inner, nonpigmented ciliary epithelium that is a continuation of the neurosensory retina. The aqueous humor is produced by the nonpigmented ciliary epithelium. The apices of both layers are attached by junctional complexes, and the basilar surfaces are covered by an inner multilaminar basement membrane and an outer (stromal) thick basal lamina.

The stroma between the ciliary epithelium and the muscle cell layer contains blood vessels, connective tissue, and nerves. Melanocytes and mast cells are seen within the stroma and between the smooth muscle fascicles. The ciliary muscle is responsible for the accommodation of the lens in near vision. It is composed of three fascicles: the outer longitudinal ciliary muscle (Brücke muscle) that extends from the scleral spur at the anterior chamber angle to the posterior ciliary body and peripheral choroid; the meridional, or radial, ciliary muscle; and the circular ciliary muscle (Müller muscle) next to the iris root. The supraciliary space, which separates the ciliary body from the sclera, is in continuity with the anterior part of the suprachoroidal space.

The Choroid

The choroid extends from the ora serrata to the optic nerve. It is a highly vascular structure, necessarily so because of the high metabolic demands of the retinal pigment epithelium and the outer retinal cell layers. The thickness varies from 0.1 mm anteriorly to 0.2 mm at the posterior pole (fig. 2-3). From the external to the internal surface, the choroid has the following layers: the lamina fusca, composed of collagen strands and long spindled-shaped melanocytes, the latter best seen when a choroidal detachment opens the suprachoroidal space, and found, also, in the scleral canals in heavily pigmented individuals; the large vessel layer (Haller layer) that contains wide-caliber arteries and veins; the medium-sized vessel layer (Sattler layer); the choriocapillaris, composed of wide, flat (40 to 50 μm), fenestrated capillaries; and the Bruch membrane, which is demonstrated by electron microscopy to be formed by the basement membrane of the retinal pigment epithelium, an inner collagenous layer, an elastic layer, an outer collagenous layer, and the basement membrane of the endothelium of the choriocapillaris.

Vascularization

The vascular supply is divided into posterior and anterior parts. The choroid is supplied by several short ciliary arteries that penetrate the sclera around the optic nerve. The ciliary body and the iris are supplied by an arterial plexus formed by the two long posterior ciliary arteries that run within the choroidal stroma associated with the long ciliary nerves, and seven anterior ciliary arteries extending from the insertions of the rectus muscles. Anteriorly, they form the major arterial circle of the iris within the ciliary body near the iris root. Radial vessels travel anteriorly from the major arterial circle within the iris stroma to form the minor arterial circle around the pupillary margin.

The venous drainage of the choroid and posterior ciliary body is through four or more vortex veins that leave the eye behind the equator, approximately one from each quadrant.

Innervation

The choroid and ciliary body are innervated by the posterior ciliary nerves (parasympathetic system). The sympathetic system is provided by anterior ciliary nerves that penetrate the eye 3 mm behind the limbus.

GENERAL CONSIDERATIONS

Melanocytic tumors are the most common primary neoplasms of the uvea. Nevi, which outnumber malignant melanomas, are present in 5 to 10 percent of enucleated eyes (1). Uveal melanoma represents less than 1 percent of cancer registration, and is therefore considered a rare tumor. Nevertheless, it accounts for 13 percent of death from malignant melanoma from all locations (2). The most frequent malignant uveal tumor is metastatic carcinoma, primarily from breast and lung, less frequently from almost any organ and tissue. Other primary uveal tumors are rare; however, they may pose clinical and sometimes histopathologic diagnostic problems. The clinical presentation, diagnosis, therapy, and prognosis vary, depending on whether the tumors arise from the iris, ciliary body, or choroid.

Although the diagnosis of intraocular tumors is often based on biomicroscopic and funduscopic findings, ancillary studies are important diagnostic tools. A- and B-scan ultrasonography of posterior choroidal tumors provide important data for the differential diagnosis of primary and metastatic tumors. Computerized tomography (CT) is useful in lesions with primary or secondary calcification. Magnetic resonance imaging (MRI) permits better visualization of intraocular tumors and determination of extraocular extension. Tumors involving the anterior segment, particularly iris tumors, are best visualized with ultrasound biomicroscopy.

One of the major controversial subjects concerning intraocular tumors is the preferred management of malignant melanoma. Enucleation, different types of brachytherapy, and other conservative modalities of therapy vary with the location and size of the tumor; the various treatments have been shown to have a very similar effect on patient survival (3). Most enucleated specimens harboring medium and some large-sized uveal melanomas had been previously treated. Most of these eyes were enucleated because of treatment failure or secondary ocular changes (e.g., radiation retinopathy) following conservative therapy.

Unlike cutaneous melanoma, dissemination, primarily to the liver, occurs mainly through the venous system into the systemic circulation. The treatment for metastatic disease has been completely ineffective (4,5).

MELANOCYTIC TUMORS OF THE UVEA

Nevi

Iris Nevi. Melanocytic nevi may arise from the iris, ciliary body, and choroid. Iris nevi occur more commonly in the lightly colored irides of white people than in pigmented individuals (6). The frequency of iris nevi from different series varies from 9.6 to 30.5 percent (7,8). Iris nevi have been associated with choroidal melanoma and cutaneous melanoma (9). Nevi account for 84 percent of suspicious malignant

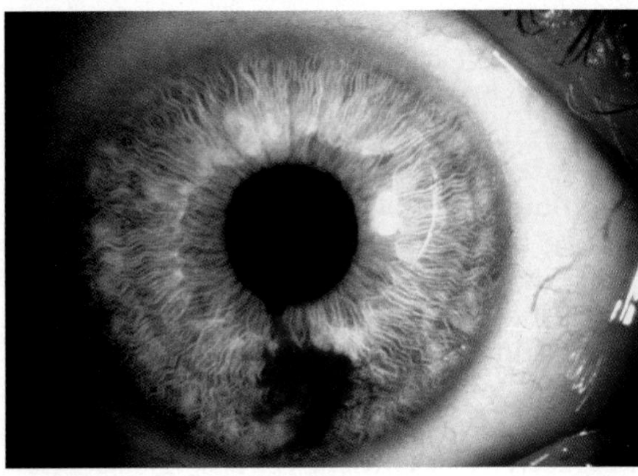

Figure 2-4

IRIS NEVUS

A circumscribed pigmented lesion of the iris is seen inferiorly.

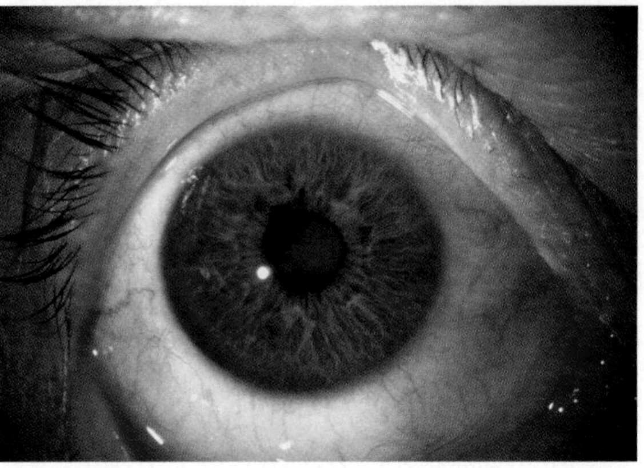

Figure 2-6

IRIS NEVUS

Small pigmented lesion with traction of the iris pigment epithelium at the pupillary margin (from 10 to 12 o'clock).

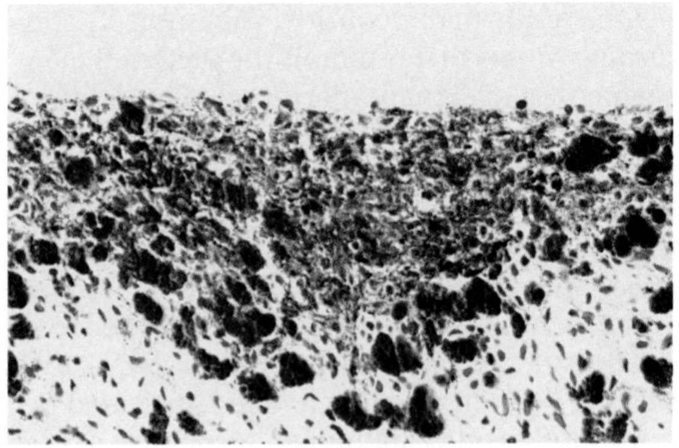

Figure 2-5

IRIS NEVUS

The iris lesion seen in figure 2-4 is composed of heavily pigmented dendritic and plump polyhedral melanocytes.

pigmented iridic lesions. Shields et al. (10) found that among 200 patients examined because of presumed iris melanomas, 31 percent had findings more consistent with nevi. In one large review of lesions involving the iris and ciliary body originally diagnosed as malignant melanoma, 87 percent of the tumors were reclassified into six benign histopathologic categories including melanocytosis, melanocytoma, epithelioid cell nevus, intrastromal spindle cell nevus, spindle cell nevus with surface plaque, and borderline spindle cell nevus (11).

Although iris nevi are seen at any age, they more commonly develop or become pigmented in the first three decades of life (figs. 2-4–2-6). Patients present with one of the following growth patterns: plaque-like lesion on the surface of the iris, intrastromal lesion or combined patterns, and diffuse stromal involvement. The management of iris nevi is observation, with periodic follow-up examination. In a series of 175 patients with suspected benign lesions of the iris that were periodically examined for a mean time of 4.7 years, only eight lesions (4.6 percent) showed clinical evidence of enlargement (12).

The lesions are composed of one or more of the following cell types: small and medium-sized spindle-shaped cells (figs. 2-5–2-7); small round or polygonal cells; large round or polygonal melanocytic cells; and sometimes, large multinucleated epithelioid cells (13). Rarely, the iris nevus is composed of balloon cells with vacuolated cytoplasm containing lipid (14). The main problem in the differential diagnosis is to exclude a low-grade spindle cell melanoma. The absence of mitotic activity and the bland cytologic features of the spindle cells favor a benign lesion. Nevi as well as melanoma may show foci of necrosis, pigment-laden macrophages, and extension onto the anterior chamber angle structures, and may result in distortion of the pupillary margin, ectropion of the iris pigment epithelium, vascularization of the iris surface (rubeosis), and glaucoma.

Ticho et al. (15) described a series of patients with bilateral, multiple, nodular nevi of the iris.

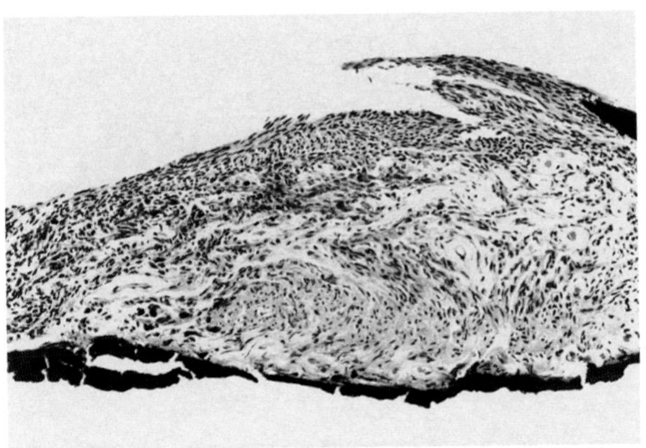

Figure 2-7

IRIS NEVUS

Iridectomy specimen from the lesion seen in figure 2-6 shows a benign, lightly pigmented, spindle cell proliferation extending along the anterior surface of the iris, with traction of the iris pigment epithelium on the right.

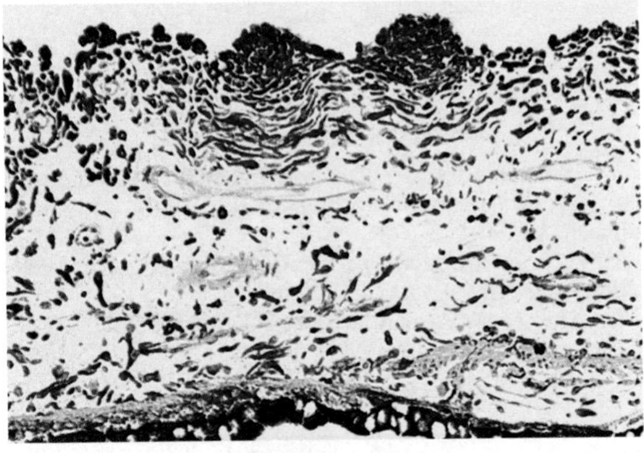

Figure 2-8

LISCH NODULES

Multiple, deeply pigmented, hamartomatous melanocytic nodules are at the anterior border layer of the iris.

Clinically, the nodules were uniform in size and were associated with other ocular abnormalities. Histopathologic examination in one case showed elevated plaques composed of aggregates of plump, lightly pigmented, nevoid cells intermixed with mature, densely pigmented, spindle-shaped uveal melanocytes.

Other lesions that may be confused with nevi are ocular melanocytosis, Lisch nodules, and Brushfield spots of the iris. Iris mamillations, an increased number of densely pigmented spindle-shaped or polygonal cells resembling normal stromal melanocytes (16), are observed in ocular melanocytosis. Lisch nodules are pigmented melanocytic iris hamartomas in patients with neurofibromatosis type 1 (fig. 2-8) (17). They usually are bilateral, superficial and deep, intrastromal nodules measuring 0.5 to 1.0 mm that are composed of spindle-shaped melanocytes (18). Brushfield spots are multiple brownish gold spots on the surface of the iris that correspond to hypercellular melanocytic foci. They are seen in 85 percent of patients with Down's syndrome and in 24 percent of normal individuals (19,20). Iris nodules, which are composed of normal-appearing melanocytes, may also be observed in patients with iris-nevus syndrome (Cogan-Reese syndrome) (21).

Ciliary Body Nevi. Nevi of the ciliary body are rare and represent approximately 3.5 percent of all uveal nevi (22). Usually, nevus cells are present at the base or around a ciliary body malignant melanoma (23). Most small ciliary body nevi are clinically undetected. Ciliary body nevi are composed of plump spindle-shaped cells without mitotic figures. They are moderately pigmented, have a slightly large nucleus with a loose chromatin pattern, and may occasionally have a small nucleolus (fig. 2-9). Some cases in which the biologic behavior is undetermined have been classified as low-grade spindle cell melanomas (see section on ciliary body melanoma). Large pigmented nevi of the ciliary body may be clinically indistinguishable from melanoma and, in such cases, are locally excised by cyclectomy with lamellar corneoscleral resection.

Choroidal Nevi. The choroid is the most common location of uveal nevi. In one histopathologic study, 94 percent of the uveal nevi were located in the choroid (23). The frequency of choroidal nevi in the adult population is 3.1 to 6.5 percent (24,25). Choroidal nevi usually do not cause symptoms and are discovered on routine ophthalmoscopic fundus examination. The size of the nevus is usually less than 5 mm in diameter; rarely are larger nevi more than 10 mm in diameter by 1.5 mm in thickness. They are circumscribed, blue-gray lesions that may have small, yellow-white drusen on their surface.

Choroidal nevi are composed of four types of cells: polyhedral small cells with oval nuclei,

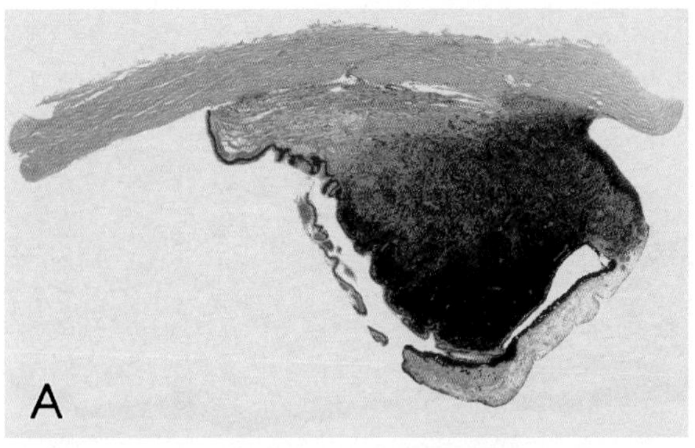

Figure 2-9

CILIARY BODY NEVUS

A: Iridocyclectomy specimen with lamellar scleral resection shows a pigmented lesion of the ciliary body and adjacent iris.

B: The melanocytic tumor is composed of heavily pigmented cells.

C: The cells have bland ovoid nuclei with small nucleoli (bleached sections).

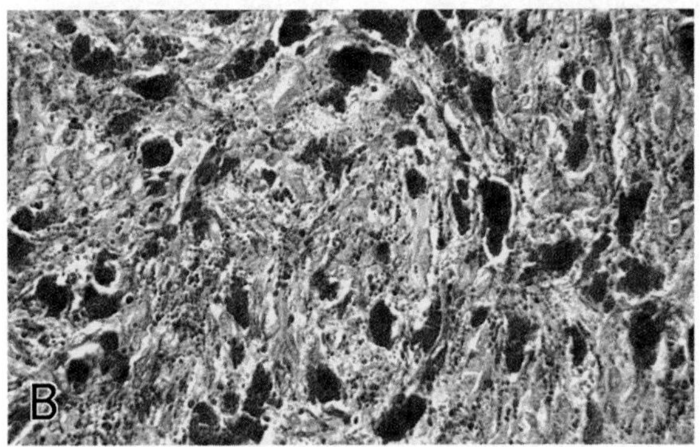

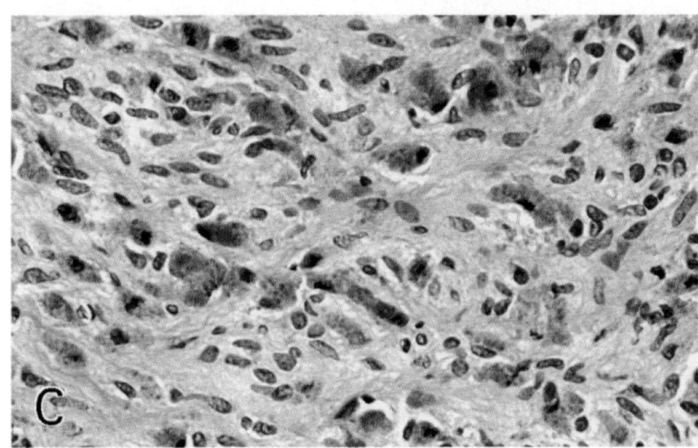

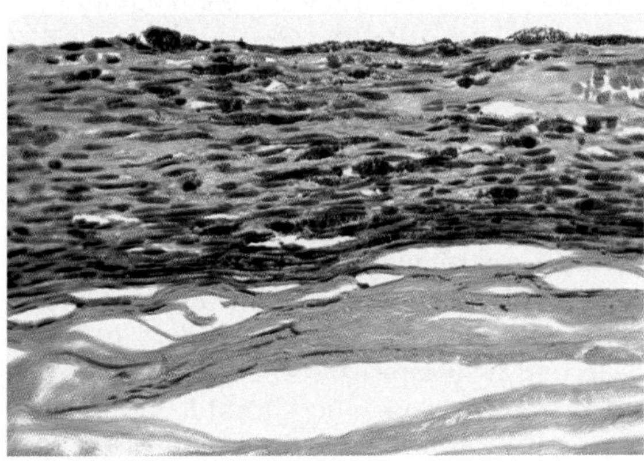

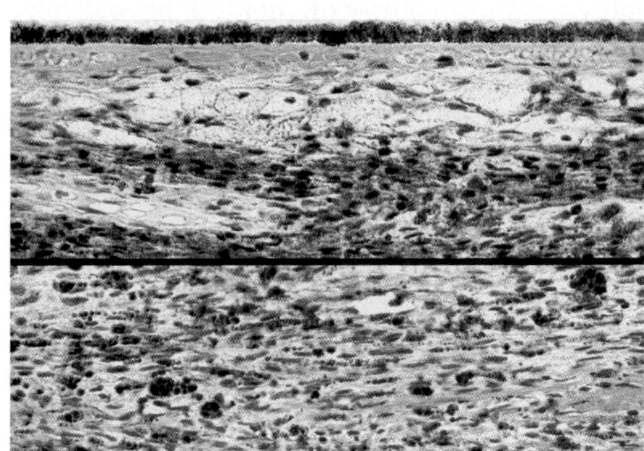

Figure 2-10

CHOROIDAL NEVUS

Left: Spindle cell nevus of the choroid.
Right: Spindle cell choroidal nevus with scattered balloon cells.

small spindle-shaped cells with oval nuclei, dendritic nevus cells, and balloon nevus cells with vacuolated cytoplasm containing lipid (fig. 2-10) (141). The degree of cell pigmentation is variable (26).

The main diagnostic challenge of choroidal melanocytic lesions is distinguishing large nevi from small melanomas. Clinical findings suggestive of malignancy are: growth or thickness greater than 2 mm, orange pigment (lipofuscin) over the lesion, pin-point detachments of the retinal pigment epithelium, serous retinal fluid, or a lesion encroaching upon the optic

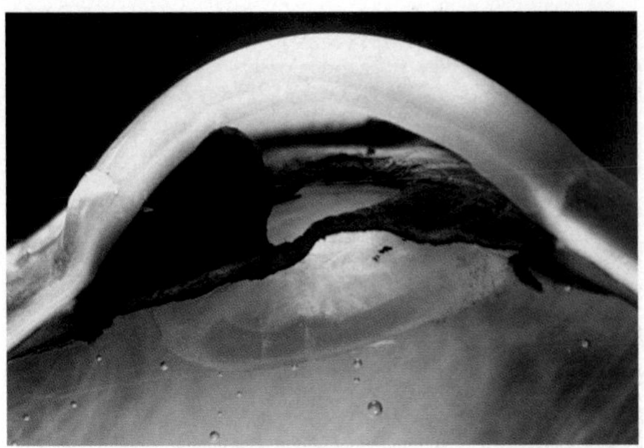

Figure 2-11

IRIS MELANOCYTOMA

A large, heavily pigmented mass is on the iridic surface.

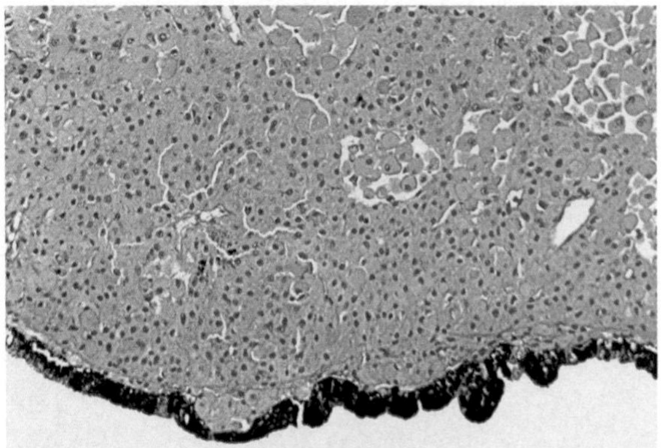

Figure 2-12

IRIS MELANOCYTOMA

Uniform populations of polygonal cells have centrally placed small round nuclei (bleached section).

disc (27). Management of choroidal nevi is by periodic observation.

Melanocytoma (Magnocellular Nevus)

Melanocytomas are a nevi variant composed of large, plump polygonal cells that have small, centrally placed, round to oval nuclei and fully melanized cytoplasm (figs. 2-11, 2-12) (28). Clinically, *melanocytomas of the iris* appear deeply pigmented to jet black and may be associated with pigment dispersion and glaucoma (melanocytomalytic glaucoma) (29). Dispersion of pigment-laden macrophages results from spontaneous foci of necrosis. Iris melanocytomas usually are stable lesions, and the documentation of growth does not necessarily represent malignant transformation (30). The development of melanoma from an iris melanocytoma is unusual (31). Management is by periodic observation. Local surgical resection by iridectomy may control transient elevations of intraocular pressure or well-established glaucoma (32).

Ciliary body and *choroidal melanocytomas* do not differ histologically from melanocytomas arising from the iris (figs. 2-13–2-15) (33,34). Because of the location and growth patterns, however, melanocytomas of the ciliary body may resemble malignant melanoma clinically. Melanocytomas of the choroid may be indistinguishable from nevi (35). Ciliary body and choroidal melanocytomas may undergo malignant transformation (36,37). Melanocytomas with progressive growth usually extend into the

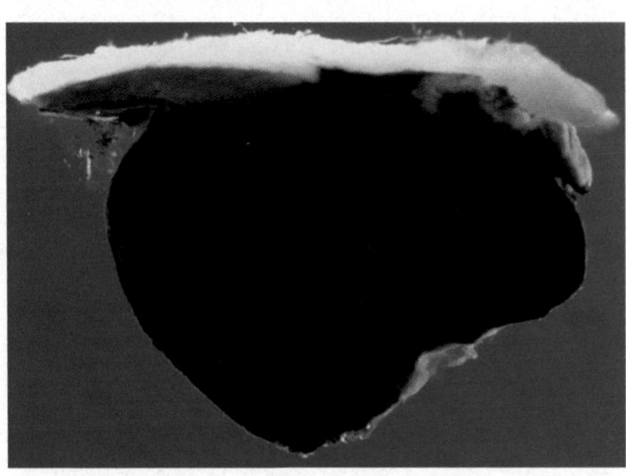

Figure 2-13

CILIARY BODY MELANOCYTOMA

Iridocyclectomy specimen demonstrates the homogeneous, jet black appearance of the mass involving the ciliary body.

anterior chamber angle structures and even extend to extrascleral areas (34,38). Pigment dispersion is common and may be secondary to spontaneous necrosis (39). Because small foci of cystic degeneration are common in ciliary body melanocytomas, these tumors may appear cystic (40).

Light and electron microscopy demonstrate two types of cells (fig. 2-16) (41). Type 1 cells are large and polyhedral, with eccentrically located round nuclei; the cytoplasm is usually packed with giant melanosomes that range in

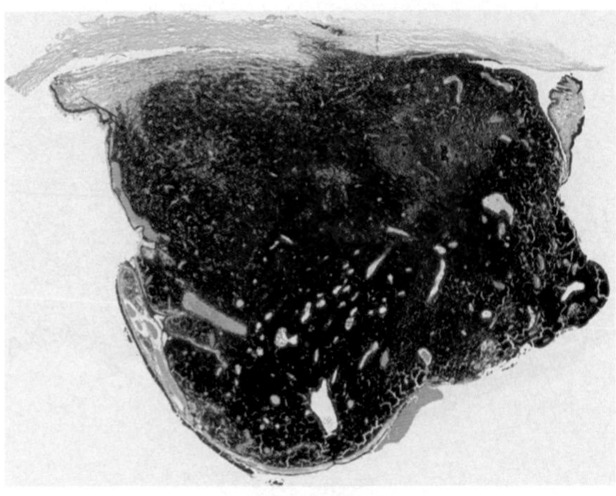

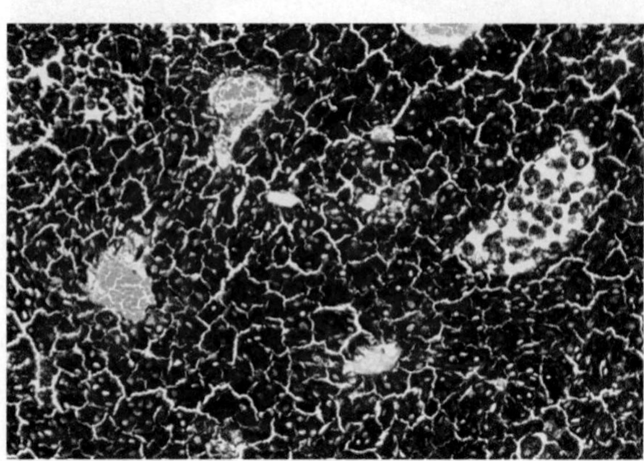

Figure 2-14

CILIARY BODY MELANOCYTOMA

Left: Low-power microscopic view of a pigmented ciliary body tumor.
Right: The tumor is composed of heavily pigmented polygonal cells with pale paracentral or eccentric nuclei.

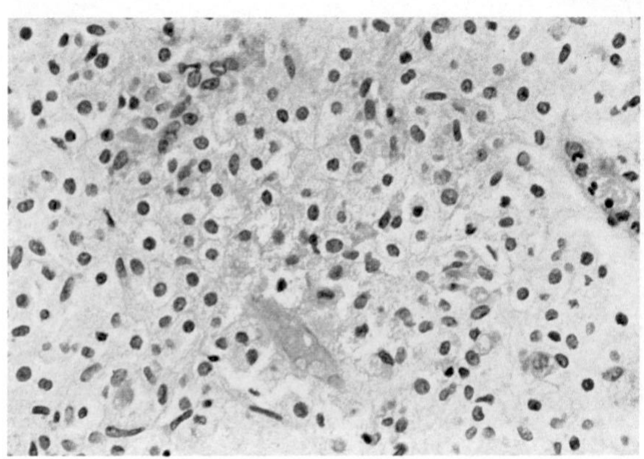

Figure 2-15

CILIARY BODY MELANOCYTOMA

Bleached preparation shows melanocytoma cells with abundant polyhedral cytoplasm.

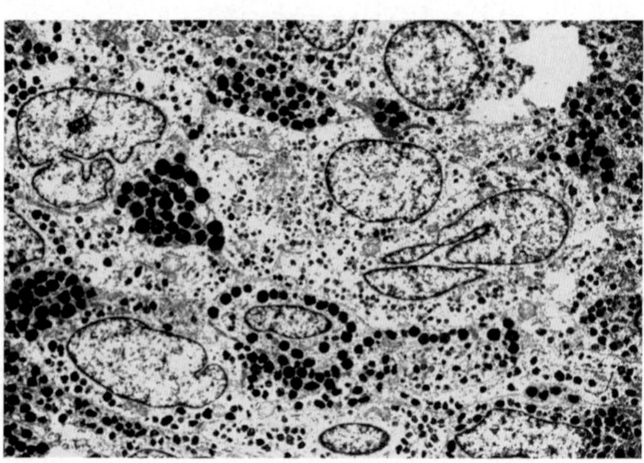

Figure 2-16

CILIARY BODY MELANOCYTOMA

Transmission electron microscopy demonstrates type 1 cells containing giant melanosomes, and spindle-shaped type 2 cells with indented nuclei and small melanosomes.

size from 1 to 4 µm in diameter. Type 2 cells have elongated cytoplasm containing small, round to oval melanin granules measuring 0.1 to 0.4 µm in length; a variable number of pigment-laden macrophages is observed. When noninvasive methods fail to support or exclude the diagnosis of malignant melanoma of the uvea, fine-needle aspiration biopsy (FNAB) may be helpful (fig. 2-17) (42). Most tumors are managed conservatively by iridocyclectomy or other combined surgical procedures.

Malignant Melanoma

Melanoma of the Iris. *Definition and General Features.* Melanomas of the iris represent 3.3 to 16.6 percent of uveal melanomas among different series (43–46). The calculated average incidence of iris melanomas in Denmark over a 25-year period was 3.2 cases/year (45). Melanomas of the iris differ from those originating in the ciliary body and choroid because they occur at an earlier age, exhibit more benign cell types, and result in a better prognosis. The average age

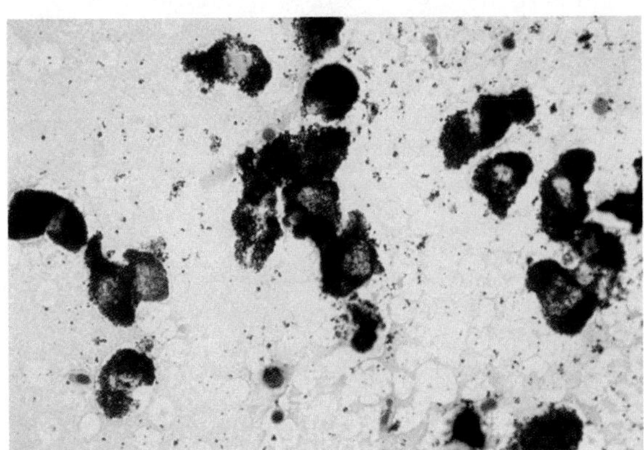

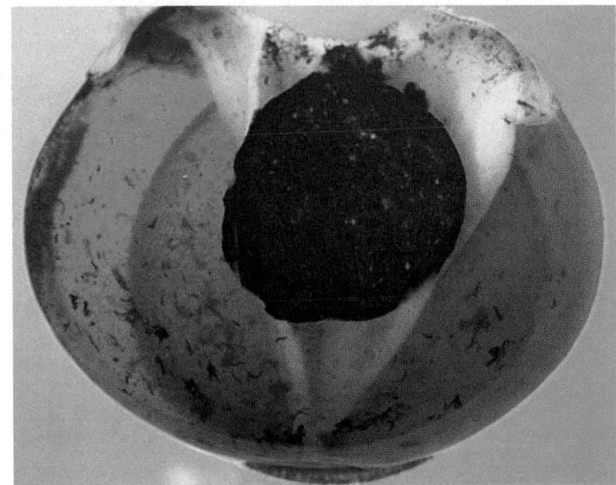

Figure 2-17

CILIARY BODY MELANOCYTOMA

Left: Fine-needle aspiration biopsy shows polyhedral cells containing large spheroidal melanin granules. The nuclei are pale and centrally located, and the nucleoli are inconspicuous.

Right: The sclera has been removed and upon sectioning discloses a heavily pigmented melanocytoma of the ciliary body.

at the time of presentation varies from 40 to 50 years (43,47–50). Iris melanomas constitute 8.5 to 10.4 percent of uveal melanomas occurring in patients younger than 20 years (43,47,49,51). Jakobiec and Silbert (52), in a review of 189 malignant melanomas from the iris and ciliary body, found that only 13 percent fulfilled the criteria for malignant melanoma (see below). It is reasonable to assume that earlier series included tumors that, according to our current knowledge, are now considered benign lesions. Iris melanomas arise in patients with ocular melanocytosis, familial atypical mole/melanoma syndrome (B-K mole syndrome), neurofibromatosis type 1, and xeroderma pigmentosum (53–56).

Clinical Features. Many patients give a history of a pigmented lesion that has been present since childhood. The duration of the lesion is longer than 1 year in almost 50 percent of cases and more than 10 years in 18 to 35 percent of cases (43,47,48). Malignant melanomas of the iris affect almost exclusively the inferior quadrants of the iris (figs. 2-18–2-20) (46). The most important clinical sign suggestive of malignancy is evidence of growth upon periodic follow-up examination of the patient (57). Another suggestive sign is prominent abnormal blood vessels within the lesion (58,59). Shields et al. (46), suggested that an iris melanoma should be suspected if the lesion is growing into the stroma, is thicker than 1 mm and at least 3 mm in diameter, or if three or more of the following findings are present: prominent vascularization, ectropion iridis, secondary glaucoma, secondary cataract, and photographic documentation of growth. Tumors with either circumscribed or diffuse involvement of the anterior chamber angle may cause secondary glaucoma. Extraocular extension occurs in 6 percent of the cases (45).

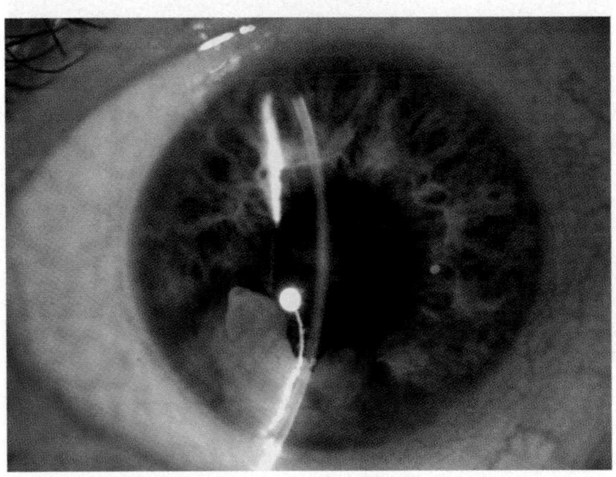

Figure 2-18

IRIS MELANOMA

Large, lightly pigmented lesion in the inferior iris. (Figs. 2-18 through 2-20 are from the same patient.)

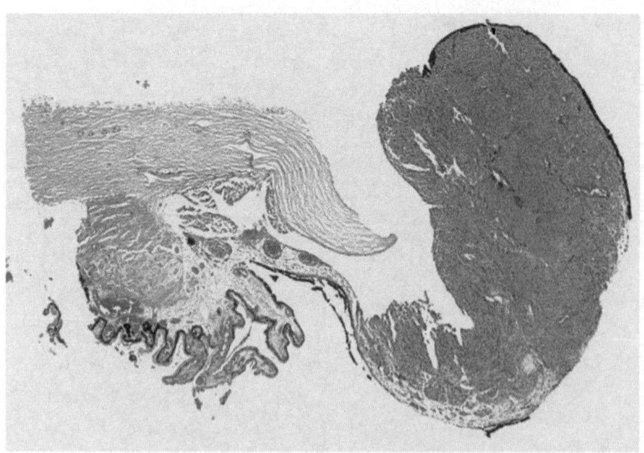

Figure 2-19

IRIS MELANOMA

Iridocyclectomy specimen from the tumor shown in figure 2-18.

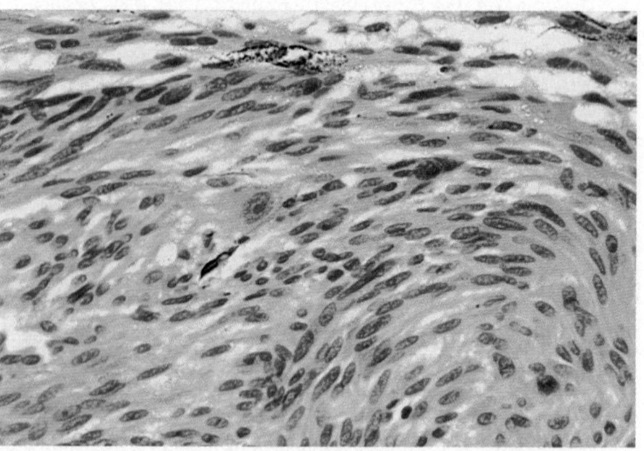

Figure 2-20

IRIS MELANOMA

The tumor is composed of spindle B type cells and a few epithelioid cells.

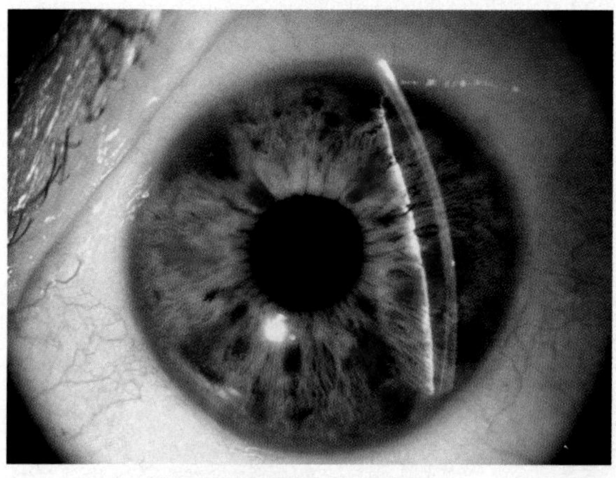

Figure 2-21

DIFFUSE MALIGNANT MELANOMA OF THE IRIS

The patient developed heterochromia iridis and secondary glaucoma.

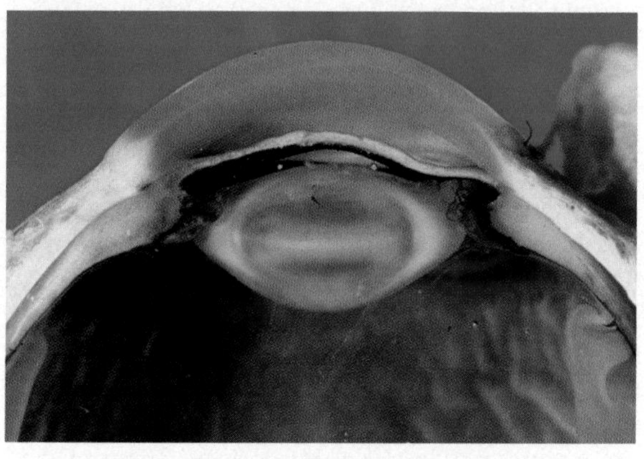

Figure 2-22

DIFFUSE MALIGNANT MELANOMA

Diffuse malignant melanoma of the iris and ciliary body (ring melanoma).

There are at least three growth patterns: nodular and circumscribed, diffuse, and tapioca melanoma. Nodular melanomas are located more frequently at the periphery, may touch the cornea, and may infiltrate the anterior chamber angle. Patients with diffuse melanomas of the iris may have heterochromia (fig. 2-21), corectopia, ectropion iridis, and glaucoma (60). This variant is frequently misdiagnosed clinically (figs. 2-22, 2-23). Tapioca melanoma is characterized by multiple nodules that project from the surface of the iris (61). Rarely, the tapioca-type growth pattern is observed in nevi. The ring melanoma type is a diffuse form of iris/ciliary body melanoma (see below).

Microscopic Findings. There are three histologic types of iris melanoma: spindle cell, mixed cell, and epithelioid cell melanomas. Spindle-shaped melanoma cells have a high nuclear to cytoplasmic ratio, oval nuclei with clumped chromatin, and prominent nucleoli. Mitotic activity usually is quite low and may vary from 1 to 3 mitoses per 20 high-power fields. Epithelioid cell melanoma is composed of noncohesive, small and large polyhedral cells with acidophilic glassy cytoplasm and large,

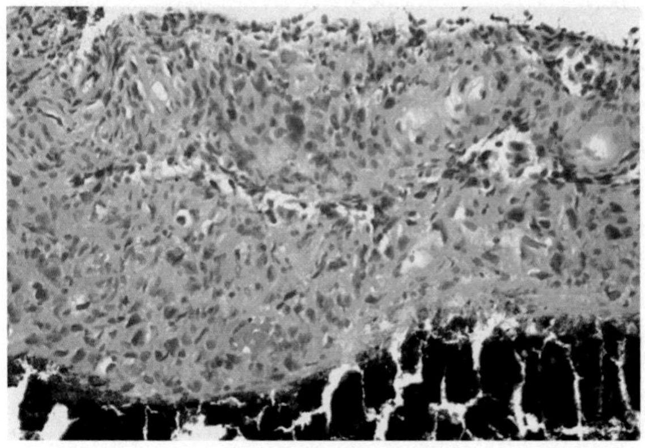

Figure 2-23

IRIS MELANOMA

Diffuse infiltration of the iris by malignant melanoma cells.

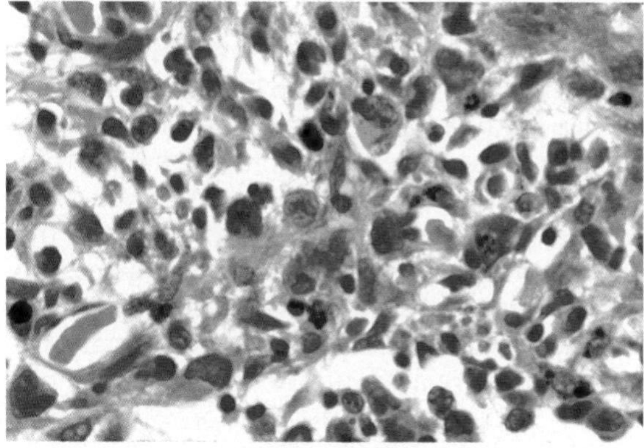

Figure 2-24

PREDOMINANT EPITHELIOID CELL MELANOMA OF THE IRIS

Small and pleomorphic epithelioid cells with eosinophilic cytoplasm and nuclear infoldings.

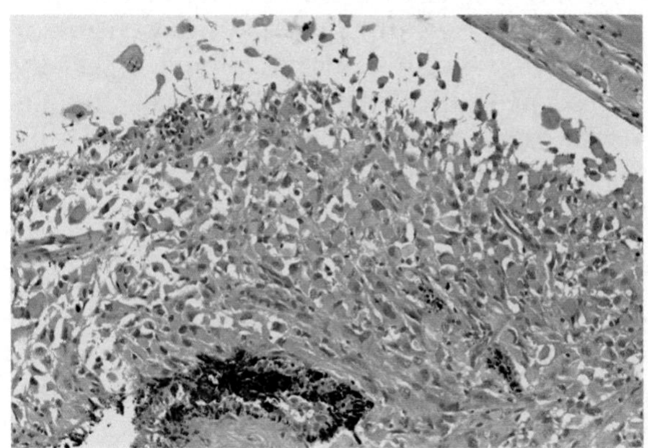

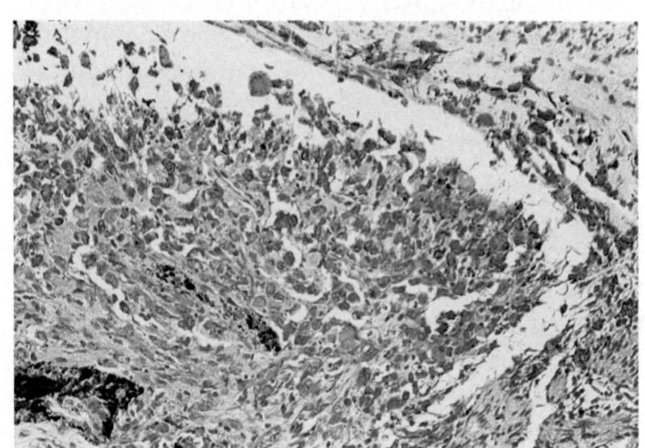

Figure 2-25

DIFFUSE EPITHELIOID MELANOMA OF THE IRIS

Left: The tumor is composed of amelanotic large epithelioid cells.
Right: The strong positivity with HMB45 antibody confirmed the diagnosis of melanoma.

round to oval vesicular nuclei with prominent eosinophilic nucleoli (fig. 2-24). Mixed cell type melanoma contains a variable number of both cell types (fig. 2-20). Another feature observed in spindle-shaped and mixed cell type melanomas is the presence of nevoid areas. Approximately 70 percent of malignant iris melanomas have a spindle-shaped cell phenotype; diffuse iris melanoma, however, has a predominance of epithelioid cells in 80 percent of the cases (43,49). Pure epithelioid cell melanomas are rare (62,63).

Immunohistochemical Findings. Immunohistochemistry is not used routinely for the diagnosis of malignant uveal melanoma. The tumor cells express Melan-A, HMB45, S-100 protein, and vimentin (fig. 2-25). In one retrospective study, the sensitivity was 100 percent for Melan-A and S-100 protein, and 55 percent for HMB45 (64).

Cytologic Findings. Cytologic smears from paracentesis and FNAB are useful in large tumors when the clinical diagnosis of malignant melanoma of the iris is uncertain (65). The aspiration of fluid with the bevel of the needle placed on the surface of the tumor may be an alternative to FNAB. In deeply pigmented tumors, it is recommended that one or two slides be examined using bleaching techniques.

Special Techniques. Silver-stained nuclear organizer regional counts are lower than 1.9 in iris nevi and greater than 2.8 in malignant melanomas (66,67). Most iris nevi and melanomas are diploid by nuclear DNA ploidy analysis (68). Studies of iris melanomas show relatively high levels of chromosomal alterations that affect numerous chromosomes (69). In a few cases, different abnormalities of chromosomes 5 and 18 as well as variations between the primary tumor and its related tumor seeding were observed, including the acquisition of an additional chromosome 15 (69).

Differential Diagnosis. The most important distinction is between a low-grade spindle-shaped melanoma and a nevus. The presence of tumor cells with large vesicular nuclei, prominent nucleoli, and mitotic activity favors a diagnosis of malignant melanoma. Large, prominent, reddish purple nucleoli are observed mainly in melanomas. Ciliary body melanomas may present as a peripheral iris tumor. Nevoid areas and extension into the anterior chamber structures may be observed in both melanomas and nevi. Nonpigmented, purely epithelioid cell melanoma may be confused with a metastatic tumor and rhabdomyosarcoma. Spindle cell tumors other than melanocytic lesions and leiomyomas are rare in the iris.

Treatment and Prognosis. Iris melanomas are invasive tumors with low-grade malignant potential. The incidence of metastases varies between 2.4 and 5.0 percent (43,49). The average interval between diagnosis and metastasis is 6.5 years (range, 1 month to 12 years) (70). The death rate from metastasis is approximately 2.3 percent (45). Metastases develop more frequently in older patients and are usually associated with glaucoma, invasion of the iris root and anterior chamber angle structures, or episcleral extension (46). Histopathologic risk factors for the occurrence of metastasis are diffuse type of growth, hyperpigmentation, and cells with prominent nucleoli. In one review, the rate of metastasis was 2.6 percent for spindle cell melanoma, 10.5 percent for mixed cell type, and 6.9 percent for epithelioid melanoma. Distant metastasis occurred in 3 of 24 (13 percent) patients with diffuse iris melanoma (60,71).

The management of patients with pigmented iris lesions should be individualized. Most lesions are managed conservatively with local resection. The only primary indication for enucleation is diffuse iris melanoma, especially if associated with ipsilateral glaucoma, although a few cases have been treated with plaque brachytherapy (60). In one study, elevated intraocular pressure was associated with enucleation in 60 percent of iris melanomas (46). Recurrences may occur many years after local excision of the primary lesion. Dedifferentiation of a low-grade malignant melanoma of the iris into a more aggressive epithelioid cell type has been described after multiple recurrences (72).

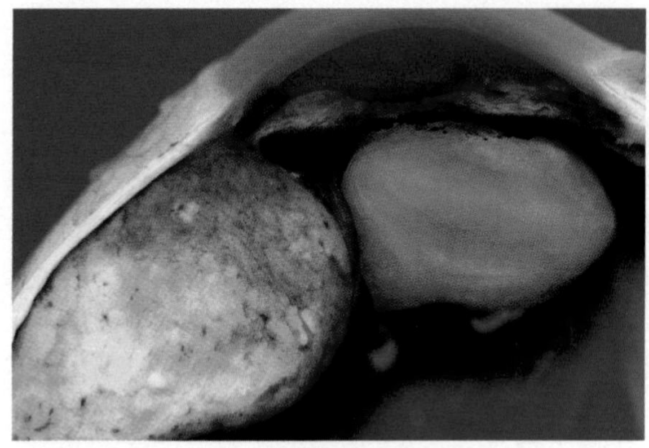

Figure 2-26

CILIARY BODY MELANOMA

Large pigmented ciliary body tumor invades the anterior chamber angle.

Melanoma of the Ciliary Body. Ciliary body melanomas account for 9 percent of all uveal melanomas (73). Primary melanomas of the ciliary body usually extend anteriorly into the iris root and the anterior chamber angle (fig. 2-26). Most commonly, however, the ciliary body is involved by progressive growth of melanomas that arise from within the choroid (fig. 2-27); these tumors should be considered choroidal tumors regarding prognosis and therapy. Patients with ciliary body melanomas present with loss of vision due to displacement or cataractous changes of the lens, a pigmented mass in the anterior chamber angle, glaucoma, or prominent episcleral vessels (sentinel vessels) over the site of the tumor. Ultrasound biomicroscopy and echography may be useful to evaluate the location, size, and extension of the mass; FNAB may provide a cytologic diagnosis to establish the appropriate management.

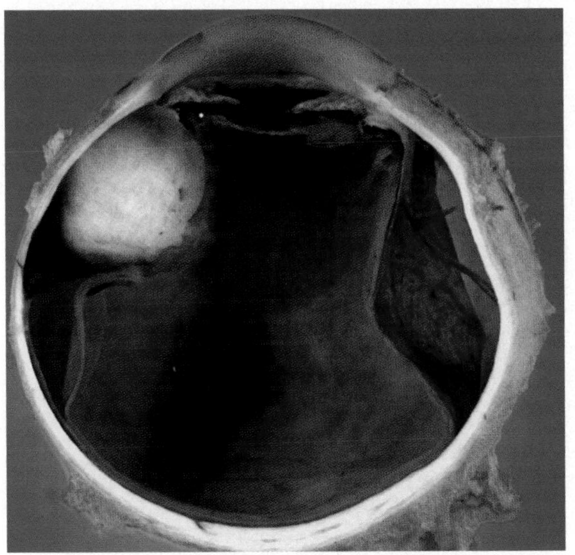

Figure 2-27

CILIARY BODY AND CHOROIDAL MELANOMA

Melanoma arising in an eye that underwent cataract surgery and intraocular lens implantation.

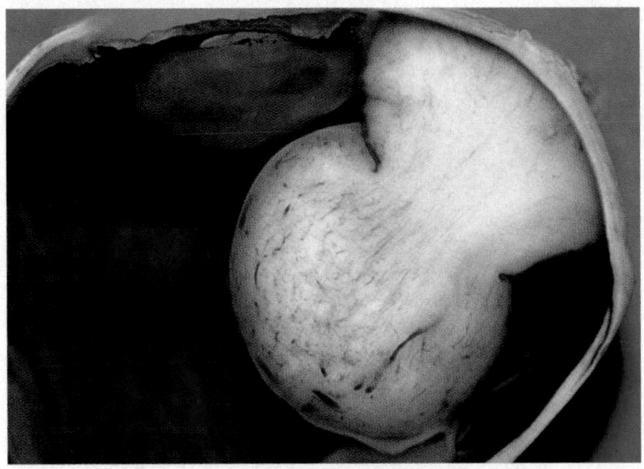

Figure 2-28

CILIARY BODY MELANOMA

Rupture of the peripheral Bruch membrane due to amelanotic melanoma results in a mushroom-shaped configuration.

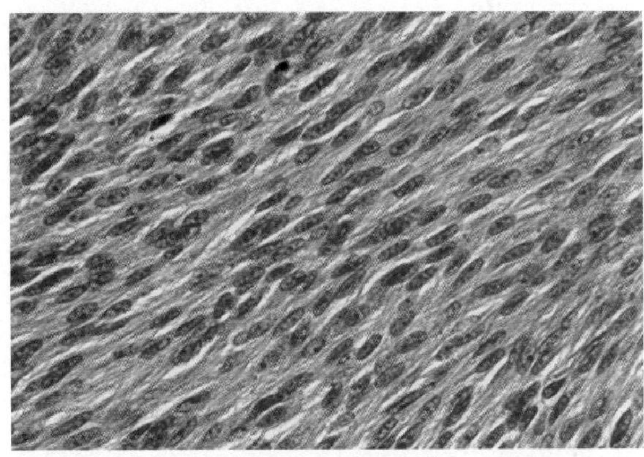

Figure 2-29

CILIARY BODY MELANOMA

The amelanotic tumor shown in figure 2-28 is composed almost exclusively of spindle B melanoma cells.

The histopathologic findings, cytologic classification, and prognostic factors of ciliary body melanoma do not differ from those of the more common choroidal melanoma (see melanoma of the choroid below) (figs. 2-28, 2-29). The management of a suspected melanoma of the ciliary body is primarily local resection of the tumor by iridocyclectomy. The 10-year survival rate is 91 percent (74,75). In one study of 49 patients, two local tumor recurrences (2.9 percent) were observed and four eyes (5.8 percent) had to be enucleated after block excision (75). Recurrences have been associated with large tumors and epithelioid cell type (76). Enucleation is indicated for the treatment of large ciliary body tumors. Tumors with episcleral invasion may have access to conjunctival lymphatic drainage and may result in metastasis to regional lymph nodes (figs. 2-30, 2-31). A few cases have been treated successfully with plaque brachytherapy or charged particle irradiation (77–79). Mortality from primary melanoma of the ciliary body is mostly limited to mixed or epithelioid cell types (80).

Ring melanoma is a variant of ciliary body and iris melanoma that invades the anterior chamber angle structures for more than 180 degrees (figs. 2-32, 2-33) (81). The tumor may extend through the drainage system of the aqueous humor, reach the intrascleral venous plexuses at the limbus, and into the conjunctiva and the venous circulation. The prognosis is poor, and patients with ring melanomas of the ciliary body are best treated by enucleation. In one recent series, metastasis developed in 12 of 23 patients (52 percent) after a mean follow-up of 55 months (82).

Melanoma of the Choroid. *General Features.* Malignant melanoma of the choroid is the most frequent primary malignant intraocular tumor

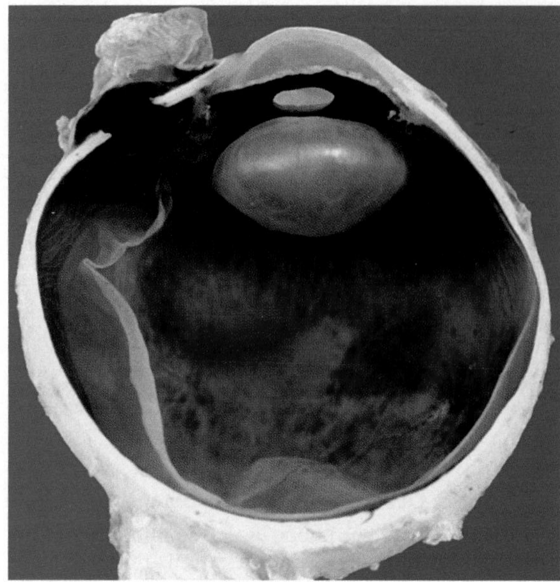

Figure 2-30

CILIARY BODY MELANOMA

Heavily pigmented melanoma of the ciliary body shows scleral invasion and episcleral extension.

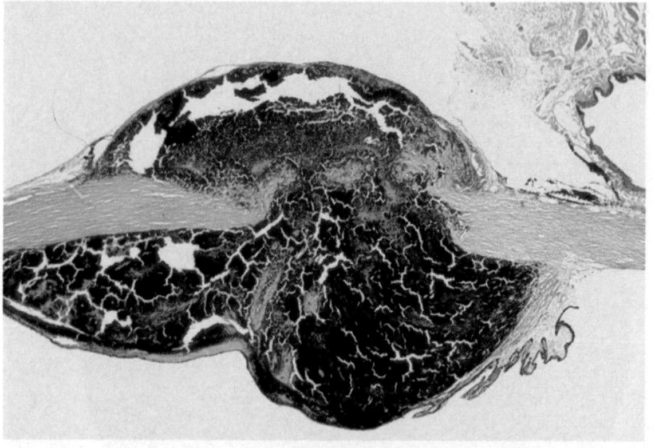

Figure 2-31

NECROTIC MELANOMA WITH EXTRASCLERAL INVASION

The episcleral nodule is close to the conjunctival lymphatic vessels on the right.

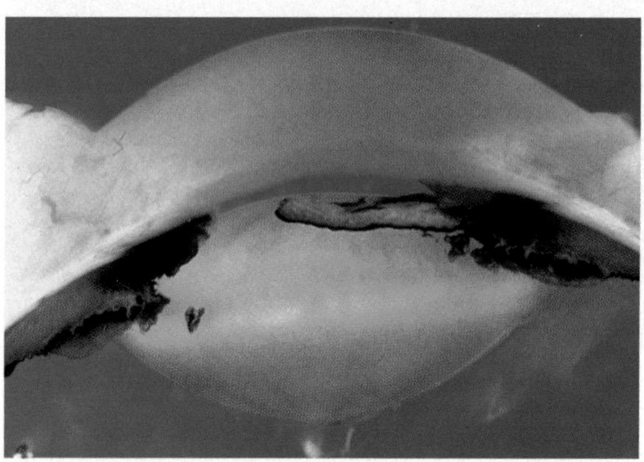

Figure 2-32

DIFFUSE IRIS AND CILIARY BODY MELANOMA

The pigmented tumor of the ciliary body extended more than 270° degrees around the anterior chamber angle.

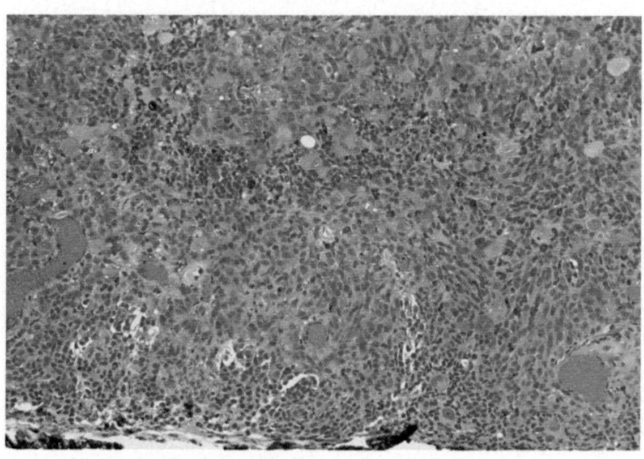

Figure 2-33

CILIARY BODY MELANOMA

Histopathologic examination of the lesion seen in figure 2-32 shows a tumor composed of epithelioid cells and scattered spindle-shaped melanoma cells.

in adults. This tumor predominately occurs in the blue-eyed, blond population of northern European ancestry; approximately 1 percent of malignant melanomas occur in African-Americans (83). The yearly incidence in whites is 6 to 8 cases/million population/year (84,85), an incidence 8.5 times greater than in African-Americans. Most studies find a higher incidence of uveal melanoma in men than women. Sun exposure is believed to be an independent risk factor for choroidal and ciliary body melanoma in Australia (86).

Congenital melanosis oculi and oculodermal melanocytosis (nevus of Ota) as well as nevi predispose to the development of uveal malignant melanoma (figs. 2-34, 2-35). Although congenital ocular melanosis is more commonly observed in pigmented races, including blacks and Asians, melanoma develops mainly in the hyperpigmented eye of whites with ocular melanocytosis. It has been estimated that 1 out

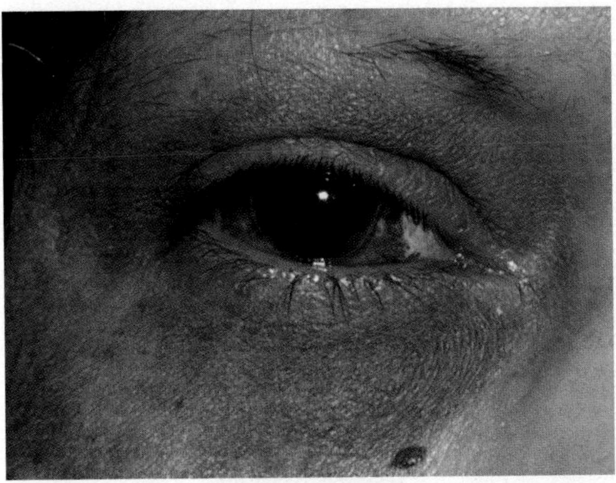

Figure 2-34

NEVUS OF OTA

Congenital hyperpigmentation of the periocular skin and eye follows the distribution of the ophthalmic branch of the trigeminal nerve.

of 400 patients with the nevus of Ota (oculodermal melanocytosis) followed for life develop a uveal melanoma (87). Because nevi are common and malignant melanomas of the uvea are rare, the calculated rate of malignant transformation of uveal nevi is estimated to be less than 1 in 15,000 nevi per year.

Most cases of uveal melanoma are sporadic. Some familiar cases have been reported in patients with the Li-Fraumeni syndrome in which mutation of the suppressor gene *p53* is observed (88). Syndromes that have been reported to be associated with uveal malignant melanoma include dysplastic nevus syndrome (B-K mole syndrome) and neurofibromatosis type 1 (89).

Clinical Features. The average age of patients at the time of diagnosis is 55 years; uveal malignant melanoma is rare in children and adolescents (90–92). In a study at the Armed Forces Institute of Pathology (AFIP) (90), 1.6 percent of uveal melanomas were seen in patients under 20 years of age. Malignant melanoma is almost always a unilateral tumor. The patients may be either asymptomatic and the tumor discovered in a routine ophthalmologic examination, or symptomatic with visual loss. Subjective findings include loss of vision, flashes, floaters, or visual field loss. Most cases of uveal melanoma are correctly diagnosed on the basis of indirect ophthalmoscopy alone. Ancillary studies include

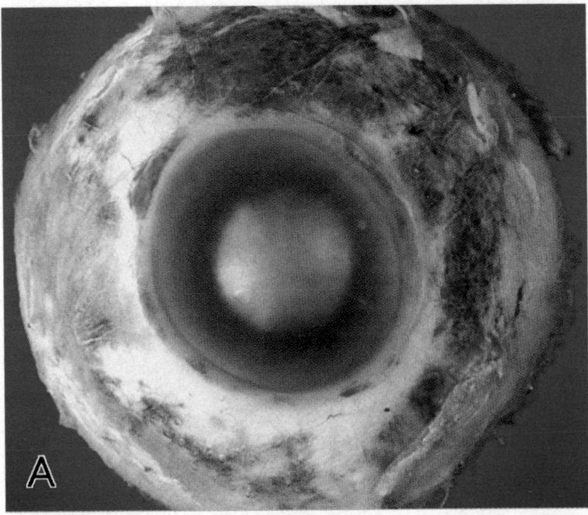

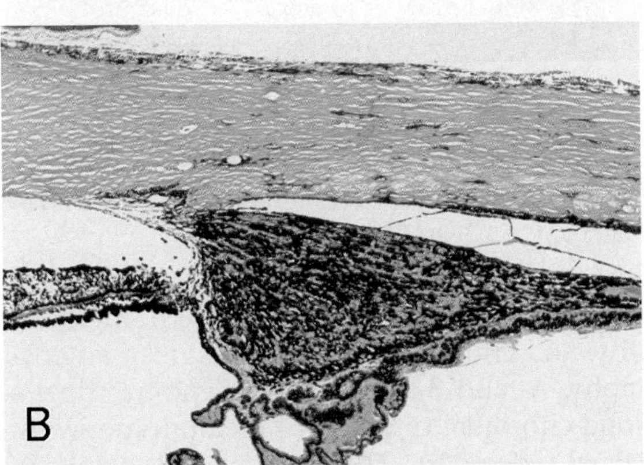

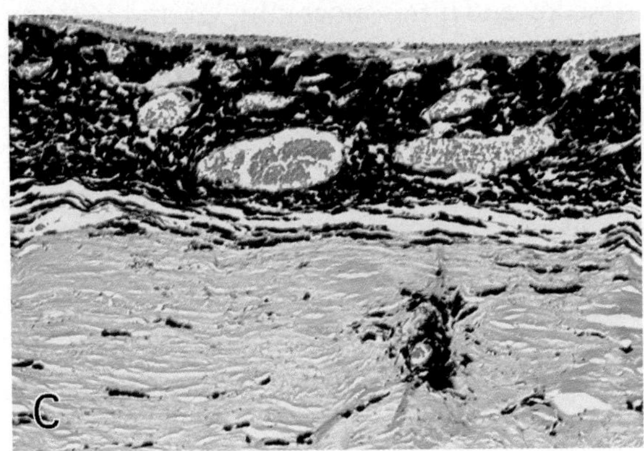

Figure 2-35

MELANOSIS OCULI

A: Congenital anterior episcleral pigmentation in a patient with a nevus of Ota (oculodermal melanocytosis).

B: Diffuse melanocytosis of ciliary body and iris.

C: Choroidal melanocytosis with intrascleral pigmentation.

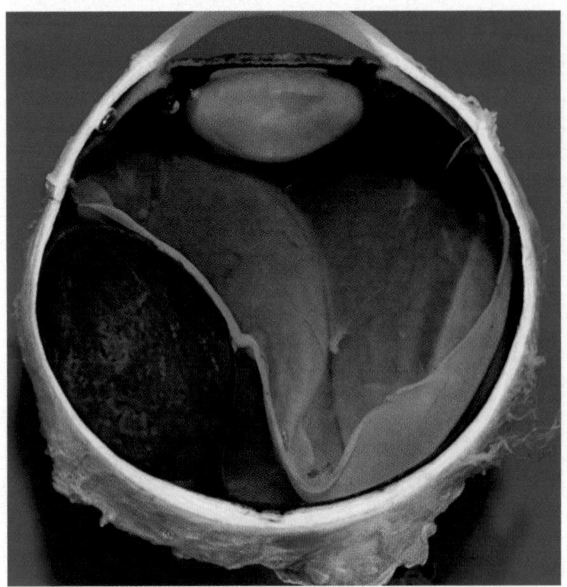

Figure 2-36

CHOROIDAL MELANOMA

Bullous detachment of the retina due to a heavily pigmented choroidal tumor.

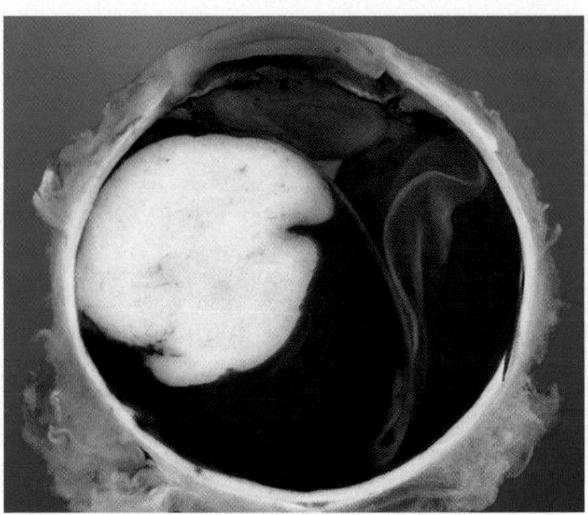

Figure 2-37

CHOROIDAL MELANOMA

Large choroidal melanoma with an amelanotic nodule within a heavily pigmented tumor.

ultrasonography, retinal fluorescein angiography, and choroidal indocyanine green angiography. A- and B-scan ultrasonography show a solid choroidal tumor with medium to low internal reflectivity. The diameter and height of the tumor are determined by indirect ophthalmoscopy and ultrasonography. CT and MRI are useful for detecting extrascleral extension. The accuracy of diagnosis in the Collaborative Ocular Melanoma Study (93) with histopathologic confirmation of the diagnosis was 99.7 percent.

Gross Findings. Choroidal melanomas are usually localized; multifocal lesions are rare. Focal malignant melanomas may adopt a variety of configurations regarding size, shape, pigmentation, and secondary ocular changes (figs. 2-36, 2-37). The size of the tumor is determined by the larger of the two perpendicular diameters at its base and the height of the mass.

Malignant melanomas of the choroid and ciliary body have been classically divided into three groups: small, measuring less than 10 x 10 x 3 mm; medium, between 10 x 10 x 3 mm and 15 x 15 x 5 mm; and large, greater than 15 x 15 x 5 mm. Diffuse malignant melanomas of the uvea extend onto more than 25 percent of the ocular fundus or a quadrant, and the maximum height usually is less than 7 mm (94). Fifty percent of uveal melanomas with a diffuse infiltrating growth pattern extend beyond the sclera at the time of enucleation (fig. 2-38). Tumors restricted to the choroid have a discoid or oval shape. Progressive growth of the mass results in extension through the overlying Bruch membrane into the subretinal space, resulting in a "collar button" or mushroom-shaped configuration (fig. 2-39). There may be infiltration by the tumor, cystoid changes, or foci of hemorrhage in the overlying retina (fig. 2-40). Total retinal detachment may be observed, especially in large tumors (fig. 2-41). Extrascleral extension occurs along the emissaries of the vortex veins, ciliary arteries, and nerves (fig. 2-42). Sections of the vortex veins at the episcleral level may be invaded by malignant melanoma cells (fig. 2-43). Rupture of the sclera as a result of direct invasion is rare. Invasion of the optic nerve is observed in less than 10 percent of enucleated eyes, and is usually associated with large tumor size, peripapillary location, and increased intraocular pressure (93).

Microscopic Findings. The combined cytologic and histopathologic classification proposed originally by Callender in 1931 (95) demonstrated prognostic significance and was the basis for subsequent modifications (96). Uveal malignant melanomas are basically composed of two main

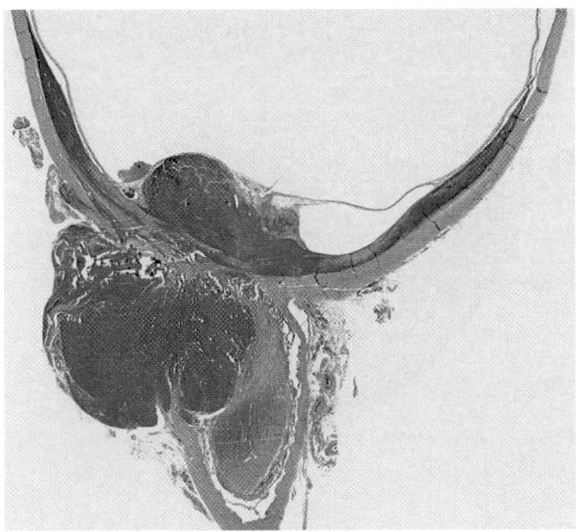

Figure 2-38

CHOROIDAL MELANOMA

Diffuse choroidal melanoma with posterior extraocular extension and optic nerve invasion.

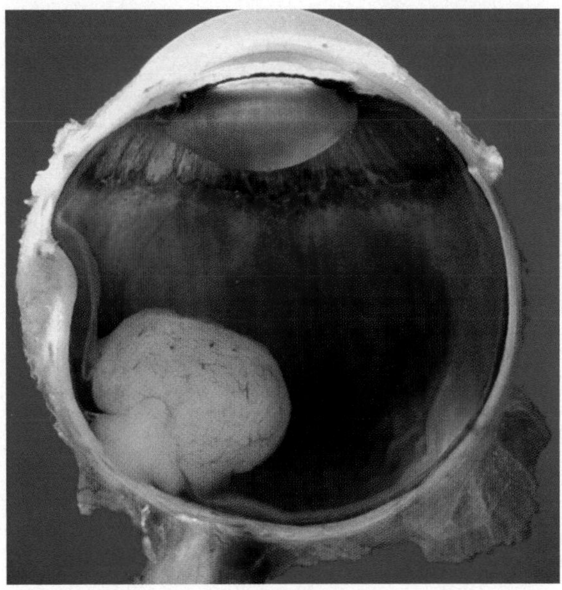

Figure 2-39

CHOROIDAL MELANOMA

Amelanotic, mushroom-shaped choroidal tumor.

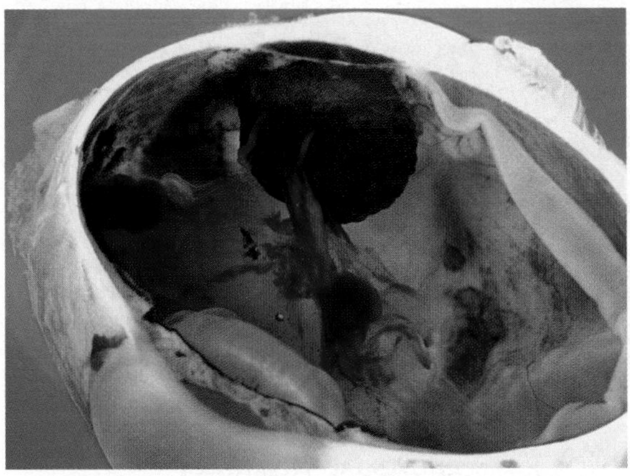

Figure 2-40

CHOROIDAL MELANOMA

Heavily pigmented, mushroom-shaped choroidal tumor has invaded the retina and caused secondary vitreous hemorrhage.

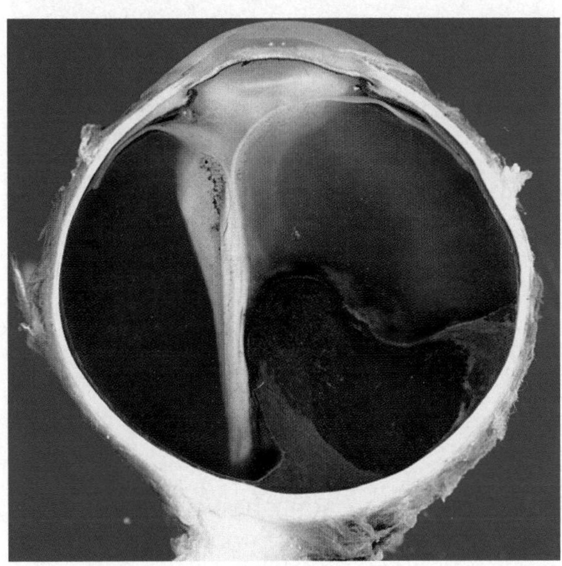

Figure 2-41

CHOROIDAL MELANOMA

Moderately pigmented, mushroom-shaped choroidal melanoma has caused total retinal detachment. A focal pigmented episcleral nodule is adjacent to the optic nerve.

cell types: spindle and epithelioid. Spindle cells have an oval, elongated nucleus and indistinct cytoplasmic border. Callender identified two types of spindle cells based on the nuclear characteristics. Spindle A cells have a slender nucleus with a small basophilic nucleolus and often have a longitudinal fold in the nucleus which is caused by invagination of the nuclear membrane. Spindle B cells have plumper nuclei, coarser chromatin, and a more prominent basophilic or eosinophilic nucleolus (fig. 2-44).

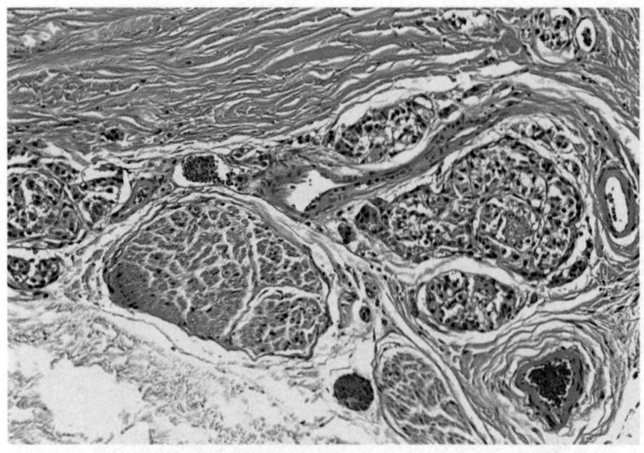

Figure 2-42

CHOROIDAL MELANOMA

Perineural and intraneural invasion of ciliary nerves at the episcleral level.

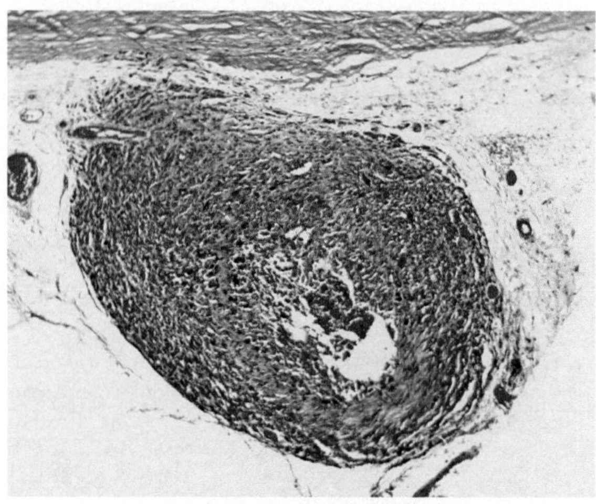

Figure 2-43

CHOROIDAL MELANOMA

Invasion of the walls and lumen of an episcleral vortex vein (trichrome stain).

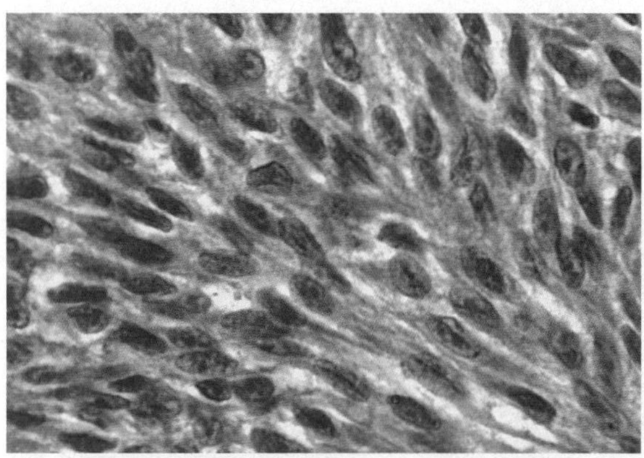

Figure 2-44

CHOROIDAL MELANOMA

Spindle cell melanoma is composed of spindle A and spindle B cells.

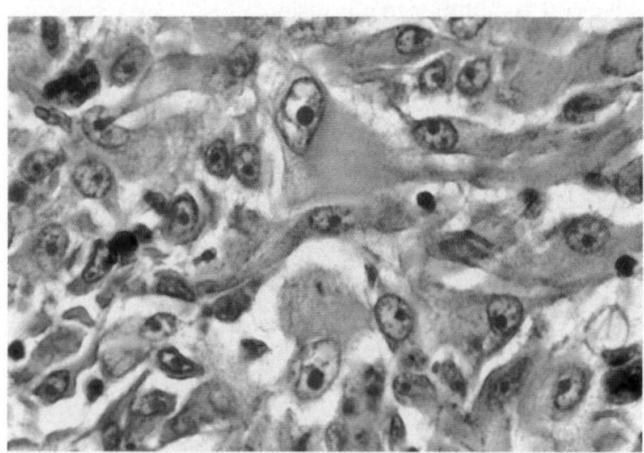

Figure 2-45

CHOROIDAL MELANOMA

The tumor is composed predominantly of large, pleomorphic, poorly cohesive epithelioid cells with prominent reddish purple nucleoli.

Epithelioid cells are noncohesive, larger, polygonal cells that have an abundant, glassy cytoplasm with a distinct cell border (fig. 2-45). The nucleus of the epithelioid cell is larger than that of the spindle cell and is round with marginated coarse chromatin. A large eosinophilic nucleolus is usually present within the clear center of the nucleus.

The Collaborative Ocular Melanoma Study Group (97) defined an intermediate cell that has features of both spindle B and epithelioid cells. Other cell types include smaller epithelioid cells with a distinct basophilic nucleolus and multinucleated and pleomorphic epithelioid cells. Some tumors may show balloon cell degeneration, characterized by abundant cytoplasm containing multiple vacuoles that stain for lipids (fig. 2-46) (98). Recently, a clear cell variant that contains glycogen has been described (99). The degree of pigmentation is highly variable and is not related to cell type. Mitotic activity usually is lower in tumors composed of spindle cells than those with epithelioid type cells. Mitotic rates are determined by counting the number

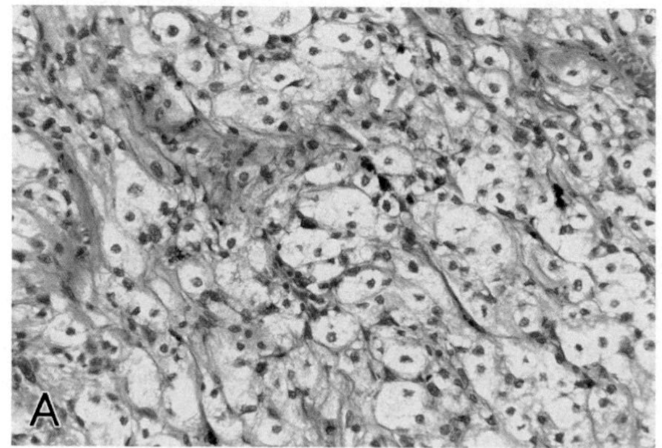

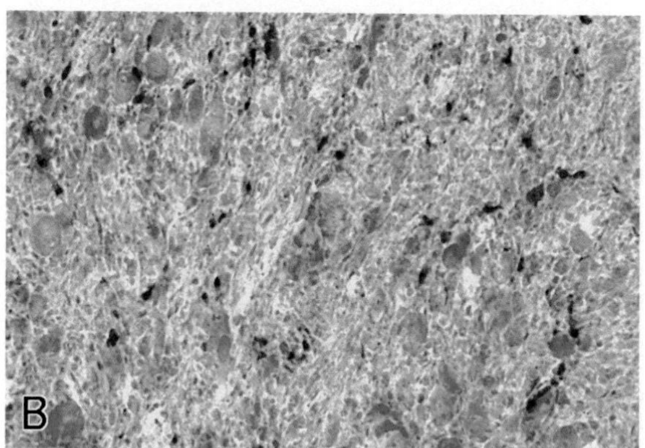

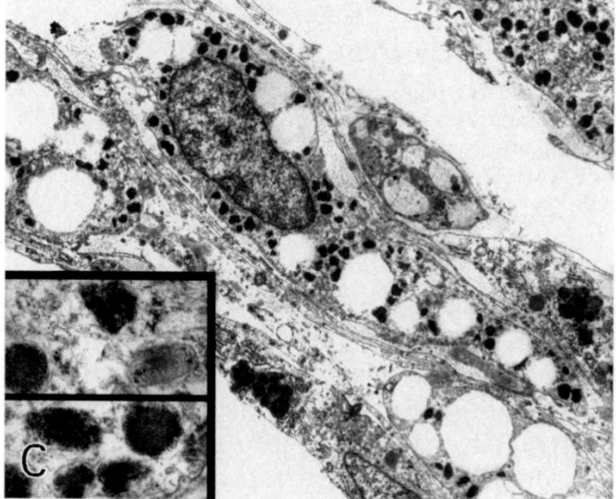

Figure 2-46

CHOROIDAL MELANOMA WITH BALLOON MELANOMA CELLS

A: Most cells have clear multivacuolated cytoplasm.

B: Frozen section stained with oil red-O shows the presence of lipid within the cytoplasm of the melanoma cells.

C: Transmission electron microscopy shows spindle-shaped cells containing melanosomes and round vacuoles (lipid). Inset: Melanosomes at different stages of maturation.

of mitotic figures per 40 high-power fields (40X objective using an 10X eyepiece).

The original Callender classification included six cell types: spindle A, spindle B, fascicular, mixed, epithelioid, and necrotic (95). The last group was composed of tumors too necrotic to classify (fig. 2-47). Tumors with a fascicular pattern are either composed of spindle B cells with nuclei arranged in columns perpendicular to a central vessel or spindle cells arranged in bundles with palisading of the nuclei. More recently, McLean and coworkers (96) made a distinction between nevus and melanoma and proposed a simplified classification. Lesions composed of spindle A cells that have a low nuclear to cytoplasmic ratio and finer, less hyperchromatic chromatin with no mitotic activity are considered benign nevi.

Currently, malignant melanomas of the uvea are divided into three cell types: 1) spindle cell (usually composed of an admixture of spindle A and spindle B cells); 2) epithelioid cell; and 3) mixed cell type (96). There is no general consensus among ophthalmic pathologists regarding the number of spindle and epithelioid cells required for the diagnosis of mixed cell type melanoma. In general, tumors with a few epithelioid cells (3 to 5 percent) are classified as mixed.

Most melanomas are well-vascularized tumors. Folberg et al. (100) found a combination of distinctive vascular patterns as demonstrated in PAS-stained slides without hematoxylin staining: 1) normal choroidal vessels, 2) silent with no tumor vessels, 3) straight vessels, 4) parallel pattern, 5) parallel with cross-linking, 6) arcs or incomplete loops, 7) arcs with branching, 8) complete loops around a lobule of tumor, and 9) networks composed of three or more back-to-back closed loops. The presence of a parallel with cross-linking pattern, arcs, and networks is associated with the presence of epithelioid cells (101,102).

Lymphocytic infiltration in malignant melanoma of the uvea is not observed as frequently

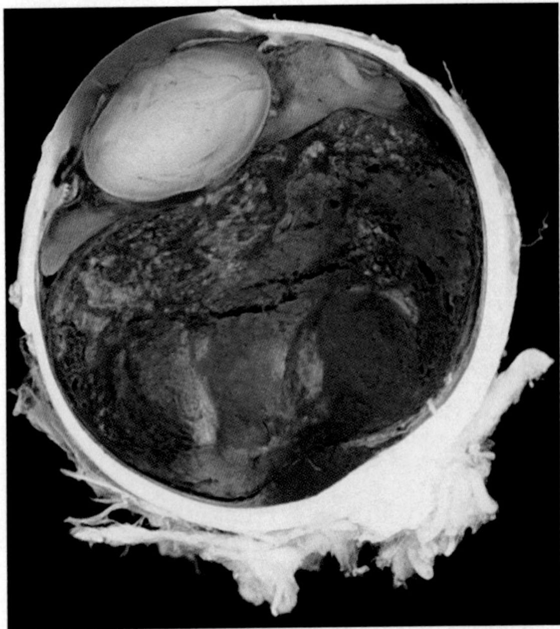

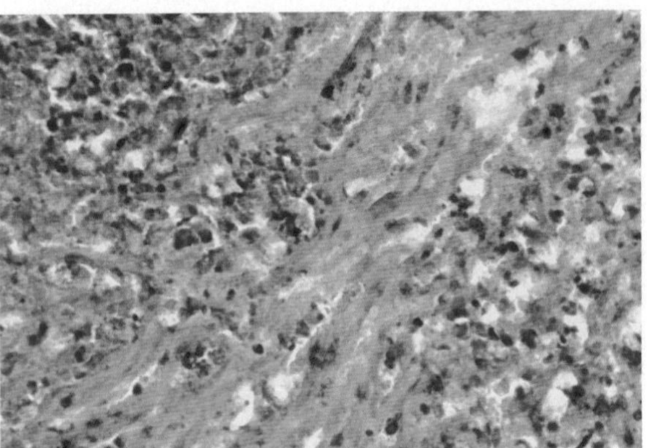

Figure 2-47

CHOROIDAL MELANOMA

Left: A large pigmented tumor fills the entire vitreous cavity. Cataract and anterior displacement of the iris diaphragm are seen.

Above: The pigmented tumor was totally necrotic. The cell type cannot be assessed.

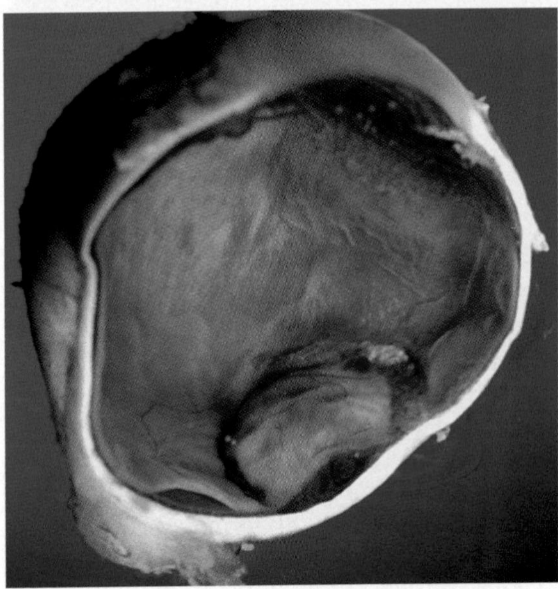

Figure 2-48

CHOROIDAL MELANOMA

This eye with malignant melanoma was enucleated after failure of plaque radiotherapy.

as in cutaneous melanoma. Two types of infiltration may be observed: patchy and diffuse lymphocytic infiltration (103). Immunohistochemically, the cells are represented by either T-cell lymphocytes or B-cell lymphocytes and plasma cells.

Microscopic Findings After Therapy. Most small, medium-sized, and a few large melanomas of the uvea are enucleated because of failure or complications following different methods of treatment, including photocoagulation, transpupillary thermotherapy, local plaque radiotherapy, proton beam therapy, and local excision. The tumor and normal ocular tissues are affected by these treatments. Besides necrosis of tumor cells, focal hemorrhages, and pigment dispersion with accumulation of pigment-laden macrophages, mitotic activity usually is greatly reduced or absent (figs. 2-48–2-50). Tumor blood vessels may show thrombosis, vascular occlusion, and fibrinous exudates. Secondary changes affecting other ocular tissues include vascular damage of the retina with lipoidal exudate, optic nerve damage, cataract, and neovascular glaucoma.

Ultrastructural Findings. The main cell types of uveal malignant melanoma are distinctive ultrastructurally (104). The spindle cells have numerous cytoplasmic filaments. Epithelioid cells have a well-developed and abundant rough-surfaced endoplasmic reticulum, free ribosomes, and numerous mitochondria.

Immunohistochemical Findings. Uveal melanoma cells are positive for HMB45, Melan-A/MART-1, S-100 protein, and vimentin (105). Melan-A and S-100 protein are 100 percent sensitive in melanocytic tumors of the iris, while

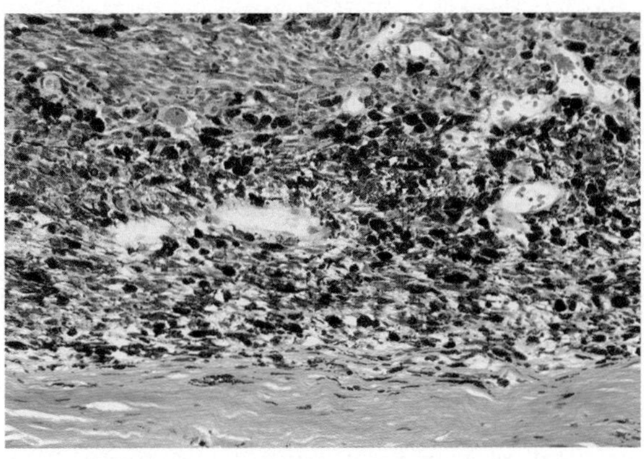

Figure 2-49

CHOROIDAL MELANOMA AFTER TREATMENT

Viable tumor cells remain and melanophages most likely represent status-postcellular necrosis.

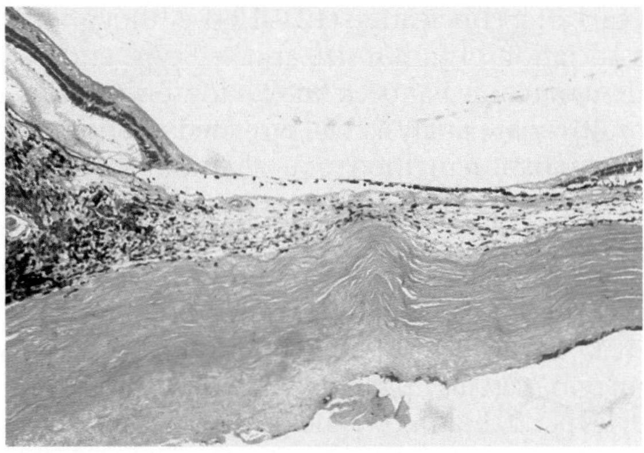

Figure 2-50

CHOROIDAL MELANOMA

Choroidal and retinal atrophy are observed near the anterior border of the tumor, and there are secondary changes of the scleral collagen after radiation therapy (I^{125} plaque).

Melan-A and HMB45 are 100 percent sensitive in epithelioid cell tumors, and 69 to 79 percent in spindle cell and mixed cell types (106). Focal reactivity for cytokeratin may be found in epithelioid cell tumors (107).

Special Studies. Several evaluation methods have been tested in search of an objective cell measurement that correlates with behavior and prognosis (108). Gamel and coworkers (109) showed that computerized mathematical models related to the size and area of the nucleolus may be used. These methods, however, are rarely used in the ophthalmic laboratory. Although the counting of nucleolar organizer regions, as disclosed with a silver stain, may distinguish between nevus and melanoma, the average counts are variable among the different cell types (97). DNA analysis has demonstrated an increased degree of aneuploidy in more highly malignant tumors (110,111). Spindle and mixed cell type tumors show prevalent diploid and near diploid/aneuploid patterns. DNA variables do not correlate with established prognosticators, nor do they reach significance by univariate and multivariate analyses (111,112). The presence of proliferating cell nuclear antigen (PCNA) and Ki-67 are associated with large tumor size and the prevalence of epithelioid cells (113). In the multivariate analysis, Ki-67 remains an important prognostic factor. Uveal melanomas may express p53 mutated proteins. Increased p53 expression is observed in epithelioid melanomas and in tumors growing in women (114,115). C-myc and bcl-2 are expressed in uveal melanoma cells (116). Improved survival is seen in patients with c-myc–positive tumors (117).

Cytologic Findings. Cytologic diagnostic evaluation of a suspected uveal malignant melanoma is undertaken when the nature of the mass cannot be established with noninvasive techniques (118, 119). The samples are preferably obtained by FNA biopsy through a transvitreal route. The identification of pigmented spindle and epithelioid melanoma cells in cytologic specimens is rather straightforward. In one study, diagnostic accuracy was 98 percent in tumors that were greater than 2 mm in thickness (120).

Differential Diagnosis. The clinical diagnostic error rate of ophthalmologists is less than 4 percent (93). Diagnostic error from pathologists is rare. Deeply pigmented melanoma cells may be difficult to differentiate from melanocytoma and tumors of the retinal pigment epithelium. Amelanotic and lightly pigmented lesions composed of spindle-shaped cells should be differentiated from rare spindle cell tumors arising within the uvea. Likewise, epithelioid amelanotic cells may be confused with metastatic carcinomas. It may be difficult to identify a totally necrotic uveal melanoma.

Treatment and Prognosis. Approximately 50 percent of patients diagnosed with a uveal melanoma develop metastases within 10 to 15 years after enucleation (121–124). Although the association of tumor size and cell type and patient outcome has been known for several years, multivariate analysis has provided a more precise statistical method for evaluation of risk factors associated with prognosis (125). The variables that are best predictive of poor patient survival are epithelioid cell type, largest tumor dimension, extrascleral extension, and mitotic activity, followed by location of the anterior tumor margin, vascular patterns, presence of lymphocytes per 20 high-power fields, greater tumor pigmentation, and foci of necrosis. Clinical risk factors for survival are older age and sex of the patients (prognosis is worse in males). Patients with massive extraocular orbital invasion at the time of diagnosis have a poor survival rate.

Melanomas of the uvea disseminate mainly through hematogenous routes. The most common site of hematogenous metastasis is the liver (93 percent) (124). It is involved initially in 85 percent and is the only site in 55 percent of patients with metastatic disease (124). Fifty percent of patients with liver metastasis also develop extrahepatic metastases, most often in the lung, bone, skin, and central nervous system (124). Spread to the regional lymph nodes is rarely observed and occurs in tumors with chamber angle or subconjunctival invasion that gain access to conjunctival or eyelid lymphatic channels. Long-term studies of survival after enucleation of uveal melanoma performed in Finland and Denmark found 5-year, 10-year, and 15-year actuarial survival rates of 65 percent, 52 percent, and 46 percent, respectively (121,122).

Zimmerman and coworkers (126) challenged the efficacy of enucleation and postulated that enucleation may cause or stimulate the development of metastasis. Although enucleation is the primary treatment for most large uveal melanomas and for tumors that have produced severe secondary glaucoma, a variety of alternative treatments have been introduced in an effort to preserve the eye and save vision (127). These include use of radioactive plaques such as cobalt 60 (Co^{60}), iodine 125 (I^{125}), ruthenium 106 (Ru^{106}), palladium 103 (Pd^{103}); charged particles (protons and helium ions); gamma knife; transpupillary thermotherapy; and local resection (128–135). Regarding short-term survival, the results after radiation therapy, corrected for tumor size, are comparable to enucleation (136). The rate of enucleation after brachytherapy is approximately 16 percent in the first 5 years (137). Orbital exenteration is only justified for very advanced uveal melanomas with massive extraocular extension.

The systemic examination of patients with uveal melanoma should include a complete physical examination with attention to the skin and subcutaneous tissues, a routine chest X ray, and determination of serum liver function studies. Serum gamma-glutamyl transpeptidase (GGT) appears to be the most sensitive blood test (138). There is no effective chemotherapy or immunotherapy for primary management of metastatic uveal melanoma, and death usually follows within a few months after diagnosis of the metastatic lesion (139,140).

Diffuse Uveal Melanocytic Proliferation

Bilateral diffuse uveal melanocytic proliferation (BDUMP) is a rare paraneoplastic syndrome (141). The simultaneous bilateral diffuse involvement of the uveal tract consists of a striking predominance of benign-appearing melanocytic cells, no evidence of metastasis from melanocytic tumors, and the presence of an associated visceral neoplasm (fig. 2-51) (142,143). BDUMP has been reported to be associated with primary carcinomas of the lung, ovary, colon, gallbladder, esophagus, pancreas, uterus, and cervix. Ophthalmoscopically, there are either multiple, pigmented, flat or slightly elevated lesions scattered throughout the fundus or flat lesions with a reticular pattern. Microscopically, the uveal tract of both eyes is diffusely infiltrated by predominantly nevoid or spindle-shaped melanocytic cells (fig. 2-51B). Although a few epithelioid cells may be present, mitotic figures are rare. Proliferative cell activity usually is present in less than 1 percent of the cells stained with Ki-67. Areas of necrosis within the tumors, invasion of emissary scleral canals, and extraocular extension are commonly observed.

These lesions, although possessing atypical cytologic and architectural features, are considered of low malignant potential. Enucleation usually is not indicated because of poor prognosis due to the associated visceral neoplasm.

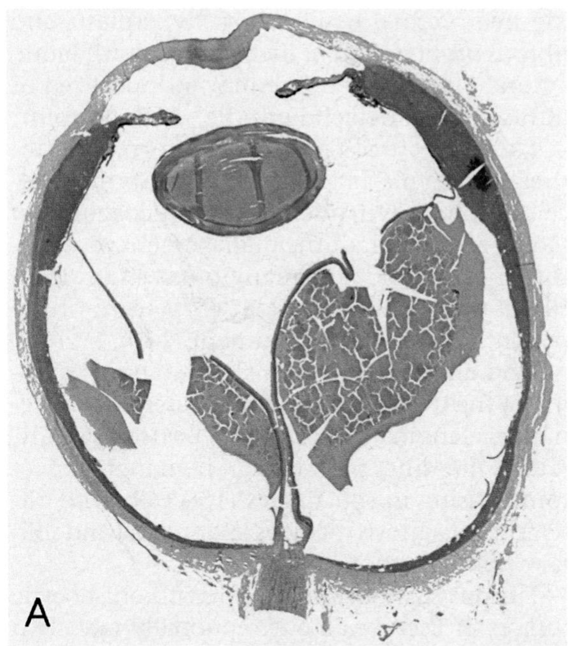

Figure 2-51

DIFFUSE UVEAL MELANOCYTIC PROLIFERATION

A: Diffuse thickening of the ciliary body and choroid, and exudative retinal detachment are seen.

B: Intrachoroidal proliferation of spindle-shaped melanocytes, with mildly hyperchromatic nuclei and a few cells with vesicular nuclei and small basophilic nucleoli.

C: Adenocarcinoma arising from the mucosa of the colon in the same patient.

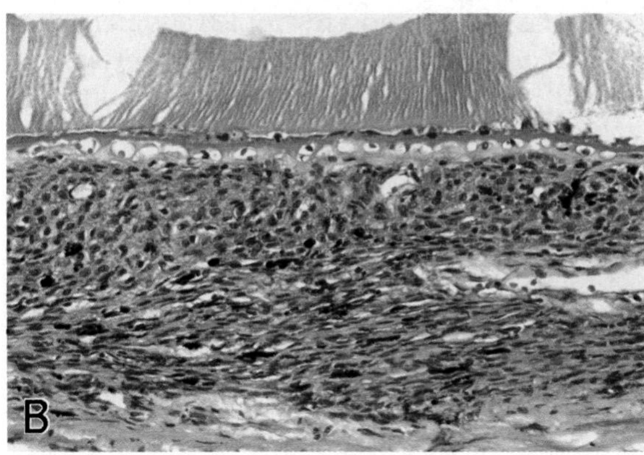

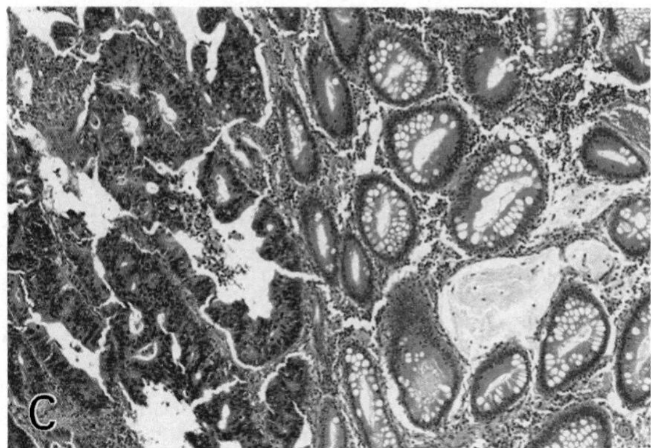

NONMELANOCYTIC TUMORS OF THE UVEA

Mesenchymal Tumors

Hemangioma. The few cases of hemangioma of the iris in the AFIP files were reviewed by Ferry, who questioned their validity (144,145). Most presumed vascular lesions were reclassified as examples of juvenile xanthogranuloma, amelanotic melanoma, and other tumors of the iris. Vascular tumors of the ciliary body appear to be exceedingly rare. A mixed *capillary-cavernous hemangioma* of the ciliary body was found in an iridocyclectomy specimen from a presumed ciliary body melanoma (146). Combined involvement of the ciliary body, iris, and choroid have been reported in cases of *congenital hemangiomatosis* (147,148).

Choroidal hemangiomas are vascular hamartomas of two types: 1) diffuse choroidal hemangiomatosis with diffuse involvement of the choroid in association with the Sturge-Weber syndrome and 2) localized (circumscribed) choroidal hemangiomas not associated with other systemic abnormalities (fig. 2-52). Witschel and Font (149), in a study of 71 cases, described several distinctive features of each type. The diffuse type is observed mainly in younger male patients. Diffuse lesions have a typical "tomato ketchup-like" fundus. Localized hemangiomas are orange-red and surrounded by a rim of displaced choroidal pigmentation (150).

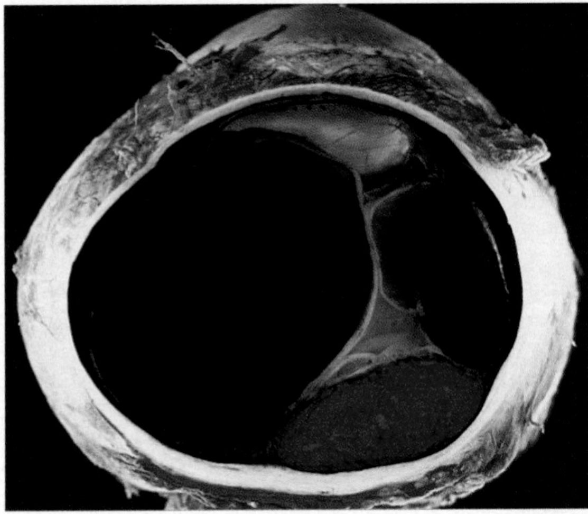

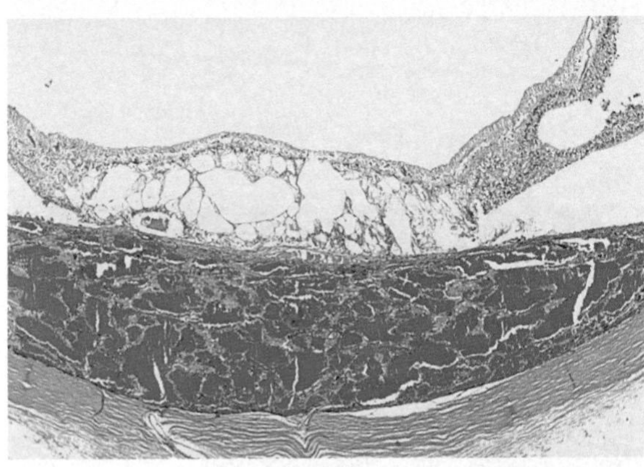

Figure 2-52

CHOROIDAL HEMANGIOMA

Top: The circumscribed choroidal vascular tumor is associated with retinal detachment.

Bottom: The choroidal hemangioma is composed of large cavernous vascular spaces. The overlying retina shows degenerative cystic changes.

Ultrasonography demonstrates typical progressive attenuation of choroidal echoes (151). Indocyanine green angiography can help determine the blood supply to these tumors (152). Histopathologic studies show that all localized lesions have clearly demarcated borders, with compressed choroidal lamellae and melanocytes (fig. 2-52, bottom) (149). In the diffuse lesions, engorgement of preexisting vessels is intermixed with the tumor blood vessels, a feature of diffuse hemangiomatosis of the choroid. Because of the predominant size of the vessels, Witschel and Font (149) classified these hemangiomas as capillary, cavernous, and mixed. The overlying neuroretinal tissues show hyperplasia and fibrous proliferation of the pigment epithelium, cystoid changes of the retina, and localized or diffuse retinal detachment (fig. 2-52, bottom).

Laser photocoagulation, external radiotherapy, plaque brachytherapy, and, more recently, photodynamic laser photocoagulation have been useful for the management of symptomatic choroidal hemangiomas (153–156). Visual acuity deteriorates in 60 percent of the patients despite local treatment (150).

Hemangiopericytoma. Hemangiopericytoma of the uvea is rare and may resemble malignant melanoma clinically (157). Histologically, it does not differ from benign hemangiopericytoma arising in soft tissues (158,159). The differential diagnosis includes leiomyoma and solitary fibrous tumor.

Fibrous Histiocytoma. Benign fibrohistiocytic tumors of the uvea are exceptionally rare. Two cases in young women have been reported (160, 161). One of the tumors resembled a solitary choroidal hemangioma or an amelanotic melanoma clinically. The patient developed total retinal detachment, and the eye was enucleated (160). The other patient underwent a FNAB; a definitive cytologic distinction from amelanotic malignant melanoma could not be made, and the eye was enucleated (161). Histopathologic examination of the enucleated eye showed a solid tumor composed of interlacing fascicles of spindle-shaped cells. Immunohistochemistry and electron microscopy revealed features of fibroblastic cells. No further postoperative recurrences or dissemination were observed.

Leiomyoma. Leiomyomas of the uvea are rare. In a retrospective review of 24 presumable leiomyomas of the iris, Fosse et al. (162) reclassified all the lesions as melanocytic using immunohistochemistry. Li et al. (163) reported a benign "leiomyoepithelioma" of the iris pigment epithelium in a 4-year-old boy. The tumor exhibited characteristics of both pigment epithelium and smooth muscle. Ciliary body leiomyomas are more common in young females; 74 percent of the patients with leiomyoma are younger than 40 years of age (164–166).

The tumors are usually located in the inferior quadrants of the eye and exhibit slow clinical progression. Transillumination is an important diagnostic tool for the differentiation of

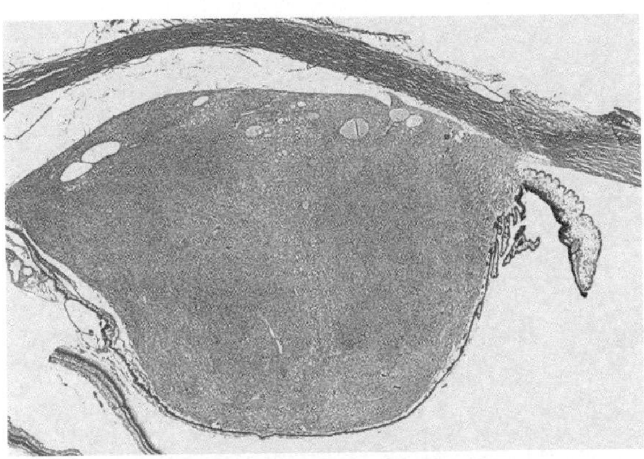

Figure 2-53

MESECTODERMAL LEIOMYOMA

Iridocyclectomy specimen contains a large, circumscribed, amelanotic tumor of the ciliary body.

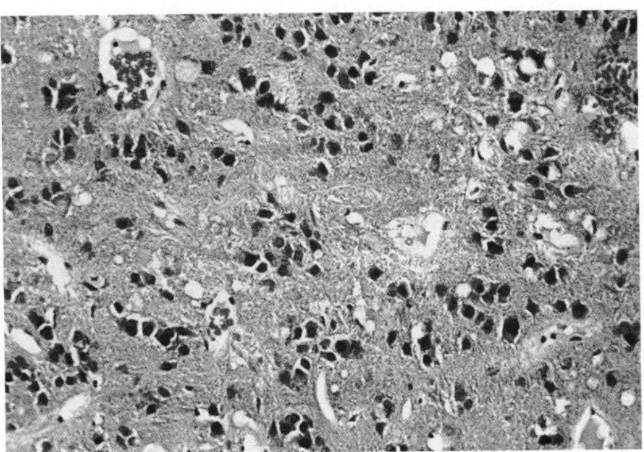

Figure 2-54

MESECTODERMAL LEIOMYOMA

The tumor displays a "neural" appearance, with clustering of tumors cells surrounded by a fibrillary background.

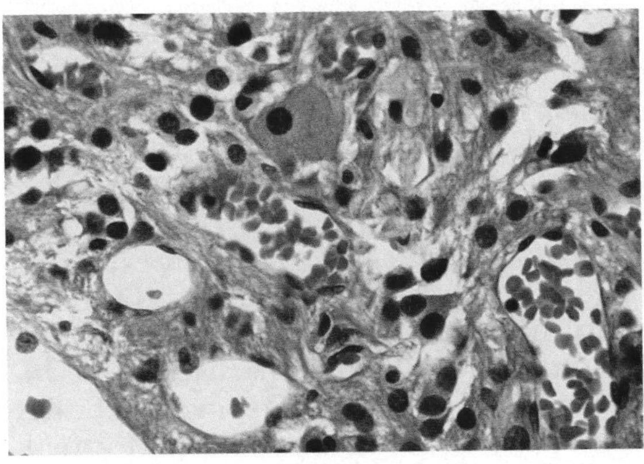

Figure 2-55

MESECTODERMAL LEIOMYOMA

Vascular spaces are surrounded by the fibrillary processes of tumor cells.

leiomyomas, which are nonpigmented tumors, from pigmented melanocytic tumors. Microscopically, the tumors are circumscribed and appear to grow from the outer muscular layers of the ciliary body into the supraciliary space. They are composed of interlacing fascicles of spindle-shaped cells with fine fibrillar cytoplasm and cigar-shaped nuclei. The diagnosis is based on the demonstration of smooth muscle actin or muscle-specific actin (167). The differential diagnosis includes amelanotic spindle cell melanoma, neurilemmoma, and neurofibroma (168,169).

Jakobiec et al. (170) described a leiomyoma found in an enucleated eye of a 57-year-old patient with a suspected uveal melanoma. The choroidal tumor was highly vascularized and composed of spindle-shaped cells with fibrillary cytoplasm. Electron microscopy demonstrated features of smooth muscle cells. The authors suggested that the tumor most likely had arisen from a perivascular smooth muscle cell.

Mesectodermal Leiomyoma. In 1976, Jakobiec et al. (171) described a benign ciliary body tumor composed of cells that exhibited slightly large, round to oval, pleomorphic nuclei with a fine fibrillary background, suggestive of a neuropil (figs. 2-53–2-55). Electron microscopy showed hybrid features of both neuroglial cells (in the perinuclear region) and smooth muscle cells in the tapering cell processes (fig. 2-56). Based on the neural crest origin of the smooth muscle of the ciliary body (head and neck mesectoderm), the authors suggested the name *mesectodermal leiomyoma* for this tumor. More recently, immunohistochemical studies have shown positive immunoreactivity for smooth muscle markers (desmin and muscle-specific actin) but negative staining for neural markers. Campbell et al. (172) showed the presence of skeinoid fibers, considered to be an ultrastructural marker of neurogenic spindle cell tumors, in mesectodermal leiomyoma. These findings clearly indicate that mesectodermal leiomyoma is unique in its histogenesis as well as in its morphology.

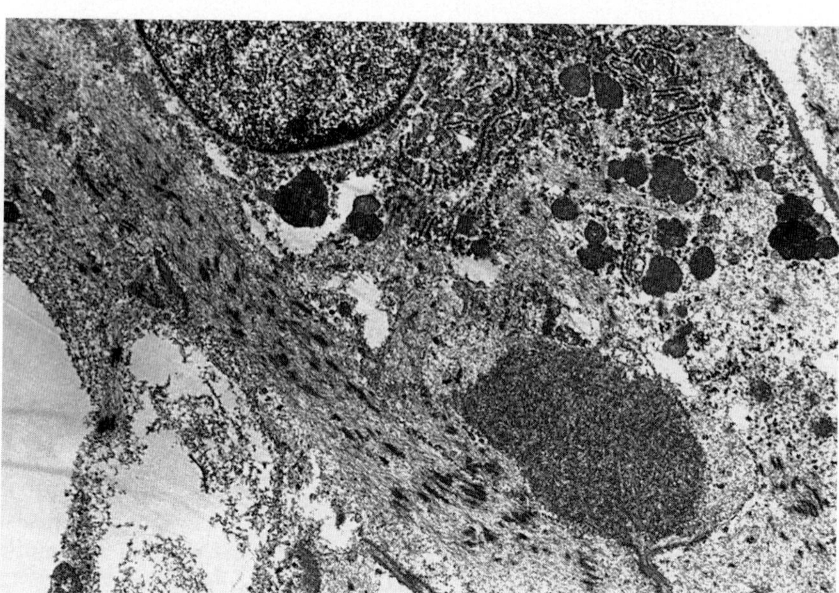

Figure 2-56

MESECTODERMAL LEIOMYOMA

The perikarion and cell processes of the tumor cells display thin cytoplasmic filaments with fusiform densities.

Other described variants of ciliary body leiomyoma include *vascular leiomyoma* and *mitochondria-rich epithelioid leiomyoma* (173). Local resection of the ciliary body mass is the preferred treatment.

Malignant Muscle Tumors. *Leiomyosarcoma* and *rhabdomyosarcoma* of the iris are extremely rare primary tumors. The diagnosis of malignancy in reported cases of leiomyosarcoma was based on the infiltrative character of the tumor; however, neither electron microscopy nor immunohistochemistry were performed. Rhabdomyosarcomas of the iris most likely arise from primitive, undifferentiated mesenchymal stromal cells. All three reported cases of rhabdomyosarcoma occurred in children (aged 4 and 5 years) (174–176). Two cases were treated initially with radiotherapy and local excision. The three eyes were ultimately enucleated, and on follow-up studies all three patients were alive and well 20 years, 5 years, and 14 months postoperatively.

Benign Peripheral Nerve Tumors

Neurofibroma. Diffuse neurofibromatous proliferations are observed in patients with neurofibromatosis type 1 (177–179). Microscopic examination of enucleated eyes show diffuse neurofibromatous thickening of the ciliary body and choroid consisting of neuronal elements, including Schwann cells, spindle-shaped cells, spindle-shaped melanocytes, ganglion cells, and occasional oval laminated neural structures ("ovoid bodies") resembling tactile end bodies. The chamber angle structure is either maldeveloped or compromised by the diffuse neurofibromatous proliferation. Other ocular findings include prominent corneal nerves, small melanocytic hamartomas of the iris (Lisch nodules), and anterior subcapsular cataracts.

Schwannoma. Uveal schwannomas (neurilemmomas) arising from the sheaths of the ciliary nerves are rare solitary tumors that may be confused clinically with amelanotic uveal malignant melanoma (180–183). Most reported cases have been associated with neurofibromatosis (184,185). Histopathologically, the intraocular tumors do not differ from schwannomas in other anatomic locations. Immunohistochemistry and electron microscopy confirm the Schwann cell origin of the tumor.

The differential diagnosis of a choroidal schwannoma includes amelanotic melanocytic tumors, leiomyoma, neurofibroma, and fibrous histiocytoma. Shields et al. (186) reported a unique choroidal tumor composed of fascicles and whorls of pigmented and nonpigmented plump spindle cells that showed light microscopic, immunohistochemical, and electron microscopic features of a melanotic schwannoma. The diagnosis is usually established histologically after enucleation of a suspected choroidal melanoma. Recurrence after primary iridocyclectomy has been reported (187).

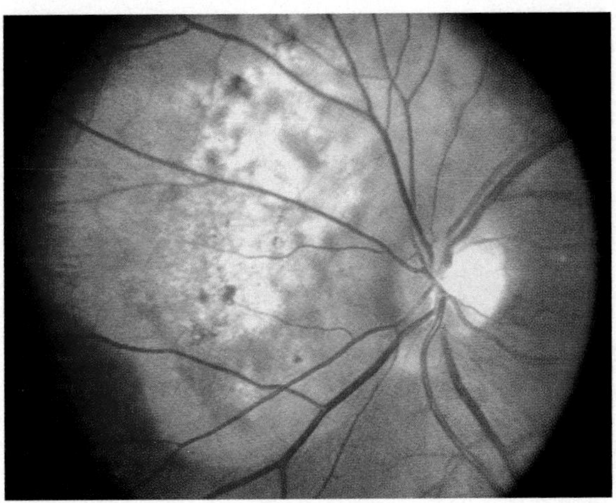

Figure 2-57

CHOROIDAL OSTEOMA

Orange-red juxtapapillary tumor in a young female.

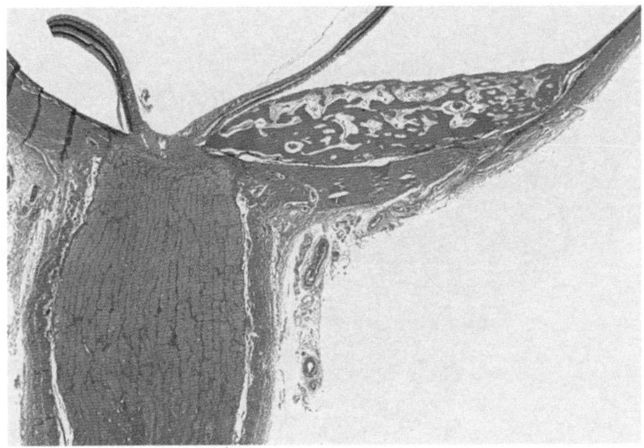

Figure 2-58

CHOROIDAL OSTEOMA

A juxtapapillary intrachoroidal mass is composed of mature bone.

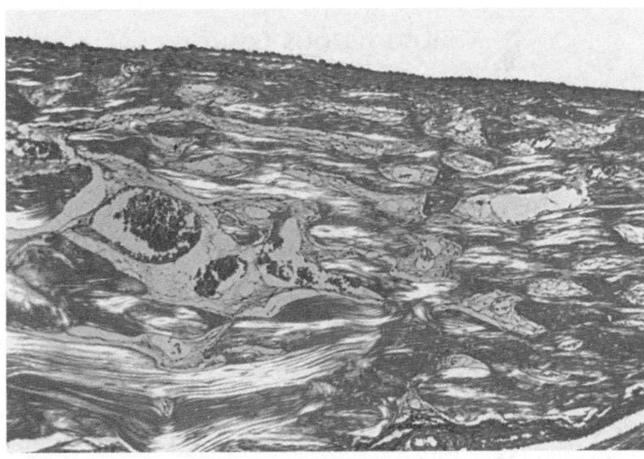

Figure 2-59

CHOROIDAL OSTEOMA

Bony trabeculae and ectatic blood vessels are seen, as well as birefringence of the lamellar bone.

Osteoma

Choroidal osteoma is a benign osseous choristoma, usually located in the peripapillary choroid and observed predominantly in young females (188,189). Since the first series studied by Gass and coworkers (188), several clinical presentations in children and elderly patients, bilateral and multifocal cases, familial cases occurring in siblings, and related ocular complications have been reported (190–193). Most patients are asymptomatic and display a typical, orange-red, juxtapapillary or peripapillary tumor with geographic, scalloped margins (fig. 2-57). Ultrasonography and CT are extremely useful for the clinical differentiation of a calcified osteoma from similar lesions.

Histopathologically, osteoma is composed of dense, bony trabeculae with large cavernous and capillary vascular spaces (figs. 2-58, 2-59). Osteoblasts, osteocytes, and occasional osteoclasts are observed. The overlying retinal pigment epithelium and retina may show degenerative changes. A choroidal osteoma should be differentiated from other types of intraocular calcification. Acquired intraocular bone formation is commonly seen in phthisical eyes, congenital anomalies, and choroidal hemangiomas, and following inflammation and trauma. Sclerochoroidal calcification is an ocular lesion characterized by typical, geographic, yellow-white fundus lesions that usually occur bilaterally in adults (194). The condition appears to represent calcium deposition in the sclera and choroid. The disease is either idiopathic or associated with Gitelman's or Bartter's syndrome in which deposition of calcium salts is seen in various tissues.

The current management for osteoma is periodic observation. Most patients with choroidal osteomas maintain good vision in at least one eye, but they have a high risk of developing choroidal neovascularization (195). Spontaneous resolution of the original tumor has been described (196).

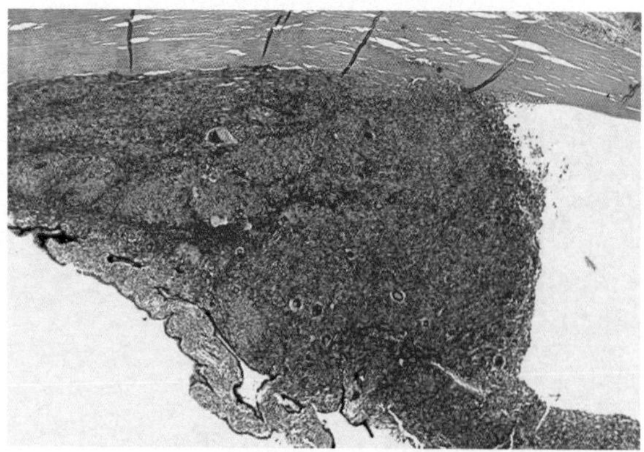

Figure 2-60

JUVENILE XANTHOGRANULOMA

The lymphohistiocytic infiltrate involves the ciliary body, iris, and anterior chamber angle. Numerous Touton giant cells are seen.

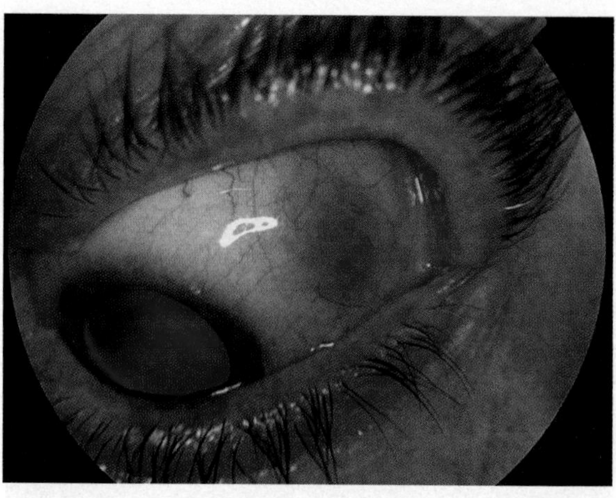

Figure 2-61

REACTIVE LYMPHOID HYPERPLASIA

The yellowish tan episcleral nodule is associated with retinal detachment and choroidal thickening.

Xanthomatous Lesions

Juvenile xanthogranuloma is a benign cutaneous disease of young children that is characterized by solitary or multiple, yellowish pink nodules of the skin, which may regress spontaneously (197). Hemorrhage into the anterior chamber (spontaneous hyphema) as a result of neovascularization of the iris may be the first clinical manifestation (198, 199). The anterior uveal involvement appears as a yellowish nodule or mass lesion with features suggestive of inflammatory disease. Similar findings are observed in adults (200). Other sites of ocular involvement include the eyelid, conjunctiva, cornea, orbit, and optic nerve (199,201).

Histologically, the involved iris and ciliary body are infiltrated by histiocytes intermixed with a variable inflammatory infiltrate composed of lymphocytes, plasma cells, eosinophils, and multinucleated giant cells (fig. 2-60). The characteristic feature is the presence of Touton giant cells. A few mitotic figures may be seen. Frozen sections stained with oil red-O show lipid droplets within the histiocytes and giant cells. Aspiration of aqueous humor from the anterior chamber or FNAB of the mass may disclose the typical, polymorphic histiocytic infiltrate and Touton giant cells (202).

Juvenile xanthogranuloma of the iris or ciliary body is usually managed with local or systemic administration of corticosteroids. Nonresponsive lesions are treated by excision or radiotherapy (203). Surgical removal is attended by a high rate of blinding complications.

Reactive Lymphoid Hyperplasia and Primary Non-Hodgkin's B-Cell Lymphoma of the Uvea

Definition and General Features. The term *reactive lymphoid hyperplasia of the uvea* was used originally to denote a particular form of unilateral lymphoid uveal infiltration composed of benign-appearing small lymphocytes, plasma cells, and lymphoid follicles with prominent germinal centers (204). In many affected eyes there was episcleral or orbital extension, the clinical course was indolent, and none of the patients died of systemic lymphoma (204). Various alternative terms have since been used for this lesion, such as *intraocular pseudotumor, massive lymphoid infiltrate,* and *uveal lymphoid neoplasia.* Immunohistochemical studies have revealed that many lesions are monoclonal, with restriction of either kappa or lambda immunoglobulin light chains. These techniques, however, cannot differentiate between tumors with benign or malignant behavior. Polymerase chain reaction amplification and immunoglobulin heavy chain gene rearrangement studies show both monoclonal and polyclonal cases. It appears that this condition encompasses a spectrum of lymphoid proliferations that vary from reactive lymphoid hyperplasia to low-grade primary B-cell lymphomas.

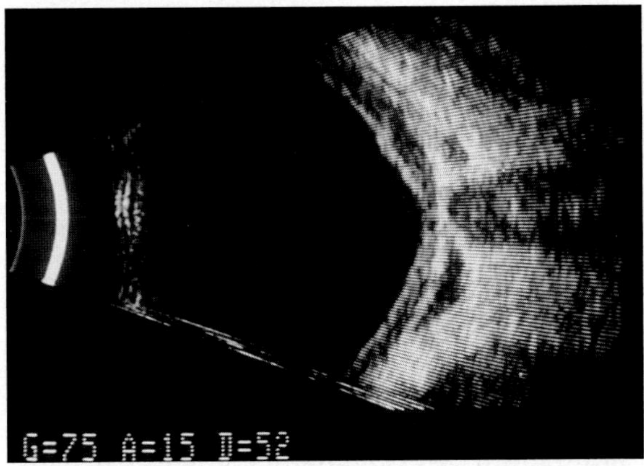

Figure 2-62

REACTIVE LYMPHOID HYPERPLASIA

Ultrasonographic study shows diffuse thickening of the choroid and a lucent episcleral nodule posteriorly.

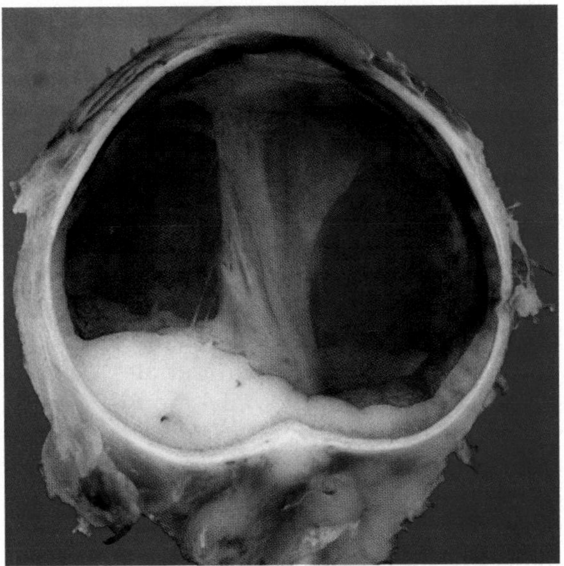

Figure 2-63

REACTIVE LYMPHOID HYPERPLASIA

Total retinal detachment and diffuse thickening of the choroid with extrascleral involvement are seen.

Clinical Features. The mean age of patients with primary lymphoid uveal infiltration is approximately 55 years. The patients usually complain of loss of vision (a result of choroidal thickening), retinal detachment, and glaucoma. Clinical examination may reveal an anterior episcleral or subconjunctival mass (fig. 2-61) (205). Ultrasonography and MRI studies demonstrate choroidal thickening and the presence of extraocular involvement (fig. 2-62) (206). Most eyes are enucleated because of secondary glaucoma, retinal detachment, or the suspicion of uveal melanoma or metastatic disease. The clinical diagnosis is usually confirmed by biopsy of the episcleral lesion, FNAB of the choroidal mass, or transscleral biopsy of the choroid.

Gross and Microscopic Findings. The enucleated eyes usually show the late stages of ocular involvement. Grossly, the uveal tract is diffusely thickened and replaced by a yellowish tan mass (fig. 2-63). Microscopically, the choroid, ciliary body, and iris show a diffuse lymphocytic infiltrate. Large lymphoid follicles with prominent germinal centers are seen with low-power microscopy (fig. 2-64). Small mature lymphocytes with scanty cytoplasm are admixed with a few plasmacytoid cells and plasma cells. There may be small lymphocytes with cleaved nuclei and nuclear atypia, consisting of small nucleoli and coarse chromatin clumping, as well as scattered mitotic figures. Cases with predominant plasmacytoid and plasma cell infiltration may show numerous Dutcher bodies, intranuclear inclusions containing periodic acid–Schiff (PAS)-positive material, and extracellular, eosinophilic, PAS-positive deposits. The lymphoid infiltrate may extend extraocularly through the posterior scleral canals. The episcleral infiltrate is usually composed of small lymphocytes and scattered plasma cells. Similarly, the anterior

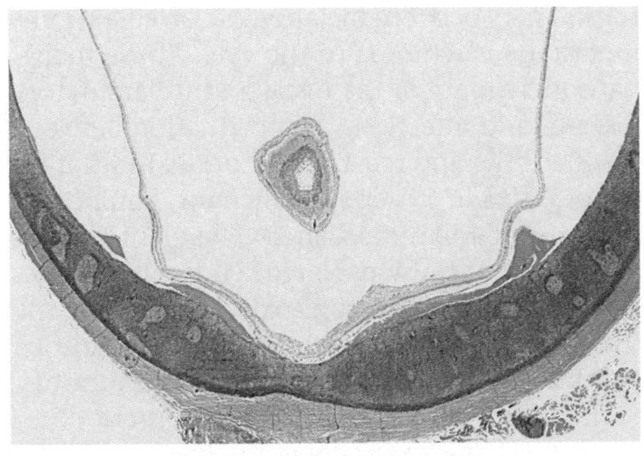

Figure 2-64

REACTIVE LYMPHOID HYPERPLASIA

The diffuse choroidal infiltrate is composed of small lymphocytes with multiple pale nodules that represent reactive lymphoid follicles.

segment shows a more mature lymphocytic infiltrate. Several secondary intraocular tissue changes may be observed, including retinal detachment, neovascularization of the iris, and peripheral anterior synechiae.

Immunohistochemical Findings. The majority of lymphoid cells (over 60 percent) express B-cell rather than T-cell markers. The monomorphic cell population usually demonstrates immunoglobulin light chain restriction (207). Cases with reactive follicles are usually polyclonal, as are episcleral infiltrates, even in the presence of intrachoroidal monoclonality.

Special Studies. In one study, the monoclonal antibody Ki-67 showed a proliferative rate of 1 to 10 percent, which is lower than the rates observed in adnexal ocular lymphomas (207). Molecular heavy chain rearrangements were monoclonal or polyclonal in three of the six cases studied. Polyclonality was seen in one case of reactive lymphoid hyperplasia and in two cases considered to be small lymphocytic lymphomas by light microscopy.

Differential Diagnosis. Diffuse uveal infiltration may occur in melanocytic proliferations, metastatic carcinoma to the eye, diffuse malignant melanoma of the uvea, and inflammatory diseases and infections. Differentiation between these entities and reactive lymphoid infiltration is not difficult. Systemic malignant lymphomas with secondary intraocular involvement are usually high-grade lesions (large cell lymphomas).

Treatment and Prognosis. Because of the small number of cases studied, no conclusions can be drawn from the results of immunohistochemical or molecular rearrangement studies and systemic extraocular involvement. In the most comprehensively studied series of 10 cases, extraocular infiltrates developed in 2 (207). The time interval between intraocular involvement and the development of extranodal infiltrates was 10 years in one of the two cases. An isolated report of mantle cell lymphoma of the uvea without systemic involvement has been published (208). Patients with uveal lymphoid infiltration should undergo staging evaluation for systemic disease including complete blood counts, serum protein electrophoresis, chest and abdominal CTs, and bone marrow biopsy.

Currently, the initial management of benign uveal lymphoid infiltrates is corticosteroids. Nonresponsive lesions and lesions consisting of low-grade lymphocytic infiltrates usually receive low-dose radiotherapy. To the best of our knowledge, no deaths from primary lymphoid infiltrates of the uvea have been reported.

SECONDARY AND METASTATIC TUMORS

Leukemia

Involvement of ocular tissues is observed in 17 percent of children with leukemia at the time of clinical presentation (209). Histopathologic examination of eyes obtained at autopsy demonstrate ocular leukemic infiltrations in 31 percent (210). The most common types of leukemia affecting the uvea are *acute lymphoblastic leukemia* and *acute lymphocytic leukemia*. *Myeloid leukemia* and *chronic lymphocytic leukemia* may also be found. The choroid is the most common intraocular site of involvement in acute and chronic leukemia and correlates with high circulating leukocyte counts and the severity of the disease (210,211). Involvement of the iris in leukemia usually occurs in association with infiltration of the ciliary body and choroid. In one study of children with ocular involvement in leukemia, 17.3 percent had anterior segment involvement (212). A study of autopsy cases of leukemia showed iris involvement in 1.5 percent of the eyes (212).

The signs and symptoms at presentation include loss of vision, heterochromia iridis, a grayish yellow mass or pseudohypopyon, and hyphema. The eye may be affected in patients after otherwise complete remission of the leukemia (213–215). In patients with a clinical history of leukemia, leukemic cells may be visualized within the lumen of blood vessels in the choriocapillaris, with secondary changes of the overlying retinal pigment epithelium and associated serous retinal detachment. The correct diagnosis is usually made by cytologic examination of samples obtained from aspiration of aqueous humor or FNAB of the uveal mass (216,217).

Lymphoma

Intraocular lymphoid proliferations occur in: 1) *primary malignant lymphoma* of the central nervous system in which involvement of the retina and vitreous may be the initial or only manifestation of the disease; 2) *lymphoid uveal infiltration,* which affects the uvea primarily, usually with episcleral extension; 3) *secondary malignant non-Hodgkin's lymphoma* in which the uveal tract is usually involved during the advanced stages of the systemic disease; 4) *angiotropic large cell lymphomas* affecting the retina and uveal blood vessels; and rarely, 5) *Hodgkin's disease* and 6) *T-cell lymphoma* and *mycosis fungoides* (218,219). Lymphoma of the iris is usually part of diffuse choroidal and ciliary body involvement (220,221).

Systemic lymphomas affecting the eye are usually high-grade B-cell non-Hodgkin's lymphomas that confer a guarded prognosis at the time of ocular involvement. In patients with intraocular involvement by systemic lymphoma, the mean interval from ocular diagnosis to death is 31 months. Intraocular involvement in Hodgkin's disease is uncommon. T-cell lymphomas with ocular involvement are highly aggressive tumors, and death follows shortly after diagnosis (221,222). Chemotherapy and radiotherapy are the recommended treatments in cases of intraocular lymphoma.

Iris masses and pseudohypopyon have been observed in children with *post-transplantation lymphoproliferative disorder* (PTLD) (223–225). The intraocular manifestation may be the first manifestation of the disease. The demonstration of Epstein-Barr virus DNA or recent seroconversion is useful for diagnosis and appropriate therapy (226). Histopathologically, the infiltrates vary from bland lymphoplasmacytic proliferations to clear-cut lymphoma. The primary management of PTLD is reduction of the immunosuppressive drug therapy.

Plasmacytoma

Uveal involvement by plasma cell proliferations is rare. Usually, the intraocular disease is part of *systemic multiple myeloma* (227). Histopathologic findings include ciliary body cysts containing abnormal immunoglobulin, secondary vascular retinal changes, hemorrhage, and retinal detachment. Rarely, cases of *solitary plasmacytoma* of the uvea occur (228). Patients with solitary plasmacytoma of the uvea have an excellent prognosis; optimal therapy is local radiotherapy. Chemotherapy is required for cases associated with systemic disease.

Metastatic Tumors

The most frequent intraocular malignancies are metastatic tumors. Most cases are seen in terminally ill patients (229,230). In one study, the overall incidence of ocular metastases among all fatal cases of cancer was 9.8 percent (229). The choroid alone is affected in approximately half of the patients with ocular involvement (230). Although almost any tumor may disseminate to the eye, the most common sites of origin are breast, lung, prostate, kidney, gastrointestinal tract, and genitourinary tract. A primary tumor cannot be demonstrated in 18 percent of uveal metastases (231,232). The temporal relationship between the primary tumor and uveal metastasis varies according with the primary location and the histopathologic classification. Among different series, ocular involvement was the initial manifestation in 30 to 45 percent of the cases (231,232).

Intraocular metastases are observed at any age but are more common between 40 and 70 years of age. Women are more frequently affected because of the high incidence of breast carcinoma. The common symptoms are blurred vision and pain. Clinical examination shows retinal detachment associated with flat lesions or nodular choroidal tumors. The lesions may be unilateral or bilateral; bilateral disease occurs in approximately 20 percent of patients. Ultrasonography is useful for differentiating metastases from primary intraocular tumors.

The iris may be the first site of metastatic disease; iris metastasis occurs in 3.5 to 9 percent of uveal metastases (233). Almost always, involvement is unilateral and the inferior quadrants are predominately affected. Although the most frequent primary tumors are from the lung and breast, almost any tumor is capable of involving the iris (232,234–236). Metastases to the iris from a renal cell carcinoma may present with hyphema. Metastatic tumors of the ciliary body usually involve the adjacent iris simultaneously (230,231). Solitary metastasis to the ciliary body is rare. Generally, metastatic tumors are composed of noncohesive cells which seed into the aqueous humor. This infiltration masquerades as a chronic iridocyclitis and results in secondary glaucoma (fig. 2-65) (237). Paracentesis followed by cytologic evaluation is useful to provide a prompt diagnosis (238).

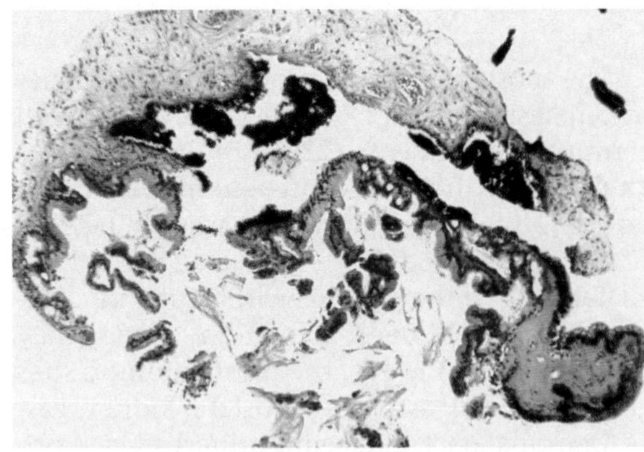

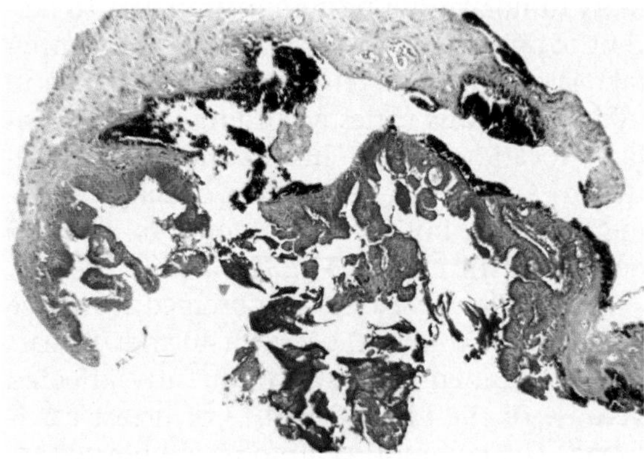

Figure 2-65

IRIS METASTASIS

Top: An adenocarcinoma of the gastrointestinal tract infiltrates the iris and ciliary body.

Bottom: Alcian blue stain discloses diffuse mucus production by the tumor cells.

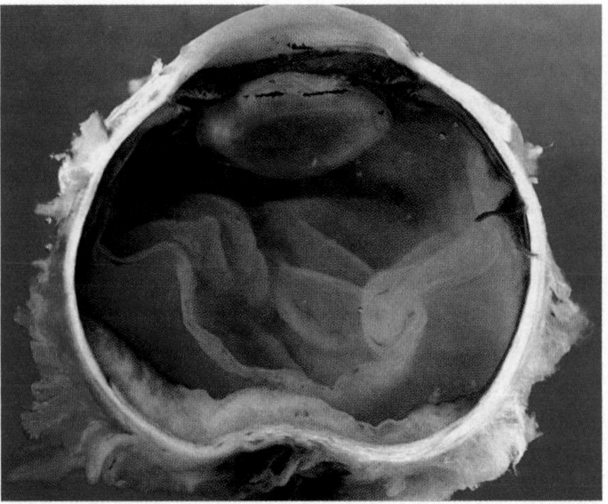

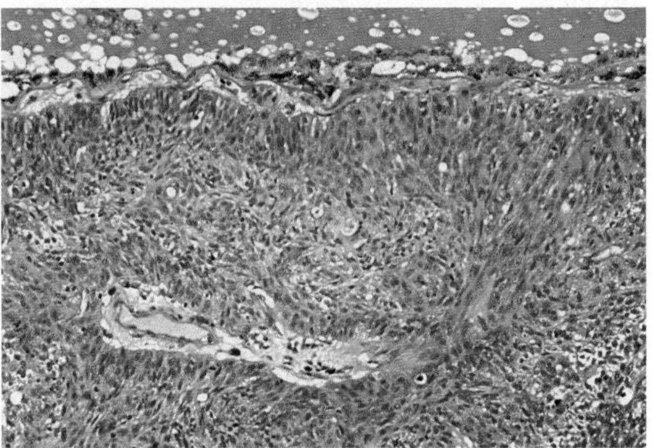

Figure 2-66

METASTATIC CARCINOMA

Top: Amelanotic flat lesion of the posterior choroid is associated with exudative retinal detachment.

Bottom: Choroidal infiltration by a poorly differentiated squamous cell carcinoma.

Gross examination of most metastatic tumors discloses a flat configuration (figs. 2-66, 2-67). The histopathologic appearance of metastases to the choroid reflects that observed in the primary tumor. A history of a documented primary tumor is important in some cases for appropriate clinicopathologic correlation. The use of immunohistochemistry and specific tumor markers usually facilitates the identification of the primary tumor. Differentiation between a primary choroidal melanoma and a metastatic melanoma to the choroid is based on the demonstration of two cell types, spindle and epithelioid, in primary melanoma; a low mitotic rate in most uveal melanomas; and the presence of bland, nevus-like cells at the base of the tumor towards the sclera. Metastatic melanomas are most commonly flat, with multiple foci and tumor emboli, which may be observed in the choroidal and retinal vessels.

Although the prognosis of patients with uveal metastasis is generally poor (234), new chemotherapy regimes have provided a longer survival period. The management of choroidal metastasis varies according to the clinical manifestation and stage of the disease. FNAB is valuable in patients with a suspicious intraocular lesion who do not have a history of primary neoplasia (fig. 2-68). Visual symptoms are ameliorated with radiation therapy.

Cysts

There are two types of iris cysts: those that originate from the iris pigment epithelium (the

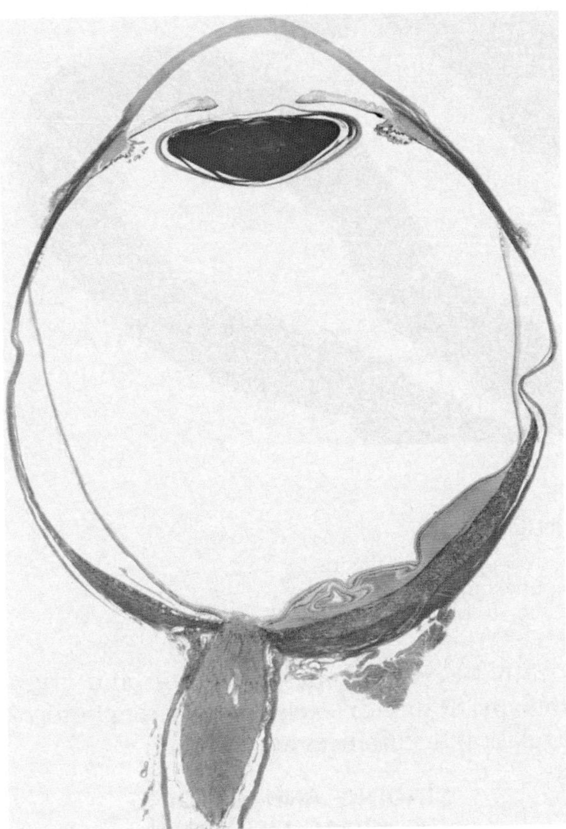

Figure 2-67

METASTATIC CARCINOMA

Low-power microscopic view shows mild choroidal thickening at the posterior pole and flat detachment of the overlying retina.

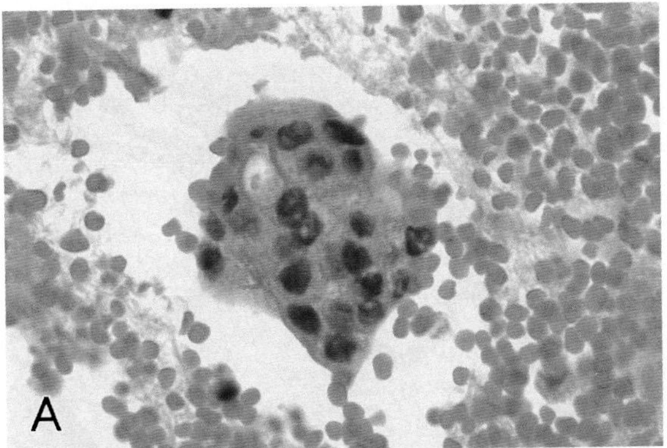

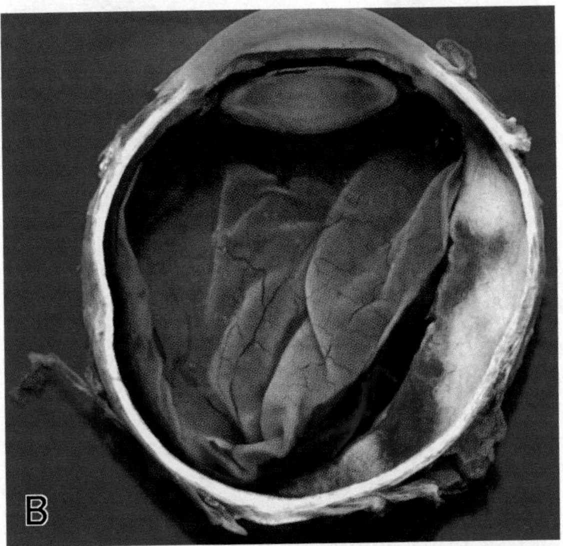

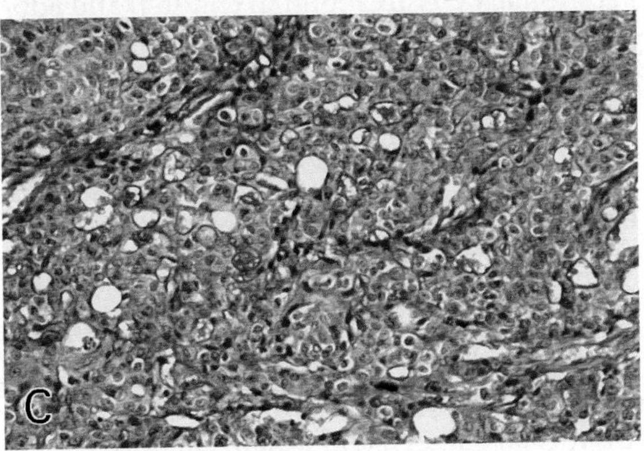

Figure 2-68

METASTATIC CARCINOMA

A: Fine-needle aspiration biopsy of a choroidal tumor shows a group of neoplastic epithelial cells forming an ill-defined glandular structure, consistent with adenocarcinoma.

B: The enucleated eye shows total retinal detachment over a white choroidal mass with foci of hemorrhage.

C: Metastatic mucus-secreting adenocarcinoma.

most common type) and those that develop within the stroma. Both types may be congenital (primary) or acquired (secondary). The main distinction between both types is the clinical appearance of either a pigmented tumor or an iris mass.

The location of primary cysts of the pigment epithelium is central (pupillary), midzonal, peripheral (iridociliary), or dislodged freely into the vitreous body or anterior chamber (239). *Primary pigmented epithelial cysts* are more common in young females. They are usually located in the horizontal meridian. Pigmented cysts in children tend to be multiple and located either in the midzonal region or pupillary margin of the iris (240). *Secondary pigmented epithelial cysts* are found near the pupillary border and may follow miotic therapy.

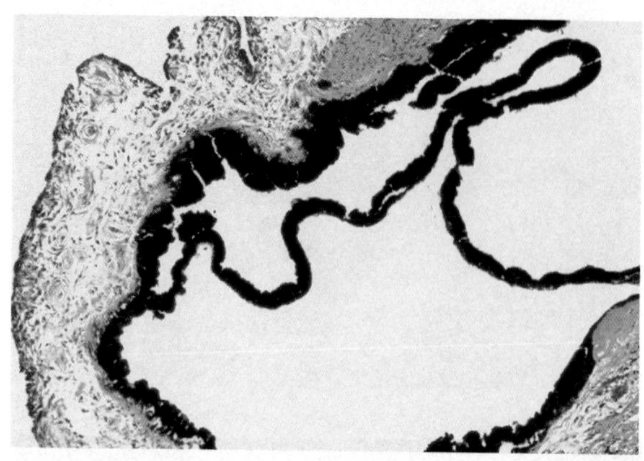

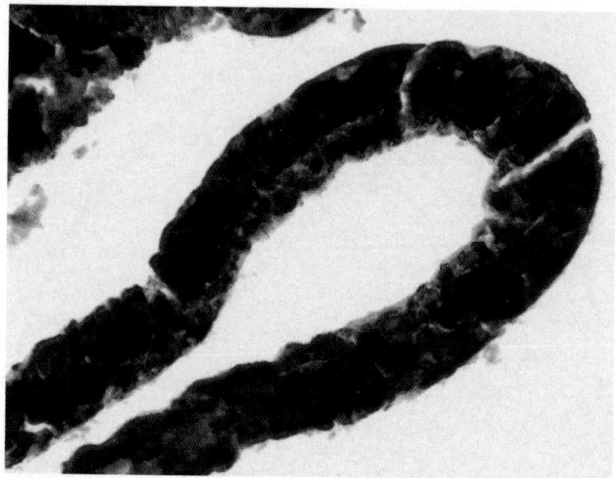

Figure 2-69

IRIS PIGMENT EPITHELIUM CYST

Left: Partially collapsed cyst at the posterior surface of the iris.
Right: The cyst is lined by pigment epithelium (high-power view).

Ultrasound biomicroscopy is useful for differentiating a cyst from a solid pigmented tumor (241). Histologically, cysts usually are lined by two layers of iris pigment epithelium (fig. 2-69). They usually remain stationary and do not require treatment.

Primary stromal cysts of the iris are rare. They are defined as an epithelium-lined cyst arising from the iris stroma in a patient with no history of prior trauma or surgery. Most primary iris stromal cysts are found in children and adolescents, and less frequently in adults (242–244). Clinically, they appear as a unilateral, smooth, round, translucent mass in the anterior chamber. Isolated case reports have been associated with a history of previous amniocentesis (245). The cysts usually are lined by stratified, nonkeratinized squamous epithelium (with or without goblet cells), which suggests a surface ectodermal origin (246). The content is usually clear but may include scanty cellular debris. Secondary epithelial cysts of the iris follow trauma or intraocular surgery, and usually are located anterior to the iris stroma. The lining of secondary epithelial cysts resembles conjunctival or corneal epithelium. Management of primary stromal cysts includes aspiration and cryotherapy, or surgical excision and laser photocoagulation; recurrences are common.

STAGING AND GRADING OF UVEAL MELANOMA

Clinical Staging

The assessment of the tumor is based on clinical examination, including slit-lamp examination and indirect ophthalmoscopy. Ultrasonography, retinography, CT scans, and MRI are used to enhance the accuracy of evaluation.

Pathologic Staging

Complete histologic study of enucleated, exenterated, or locally resected specimens is indicated. Study of the surgical margins, optic nerve, and vortex vein is necessary when appropriate. FNAB of enlarged lymph nodes or orbital masses is desirable.

The system presented in Table 2-1 is recommended by the Task Force for Staging of Cancer of the Eye of the American Joint Committee on Cancer (247).

Table 2-1

DEFINITION OF TNM (APPLIED TO BOTH CLINICAL AND PATHOLOGIC STAGING)

Iris

Primary Tumor (T)

TX Primary tumor cannot be assessed
T0 No evidence of primary tumor
T1 Tumor limited to the iris
T2 Tumor involves one quadrants or less, with invasion into the anterior chamber angle
T3 Tumor involves more than one quadrant, with invasion into the anterior chamber angle, ciliary body, and/or choroid
T4 Tumor with extraocular extension

Regional Lymph Nodes (N)

NX Regional lymph nodes cannot be assessed
N0 No regional lymph node metastasis
N1 Regional lymph node metastasis

Distant Metastasis (M)

MX Distant metastasis cannot be assessed
M0 No distant metastasis
M1 Distant metastasis

Ciliary Body

Primary Tumor (T)

TX Primary tumor cannot be assessed
T0 No evidence of primary tumor
T1 Tumor limited to the ciliary body
T2 Tumor invades into the anterior chamber and/or iris
T3 Tumor invades choroid
T4 Tumor with extraocular extension

Regional Lymph Nodes (N)

NX Regional lymph nodes cannot be assessed
N0 No regional lymph node metastasis
N1 Regional lymph node metastasis

Distant Metastasis (M)

MX Distant metastasis cannot be assessed
M0 No distant metastasis
M1 Distant metastasis

Choroid

Primary Tumor (T)

TX Primary tumor cannot be assessed
T0 No evidence of primary tumor
T1 Tumor 10 mm or less in greatest dimension with an elevation of 3 mm or less[a]
T1a Tumor 7 mm or less in greatest dimension with an elevation of 2 mm or less
T1b Tumor more than 7 mm but not more than 10 mm in greatest dimension with an elevation of more than 2 mm but not more than 3 mm
T2 Tumor more than 10 mm but not more than 15 mm in greatest dimension with an elevation of more than 3 mm but not more than 5 mm
T3 Tumor more than 15 mm in greatest dimension or with an elevation more than 5 mm
T4 Tumor with extraocular extension

Regional Lymph Nodes (N)

NX Regional lymph nodes cannot be assessed
N0 No regional lymph node metastasis
N1 Regional lymph node metastasis

Distant Metastasis (M)

MX Distant metastasis cannot be assessed
M0 No distant metastasis
M1 Distant metastasis

Stage Grouping

Iris and Ciliary Body

Stage I	T1	N0	M0
Stage II	T2	N0	M0
Stage III	T3	N0	M0
Stage IVA	T4	N0	M0
Stage IVB	Any T	N1	M0
	Any T	Any N	M1

Choroid

Stage IA	T1a	N0	M0
Stage IB	T1b	N0	M0
Stage II	T2	N0	M0
Stage III	T3	N0	M0
Stage IVA	T4	N0	M0
Stabe IVB	Any T	N1	M0
	Any T	Any N	M1

Histopathologic Type

Spindle cell melanoma
Mixed cell melanoma
Epithelioid cell melanoma

Histopathologic Grade (G)

GX Grade cannot be assessed
G1 Spindle cell melanoma
G2 Mixed cell melanoma
G3 Epithelioid cell melanoma

Venous Invasion (V)

VX Venous invasion cannot be assessed
V0 Veins do not contain tumor
V1 Veins in melanoma contain tumor
V2 Vortex veins contain tumor

Scleral Invasion (S)

SX Scleral invasion cannot be assessed
S0 Sclera does not contain tumor
S1 Intrascleral invasion of the tumor (includes perineural and perivascular tumor invasion of the scleral canals)
S2 Extrascleral extension of the tumor

[a]When dimension and elevation show difference in classification, the highest category should be used for classification. In clinical practice, one optic disc diameter averages 1.5 mm. The elevation may be estimated in diopters, where 3 diopters = 1 mm. Ultrasonography may provide a more accurate assessment.

REFERENCES

General Considerations

1. Hale PN, Allen RA, Straatsma BR. Benign melanomas (nevi) of the choroid and ciliary body. Arch Ophthalmol 1965;74:532–8.
2. Davidorf FH. The melanoma controversy. A comparison of choroidal, cutaneous, and iris melanomas. Surv Ophthalmol 1981;25:373–7.
3. Diener-West M, Earle JD, Fine SL, et al. The COMS randomized trial of iodine 125 brachytherapy for choroidal melanoma, III: initial mortality findings. COMS Report No. 18. Arch Ophthalmol 2001;119:969–82.
4. Albert DM, Niffenegger AS, Willson JK. Treatment of metastatic uveal melanoma: review and recommendations. Surv Ophthalmol 1992;36: 429–38.
5. Bedikian AY, Legha SS, Mavligit G, et al. Treatment of uveal melanoma metastatic to the liver: a review of the MD Anderson Cancer Center experience and prognostic factors. Cancer 1995;76:1665–70.

Nevi

6. Kliman GH, Augsburger JJ, Shields JA. Association between iris color and iris melanocytic lesions. Am J Ophthalmol 1985;100:547–8.
7. Ashton N. Primary tumours of the iris. Br J Ophthalmol 1964;48:650–68.
8. Duke JR, Dunn SN. Primary tumors of the iris. Arch Ophthalmol 1958;59:204–14.
9. Albert DM, Searl SS, Forget B, Lavin PT, Kirkwood J, Nordlund JJ. Uveal findings in patients with cutaneous melanoma. Am J Ophthalmol 1983;95:474–9.
10. Shields JA, Sanborn GE, Augsburger JJ. The differential diagnosis of malignant melanoma of the iris. A clinical study of 200 patients. Ophthalmology 1983;90:716–20.
11. Jakobiec FA, Silbert G. Are most iris "melanomas" really nevi? A clinicopathologic study of 189 lesions. Arch Ophthalmol 1981;99:2117–32.
12. Territo C, Shields CL, Shields JA, Augsburger JJ, Schroeder RP. Natural course of melanocytic tumors of the iris. Ophthalmology 1988;95:1251–5.
13. Shields JA, Karan DS, Perry HD, Donoso LA. Epithelioid cell nevus of the iris. Arch Ophthalmol 1985;103:235–7.
14. Margo CE, Groden L. Balloon cell nevus of the iris. Am J Ophthalmol 1986;102:282–3.
15. Ticho BH, Rosner M, Mets MB, Tso MO. Bilateral diffuse iris nodular nevi. Clinical and histopathologic characterization. Ophthalmology 1995;102:419–25.
16. Ragge NK, Acheson J, Murphree AL. Iris mammillations: significance and associations. Eye 1996;10(Pt 1):86–91.
17. Lewis RA, Riccardi VM. Von Recklinghausen neurofibromatosis. Incidence of iris hamartomata. Ophthalmology 1981;88:348–54.
18. Williamson TH, Garner A, Moore AT. Structure of Lisch nodules in neurofibromatosis type 1. Ophthalmic Paediatr Genet 1991;12:11–7.
19. Brushfield T. Mongolism. Br J Child Dis 1924;21:241–58.
20. Donaldson DD. The significance of spotting of the iris in Mongoloids. Brushfield spots. Arch Ophthalmol 1961;4:26–31.
21. Eagle RC Jr, Font RL, Yanoff M, Fine BS. The iris naevus (Cogan-Reese) syndrome: light and electron microscopic observations. Br J Ophthalmol 1980;64:446–52.
22. Naumann GO. [Pigmented nevi of the choroid and ciliary bodies. A clinical and histopathological study.] Adv Opthalmol 1970;23:187–272. (German.)
23. Naumann G, Yanoff M, Zimmerman LE. Histogenesis of malignant melanomas of the uvea. I. Histopathologic characteristics of nevi of the choroid and ciliary body. Arch Ophthalmol 1966;76:784–96.
24. Ganley JP, Comstock GW. Benign nevi and malignant melanomas of the choroid. Am J Ophthalmol 1973;76:19–25.
25. Sumich P, Mitchell P, Wang JJ. Choroidal nevi in a white population: the Blue Mountains Eye Study. Arch Ophthalmol 1998;116:645–50.

25a. Barr CC, Zimmerman LE, Curtin VT, Font RL. Bilateral diffuse melanocytic uveal tumors associated with systemic malignant neoplasms. A recently recognized syndrome. Arch Ophthalmol 1982;100:249–55.

26. Brown GC, Shields JA, Augsburger JJ. Amelanotic choroidal nevi. Ophthalmology 1981;88: 1116–21.
27. Butler P, Char DH, Zarbin M, Kroll S. Natural history of indeterminate pigmented choroidal tumors. Ophthalmology 1994;101:710–6.

Melanocytoma

28. Zimmerman LE. Melanocyes, melanocytic nevi, and melanocytomas. The Jonas S. Friedenwald Memorial Lecture. Invest Ophthalmol 1965;4: 11–41.

29. Fineman MS, Eagle RC Jr, Shields JA, Shields CL, De Potter P. Melanocytomalytic glaucoma in eyes with necrotic iris melanocytoma. Ophthalmology 1998;105:492–6.
30. Shields JA, Eagle RC Jr, Shields CL, Nelson LB. Progressive growth of an iris melanocytoma in a child. Am J Ophthalmol 2002;133:287–9.
31. Cialdini AP, Sahel JA, Jalkh AE, Weiter JJ, Zakka K, Albert DM. Malignant transformation of an iris melanocytoma. A case report. Graefes Arch Clin Exp Ophthalmol 1989;227:348–54.
32. Kiratli H, Bilgic S, Gedik S. Late normalization of melanocytomalytic intraocular pressure elevation following excision of iris melanocytoma. Graefes Arch Clin Exp Ophthalmol 2001; 239:712–5.
33. Frangieh GT, el Baba F, Traboulsi EI, Green WR. Melanocytoma of the ciliary body: presentation of four cases and review of nineteen reports. Surv Ophthalmol 1985;29:328–34.
34. LoRusso FJ, Boniuk M, Font RL. Melanocytoma (magnocellular nevus) of the ciliary body: report of 10 cases and review of the literature. Ophthalmology 2000;107:795–800.
35. Brownstein S, Dorey MW, Mathew B, Little JM, Lindley JI. Melanocytoma of the choroid: atypical presentation and review of the literature. Can J Ophthalmol 2002;37:247–52.
36. Heitman KF, Kincaid MC, Steahly L. Diffuse malignant change in a ciliochoroidal melanocytoma in a patient of mixed racial background. Retina 1988;8:67–72.
37. Shields JA, Shields CL, Eagle RC Jr, Santos C, Singh AD. Malignant melanoma arising from a large uveal melanocytoma in a patient with oculodermal melanocytosis. Arch Ophthalmol 2000;118:990–3.
38. Rummelt V, Naumann GO, Folberg R, Weingeist TA. Surgical management of melanocytoma of the ciliary body with extrascleral extension. Am J Ophthalmol 1994;117:169–76.
39. Robertson DM, Campbell RJ, Salomao DR. Mushroom-shaped choroidal melanocytoma mimicking malignant melanoma. Arch Ophthalmol 2002;120:82–5.
40. Croxatto JO, Malbran ES, Lombardi AA. Cavitary melanocytoma of the ciliary body. Ophthalmologica 1984;189:130–4.
41. Juarez CP, Tso MO. An ultrastructural study of melanocytomas (magnocellular nevi) of the optic disk and uvea. Am J Ophthalmol 1980; 90:48–62.
42. El-Harazi SM, Kellaway J, Font RL. Melanocytoma of the ciliary body diagnosed by fineneedle aspiration biopsy. Diagn Cytopathol 2000;22:394–7.

Malignant Melanoma

43. Rones B, Zimmerman LE. The prognosis of primary tumors of the iris treated by iridectomy. AMA Arch Ophthalmol 1958;60:193–205.
44. Holland G. [On the clinical features and pathology of pigment tumors of the iris.] Klin Monatsbl Augenheilkd 1967;150:359–70. (German.)
45. Jensen OA. Malignant melanoma of the iris. A 25-year analysis of Danish cases. Eur J Ophthalmol 1993;3:181–8.
46. Shields CL, Shields JA, Materin M, Gershenbaum E, Singh AD, Smith A. Iris melanoma: risk factors for metastasis in 169 consecutive patients. Ophthalmology 2001;108:172–8.
47. Duke JR, Dunn SN. Primary tumors of the iris. AMA Arch Ophthalmol 1958;59:204–14.
48. Ashton N. Primary tumours of the iris. Br J Ophthalmol 1964;48:650–68.
49. Arentsen JJ, Green WR. Melanoma of the iris: report of 72 cases treated surgically. Ophthalmic Surg 1975;6:23–37.
50. Cleasby GW. Malignant melanomas of the iris. AMA Arch Ophthalmol 1958;60:403–17.
51. Lerner HA. Malignant melanoma of the iris in children. A report of a case in a 9-year-old girl. Arch Ophthalmol 1970;84:754–7.
52. Jakobiec FA, Silbert G. Are most iris "melanomas" really nevi? A clinicopathologic study of 189 lesions. Arch Ophthalmol 1981;99:2117–32.
53. Cu-Unjieng AB, Shields CL, Shields JA, Eagle RC Jr. Iris melanoma in ocular melanocytosis. Cornea 1995;14:206–9.
54. Singh AD, Shields JA, Eagle RC, Shields CL, Marmor M, De Potter P. Iris melanoma in a ten-year-old boy with familial atypical mole-melanoma (FAM-M) syndrome. Ophthalmic Genet 1994;15:145–9.
55. Honavar SG, Singh AD, Shields CL, Shields JA, Eagle RC Jr. Iris melanoma in a patient with neurofibromatosis. Surv Ophthalmol 2000;45: 231–6.
56. Johnson MW, Skuta GL, Kincaid MC, Nelson CC, Wolter JR. Malignant melanoma of the iris in xeroderma pigmentosum. Arch Ophthalmol 1989;107:402–7.
57. Harbour JW, Augsburger JJ, Eagle RC Jr. Initial management and follow-up of melanocytic iris tumors. Ophthalmology 1995;102:1987–93.
58. Dart JK, Marsh RJ, Garner A, Cooling RJ. Fluorescein angiography of anterior uveal melanocytic tumours. Br J Ophthalmol 1988;72:326–37.
59. Bandello F, Brancato R, Lattanzio R, Carnevalini A, Rossi A, Coscas G. Biomicroscopy and fluorescein angiography of pigmented iris tumors. A retrospective study of 44 cases. Int Ophthalmol 1994;18:61–70.

60. Demirci H, Shields CL, Shields JA, Eagle RC Jr, Honavar SG. Diffuse iris melanoma: a report of 25 cases. Ophthalmology 2002;109:1553–60.
61. Hassenstein A, Bialasiewicz AA, von Domarus D, Schafer H, Richard G. Tapioca melanomas of the iris: immunohistology and report of two cases. Graefes Arch Clin Exp Ophthalmol 1999; 237:424–8.
62. Geisse LJ, Robertson DM. Iris melanomas. Am J Ophthalmol 1985;99:638–48.
63. Workman DM, Weiner JW. Melanocytic lesions of the iris—a clinocopathological study of 100 cases. Aust N Z J Ophthalmol 1990;18:381–4.
64. Heegaard S, Jensen OA, Prause JU. Immunohistochemical diagnosis of malignant melanoma of the conjunctiva and uvea: comparison of the novel antibody against melan-A with S100 protein and HMB-45. Melanoma Res 2000;10:350–4.
65. Grossniklaus HE. Fine-needle aspiration biopsy of the iris. Arch Ophthalmol 1992;110:969–76.
66. Deuble K, McCartney A. Nucleolar organiser regions in iris melanocytic tumours: an accurate predictor? Eye 1990;4(Pt 5):743–50.
67. Marcus DM, Mawn LA, Egan KM, Albert DM. Nucleolar organizer regions in iris nevi and melanomas. Am J Ophthalmol 1992;114:202–7.
68. Grossniklaus HE, Oakman JH, Cohen C, Calhoun FP Jr, DeRose PB, Drews-Botsch C. Histopathology, morphometry, and nuclear DNA content of iris melanocytic lesions. Invest Ophthalmol Vis Sci 1995;36:745–50.
69. Sisley K, Brand C, Parsons MA, Maltby E, Rees RC, Rennie IG. Cytogenetics of iris melanomas: disparity with other uveal tract melanomas. Cancer Genet Cytogenet 1998;101:128–33.
70. Geisse LJ, Robertson DM. Iris melanomas. Am J Ophthalmol 1985;99:638–48.
71. Brown D, Boniuk M, Font RL. Diffuse malignant melanoma of iris with metastases. Surv Ophthalmol 1990;34:357–64.
72. Bechrakis NE, Lee WR. Dedifferentiation potential of iris melanomas. Fortschr Ophthalmol 1991;88:651–6.
73. Duke-Elder S, Perkins ES. Diseases of the uveal tract. In: Duke-Elder S, ed. System of ophthalmology. Vol IX. St. Louis: CV Mosby; 1966:285–94.
74. Shields JA, Shields CL, Shah P, Sivalingam V. Partial lamellar sclerouvectomy for ciliary body and choroidal tumors. Ophthalmology 1991;98:971–83.
75. Naumann GO, Rummelt V. Block excision of tumors of the anterior uvea. Report on 68 consecutive patients. Ophthalmology 1996;103:2017–27.
76. Damato BE, Paul J, Foulds WS. Risk factors for residual and recurrent uveal melanoma after trans-scleral local resection. Br J Ophthalmol 1996;80:102–8.
77. Decker M, Castro JR, Linstadt DE, et al. Ciliary body melanoma treated with helium particle irradiation. Int J Radiat Oncol Biol Phys 1990;19: 243–7.
78. Gunduz K, Shields CL, Shields JA, Cater J, Freire JE, Brady LW. Plaque radiotherapy of uveal melanoma with predominant ciliary body involvement. Arch Ophthalmol 1999;117:170–7.
79. Finger PT. Plaque radiation therapy for malignant melanoma of the iris and ciliary body. Am J Ophthalmol 2001;132:328–35.
80. Memmen JE, McLean IW. The long-term outcome of patients undergoing iridocyclectomy. Ophthalmology 1990;97:429–32.
81. Manschot WA. Ring melanoma. Arch Ophthalmol 1964;17:625–32.
82. Demirci H, Shields CL, Shields JA, Honavar SG, Eagle RC Jr. Ring melanoma of the ciliary body: report on twenty-three patients. Retina 2002; 22:698–706.
83. Margo CE, McLean IW. Malignant melanoma of the choroid and ciliary body in black patients. Arch Ophthalmol 1984;102:77–9.
84. Scotto J, Fraumeni JF, Lee JA. Melanomas of the eye and other noncutaneous sites: epidemiologic aspects. J Natl Cancer Inst 1976;56:489–91.
85. Bergman L, Seregard S, Nilsson B, Ringborg U, Lundell G, Ragnarsson-Olding B. Incidence of uveal melanoma in Sweden from 1960 to 1998. Invest Ophthalmol Vis Sci 2002;43:2579–83.
86. Vajdic CM, Kricker A, Giblin M, et al. Sun exposure predicts risk of ocular melanoma in Australia. Int J Cancer 2002;101:175–82.
87. Singh AD, De Potter P, Fijal BA, Shields CL, Shields JA, Elston RC. Lifetime prevalence of uveal melanoma in white patients with oculo (dermal) melanocytosis. Ophthalmology 1998;105:195–8.
88. Jay M, McCartney AC. Familial malignant melanoma of the uvea and p53: a Victorian detective story. Surv Ophthalmol 1993;37:457–62.
89. Vink J, Crijns MB, Mooy CM, Bergman W, Oosterhuis JA, Went LN. Ocular melanoma in families with dysplastic nevus syndrome. J Am Acad Dermatol 1990;23(Pt 1):858–62.
90. Barr CC, McLean IW, Zimmerman LE. Uveal melanoma in children and adolescents. Arch Ophthalmol 1981;99:2133–6.
91. Gailloud C, Zografos L, Bercher L, Uffer S, Egger E. [Uveal melanomas in patients less than 20 years of age.] Klin Monatsbl Augenheilkd 1992; 200:428–30. (French.)
92. Singh AD, Shields CL, Shields JA, Sato T. Uveal melanoma in young patients. Arch Ophthalmol 2000;118:918–23.

93. Histopathologic characteristics of uveal melanomas in eyes enucleated from the Collaborative Ocular Melanoma Study. COMS report no. 6. Am J Ophthalmol 1998;125:745–66.
94. Font RL, Spaulding AG, Zimmerman LE. Diffuse malignant melanoma of the uveal tract: a clinicopathologic report of 54 cases. Trans Am Acad Ophthalmol Otolaryngol 1968;72:877–94.
95. Callender GR. Malignant melanotic tumors of the eye: a study of histologic types in 111 cases. Trans Am Acad Ophthalmol Otolaryngol 1931;36:131–42.
96. McLean IW, Foster WD, Zimmerman LE, Gamel JW. Modifications of Callender's classification of uveal melanoma at the Armed Forces Institute of Pathology. Am J Ophthalmol 1983;96: 502–9.
97. Marcus, DM, Minkovitz, JB, Wardwell SD, et al. The value of nucleolar organizer regions in uveal melanoma. Collaborative Ocular Melanoma Study Group. Am J Ophthalmol 1990; 110:527–34.
98. Khalil MK. Balloon cell malignant melanoma of the choroid: ultrastructural studies. Br J Ophthalmol 1983;67:579–84.
99. Grossniklaus HE, Albert DM, Green WR, Conway BP, Hovland KR. Clear cell differentiation in choroidal melanoma. COMS report no. 8. Collaborative Ocular Melanoma Study Group. Arch Ophthalmol 1997;115:894–8.
100. Folberg R, Pe'er J, Gruman LM, et al. The morphologic characteristics of tumor blood vessels as a marker of tumor progression in primary uveal melanoma: a matched case-control study. Hum Pathol 1992;23:1298–305.
101. Folberg R, Rummelt V, Parys-Van Ginderdeuren R, et al. The prognostic value of tumor blood vessel morphology in the primary uveal melanoma. Ophthalmology 1993;100:1389–98.
102. Folberg R, Pe'er J, Gruman LM, et al. The morphologic characteristics of tumor blood vessels as a marker of tumor progression in primary human uveal melanoma: a matched case-control study. Hum Pathol 1992;23:1298–305.
103. de la Cruz PO Jr, Specht CS, McLean IW. Lymphocytic infiltration in uveal malignant melanoma. Cancer 1990;65:112–5.
104. Iwamoto T, Jones IS, Howard GM. Ultrastructural comparison of spindle A, spindle B, and epithelioid-type cells in uveal malignant melanoma. Invest Ophthalmol 1972;11:873–89.
105. Burnier MN Jr, McLean IW, Gamel JW. Immunohistochemical evaluation of uveal melanocytic tumors. Expression of HMB-45, S-100 protein, and neuron-specific enolase. Cancer 1991;68:809–14.
106. Heegaard S, Jensen OA, Prause JU. Immunohistochemical diagnosis of malignant melanoma of the conjunctiva and uvea: comparison of the novel antibody against melan-A with S100 protein and HMB-45. Melanoma Res 2000;10:350–4.
107. Fuchs U, Kivela T, Summanen P, Immonen I, Tarkkanen A. An immunohistochemical and prognostic analysis of cytokeratin expression in malignant uveal melanoma. Am J Pathol 1992;141:169–81.
108. McLean IW, Gamel JW. Prediction of metastasis of uveal melanoma: comparison of morphometric determination of nucleolar size and spectrophotometric determination of DNA. Invest Ophthalmol Vis Sci 1988;29:507–11.
109. Gamel JW, McLean I, Greenberg RA, et al. Objective assessment of the malignant potential of intraocular melanomas with standard microslides stained with hematoxylin-eosin. Hum Pathol 1985;16:689–92.
110. Meecham WJ, Char DH. DNA content abnormalities and prognosis in uveal melanoma. Arch Ophthalmol 1986;104:1626–9.
111. Toti P, Greco G, Mangiavacchi P, Bruni A, Palmeri ML, Luzi P. DNA ploidy pattern in choroidal melanoma: correlation with survival. A flow cytometry study on archival material. Br J Ophthalmol 1998;82:1433–7.
112. Coleman K, Baak JP, van Diest PJ, Curran B, Mullaney J, Fenton M, Leader M. DNA ploidy status in 84 ocular melanomas: a study of DNA quantitation in ocular melanomas by flow cytometry and automatic and interactive static image analysis. Hum Pathol 1995;26:99–105.
113. Karlsson M, Boeryd B, Carstensen J, et al. Correlations of Ki-67 and PCNA to DNA ploidy, S-phase fraction and survival in uveal melanoma. Eur J Cancer 1996;32A:357–62.
114. Tobal K, Warren W, Cooper CS, McCartney A, Hungerford J, Lightman S. Increased expression and mutation of p53 in choroidal melanoma. Br J Cancer 1992;66:900–4.
115. Sulkowski S, Sulkowska M, Famulski W, Chyczewski L, Bakunowicz-Lazarczyk A. Expression of P53 protein in primary uveal melanoma. Folia Histochem Cytobiol 2001;39:159–60.
116. Chana JS, Wilson GD, Cree IA, et al. c-myc, p53, and Bcl-2 expression and clinical outcome in uveal melanoma. Br J Ophthalmol 1999;83: 110–4.
117. Chana JS, Cree IA, Foss AJ, Hungerford JL, Wilson GD. The prognostic significance of c-myc oncogene expression in uveal melanoma. Melanoma Res 1998;8:139–44.

118. Augsburger JJ, Shields JA, Folberg R, Lang W, O'Hara BJ, Claricci JD. Fine needle aspiration biopsy in the diagnosis of intraocular cancer. Cytologic-histologic correlations. Ophthalmology 1985;92:39–49.
119. Folberg R, Augsburger JJ, Gamel JW, Shields JA, Lang WR. Fine-needle aspirates of uveal melanomas and prognosis. Am J Ophthalmol 1985;100:654–7.
120. Cohen VM, Dinakaran S, Parsons MA, Rennie IG. Transvitreal fine needle aspiration biopsy: the influence of intraocular lesion size on diagnostic biopsy result. Eye 2001;15(Pt 2):143–7.
121. Raivio I. Uveal melanoma in Finland. An epidemiological, clinical, histological and prognostic study. Acta Ophthalmol Suppl 1977;133:1–64.
122. Jensen OA. Malignant melanomas of the human uvea: 25-year follow-up of cases in Denmark, 1943-1952. Acta Ophthalmol (Copenh) 1982;60:161–82.
123. Diener-West M, Hawkins BS, Markowitz JA, Schachat AP. A review of mortality from choroidal melanoma. II. A meta-analysis of 5-year mortality rates following enucleation, 1996 through 1988. Arch Ophthalmol 1992; 110: 245–50.
124. Collaborative Ocular Melanoma Study Group. Assessment of metastatic disease status at death in 435 patients with large choroidal melanoma in the Collaborative Ocular Melanoma Study (COMS). COMS report no. 15. Arch Ophthalmol 2001;119:670–6.
125. McLean MJ, Foster WD, Zimmerman LE. Prognostic factors in small malignant melanomas of choroid and ciliary body. Arch Ophthalmol 1977;95:48–58.
126. Zimmerman LE, McLean IW, Foster WD. Does enucleation of the eye containing a malignant melanoma prevent or accelerate the dissemination of tumor cells? Br J Ophthalmol 1978;62:420–5.
127. Augsburger JJ, Gamel JW, Sardi VF, Greenberg RA, Shields JA, Brady LW. Enucleation vs cobalt plaque radiotherapy for malignant melanomas of the choroid and ciliary body. Arch Ophthalmol 1986;104:655–61.
128. Garretson BR, Robertson DM, Earle JD. Choroidal melanoma treatment with iodine 125 brachytherapy. Arch Ophthalmol 1987; 105:1394–7.
129. Lommatzsch PK. Results after beta-irradiation (106Ru/106Rh) of choroidal melanomas: 20 years' experience. Br J Ophthalmol 1986;70: 844–51.
130. Augsburger JJ, Gamel JW, Lauritzen K, Brady LW. Cobalt-60 plaque radiotherapy vs enucleation for posterior uveal melanoma. Am J Ophthalmol 1990;109:585–92.
131. Finger PT, Moshfeghi DM, Ho TK. Palladium 103 ophthalmic plaque radiotherapy. Arch Ophthalmol 1991;109:1610–3.
132. Gragoudas ES, Seddon JM, Egan KM, et al. Metastasis from uveal melanoma after proton beam irradiation. Ophthalmology 1988;95:992–9.
133. Logani S, Helenowski TK, Thakrar H, Pothiawala B. Gamma knife radiosurgery in the treatment of ocular melanoma. Stereotact Funct Neurosurg 1993;61(Suppl 1):38–44.
134. Oosterhuis JA, Journee-de Korver HG, Keunen JE. Transpupillary thermotherapy: results in 50 patients with choroidal melanoma. Arch Ophthalmol 1998;116:157–62.
135. Peyman GA, Juarez CP, Diamond JG, Raichand M. Ten years experience with eye wall resection for uveal malignant melanomas. Ophthalmology 1984;91:1720–5.
136. Diener-West M, Earle JD, Fine SL, et al. The COMS randomized trial of iodine 125 brachytherapy for choroidal melanoma, III: initial mortality findings. COMS Report No. 18. Arch Ophthalmol 2001;119:969–82.
137. Jampol LM, Moy CS, Murray TG, et al. The COMS randomized trial of iodine 125 brachytherapy for choroidal melanoma: IV. Local treatment failure and enucleation in the first 5 years after brachytherapy. COMS report no. 19. Ophthalmology 2002;109:2197–206.
138. Felberg NT, Shields JA, Maguire J, Piperata S, Amsel J. Gamma-glutamyl transpeptidase in the prognosis of patients with uveal malignant melanoma. Am J Ophthalmol 1983;95:467–73.
139. Leyvraz S, Spataro V, Bauer J, et al. Treatment of ocular melanoma metastatic to the liver by hepatic arterial chemotherapy. J Clin Oncol 1997;15:2589–95.
140. Becker JC, Terheyden P, Kampgen E, et al. Treatment of disseminated ocular melanoma with sequential fotemustine, interferon alpha, and interleukin 2. Br J Cancer 2002;87:840–5.

Diffuse Uveal Melanocytic Proliferation

141. Barr CC, Zimmerman LE, Curtin VT, Font RL. Bilateral diffuse melanocytic uveal tumors associated with systemic malignant neoplasms. A recently recognized syndrome. Arch Ophthalmol 1982;100:249–55.
142. Rohrbach JM, Roggendorf W, Thanos S, Steuhl KP, Thiel HJ. Simultaneous bilateral diffuse melanocytic uveal hyperplasia. Am J Ophthalmol 1990;110:49–56.

143. Margo CE, Pavan PR, Gendelman D, Gragoudas E. Bilateral melanocytic uveal tumors associated with systemic non-ocular malignancy. Malignant melanomas or benign paraneoplastic syndrome? Retina 1987;7:137–41.

Hemangioma

144. Amasio E, Brovarone FV, Musso M. Angioma of the iris. Ophthalmologica 1980;180:15–8.
145. Ferry AP. Hemangiomas of the iris and ciliary body. Do they exist? A search for a histologically proved case. Int Ophthalmol Clin 1972;12:177–94.
146. Isola VM. Hemangioma of the ciliary body: a case report and review of the literature. Ophthalmologica 1996;210:239–43.
147. Weiss MJ, Ernest JT. Diffuse congenital hemangiomatosis with infantile glaucoma. Am J Ophthalmol 1976;81:216–8.
148. Chang CW, Rao NA, Stout JT. Histopathology of the eye in diffuse neonatal hemangiomatosis. Am J Ophthalmol 1998;125:868–70.
149. Witschel H, Font RL. Hemangioma of the choroid. A clinicopathologic study of 71 cases and a review of the literature. Surv Ophthalmol 1976;20:415–31.
150. Shields CL, Honavar SG, Shields JA, Cater J, Demirci H. Circumscribed choroidal hemangioma: clinical manifestations and factors predictive of visual outcome in 200 consecutive cases. Ophthalmology 2001;108:2237–48.
151. Verbeek AM, Koutentakis P, Deutman AF. Circumscribed choroidal hemangioma diagnosed by ultrasonography. A retrospective analysis of 40 cases. Int Ophthalmol 1995-96;19:185–9.
152. Piccolino FC, Borgia L, Zinicola E. Indocyanine green angiography of circumscribed choroidal hemangiomas. Retina 1996;16:19–28.
153. Schilling H, Sauerwein W, Lommatzsch A, et al. Long-term results after low dose ocular irradiation for choroidal haemangiomas. Br J Ophthalmol 1997;81:267–73.
154. Zografos L, Egger E, Bercher L, Chamot L, Munkel G. Proton beam irradiation of choroidal hemangiomas. Am J Ophthalmol 1998;126:261–8.
155. Garcia-Arumi J, Ramsay LS, Guraya BC. Transpupillary thermotherapy for circumscribed choroidal hemangiomas. Ophthalmology 2000;107:351–6.
156. Schmidt-Erfurth UM, Michels S, Kusserow C, Jurklies B, Augustin AJ. Photodynamic therapy for symptomatic choroidal hemangioma: visual and anatomic results. Ophthalmology 2002;109:2284–94.

Hemangiopericytoma

157. Papale JJ, Frederick AR, Albert DM. Intraocular hemangiopericytoma. Arch Ophthalmol 1983;101:1409–11.
158. Gieser SC, Hufnagel TJ, Jaros PA, MacRae D, Khodadoust AA. Hemangiopericytoma of the ciliary body. Arch Ophthalmol 1988;106:1269–72.
159. Brown HH, Brodsky MC, Hembree K, Mrak RE. Supraciliary hemangiopericytoma. Ophthalmology 1991;98:378–82.

Fibrous Histiocytoma

160. Croxatto JO, D'Alessandro C, Lombardi A. Benign fibrous tumor of the choroid. Arch Ophthalmol 1989;107:1793–6.
161. Lam DS, Chow LT, Gandhi SR, Cheng MF, Chan DH, Tso MO. Benign fibrous histiocytoma of the choroid. Eye 1998;12(Pt 2):208–11.

Leiomyoma

162. Foss AJ, Pecorella I, Alexander RA, Hungerford JL, Garner A. Are most intraocular "leiomyomas" really melanocytic lesions? Ophthalmology 1994;101:919–24.
163. Li ZY, Tso MO, Sugar J. Leiomyoepithelioma of iris pigment epithelium. Arch Ophthalmol 1987;105:819–24.
164. Shields JA, Shields CL, Eagle RC Jr, De Potter P. Observations on seven cases of intraocular leiomyoma. The 1993 Byron Dermorest Lecture. Arch Ophthalmol 1994;112:521–8.
165. Croxatto JO, Malbran ES. Unusual ciliary body tumor. Mesectodermal leiomyoma. Ophthalmology 1982;89:1208–12.
166. Heegaard S, Jensen PK, Scherfig E, Prause JU. Leiomyoma of the ciliary body. Report of 2 cases. Acta Ophthalmol Scand 1999;77:709–12.
167. Eide N, Farstad IN, Roger M. A leiomyoma of the iris documented by immunohistochemistry and electron microscopy. Acta Ophthalmol Scand 1997;75:470–3.
168. Okamoto N, Sotani T, Shimo-Oku M, Sashikata T. A case with leiomyoma of iris extirpated with cryosurgery and its pathological findings. Acta Ophthalmol (Copenh) 1982;60:183–9.
169. Jellie HG, Gonder JR, Willis NR, Green L, Tokarewicz AC. Leiomyoma of the iris. Can J Ophthalmol 1989;24:169–71.
170. Jakobiec FA, Witschel H, Zimmerman LE. Choroidal leiomyoma of vascular origin. Am J Ophthalmol 1976;82:205–12.

Mesectodermal Leiomyoma

171. Jakobiec FA, Font RL, Tso MO, Zimmerman LE. Mesectodermal leiomyoma of the ciliary body: a tumor of presumed neural crest origin. Cancer 1977;39:2102–13.
172. Campbell RJ, Min KW, Bolling JP. Skeinoid fibers in mesectodermal leiomyoma of the ciliary body. Ultrastruct Pathol 1997;21:559–67.
173. Schlotzer-Schrehardt U, Junemann A, Naumann GO. Mitochondria-rich epithelioid leiomyoma of the ciliary body. Arch Ophthalmol 2002;120:77–82.

Malignant Muscle Tumors

174. Woyke S, Chwirot R. Rhabdomyosarcoma of the iris. Report of the first recorded case. Br J Ophthalmol 1972;56:60–4.
175. Font RL, Zimmerman LE. Electron microscopic verification of primary rhabdomyosarcoma of the iris. Am J Ophthalmol 1972;74:110–7.
176. Elsas FJ, Mroczek EC, Kelly DR, Specht CS. Primary rhabdomyosarcoma of the iris. Arch Ophthalmol 199;109:982–4.

Neurofibroma

177. Font RL, Ferry AP. The phakomatoses. Int Ophthalmol Clin 1972;12:1–50.
178. Brownstein S, Little JM. Ocular neurofibromatosis. Ophthalmology 1983;90:1595–9.
179. Burke JP, Leitch RJ, Talbot JF, Parsons MA. Choroidal neurofibromatosis with congenital iris ectropion and buphthalmos: relationship and significance. J Pediatr Ophthalmol Strabismus 1991;28:265–7.

Schwannoma

180. Donovan BF. Neurilemmoma of the ciliary body. Arch Ophthalmol 1956;55:672–5.
181. Rosso R, Colombo R, Ricevuti G. Neurilemmoma of the ciliary body: report of a case. Br J Ophthalmol 1983;67:585–7.
182. Smith PA, Damato BE, Ko MK, Lyness RW. Anterior uveal neurilemmoma—a rare neoplasm simulating malignant melanoma. Br J Ophthalmol 1987;71:34–40.
183. Freedman SF, Elner VM, Donev I, Gunta R, Albert DM. Intraocular neurilemmoma arising from the posterior ciliary nerve in neurofibromatosis. Pathologic findings. Ophthalmology 1988;95:1559–64.
184. Shields JA, Sanborn GE, Kurz GH, Augsburger JJ. Benign peripheral nerve tumor of the choroid. A clinicopathologic correlation and review of the literature. Ophthalmology 1981;88: 1322–9.
185. Fan JT, Campbell RJ, Robertson DM. A survey of intraocular schwannoma with a case report. Can J Ophthalmol 1995;30:37–41.
186. Shields JA, Font RL, Eagle RC Jr, Shields CL, Gass JD. Melanotic schwannoma of the choroid. Immunohistochemistry and electron microscopic observations. Ophthalmology 1994; 101:843–9.
187. Hufnagel TJ, Sears ML, Shapiro M, Kim JH. Ciliary body neurilemoma recurring after 15 years. Graefes Arch Clin Exp Ophthalmol 1988;226: 443–6.

Osteoma

188. Gass JD, Guerry RK, Jack RL, Harris G. Choroidal osteoma. Arch Ophthalmol 1978;96:428–35.
189. Shields CL, Shields JA, Augsburger JJ. Choroidal osteoma. Surv Ophthalmol 1988;33:17–27.
190. Kelinske M, Weinstein GW. Bilateral choroidal osteomas. Am J Ophthalmol 1981;92:676–80.
191. Noble KG. Bilateral choroidal osteoma in three siblings. Am J Ophthalmol 1990;109:656–60.
192. Kida Y, Shibuya Y, Oguni M, et al. Choroidal osteoma in an infant. Am J Ophthalmol 1997; 124:119–20.
193. Wiesner PD, Nofsinger K, Jackson WE. Choroidal osteoma: two case reports in elderly patients. Ann Ophthalmol 1987;19:19–23.
194. Shields JA, Shields CL. CME review: sclerochoroidal calcification: the 2001 Harold Gifford Lecture. Retina 2002;22:251–61.
195. Aylward GW, Chang TS, Pautler SE, Gass JD. A long-term follow-up of choroidal osteoma. Arch Ophthalmol 1998;116:1337–41.
196. Trimble SN, Schatz H, Schneider GB. Spontaneous decalcification of a choroidal osteoma. Ophthalmology 1988;95:631–4.

Xanthomatous Lesions

197. Tahan SR, Pastel-Levy C, Bhan AK, Mihm MC Jr. Juvenile xanthogranuloma. Clinical and pathologic characterization. Arch Pathol Lab Med 1989;113:1057–61.
198. Sanders TE. Intraocular juvenile xanthogranuloma (nevoxanthogranuloma): a survey of 20 cases. Trans Am Ophthalmol Soc 1960;58:59–74.
199. Zimmerman LE. Ocular lesions of juvenile xanthogranuloma (nevoxanthogranuloma). Trans Am Acad Ophthalmol Otolaryngol 1965;69: 412–39.
200. Brenkman RF, Oosterhuis JA, Manschot WA. Recurrent hemorrhage in the anterior chamber caused by a (juvenile) xanthogranuloma of the iris in an adult. Doc Ophthalmol 1977;42:329–33.
201. Wertz FD, Zimmerman LE, McKeown CA, Croxatto JO, Whitmore PV, LaPiana FG. Juvenile xanthogranuloma of the optic nerve, disc, retina, and choroid. Ophthalmology 1982;89: 1331–5.

202. Schwartz LW, Rodrigues MM, Hallett JW. Juvenile xanthogranuloma diagnosed by paracentesis. Am J Ophthalmol 1974;77:243–6.
203. Hadden OB. Bilateral juvenile xanthogranuloma of the iris. Br J Ophthalmol 1975;59:699–702.

Reactive Lymphoid Hyperplasia/ Primary Uveal Lymphoma

204. Ryan SJ, Zimmerman LE, King FM. Reactive lymphoid hyperplasia. An unusual form of intraocular pseudotumor. Trans Am Acad Ophthalmol Otolaryngol 1972;76:652–71.
205. Jakobiec FA, Sacks E, Kronish JW, Weiss T, Smith M. Multifocal static creamy choroidal infiltrates. An early sign of lymphoid neoplasia. Ophthalmology 1987;94:397–406.
206. Lombardi A, Croxatto JO, Zambrano A. Diffuse lymphoid infiltration of the uvea and periocular tissues. In: Sampaolesi R, ed. Ultrasonography in ophthalmology 12. Dordrecht, the Netherlands: Kluver Academic Pub.; 1990:427–37.
207. Cockerham GC, Hidayat AA, Bijwaard KE, Sheng ZM. Re-evaluation of "reactive lymphoid hyperplasia of the uvea": an immunohistochemical and molecular analysis of 10 cases. Ophthalmology 2000;107:151–8.
208. Rowley SA, Fahy GT, Brown LJ. Mantle cell lymphoma presenting as a choroidal mass: part of the spectrum of uveal lymphoid infiltration. Eye 2000;14(Pt 2):241–4.

Leukemia

209. Reddy SC, Menon BS. A prospective study of ocular manifestations in childhood acute leukaemia. Acta Ophthalmol Scand 1998;76:700–3.
210. Leonardy NJ, Rupani M, Dent G, Klintworth GK. Analysis of 135 autopsy eyes for ocular involvement in leukemia. Am J Ophthalmol 1990;109:436–44.
211. Kincaid MC, Green WR. Ocular and orbital involvement in leukemia. Surv Ophthalmol 1983;27:211–32.
212. Ridgway EW, Jaffe N, Walton DS. Leukemic ophthalmopathy in children. Cancer 1976; 38:1744–9.
213. Uozumi K, Takatsuka Y, Ohno N, et al. Isolated choroidal leukemic infiltration during complete remission. Am J Hematol 1997;55:164–5.
214. Decker EB, Burnstine RA. Leukemic relapse presenting as acute unilateral hypopyon in acute lymphocytic leukemia. Ann Ophthalmol 1993;25:346–9.
215. Sahdev I, Weinblatt ME, Lester H, Finger PT, Kochen J. Primary ocular recurrence of leukemia following bone marrow transplant. Pediatr Hematol Oncol 1993;10:279–82.
216. Zakka KA, Yee RD, Shorr N, Smith GS, Pettit TH, Foos RY. Leukemic iris infiltration. Am J Ophthalmol 1980;89:204–9.
217. Schachat AP, Jabs DA, Graham ML, Ambinder RF, Green WR, Saral R. Leukemic iris infiltration. J Pediatr Ophthalmol Strabismus 1988;25: 135–8.

Lymphoma

218. al-Hazzaa SA, Green WR, Mann RB. Uveal involvement in systemic angiotropic large cell lymphoma. Microscopic and immunohistochemical studies. Ophthalmology 1993;100: 961–5.
219. Erny BC, Egbert PR, Peat IM, Shorrock K, Rosenthal AR. Intraocular involvement with subretinal pigment epithelium infiltrates by mycosis fungoides. Br J Ophthalmol 1991;75: 698–701.
220. Jensen OA, Johansen S, Kiss K. Intraocular T-cell lymphoma mimicking a ring melanoma. First manifestation of systemic disease. Report of a case and survey of the literature. Graefes Arch Clin Exp Ophthalmol 1994;232:148–52.
221. Velez G, de Smet MD, Whitcup SM, Robinson M, Nussenblatt RB, Chan CC. Iris involvement in primary intraocular lymphoma: report of two cases and review of the literature. Surv Ophthalmol 2000;44:518–26.
222. Cochereau I, Hannouche D, Geoffray C, Toublanc M, Hoang-Xuan T. Ocular involvement in Epstein-Barr virus-associated T-cell lymphoma. Am J Ophthalmol 1996;121:322–4.
223. Brodsky MC, Casteel H, Barber LD, Kletzl M, Roloson GJ. Bilateral iris tumors in an immunosuppressed child. Surv Ophthalmol 1991;36: 217–22.
224. Chan SM, Hutnik CM, Heathcote JG, Orton RB, Banerjee D. Iris lymphoma in a pediatric cardiac transplant recipient: clinicopathologic findings. Ophthalmology 2000;107:1479–82.
225. Cho AS, Holland GN, Glasgow BJ, Isenberg SJ, George BL, McDiarmid SV. Ocular involvement in patients with posttransplant lymphoproliferative disorder. Arch Ophthalmol 2001; 119:183–9.
226. O'hara M, Lloyd WC 3rd, Scribbick FW, Gulley ML. Latent intracellular Epstein-Barr virus DNA demonstrated in ocular posttransplant lymphoproliferative disorder mimicking granulomatous uveitis with iris nodules in a child. J AAPOS 2001;5:62–3.

Plasmacytoma

227. Honavar SG, Shields JA, Shields CL, Demirci H, Ehya H. Extramedullary plasmacytoma confined to the choroid. Am J Ophthalmol 2001; 131:277–8.

228. Khouri GG, Murphy RP, Kuhajda FP, Green WR. Clinicopathologic features in two cases of multiple myeloma. Retina 1986;6:169–75.

Metastatic Tumors

229. Nelson CC, Hertzberg BS, Klintworth GK. A histopathologic study of 716 unselected eyes in patients with cancer at the time of death. Am J Ophthalmol 1983;95:788–93.
230. Block RS, Gartner S. The incidence of ocular metastatic carcinoma. Arch Ophthalmol 1971; 85:673–5.
231. Ferry AP, Font RL. Carcinoma metastatic to the eye and orbit. I. A clinicopathologic study of 227 cases. Arch Ophthalmol 1974;92:276–86.
232. Shields CL, Shields JA, Gross NE, Schwartz GP, Lally SE. Survey of 520 eyes with uveal metastases. Ophthalmology 1997;104:1265–76.
233. Sunba MS, Rahi AH, Morgan G. Tumors of the anterior uvea. I. Metastasizing malignant melanoma of the iris. Arch Ophthalmol 1980;98:82–5.
234. Shields JA, Shields CL, Kiratli H, de Potter P. Metastatic tumors to the iris in 40 patients. Am J Ophthalmol 1995;119:422–30.
235. Woog JJ, Chess J, Albert DM, Dueker DK, Berson FG, Craft J. Metastatic carcinoma of the iris simulating iridocyclitis. Br J Ophthalmol 1984; 68:167–73.
236. Viestenz A, Berger T, Kuchle M. Cutaneous melanoma metastasizing to the iris and choroid: a case report. Graefes Arch Clin Exp Ophthalmol 2002;240:1036–8.
237. Morgan WE 3rd, Malmgren RA, Albert DM. Metastatic carcinoma of the ciliary body simulating uveitis. Diagnosis by cytologic examination of aqueous humor. Arch Ophthalmol 1970;83:54–8.
238. Gupta M, Puri P, Jacques R, Rennie IG. Fine needle aspiration biopsy: an investigative tool for iris metastasis. Eye 2001;15(Pt 4):541–2.

Cysts

239. Lois N, Shields CL, Shields JA, Mercado G. Primary cysts of the iris pigment epithelium. Clinical features and natural course in 234 patients. Ophthalmology 1998;105:1879–85.
240. Shields JA, Shields CL, Lois N, Mercado G. Iris cysts in children: classification, incidence, and management. The 1998 Torrence A Makley Jr Lecture. Br J Ophthalmol 1999;83:334–8.
241. Marigo FA, Esaki K, Finger PT, et al. Differential diagnosis of anterior segment cysts by ultrasound biomicroscopy. Ophthalmology 1999; 106:2131–5.
242. Naumann G, Green WR. Spontaneous nonpigmented iris cysts. Arch Ophthalmol 1967;78: 496–500.
243. Brooks SE, Baerveldt G, Rao NA, Smith RE. Primary iris stromal cysts. J Pediatr Ophthalmol Strabismus 1993;30:194–8.
244. Lois N, Shields CL, Shields JA, Mercado G, De Potter P. Primary iris stromal cysts. A report of 17 cases. Ophthalmology 1998;105:1317–22.
245. Rummelt V, Rummelt C, Naumann GO. Congenital nonpigmented epithelial iris cysts after amniocentesis. Clinicopathologic report on two children. Ophthalmology 1993;100:776–81.
246. Coburn A, Messmer EP, Boniuk M, Font RL. Spontaneous intrastromal iris cyst. A case report with immunohistochemical and ultrastructural observations. Ophthalmology 1985; 92:1691–5.

Staging and Grading

247. AJCC cancer staging manual, 5th ed. American Joint Committee on Cancer. Philadelphia: Lippincott, Williams & Wilkins; 1997.

3 TUMORS OF THE RETINA

ANATOMY AND HISTOLOGY

The retina is formed from two layers of ectodermal cells of the optic vesicle; the optic vesicle itself is derived from cells lining the floor of the primitive forebrain. The outer layer of the vesicle contributes to the formation of retinal pigment epithelium (RPE), and the inner layer forms the sensory retina. The polygonal cells of the RPE produce melanin, but differ morphologically from choroidal melanocytes, which are derived from neural crest and are dendritic or spindle shaped. The melanosomes of uveal melanocytes are small and round; RPE melanosomes are large and oval.

The RPE extends from the margin of the optic disc to the ora serrata; it is then continuous with the pigment epithelium of the ciliary body. Although RPE cells are uniform in appearance, the epithelial cells in the macular region are taller, narrower, and more pigmented. The apical surface of each RPE cell has long microvilli, which interdigitate with the photoreceptor outer segments. The basal surface of each cell has a convoluted membrane that has several infoldings and is firmly attached to the Bruch membrane. Near the apical surface, adjacent RPE cells are joined by junctional complexes, which prevent diffusion of substances between the choriocapillaris and subretinal space. These junctional complexes form the outer component of the blood-retinal barrier.

The RPE is metabolically active, scavenging the shed discs of photoreceptor outer segments. The lysosomal system of the RPE cells digests the phagocytosed outer segments. The cytoplasm of the cells contains abundant smooth endoplasmic reticulum; with increasing age, there is an accumulation of lipofuscin.

The sensory retina is a thin, multilayered, transparent structure that extends from the margin of the optic disc to the ora serrata. From there, it is continuous with the nonpigmented ciliary epithelium.

The retina is subdivided into nine histologically distinct layers (1). Starting on the outside and moving toward the vitreous body, these layers are the photoreceptors of the rods and cones, the external limiting membrane, the outer nuclear layer, the outer plexiform layer, the inner nuclear layer, the inner plexiform layer, the ganglion cell layer, the nerve fiber layer, and the internal limiting membrane (fig. 3-1). This last layer is adjacent to the vitreous body.

The layer of rods and cones has a palisaded arrangement. The rods are slender and cylindrical, whereas the cones are flask-shaped and shorter than the rods. Both types of cells are made up of inner and outer segments. The inner segments of both contain numerous mitochondria, more in cones than in rods. The outer segments contain discs. The posterior pole of the retina is known as the macula; the center of this structure is the fovea. The fovea contains only cones. The rod and cone outer and inner segments are surrounded by glycosaminoglycans which are resistant to digestion with hyaluronidase.

The external limiting membrane is not a true membrane; rather, it is a continuous layer of junctional complexes uniting photoreceptor cell inner segments to the Müller cells, specialized glial cells. The outer nuclear layer is made up of eight to nine layers of photoreceptor cell nuclei, which stain densely with hematoxylin. The outer plexiform layer represents the synapses between the cells of the outer and inner nuclear layer. The inner nuclear layer consists of the nuclei of Müller cells and three types of neurons: bipolar cells, horizontal cells, and amacrine cells. The inner plexiform layer is composed of the synapses of the bipolar cells, the amacrine cells, and ganglion cells.

The ganglion cell layer is made up of a row of ganglion cells separated from each other by the cytoplasmic extensions of the cells, astrocytes, and blood vessels. The ganglion cells have large nuclei and prominent Nissl granules.

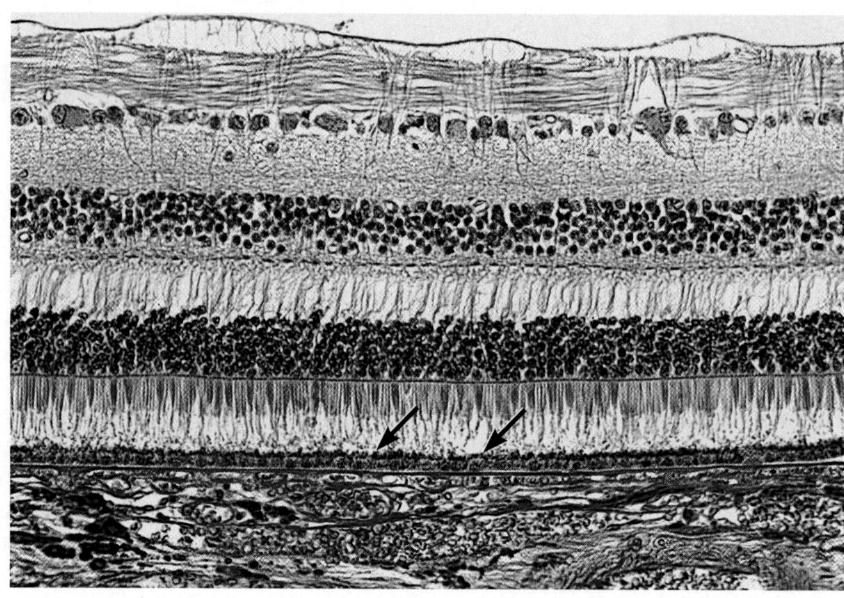

Figure 3-1

NORMAL SENSORY RETINA AND RETINAL PIGMENT EPITHELIUM

The sensory retina is composed of eight layers. The retinal pigment epithelium (RPE) is a distinct layer containing melanin pigment. Arrows indicate retinal pigment epithelium.

These cells are numerous and are arranged in several layers in the macula. In the extramacular retina, however, they form a single layer. The axons of the ganglion cells form the nerve fiber layer and extend to form the optic nerve. The internal limiting membrane is formed from footplate-like extensions of the Müller cells. This membrane represents the basal lamina of the Müller cells, which spans the entire thickness of the sensory retina.

The central retinal artery enters through the optic nerve head and divides into four branches that supply blood to the inner retina through a capillary network. These capillaries are absent in the fovea. Tight junctions between the retinal vascular endothelial cells form the inner blood-retinal barrier. The retinal vascular system extends into the retina as far as the inner portion of the inner nuclear layer. The remaining outer layers, including the outer portion of the inner nuclear layer, derive their nutrition from the choriocapillaris.

CLASSIFICATION AND FREQUENCY

A variety of benign and malignant tumors involve the retina. Retinoblastoma is a common primary malignancy that occurs mainly in young children; primary intraocular large B-cell lymphoma has been diagnosed more often in adults in recent years. Both of these malignancies, however, are relatively rare. The retina and RPE are rare sites for either benign or malignant primary tumors (2,3).

The relative frequency of retinoblastoma or other retinal and RPE tumors varies from one series to another. The series from the Armed Forces Institute of Pathology (AFIP) (4) and the Doheny Eye Institute revealed that the most common tumor was retinoblastoma, followed by primary intraocular lymphoma. In both series, angiomatosis retinae (capillary hemangioma of von Hippel) was the third most common tumor (Tables 3-1, 3-2).

RETINOBLASTOMA

Definition. *Retinoblastoma*, the most common primary intraocular tumor of childhood, arises from the sensory retina. It is composed of cells with large basophilic nuclei and scanty cytoplasm, displaying areas of necrosis and numerous mitotic figures. Although histologic sections may suggest that the tumor arises in any of the nucleated retinal cells, it appears that the tumor derives from immature neural epithelium (the inner lay of the optic cup). This epithelium has the potential to differentiate into photoreceptor cells and Müller cells (5). Moreover, retinoblastoma has been shown to differentiate along the cone cell lineage (6).

General Features. In the United States, the incidence of retinoblastoma is 1/18,000 live births or approximately 11 cases/million children

Table 3-1

TUMORS AND PSEUDOTUMORS OF THE NEUROSENSORY RETINA[a]

Type of Tumor	Number of Cases
Retinoblastoma	188
Pseudoretinoblastoma	
Coats' disease	17
Toxocara endophthalmitis	5
Persistent hyperplastic primary vitreous	6
Capillary hemangioma of von Hippel	4
Cavernous hemangioma	1
Astrocytoma	1
Astrocytic hamartoma (tuberous sclerosis)	1
Malignant lymphoma	14
Leukemia	3

[a]Frequency distribution of 240 tumors from the Armed Forces Institute of Pathology (AFIP) Registry of Ophthalmic Pathology collected between 1984 and 1989.

Table 3-2

TUMORS OF THE RETINA[a]

Type of Tumor	Number of Cases
Neurosensory retina	
Retinoblastoma	408
Lymphoma (primary intraocular lymphoma)	32
Capillary hemangioma of von Hippel	10
Astrocytoma	2
Leukemia	2
Metastasis	2
Retinal pigment epithelium	
Adenocarcinoma	4
Adenoma	2

[a]Frequency distribution of 462 tumors from the Doheny Eye Institute files collected between 1970 and 2000.

under 5 years (7). Studies from Australia, New Zealand, and Sweden show incidence rates of 1/17,000 to 18,000 live births. In Japan, the incidence is 1/23,829 live births (8). The incidence of retinoblastoma appears to be constant among the various populations of the world, suggesting that environmental influences play little role in its etiology (8).

There are two forms of retinoblastoma: an inherited autosomal dominant type, which constitutes 30 to 40 percent of the cases, and a noninheritable sporadic form, which constitutes the remaining 60 to 70 percent. A subclass of heritable retinoblastoma is seen in patients with a chromosomal deletion, but this is the least common form of retinoblastoma. One third of heritable cases result from the inheritance of a retinoblastoma-predisposing mutation (mutation on the retinoblastoma gene). The remaining two thirds are caused by new germline mutations that were not present in the parents but can be transmitted to future offspring (9). Heritable retinoblastomas may be bilateral or multiple in one eye (multicentric retinoblastoma). Familial cases of heritable retinoblastoma affect several family members.

Patients with chromosomal deletion retinoblastoma show a measurable defect in one of the long arms of chromosome 13, involving the 14 band. These children also have various somatic and mental developmental abnormalities, unlike children with other forms of retinoblastoma. It appears that a single locus exists for all the forms of retinoblastoma in the region 13q14 (8). The heritable retinoblastomas, including those associated with the chromosomal deletion and sporadic cases, show virtually identical histopathologic changes; however, in the chromosomal deletion cases, the enucleated globes harboring the tumor may reveal proliferation of pars plana ciliaris epithelium (10).

In 1809, Wardrop established retinoblastoma as an entity and advocated enucleation as treatment. Virchow considered the tumor to be a glioma of the retina, whereas Flexner, in 1881, proposed the term "neuroepithelioma of the retina" based on the characteristic rosettes seen on histologic evaluation. Although many names have been proposed for the retinal tumor, Verhoeff suggested "retinoblastoma" in 1922. This name was adopted by the American Ophthalmologic Society and, recently, by the World Health Organization (11).

The rosettes described and illustrated by Flexner in 1881 and by Wintersteiner in 1897 were given their names, and the presence of such rosettes in a tumor was considered to be the highest degree of differentiation. In 1969, however, Tso et al. (12–14) described further differentiated tumor cells that were cytologically benign appearing and showed clear photoreceptor differentiation. These cells were called "fleurettes," and were seen as a small component within a tumor otherwise showing typical histologic features of retinoblastoma (13,14). In 1983, Margo and coworkers (15) described tumors that were entirely benign appearing with numerous fleurettes. Based on the histologic features and on follow-up examinations conducted from 3 to 16 years after the diagnosis, they concluded that these tumors were a benign variant of retinoblastoma, and named them *retinocytomas*. In 1982, based on clinical observations, Gallie et al. (16) introduced the term *retinoma* for the benign counterpart of retinoblastoma. It is possible that retinomas and retinocytomas are identical tumors. Although clinically and histologically retinocytoma/ retinomas are distinct from retinoblastomas, the benign retinal tumor appears to carry the same genetic implications as retinoblastoma.

Molecular Biology. There are two distinct gene families that either promote (proto-oncogenes) or suppress (antioncogenes) cell proliferation. The retinoblastoma susceptibility gene (*RB1*) is an antioncogene (8). Antioncogenes, also known as growth-suppressor genes, actively inhibit cell proliferation and are temporarily inactivated in normal cell growth and proliferation. Loss of function in these growth-suppressor genes results in uncontrolled proliferation of the affected cells and development of malignancy. The oncogenic effect of these genes can result from such mechanisms as recessive loss-of-function mutations, wherein both copies of the gene are inactivated or lost.

Antioncogene mutations in germ cells (gametes) or in somatic cells may result in cancer. Germline mutations may occur de novo in the gamete, or the mutation may pass from one generation to another in a family as an autosomal dominant trait. Somatic mutations in antioncogenes *(RB1)* may take place preferentially in tissue such as embryonic retina (8).

The *RB1* gene contains 27 exons and 26 introns, with a total gene size of over 200 kb (17). The gene is located in the region of q14 of chromosome 13. The *RB1* gene encodes a 110-kDa nuclear phosphoprotein made up of 928 amino acids (pRB). It negatively regulates the progression of the cell cycle, and its function is determined by its phosphorylation state. In its hypophosphorylated (active) form, the protein binds to transcription factors, which are required to initiate the genes that control DNA synthesis and cell proliferation. Active pRB blocks the G1 phase of the cell cycle. In the hyperphosphorylated (inactive) form, the protein releases transcription factors so that DNA synthesis and cell proliferation can take place without hindering the progression of the G1 phase. The phosphorylation requires enzyme complexes 4-6/cyclin-dependent kinases. These kinases in turn are regulated by cyclin-dependent kinase inhibitors. Although several genes and their products control cell proliferation, current experimental evidence suggests that pRB is a master regulator of the cell cycle, differentiation, and apoptosis (18).

The *RB1* gene is a recessive human cancer gene. Retinoblastoma development requires loss or inactivation of both the alleles. Inheritance of one inactive copy of one *RB1* locus is associated with predisposition to the development of retinoblastoma. Inactivation of the second allele initiates formation of the retinal tumor. The inactivation of the second allele is a product of the random background mutation rate. Based on mathematical analysis, Knudson (19) proposed the two-hit hypothesis for the development of retinoblastoma: two mutations are required. The first mutation (first hit) takes place in the germline of patients with hereditary retinoblastoma and in a somatic cell (retinal cells) in patients with the nonhereditary form. In both forms of the tumor, the second mutation (second hit) occurs in the somatic cell, causing the somatic cell with the two mutations to become malignant.

Different types of mutations are found in the *RB1* gene, including frameshift and nonsense mutations, inframe and missense mutations, splicing mutations, mutations in the noncoding regions, and point mutations of codon 661 (8). Such mutations usually result in the absence of RB protein in tumor cells (20). The germline mutations arise mainly during spermatogenesis rather than during oogenesis. Both advanced maternal and advanced paternal age are significant risk factors for the development of sporadic hereditary retinoblastoma (21). Unlike the first mutation, the second (second hit) is almost always due to a chromosomal aberration. This occurs at a higher rate than the first mutation and is sensitive to environmental factors such as therapeutic exposure to ionizing radiation. The second hit frequently results in a loss of heterozygosity. With loss of heterozygosity, the retinoblastoma is usually differentiated, without choroidal invasion (22).

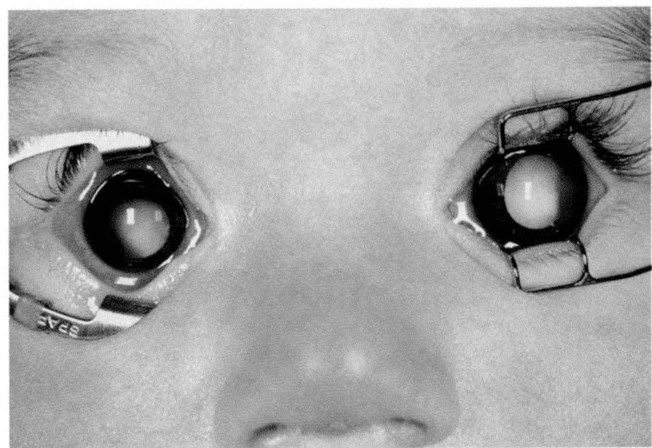

Figure 3-2

BILATERAL RETINOBLASTOMA

A child with heritable retinoblastoma presented with bilateral leukocoria.

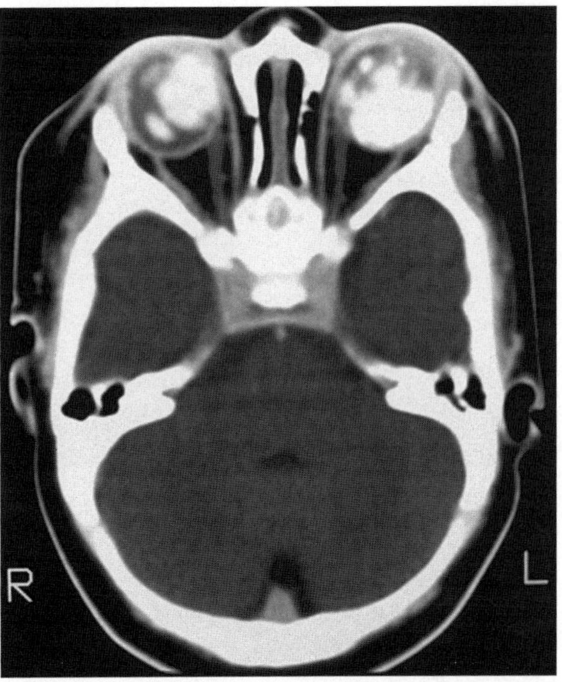

Figure 3-3

BILATERAL RETINOBLASTOMA

Computerized tomography (CT) shows bilateral intraocular mass lesions.

The occurrence of somatic mutations of both *RB1* alleles is not unique to retinoblastoma. Such mutations also occur in other malignant tumors, such as osteosarcoma, breast carcinoma, small cell lung carcinoma, alveolar rhabdomyosarcoma, and others (23–30). In these nonocular malignancies, the loss of alleles appears to be environmentally induced.

Clinical Features. Retinoblastoma is diagnosed in children during the first 3 years of age; however, these tumors can be congenital or they can develop in older children and, rarely, in adults (8,31,32). Presenting signs and symptoms in children depend to a large extent on the location, size, and extraocular spread of the tumor (figs. 3-2–3-6). The most common signs and symptoms include leukocoria (white pupil) in about 50 percent of the cases and strabismus in about 24 percent of cases (8). Less common manifestations include red painful eye with glaucoma, poor vision, and clinical findings simulating orbital cellulitis.

Leukocoria results when the mass is located behind the lens or when a discrete intraretinal mass is situated at the posterior pole (8,31). Frequently, leukocoria is noted by a family member or a primary care physician. The family members usually notice the white pupil at dusk or in a darkened room when the pupil dilates naturally because of a low ambient light level (8). Tumors located in the macula may present with strabismus. Extraocular extension, presenting as a fungating mass or proptosis with signs simulating orbital inflammation (8,31), is rare in the United States.

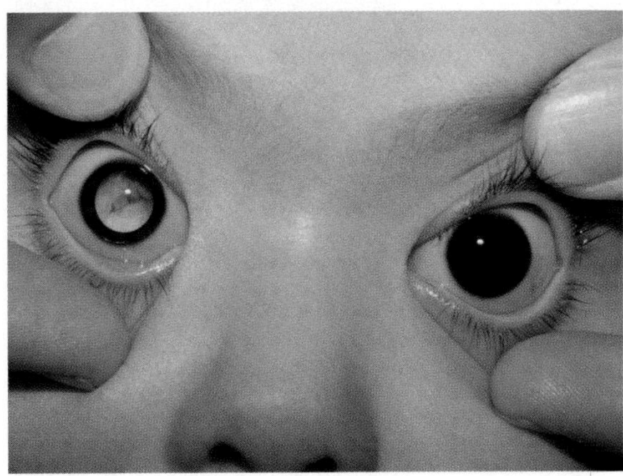

Figure 3-4

UNILATERAL RETINOBLASTOMA

A child presented with unilateral leukocoria. Exophytic growth of the intraocular tumor produced retinal detachment.

Clinically, retinoblastoma is a relatively transparent lesion (fig. 3-5) in the sensory retina

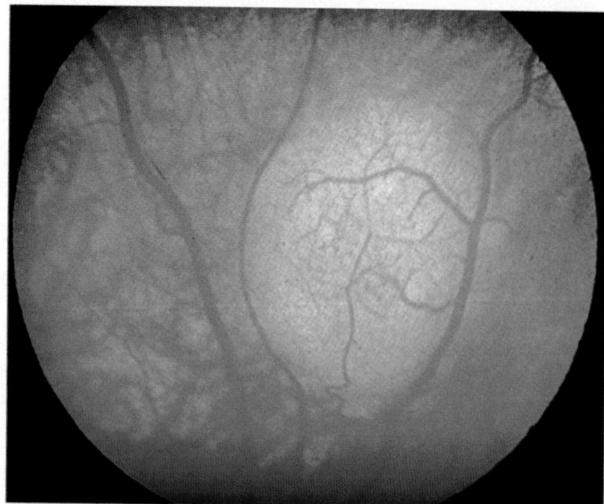

Figure 3-5

RETINOBLASTOMA

Funduscopic examination shows a relatively small retinoblastoma with an abnormal vascular pattern.

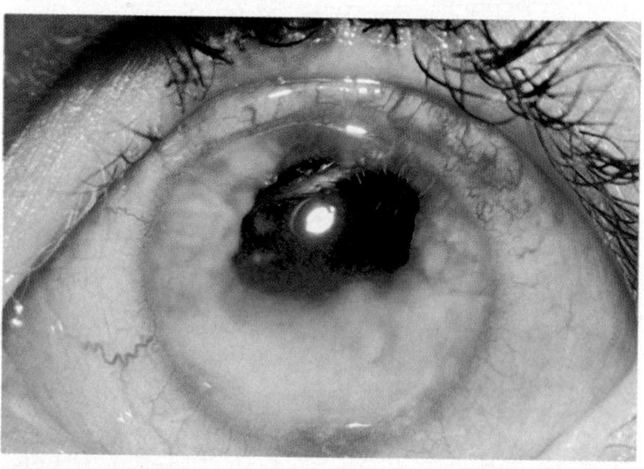

Figure 3-6

RETINOBLASTOMA

The pseudohypopyon results from tumor seeding the anterior chamber. Multiple iris nodules are observed.

that enlarges to become an opaque white mass containing vascular channels supplied by a dilated feeding arteriole (31). The tumor can cause retinal detachment. It can grow into the subretinal space (exophytic growth) or towards the vitreous body and involve the vitreous body with tumor seedings (endophytic growth). Spread of tumor seedings into the anterior chamber may produce a collection of neoplastic cells in the inferior part of the chamber (pseudohypopyon), simulating inflammation (fig. 3-6). A less common pattern is diffuse, flat growth of the tumor.

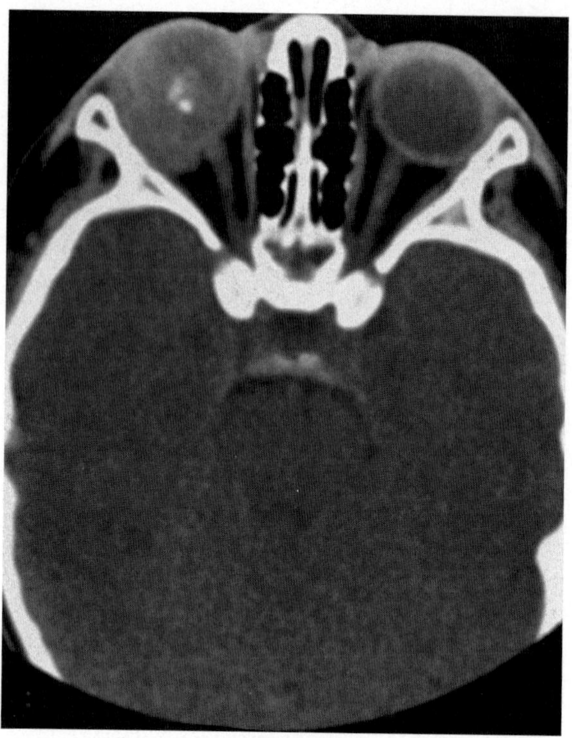

Figure 3-7

RETINOBLASTOMA

CT scan reveals a calcified intraocular mass.

Helpful diagnostic tools include computerized tomography (CT) scans and ultrasonography (8). CT scan reveals calcification in a solid mass (fig. 3-7) or in multifocal lesions. Although most endophytic and exophytic tumors show calcification, such a finding may be absent in diffuse tumors. CT and magnetic resonance imaging (MRI) can detect gross extension of the tumor into the optic nerve and extraocular extension; however, these imaging techniques may not detect microscopic spread within the optic nerve beyond lamina cribrosa (3,4).

Gross and Microscopic Findings. Grossly, retinoblastoma can present with different growth patterns, including exophytic (fig. 3-8), endophytic (fig. 3-9), endophytic mixed with exophytic (fig. 3-10), and diffuse growth (fig. 3-11A); complete spontaneous regression is also possible (3,4). Endophytic retinoblastomas are friable tumors that grow and seed the vitreous body. Vitreous seedings grow into separate, small, spheroidal masses, which on clinical examination appear as fluff balls or cotton balls.

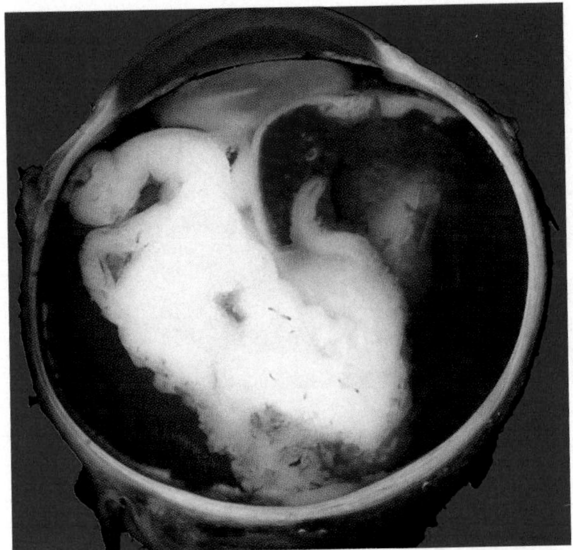

Figure 3-8

RETINOBLASTOMA

Exophytic growth of the tumor.

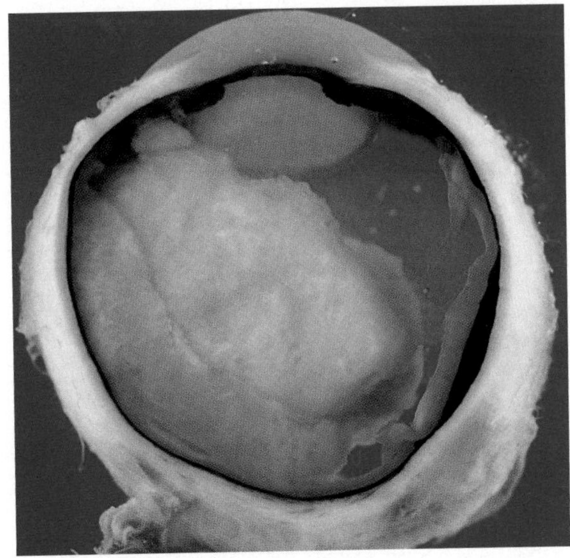

Figure 3-9

RETINOBLASTOMA

Endophytic growth pattern.

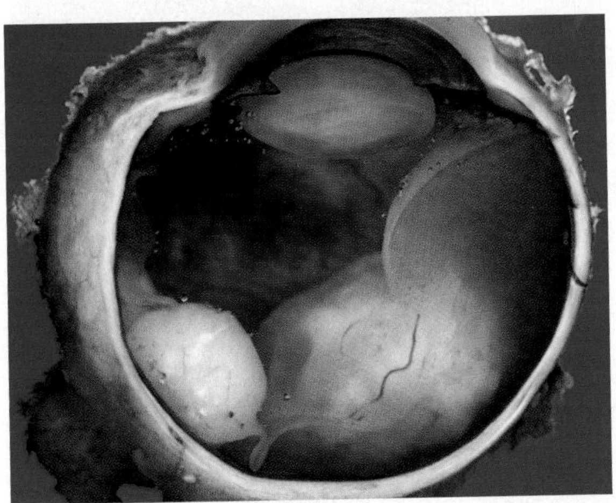

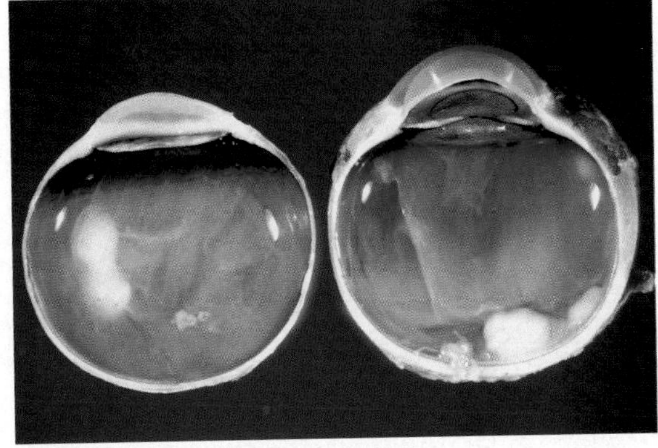

Figure 3-10

RETINOBLASTOMA

Left: Mixed endophytic tumor associated with an exophytic mass.
Right: Multiple retinal tumors are present in an eye from a child with heritable retinoblastoma.

Such tumor seedings may grow along the inner surface of the retina (fig. 3-11B,C) and invade the retina away from the site of the main mass. The seedings are often difficult to distinguish from a retinoblastoma with a multicentric origin (4); however, the seedings are mostly seen on the inner surface of the retina rather than within it. They are usually seen in association with tumor cell clusters within the vitreous body (4). The neoplastic seeds in the vitreous body may spread into the posterior and anterior chambers and deposit on the lens, zonular fibers, ciliary epithelium, iris, corneal endothelium, and trabecular meshwork. Through the meshwork, the tumor cells gain access to the aqueous outflow pathways to reach an extraocular site.

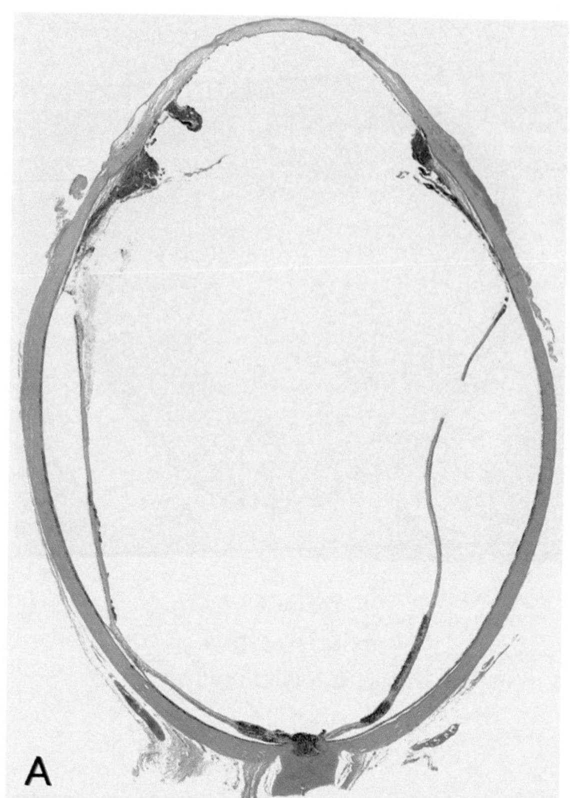

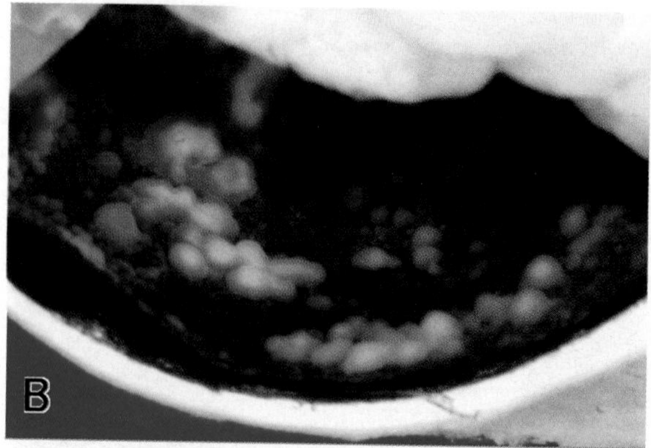

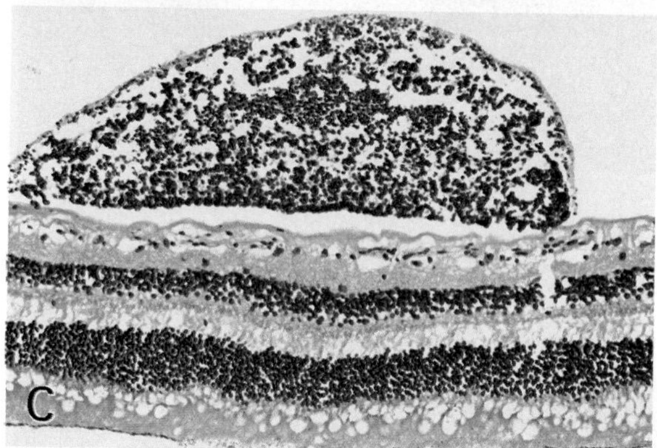

Figure 3-11

DIFFUSE INFILTRATING RETINOBLASTOMA

A: Diffuse tumor involves the retina, ciliary body, and optic nerve, with tumor seedings in the anterior chamber.
B: Tumor seedings along the inner surface of the retina.
C: A tumor nodule rests on the internal limiting membrane.

Exophytic retinoblastomas grow mainly toward the choroid, growing first into the subretinal space and causing retinal detachment. Subretinal tumor cells can invade the RPE, growing under and replacing these pigmented cells. The tumor can subsequently extend into the choroid (figs. 3-12–3-14), infiltrating through the Bruch membrane. From the choroid, the tumor spreads along ciliary vessels and nerves into the orbit and conjunctiva. From these sites the tumor may metastasize by gaining access to lymphatic and vascular channels.

Mixed endophytic-exophytic tumor growth shows the above-described features of both endophytic and exophytic tumors. Such a mixed pattern is observed in large tumors. In fact, a mixed pattern of growth may be more common than other gross appearances of retinoblastoma (3,4).

The diffuse infiltrating growth pattern is rarely seen in retinoblastomas. This growth pattern causes diffuse thickening of the retina (fig. 3-11A). The neoplastic cells may invade the vitreous body and seed the anterior chamber to form a pseudohypopyon. These tumors, which occur in older children, can be devoid of calcium deposits. Occasionally, diffuse retinoblastomas arise from the anterior retina, and seed the vitreous body and anterior chamber (33).

Retinoblastomas may undergo complete spontaneous regression. Regression follows severe intraocular inflammation in the eye harboring the tumor and is followed by the eye becoming phthisical (3). The mechanism by which the tumor spontaneously regresses is not clearly understood. Various mechanisms have been proposed for this regression, including vascular occlusion, calcium toxicity, and inflammation.

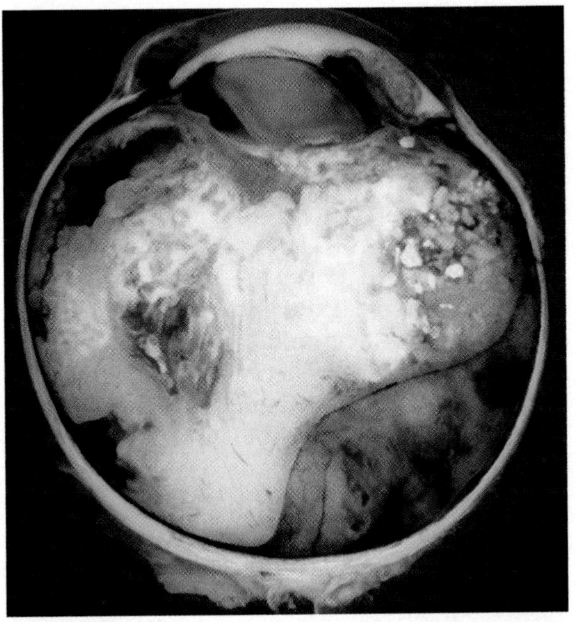

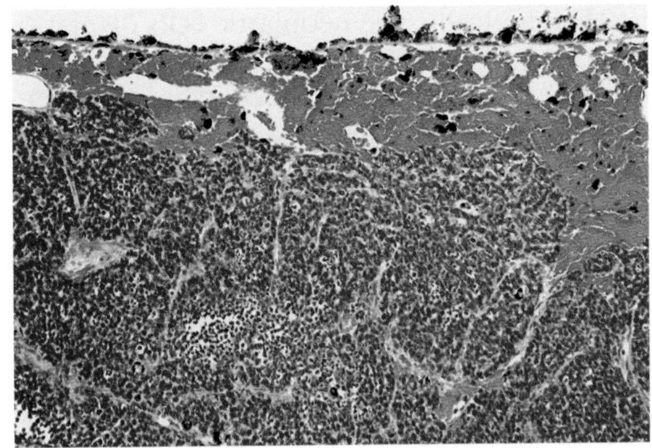

Figure 3-12

RETINOBLASTOMA

Left: The tumor has invaded the choroid.
Above: Massive choroidal invasion is present.

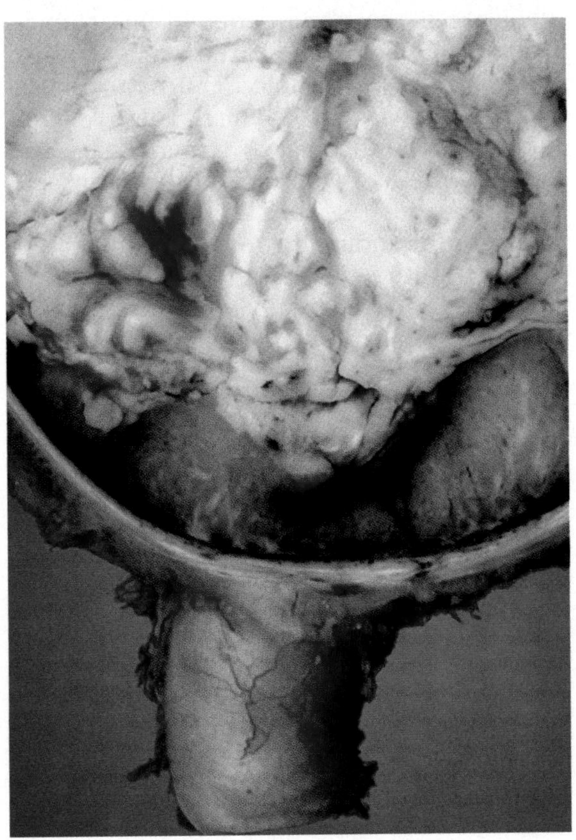

Figure 3-13

RETINOBLASTOMA

The tumor invaded the choroid and optic nerve.

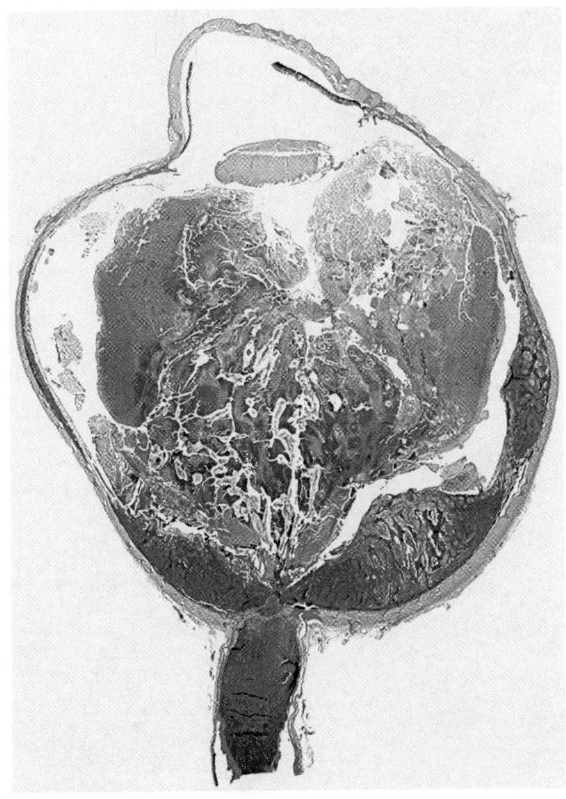

Figure 3-14

RETINOBLASTOMA

Large choroidal and optic nerve invasion by the tumor. The tumor cells are present at the line of surgical transection of the nerve.

Histologically, the neoplastic cells display a large basophilic nucleus and scanty cytoplasm. Areas of necrosis and calcification are common (fig. 3-15), as is the presence of numerous mitotic figures. Vascularity is prominent, and the vessels are surrounded by viable tumor cells (fig. 3-16). Malignant cells located 90 to 110 µm from the vessels may reveal ischemic coagulative necrosis (4). Several apoptotic neoplastic cells may be present in the tumor.

The foci of calcification are seen in the areas of necrosis. Tumors with extensive necrosis may liberate DNA from the tumor cells. The DNA is deposited as a basophilic material, preferentially in the walls of tumor blood vessels (fig. 3-17) and iris vessels, along the internal limiting membrane of the retina, in the outer layers of the trabecular meshwork, and in the Schlemm canal. The deposits are positive with the Feulgen stain, and the staining diminishes with deoxyribonuclease (DNase) pretreatment (34). Ultrastructurally, the deposits have an affinity for collagen and basal lamina, are electron dense, and contain vacuoles (34). Such deposits are seen primarily in tumors devoid of Flexner-Wintersteiner rosettes (undifferentiated retinoblastomas).

The formation of Flexner-Wintersteiner rosettes (fig. 3-18) and fleurettes (fig. 3-19) is a highly characteristic histologic feature of well-differentiated retinoblastoma. The rosette-forming cells are malignant cells that may exhibit mitotic activity; they are mixed with nonrosette-forming tumor cells (undifferentiated tumor cells). Some incompletely formed rosettes blend with undifferentiated tumor cells. Flexner-Wintersteiner rosettes are typically made up of cuboidal cells that circumscribe an apical lumen (fig. 3-18). The basal end of these cells contains the nucleus, and the apical end has cytoplasmic projections into the lumen. These cells appear to be held together by terminal bars. The lumen contains hyaluronidase-resistant acid mucopolysaccharides (fig. 3-20), similar to the material surrounding the rods and cones of the retina (3). Although Flexner-Wintersteiner rosettes are characteristically seen in retinoblastomas, they have been observed as well in pinealoblastomas and medulloepitheliomas (4).

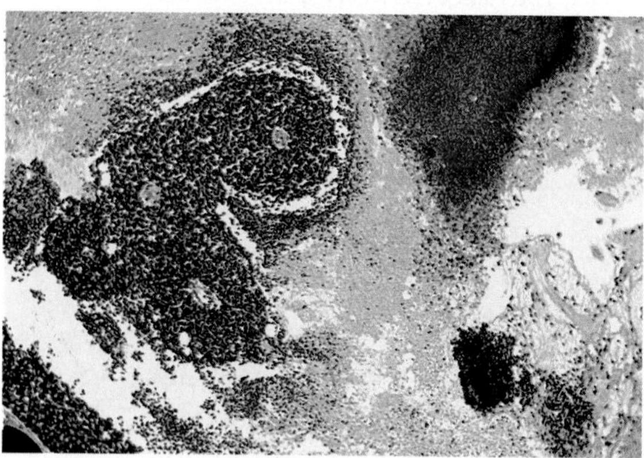

Figure 3-15

RETINOBLASTOMA

The tumor is composed of basophilic cells. Areas of necrosis and foci of calcification are seen.

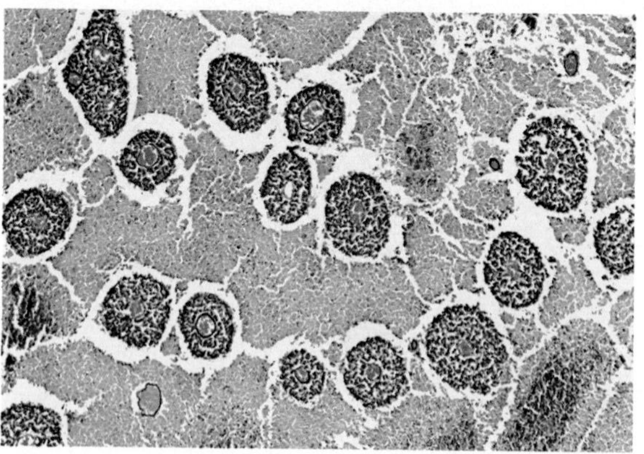

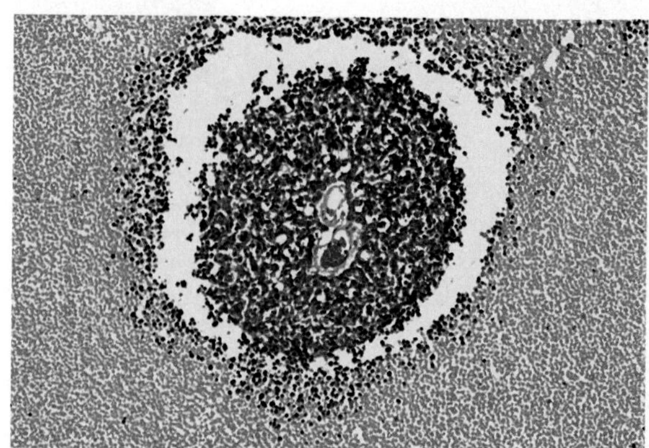

Figure 3-16

RETINOBLASTOMA

Left: Vessels are surrounded by viable neoplastic cells forming perivascular sleeves.
Right: High-power view shows perivascular cuffing of tumor cells.

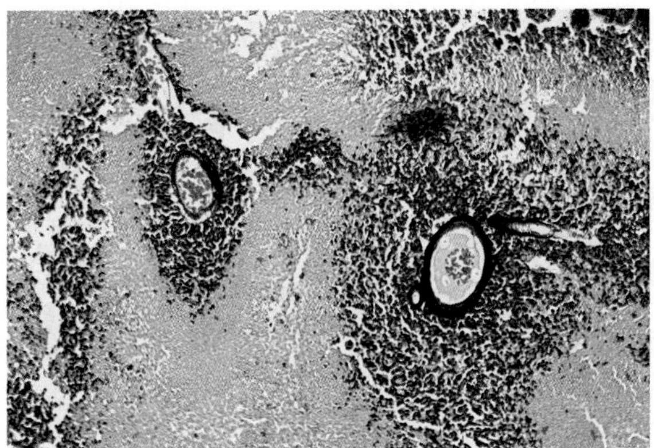

Figure 3-17

RETINOBLASTOMA

Deposits of basophilic material represent DNA released from the necrotic tumor cells. The basophilic material is present in the vessel walls of the tumor.

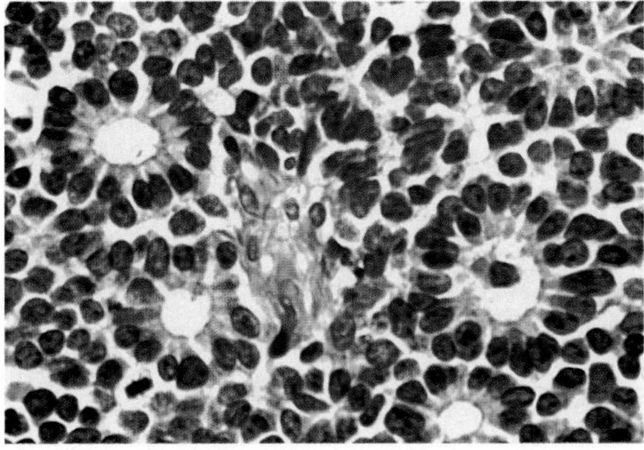

Figure 3-18

RETINOBLASTOMA

Flexner-Wintersteiner rosettes are seen in a well-differentiated retinoblastoma. The rosettes are made up of cuboidal cells; occasional cytoplasmic projections extend into the lumen of the rosettes.

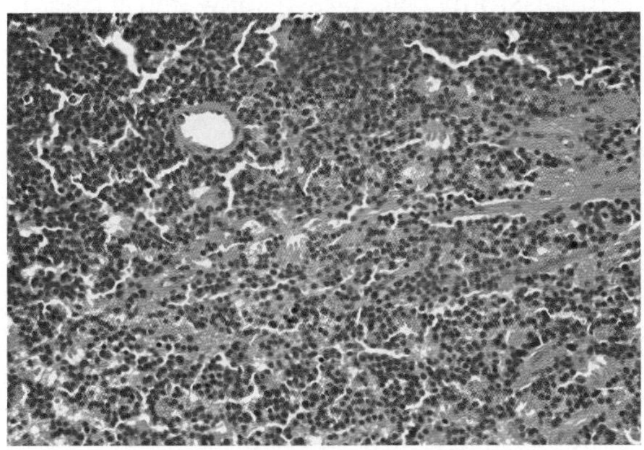

Figure 3-19

RETINOBLASTOMA

Undifferentiated cells (mostly left upper corner) are intermixed with well-differentiated areas displaying fluerettes (lower half of the field).

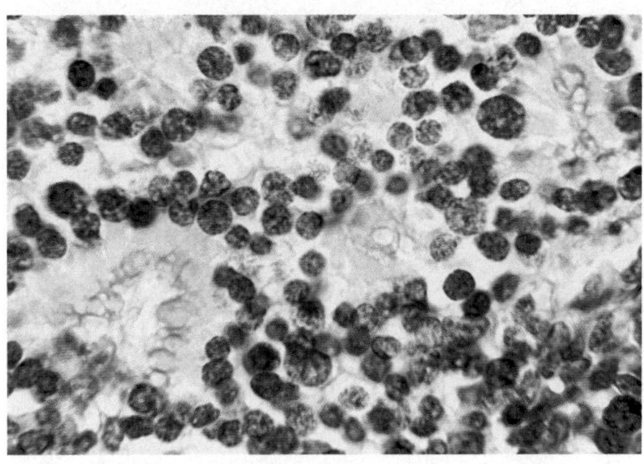

Figure 3-20

RETINOBLASTOMA

The lumens of Flexner-Wintersteiner rosettes contain Alcian blue–positive material that is resistant to hyaluronidase digestion.

Further differentiated retinoblastomas have areas of benign-appearing cells known as fleurettes, with features of photoreceptor differentiation that resemble cone inner segments (fig. 3-21) (12–14). These areas are easily spotted as discrete, comparatively eosinophilic islands, in contrast to the intensely basophilic portion of the tumor. In the benign-appearing area, the neoplastic cells have abundant cytoplasm and smaller nuclei. Mitotic figures are rare, and necrosis may be absent. There may be scattered deposits of calcium. The benign-appearing cells, in groups or individually, have long cytoplasmic processes, which extend through a fenestrated membrane and commonly fan out like a bouquet of flowers (fig. 3-21) (12–14). The fleurettes are resistant to radiation and are seen both in tumors with malignant features and in the benign counterpart of retinoblastoma, retinocytoma (15,35).

Even though they are not specific for retinoblastoma, Homer-Wright rosettes (fig. 3-22) are seen in both undifferentiated and differentiated retinoblastomas. These rosettes resemble

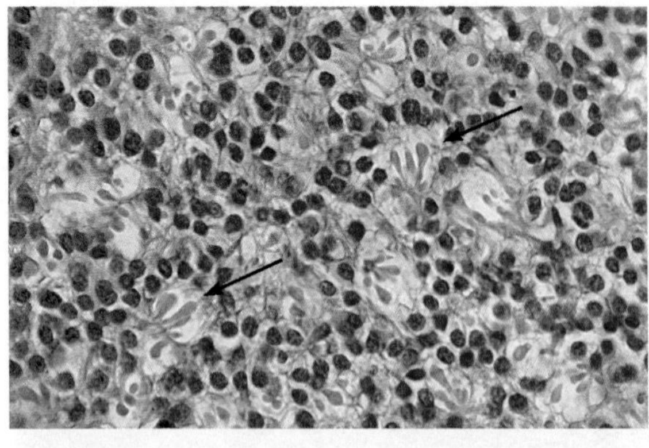

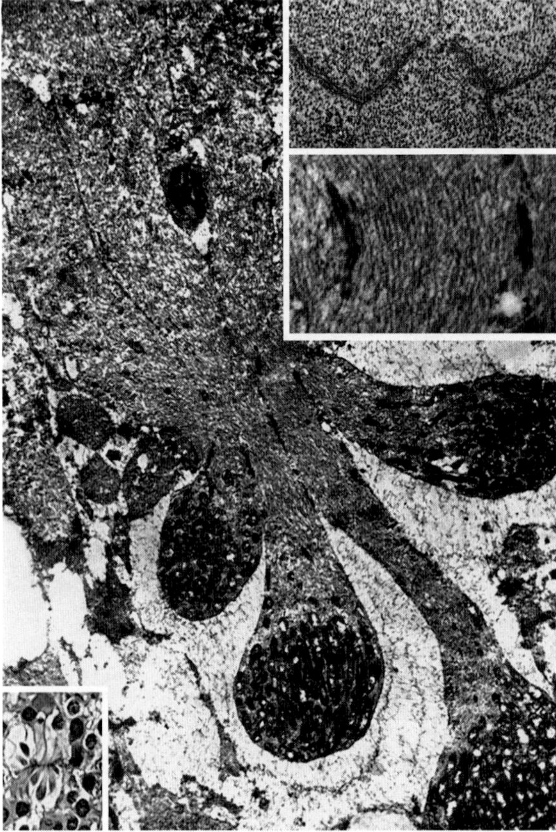

Figure 3-21

RETINOBLASTOMA

Top: Fleurettes (arrows) are seen among tumor cells. Bottom: Ultrastructurally, the fleurettes reveal photoreceptor differentiation resembling cone inner segments.

Flexner-Wintersteiner rosettes, but they lack a lumen. Instead, extensions of cytoplasmic processes form a tangle of neurofibrillary structures in the center of the rosette.

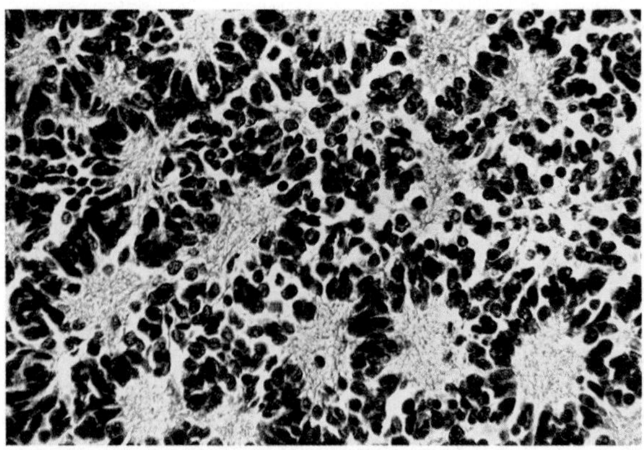

Figure 3-22

RETINOBLASTOMA

Neurofibrillary structures are seen in the center of the Homer-Wright rosettes.

Phthisical globes harboring totally necrotic retinoblastoma (fig. 3-23A) show dense calcification and complete coagulative necrosis of the tumor cells. There is exuberant proliferation of RPE cells and ciliary epithelium, gliosis, and ossification. In such cases, the histologic diagnosis of retinoblastoma may be difficult (3). Calcification may outline the tumor cells. Similar gross and microscopic features are seen in tumors treated with radiation (fig. 3-23B,C).

Extraocular Extension and Metastasis. The most common method of extraocular spread of retinoblastoma is by invasion through the optic disc into the optic nerve (fig. 3- 24). From the retrobulbar nerve the tumor spreads along the nerve fibers into the optic chiasm or infiltrates through the pia into the subarachnoid space. From this site the tumor cells gain access to cerebrospinal fluid and spread to the brain and spinal cord. Tumors that invade the choroid may gain access to the sclera and orbit (fig. 3-25). Extraocular extension increases the risk of metastasis by lymphatic or hematogenous dissemination.

Hematogenous spread of retinoblastoma leads to widespread metastasis to lung, bone, brain, and other viscera. Lymphatic spread occurs with retinoblastomas that extend to the bulbar conjunctiva and eyelids. The metastatic lesions are typically less differentiated than the primary tumor, and rosettes are rarely observed. Fleurettes have not been noted at metastatic sites. Intracranial metastasis can be confused with *trilateral retinoblastoma*; the latter entity

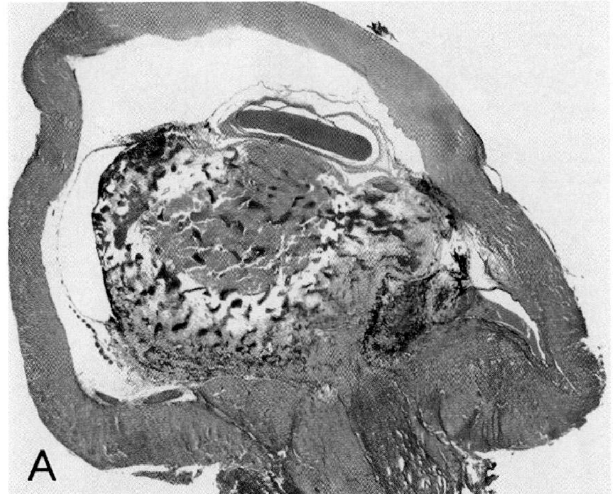

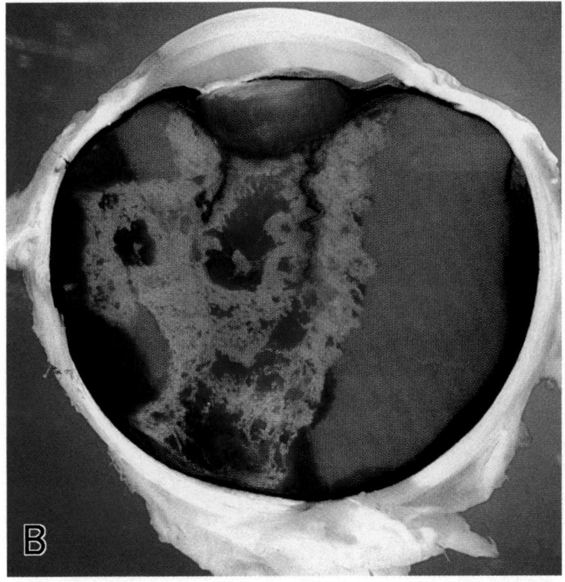

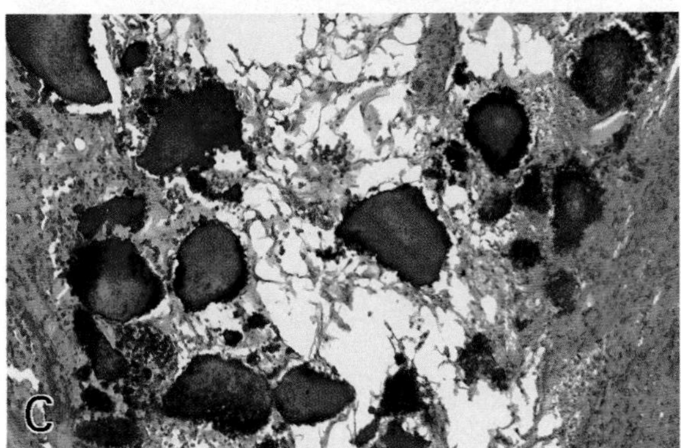

Figure 3-23

RETINOBLASTOMA

A: Phthisical globe harbors a regressed retinoblastoma with foci of calcification.

B: Gross appearance of necrotic retinoblastoma with foci of hemorrhage following radiation.

C: The regressed tumor has extensive areas of calcification.

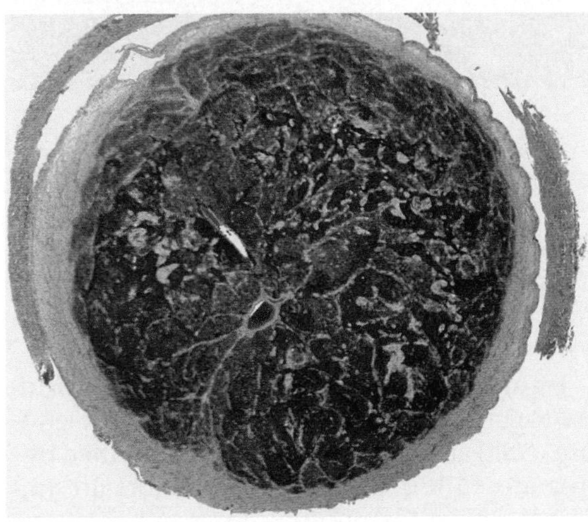

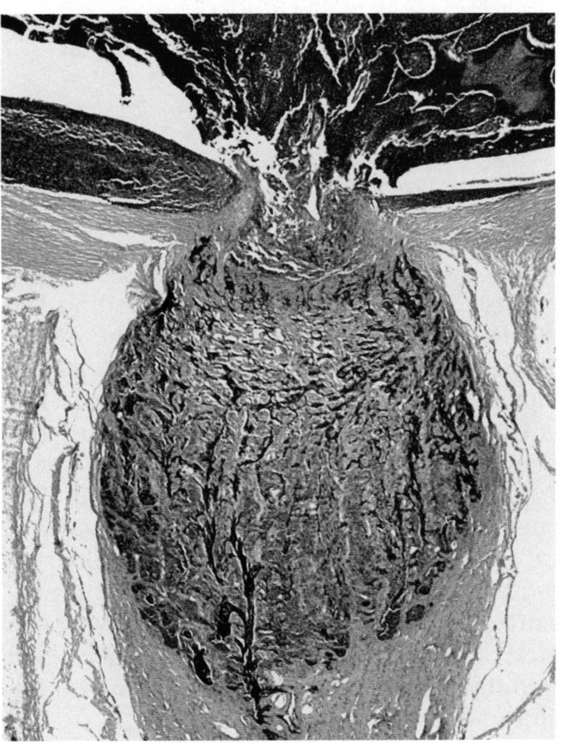

Figure 3-24

RETINOBLASTOMA

Above: The tumor invades the optic nerve along the nerve fiber bundles.

Right: Transverse section of the nerve shows invasion by retinoblastoma cells.

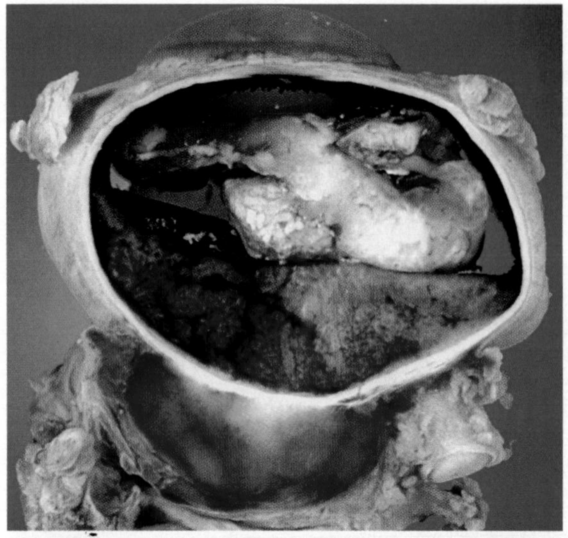

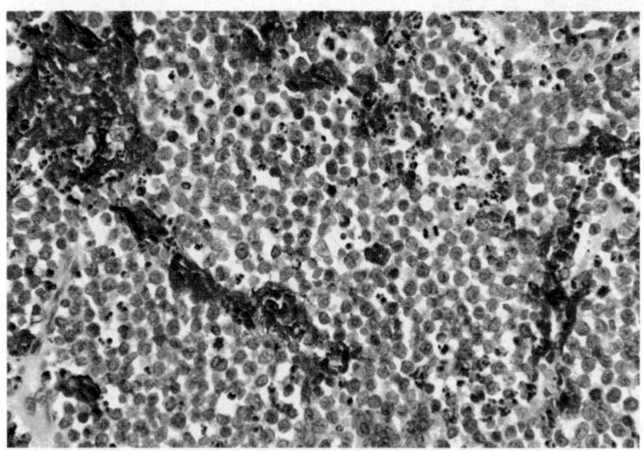

Figure 3-25

RETINOBLASTOMA

Top: Massive choroidal and orbital invasion.
Bottom: There is diffuse infiltration by undifferentiated tumor cells.

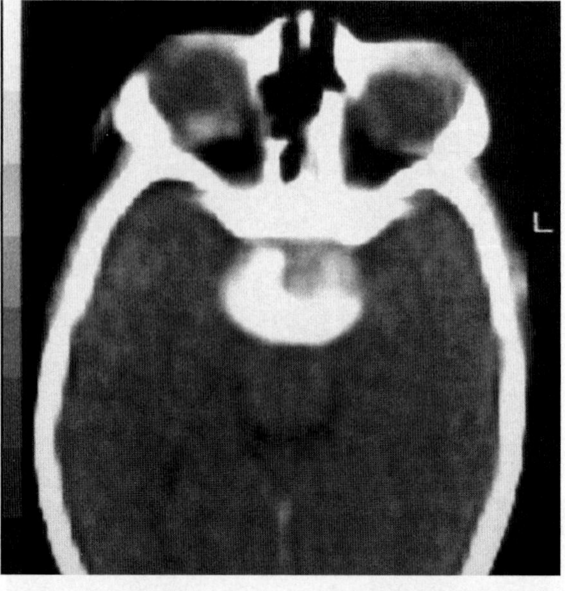

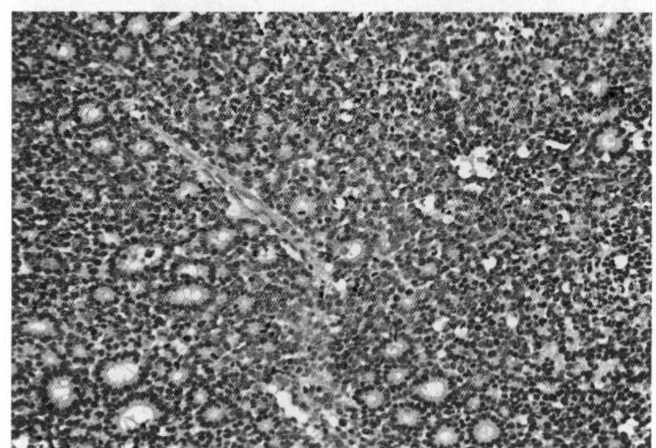

Figure 3-26

TRILATERAL RETINOBLASTOMA

Top: CT scan shows bilateral intraocular tumors and a mass in the region of the pineal gland.
Bottom: Low magnification of the pineal tumor shows Flexner-Wintersteiner rosettes.

consists of bilateral retinoblastomas and the occurrence of a similar tumor in the pineal gland (fig. 3-26) and parasellar sites. Unlike the metastasis, the intracranial component of trilateral retinoblastoma does have rosettes and fleurettes (3,4).

Retinoblastoma can recur in the orbit after enucleation of the globe as a result of subclinical involvement of the orbit, incomplete removal of the orbital component, and/or invasion of the optic nerve beyond the plane of surgical transection. Usually recurrent tumors show undifferentiated features. They rarely reveal calcification and necrosis.

Immunohistochemical Findings. Retinoblastoma cells react with neuron-specific enolase (NSE) at the differentiated and undifferentiated areas (36). Differentiated tumors are immunoreactive for photoreceptor proteins, primarily cone opsin, although some tumors are reactive to the rod opsin, interphotoreceptor retinol-binding protein (IRBP), and S-antigen (5, 6,36,37). These immunohistochemical findings indicate the neuronal nature of retinoblastoma with photoreceptor-like features. Staining for focal glial cell differentiation with glial fibrillary acidic protein (GFAP), along with staining with NSE, has been reported (fig. 3-27) (38). The GFAP-positive glial cells may be reactive astrocytes (36,37).

Immunolocalization of Rb protein (pRB) using various monoclonal and polyclonal antibodies developed against pRB reveals staining in the cytoplasm and nucleus of the tumor cells. This positive immunoreaction is believed to be caused by the presence of mutant *RB1* gene transcripts in the neoplastic cells (39).

Ultrastructural Findings. Ultrastructural examination of a well-differentiated tumor with Flexner-Wintersteiner rosettes shows photoreceptor-like differentiation. The cytoplasm of the cells forming the rosettes has prominent mitochondria, microtubules, and zonula adherens-like junctions similar to those noted in the inner segments of photoreceptor cells. The cytoplasmic projections found in the Flexner-Wintersteiner rosettes may also show cilia with a 9+0 pattern and lamellated membrane structures that resemble discs of photoreceptor outer segments. The neoplastic cells forming fleurettes also show photoreceptor differentiation (see fig. 3-21), displaying more abundant cytoplasm and bulbous processes containing numerous mitochondria which resemble cone inner segments (14). The foci of calcification show needle-like structures within the mitochondrial membranes of the neoplastic cells, with disrupted plasmalemma (40).

Cytologic Findings. Cytologic examination of aqueous and vitreous humor is useful for diagnosing retinoblastomas with atypical clinical features that present with cells in the intraocular cavities. The neoplastic cells are seen singly or in clusters, display prominent nuclei with scanty cytoplasm, and are associated with necrotic debris (fig. 3-28). Capillaries surrounded by viable tumor cells may be found.

Fine-needle aspiration biopsy material reveals two types of cells: cells with prominent nuclei and scanty cytoplasm and cells with striking cytoplasmic processes. The latter may form Flexner-Wintersteiner rosettes; however, such rosettes may not be common, and occasionally, Homer-Wright rosettes are seen. Along with necrotic debris, calcific deposits may be observed (41).

Differential Diagnosis. Medulloepithelioma may be mistaken for retinoblastoma. Similar to retinoblastoma, the former tumor occurs mainly in children; however, medulloepithelioma, which is clinically diagnosed at about 5 years of age, generally arises from ciliary epithelium. Histologically, medulloepithelioma has proliferating medullary epithelium arranged in cords and sheets. The cords show single or multilayered columnar epithelium that may resemble embryonic retina. Cystic spaces lined by the neoplastic cells and containing hyaluronic acid are a common feature. Heterotopic elements such as blasts may be present in some. Malignant medulloepithelioma may show Flexner-Wintersteiner rosettes and sheets of basophilic cells similar to retinoblastoma.

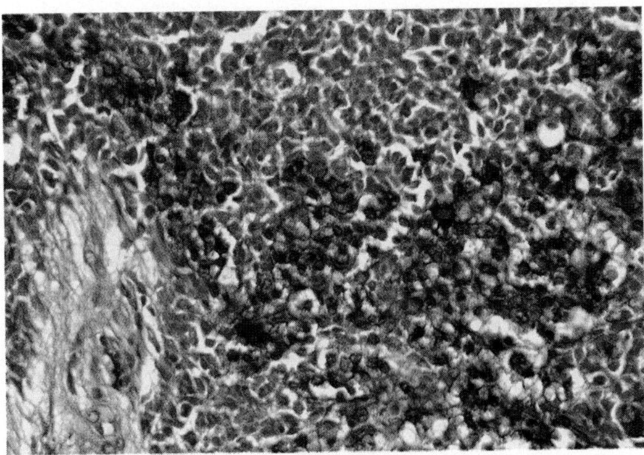

Figure 3-27

RETINOBLASTOMA

Tumor cells are immunoreactive for neuron-specific enolase.

Although nematode endophthalmitis (fig. 3-29), persistent hyperplastic primary vitreous (fig. 3-30), and Coats' disease (fig. 3-31) may be clinically mistaken for retinoblastoma, these lesions are diagnosed without difficulty by their characteristic histopathologic features. Nematode endophthalmitis is a sclerosing, chronic vitreous body inflammation caused by *Toxocara* larva (fig. 3-29). Persistent hyperplastic primary vitreous shows a retrolental fibrovascular mass, ruptured posterior lens capsule, and elongated ciliary processes that are drawn into the mass (fig. 3-30). Clinically, Coats' disease may mimic exophytic retinoblastoma; histologically, however, the retina shows telangiectatic vessels with accumulations of eosinophilic exudate in the outer retinal layers and subretinal space (fig. 3-31).

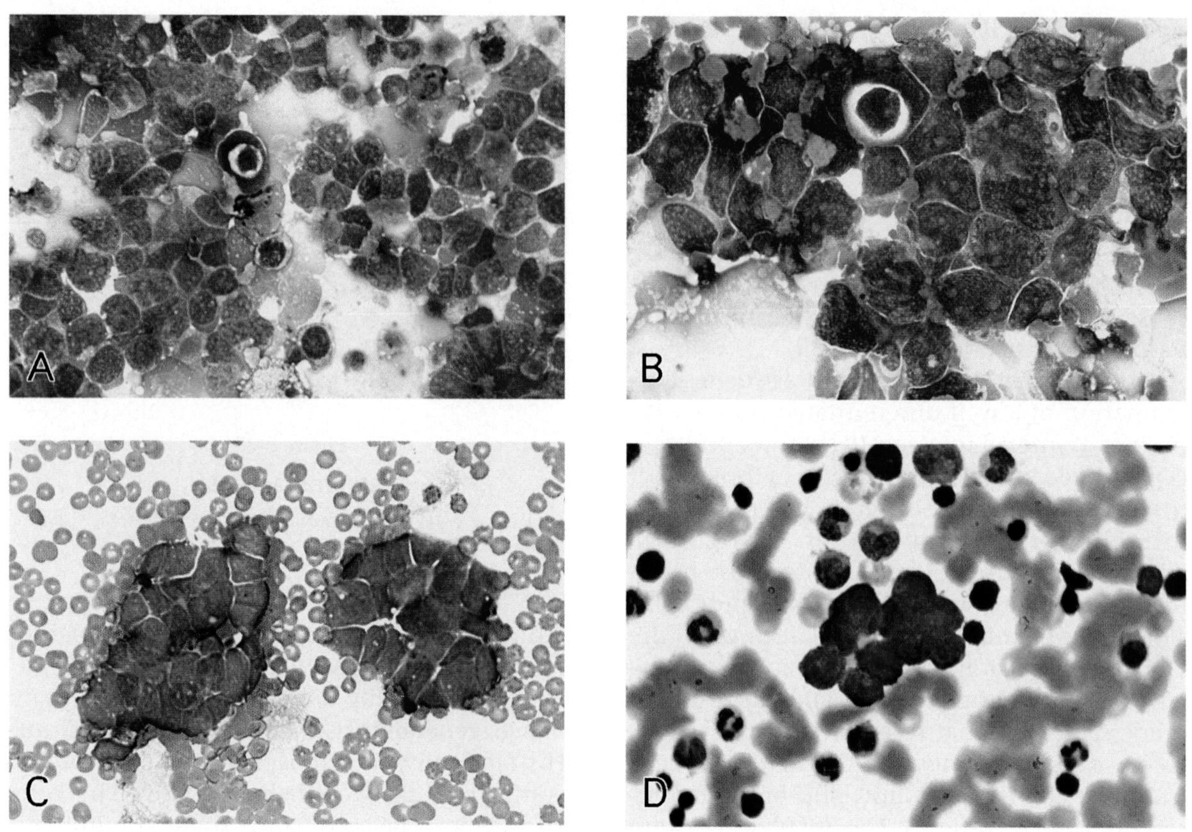

Figure 3-28

RETINOBLASTOMA

Cytologic preparations show clusters of tumor cells with prominent pleomorphic nuclei and scanty cytoplasm in aspirates from the anterior chamber (A), the vitreous (B), the cerebrospinal fluid (C), and the bone marrow (D).

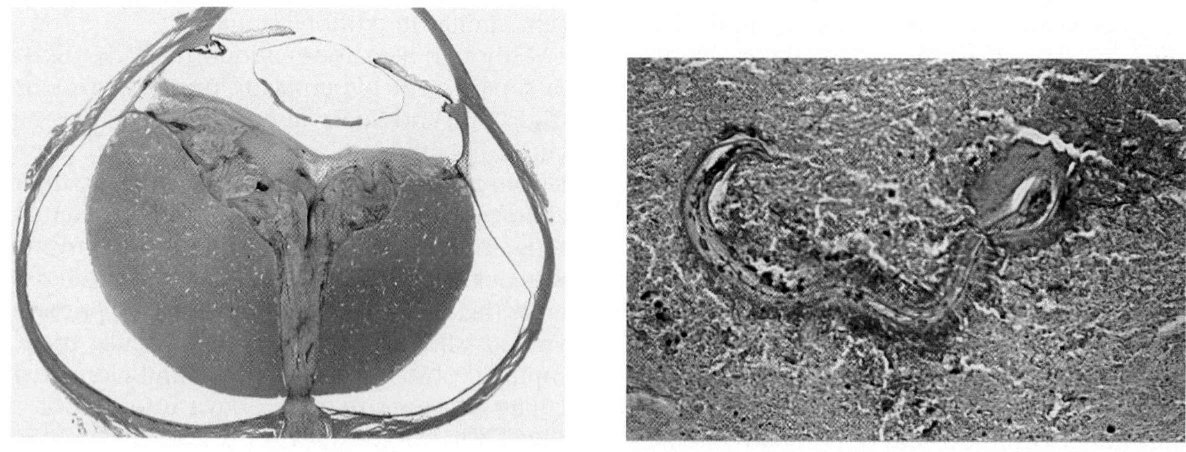

Figure 3-29

NEMATODE ENDOPHTHALMITIS

Left: A sclerosing inflammatory mass is present behind the lens, leading to total retinal detachment.
Right: A degenerated nematode larva is seen in the retrolental mass.

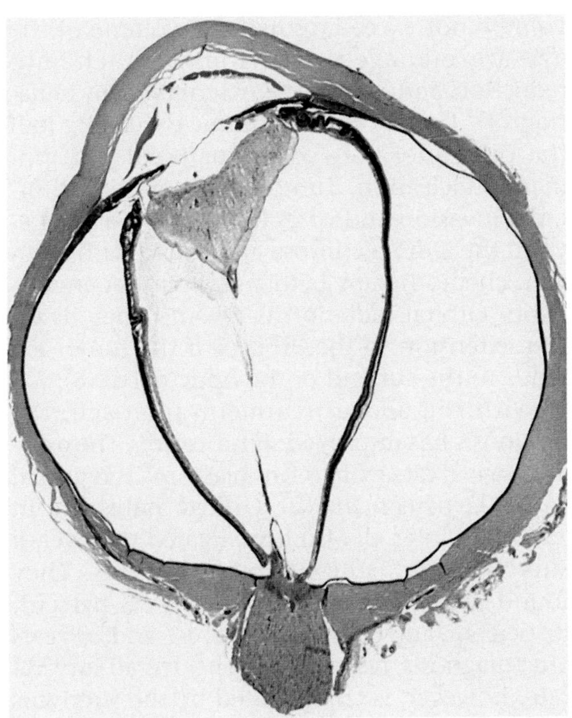

Figure 3-30

PERSISTENT HYPERPLASTIC PRIMARY VITREOUS

A retrolental mass and a persistent hyaloid vessel are present in the vitreous cavity.

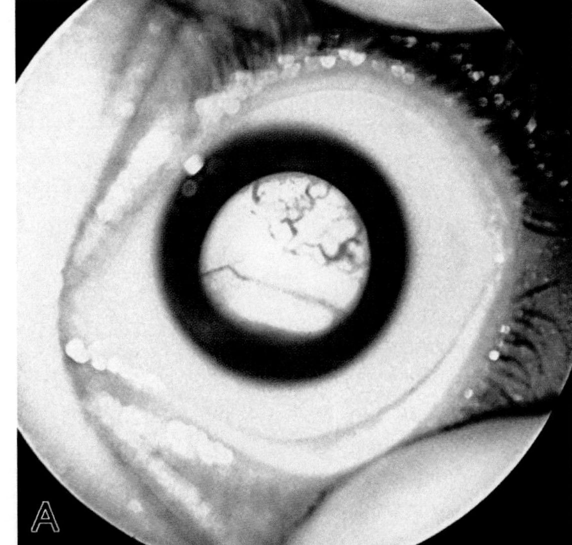

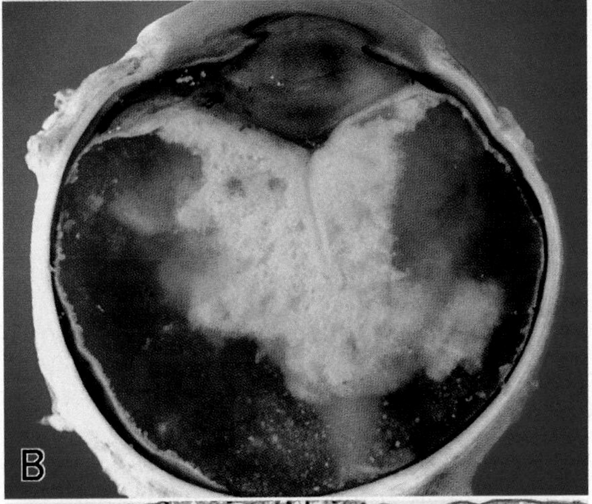

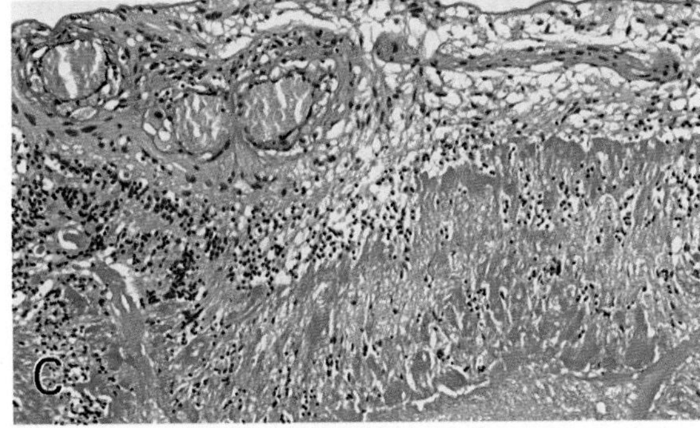

Figure 3-31

COATS' DISEASE

A: Coats' disease presenting with leukocoria.

B: Gross examination of the enucleated globe reveals retinal detachment and accumulation of lipid-rich exudates in the subretinal space.

C: There are dilated vessels and accumulation of PAS-positive exudates in the outer retina and subretinal space.

The subretinal exudates contain lipids and stain with the periodic acid–Schiff (PAS) stain.

Treatment and Prognosis. The risk factors for metastasis in patients with retinoblastoma have been studied extensively. In a current study (42), the following factors were found to be independently associated with the development of metastases: optic nerve invasion, with or without extension of the tumor to the resection site; choroidal invasion; and enucleation of an affected eye more than 120 days after initial diagnosis.

Since the management of retinoblastoma depends on staging, Reese and Ellsworth (43) proposed criteria for suitability for treatment. They grouped the findings into patients with very favorable, favorable, doubtful, unfavorable, or very unfavorable prognoses (Table 3-3). In recent years, other staging systems have been introduced (Table 3-4); however, none of these schemes significantly correlate with progression-free survival (44,45). Staging, however, may

Table 3-3

REESE-ELLSWORTH CLASSIFICATION OF RETINOBLASTOMA CRITERIA FOR SUITABILITY FOR TREATMENT[a]

Group I: Very favorable prognosis
A. Solitary tumor, less than 4 dd[b] in size, at or behind the equator
B. Multiple tumors, none over 4 dd in size, all at or behind the equator
Group II: Favorable prognosis
A. Solitary lesions 4-10 dd in size, at or behind the equator
B. Multiple tumors, 4-10 dd in size, behind the equator
Group III: Doubtful prognosis
A. Any lesion anterior to the equator
B. Solitary tumors larger than 10 dd behind the equator
Group IV: Unfavorable prognosis
A. Multiple tumors, some larger than 10 dd
B. Any lesion extending anteriorly to the ora serrata
Group V: Very unfavorable prognosis
A. Massive tumors involving over half the retina
B. Vitreous seeding

[a]Modified from reference 45.
[b]dd = optic disc diameter.

identify patients at higher risk and may be useful in selecting appropriate treatment (44,45).

Retinoblastoma management varies from cryodestruction of the tumor to enucleation of the globe harboring the mass. In some cases, enucleation is followed by adjuvant chemotherapy (8). Factors such as location and size of the tumor, diffuse intraocular spread of the mass, massive choroidal involvement and/or invasion of the optic nerve posterior to the lamina cribrosa, and extraocular extension determine whether the patient receives the local treatment only or adjuvant chemotherapy. Peripheral, small retinoblastomas are usually treated by cryotherapy, and posterior tumors are managed by direct laser photocoagulation. Tumors located away from the disc and macula, measuring 10 mm or less and without diffuse vitreous seedings, are usually treated by brachytherapy. Larger tumors not exceeding 15 mm are managed with multidrug (three chemotherapeutic agents) chemoreduction combined with cryotherapy, brachytherapy, or laser therapy. Patients with diffuse intraocular disease, vitreous seeding, and tumor volume not exceeding half the volume of the eye are managed with four-drug chemoreduction and whole eye external beam radiation (8). Tumors with a volume exceeding half the volume of the eye are managed with primary enucleation. Tumors with massive choroidal invasion and/or optic nerve invasion beyond the lamina cribrosa are treated with adjuvant chemotherapy before and/or after enucleation. Orbital radiation is given if there is direct extension to the orbit or if the tumor extends to the cut end of the optic nerve (8).

With the above treatment approach, the prognosis has improved significantly. The overall survival rate from retinoblastoma is reported to be 92 percent in the United States (8). In 1985, Rubin et al. (46) investigated the overall survival data using life-table analysis. They found predicted survival rates of 93 percent, 82 percent, and 66 percent at 5, 10, and 20 years after diagnosis, respectively. The overall survival rate, however, is complicated by the survivors of bilateral retinoblastoma, who have a high risk of developing a second malignant neoplasm. Eng et al. (47) found that 35 percent of bilaterally affected patients who were treated with external beam radiation died within 40 years after the diagnosis of retinoblastoma from a second malignant tumor, whereas only 6 percent of bilaterally affected individuals who were not treated with external beam radiation died from such second malignancies. A study by the AFIP (48) showed the 30-year cumulative incidence of second malignant neoplasms was 35 percent for patients receiving radiotherapy, compared to 6 percent for those who did not receive such therapy. Moreover, the incidence rate of such second malignancies was 29 percent inside the radiation field and 8 percent outside the field. The latter figure was not significantly different from the rate reported for patients who did not receive radiotherapy. The most common second tumor developing in and out of the field of irradiation in retinoblastoma survivors is sarcoma, followed by melanoma and epithelial malignancies such as sebaceous carcinoma, squamous cell carcinoma, and transitional cell carcinoma. Among the sarcomas, osteogenic sarcoma was most common, followed by spindle cell sarcoma, chondrosarcoma, and leiomyosarcoma (48–50). Survivors

Table 3-4

A: STAGING AND GROUPING OF RETINOBLASTOMA—ST. JUDE STAGING SCHEMA[a]

Stage I:	Tumor (unifocal or multifocal) confined to retina
	A. Occupying 1 quadrant or less
	B. Occupying 2 quadrants or less
	C. Occupying more than 50 percent of retinal surface
Stage II:	Tumor (unifocal or multifocal) confined to globe
	A. With vitreous seeding
	B. Extending to optic nerve head
	C. Extending to choroid
	D. Extending to choroid and optic nerve head
	E. Extending to emissaries
Stage III:	Extraocular extension of tumor (regional)
	A. Extending beyond cut end of optic nerve (including subarachnoid extension)
	B. Extending through sclera into orbital contents
	C. Extending to choroid and beyond cut end of optic nerve (including subarachnoid extension)
	D. Extending through sclera into orbital contents and beyond cut end of optic nerve (including subarachnoid extension)
Stage IV:	Distant Metastases
	A. Extending through optic nerve to brain
	B. Blood-borne metastases to soft tissues and bone
	C. Bone marrow metastases

B: MODIFIED ST. JUDE STAGING AND GROUPING OF RETINOBLASTOMA[a]

Stage I:	Tumor confined to the retina
	A. Solitary: <6 dd[b]
	B. Multiple; all <6 dd
	C. Solitary or multiple lesions involving < 50 percent of retinal surface behind equator
	D. > 50 percent retinal involvement, behind equator
	E. > 50 percent retinal involvement, or with involvement anterior to equator
Stage II:	Tumor confined to globe/extraretinal
	A. Extends to optic nerve head
	B. 1. Extends to choroid
	2. Extends to choroid with replacement
	C. Anterior chamber involvement
	D. Extends to choroid (1 or 2) and optic nerve
Stage III:	Extrachoroidal extension
	A. Extends to emissaries
	B. Extends beyond cut end of optic nerve (including subarachnoid)
	C. Extends through sclera into orbit
	D. Extends to choroid (1 or 2) and beyond cut end of optic nerve (includes subarachnoid)
	E. Extends through sclera and cut end of optic nerve
Stage IV:	Distant disease
	A. Extends through optic nerve into brain (includes positive cerebrospinal fluid)
	B. Blood-borne metastases to soft tissue, nodes, or bone
	C. Bone marrow metastases

[a]Modified from reference 45.
[b]dd = optic disc diameter.

of heritable retinoblastomas may develop pinealoblastoma. Survivors of retinoblastoma, particularly those receiving radiation therapy, are also found to have a higher risk for developing additional nonocular tumors, usually of the soft tissues of the head and skin (50).

Retinocytoma

Retinocytoma is composed of totally benign-appearing cells and fleurettes (15). The neoplastic cells form plaquoid noninvasive lesions, and they do not exhibit necrosis or mitotic figures (fig. 3-32). These tumors may contain glial cells,

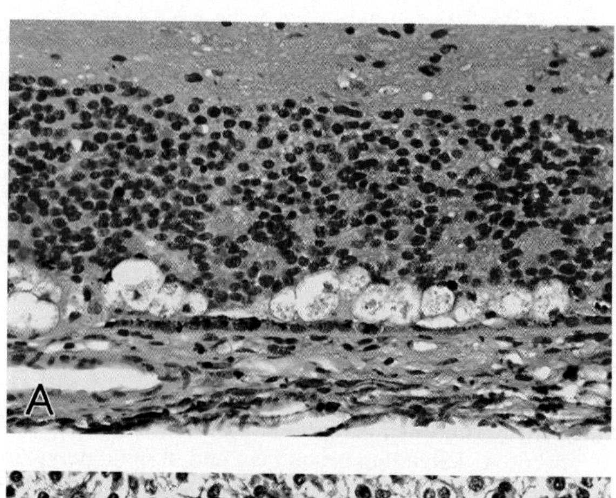

Figure 3-32

RETINOCYTOMA

A: Benign-appearing tumor cells form numerous fleurettes.

B: Areas of calcification.

C: The tumor cells have benign cytologic features.

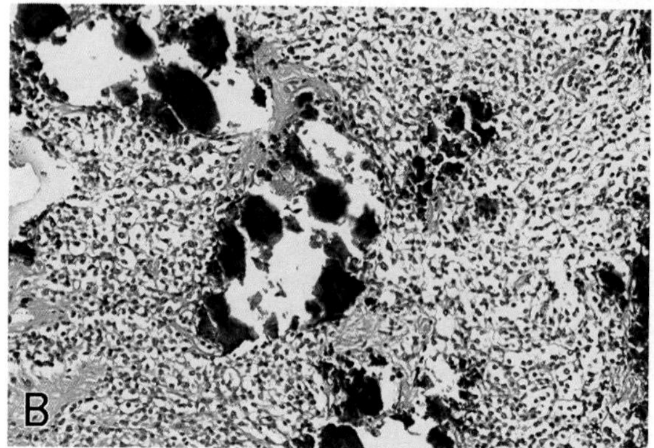

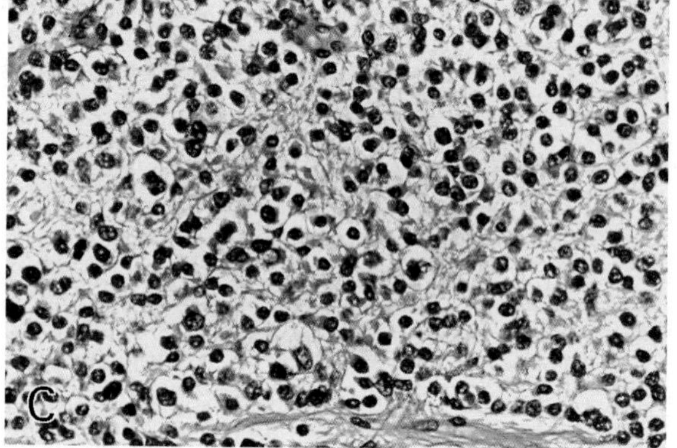

which likely represent reactive gliosis. Although most retinocytomas follow a benign clinical course, malignant transformation has been reported in a few (51).

GLIAL TUMORS AND TUMOR-LIKE CONDITIONS

Astrocytoma

Astrocytic tumors of the retina are rare. These tumors can be solitary in individuals without the stigmata of phakomatosis, or they can be multiple in individuals with tuberous sclerosis or neurofibromatosis (52,53). In such phakomatoses, the glial tumors are mostly hamartomas. A review of 42 histologically documented astrocytic tumors showed that 29 percent occurred in individuals without tuberous sclerosis or neurofibromatosis; the remaining 71 percent occurred in individuals with tuberous sclerosis (57 percent) or neurofibromatosis (14 percent) (53).

Histologically, there are elongated, fibrous astrocytes with small oval nuclei and an interlacing cytoplasmic process that forms a fine meshwork. The tumor cells are immunoreactive to GFAP. Rarely, the tumors are made up of giant astrocytes that may show Müller cell differentiation (54,55). Astrocytomas have a benign course; the entire lesion is localized to the retina without infiltrative margins or destruction of the internal limiting membrane and Bruch membrane.

Astrocytic Hamartoma

Astrocytic hamartoma, which is similar to astrocytoma, occurs in patients with tuberous sclerosis and neurofibromatosis (56,57). The hamartomas contain giant astrocytes, are often multiple, and are located peripherally in patients with tuberous sclerosis. They can also be seen in the peripapillary retina (58). Early lesions are flat and translucent; older lesions may show calcification. Occasional peripapillary astrocytic hamartomas present with vitreous body seeding (58). Clinically, astrocytomas and astrocytic hamartomas may be confused with retinoblastoma.

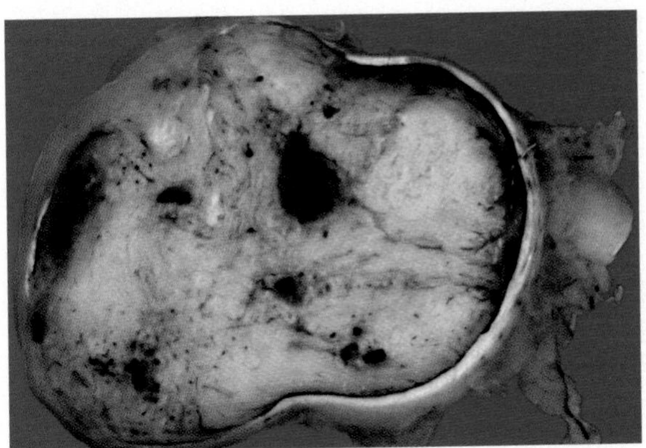

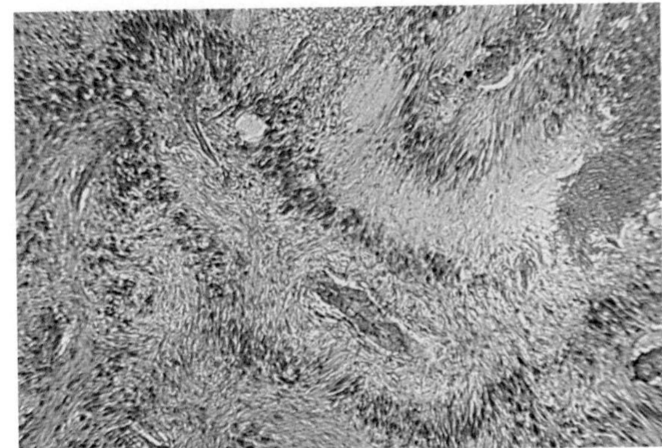

Figure 3-33

RETINAL MASSIVE GLIOSIS

Left: Gross appearance of massive gliosis of the retina.
Right: Reactive astrocytes with abundant pale eosinophilic cytoplasm form bundles of spindle-shaped cells.

Massive Gliosis of the Retina

Massive glial proliferation simulating a neoplasm occurs in eyes with underlying pathologic processes such as retinitis, longstanding retinal detachment, or central retinal vein occlusion during childhood (59–62). Histologically, the massive gliosis is made up of interweaving bundles of spindle-shaped astrocytes (fig. 3-33). Such astrocytes contain small nuclei and abundant, pale, eosinophilic cytoplasm. The glial mass also shows numerous, dilated, thick-walled blood vessels. Foci of calcification and ossification may be present in longstanding lesions. Immunohistochemical and electron microscopic studies reveal that the glial cells are of Müller cell origin (62).

VASCULAR TUMORS

Angiomatosis Retinae

This benign angioblastic tumor, which develops in about 60 percent of patients with von Hippel-Lindau (VHL) disease, is also known as *capillary hemangioma of von Hippel* or *hemangioblastoma of the retina* (63–65). VHL disease is dominantly inherited and confers a predisposition for the development of angiomatosis retinae and various nonocular tumors (63). The latter include hemangioblastomas of the central nervous system (CNS), renal cell carcinoma, pheochromocytoma, and pancreatic tumors.

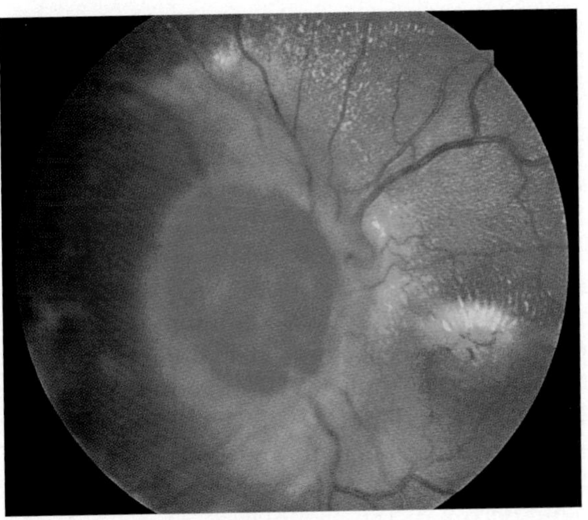

Figure 3-34

ANGIOMATOSIS RETINAE

Ophthalmoscopic examination shows a reddish pink mass at the juxtapapillary retina. Prominent intraretinal lipoidal exudates surround the mass.

Ophthalmoscopic examination shows pink (fig. 3-34) or yellow retinal tumors supplied by a large artery and vein. Secondary retinal detachment due to exudation may develop, and sometimes there is hemorrhage, fibrosis, and gliosis. Histopathologically, the tumor is made up of small vascular channels of different sizes (fig. 3-35) interposed by vacuolated or foamy stromal cells (66). The origin of these stromal cells is not clear; they may represent histiocytes, endothelial cells, or astrocytes.

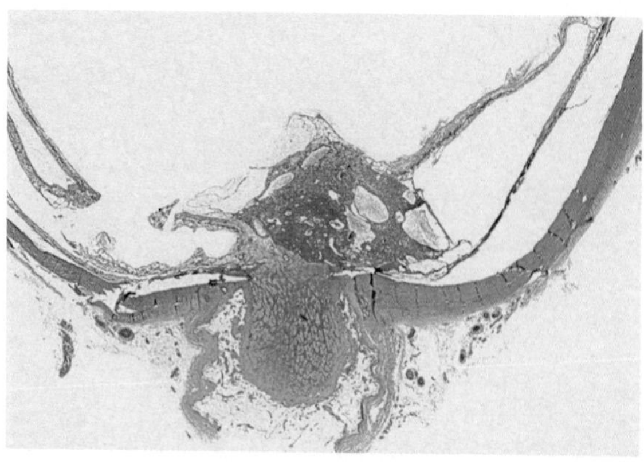

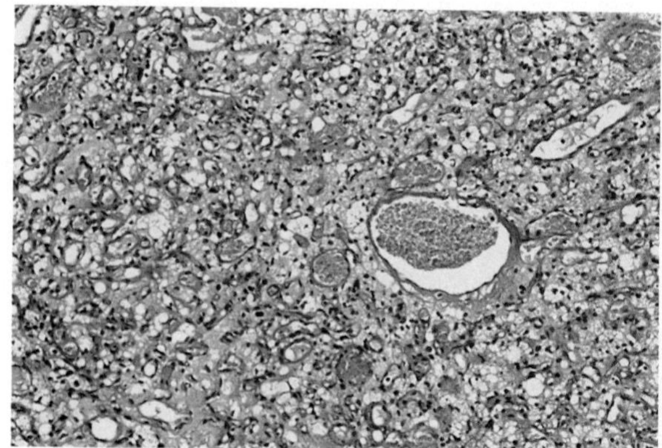

Figure 3-35

ANGIOMATOSIS RETINAE

Left: A juxtapapillary angioma, composed of vascular channels of variable size, in an enucleated eye.

Right: Higher magnification reveals numerous vascular channels and lipidized stromal cells that exhibit prominent foamy cytoplasm (periodic acid–Schiff [PAS] stain).

The *VHL* gene is localized to the short arm of chromosome 3 (3P25.5) and is characterized as a tumor suppressor gene. The development of various tumors associated with VHL disease may require, in most instances, inactivation of both the alleles: the first involving a germline mutation, and the second at the somatic level (67,68). Moreover, the *VHL* gene product, VHL protein, has been shown to inhibit vascular endothelial growth factor (VEGF) under normoxic conditions. The mutant VHL protein cannot regulate the transcription of VEGF mRNA, resulting in vascular proliferation and formation of new blood vessels. Loss of heterozygosity of the *VHL* gene occurs in the vacuolated stromal cells of angiomatosis retinae. These stromal cells also express VEGF mRNA and VEGF protein, suggesting that stromal cells could be the true neoplastic cells of retinal angioma and that the vascular component may result from VEGF expressed by these neoplastic stromal cells (68).

Retinal tumors are usually managed by photocoagulation or cryotherapy. Larger angiomas are treated by plaque therapy or external beam radiation.

Cavernous Hemangioma

Rarely, *cavernous hemangiomas* develop in the retina, usually bilaterally as a manifestation of a probably autosomal dominant inheritance pattern with incomplete penetrance (69,70). Retinal angiomas may be observed in conjunction with CNS and/or cutaneous angiomas (70,71). Such findings suggest that the entity could be considered as a phakomatosis (70). Cavernous, the hemangioma presents as clusters of dark-red saccular aneurysms. Histopathologically, large vascular channels with normal walls are seen. Angiographically, these vascular channels do not leak fluorescein dye (71).

MELANOGENIC NEUROECTODERMAL TUMOR OF THE RETINA

Melanogenic neuroectodermal tumor of the retina, also known as *primary malignant melanoma of the retina*, is a rare neoplasm arising from the retina. These tumors display poorly differentiated neuroblastic cells and anaplastic epithelioid cells. The tumor cells are immunoreactive for HMB45. Electron microscopy reveals premelanosomes in the tumor cells (72).

LYMPHOID MALIGNANCIES

Primary Intraocular Lymphoma

Definition. Approximately 98 percent of *primary intraocular lymphomas* are extranodal, non-Hodgkin's B-cell lymphomas, which, as the name implies, are localized to the intraocular structures: vitreous body, retina, and subretinal and sub-RPE spaces. This is in contrast to secondary involvement of the eye by nodal lymphoma, in which mainly the uvea is infiltrated by the tumor cells. Primary intraocular lymphoma may occur in isolation, without CNS involvement; however, since the ocular and CNS components have identical cytologic features and phenotypic expression, these two entities are lumped under the heading *primary central nervous system lymphoma* (PCNSL). Approximately 2 percent of these are *T-cell lymphomas*. Others, such as *Ki-1 lymphoma, lymphomatoid granulomatosis, T-cell–rich B-cell lymphoma, signet ring cell lymphoma, angiotrophic lymphoma,* and *plasmacytoma*, occur even more rarely (73,74).

General Features. Many names have been applied to the entity that is now referred to as PCNSL, including reticulum cell sarcoma, microglioma, perithelial sarcoma, and lymphosarcoma. These former labels were based on the lack of a clear understanding of the nature of PCNSL. After the introduction of cell surface markers, the infiltrating cells in the vitreous body and the CNS were found to express phenotypic markers for B cells (75–79).

PCNSL most commonly affects individuals in the fifth to seventh decades of life. It is generally considered a rare condition, but its incidence is increasing. Data from the National Cancer Institute reveal that 2.7 cases/10 million people were reported from 1972 to 1974, compared with 7.5 cases/10 million people from 1982 to 1984 (80). This increase was seen in both sexes, even after the exclusion of acquired immunodeficiency syndrome (AIDS) as a risk factor. A continuing increase has been reported during the subsequent years, with 30 cases/10 million people reported in 1991 (81). The reasons for this increase are unknown. Part of the increase is likely due to increased awareness and improved diagnostic techniques, but most of the increase reported in the 1970s to 1980s occurred before the widespread availability of CT. Despite this increase, the risk of an immunocompetent individual developing PCNSL is low.

It is generally held that neither the CNS nor the eye normally contains lymphatic tissue. This fact, combined with the definition of PCNSL as occurring only in the CNS or the eye, raises the issue of the origin of the tumor cells. Different hypotheses exist, but none has been proven unequivocally. It may be that the lymphoma cells arise in a site external to the CNS or retina but are only able to grow unabated in these immunologically sequestered locations (74,82). Another possibility is that these cells may express CNS- and/or retina-specific cell adhesion molecules. There is no evidence, however, that PCNSL cells express cell adhesion molecules that are not present on nodal lymphomas as well (80–83). A separate theory supposes a preexisting polyclonal inflammatory lesion in which a monoclonal proliferation subsequently develops. This theory has been supported by the demonstration of inflammatory lesions preceding the onset of PCNSL in intraocular lymphoma (84).

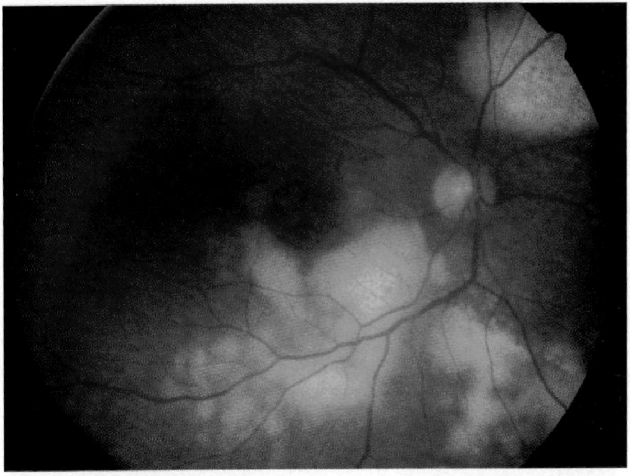

Figure 3-36

PRIMARY INTRAOCULAR LYMPHOMA OF THE RETINA

Lymphoma presents with subretinal and sub-RPE yellowish deposits.

Clinical Features. Involvement of the CNS, vitreous, and retina varies in PCNSL, with evidence of ocular disease reported in 12 to 25 percent of patients (74,85–88). Patients may present with either CNS or ocular complaints or with both. The clinical features vary depending on the site of tumor cell infiltration. These sites include vitreous body, vitreous and retina, sub-RPE (fig. 3-36), CNS, or any combination of these sites.

When ocular findings present first, decreased visual acuity and floaters are typically present. In these cases, the finding of a vitreous body cellular infiltration is the only evidence of the disease. Ocular lesions are described as creamy yellow subretinal infiltrates with overlying RPE detachments; but they may take on many forms, such as discrete white lesions, suggestive of acute retinal necrosis, toxoplasmosis, and other uveitis entities.

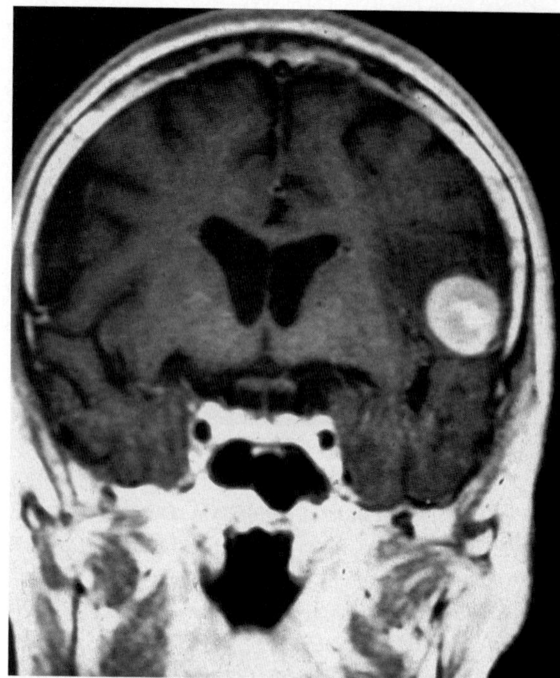

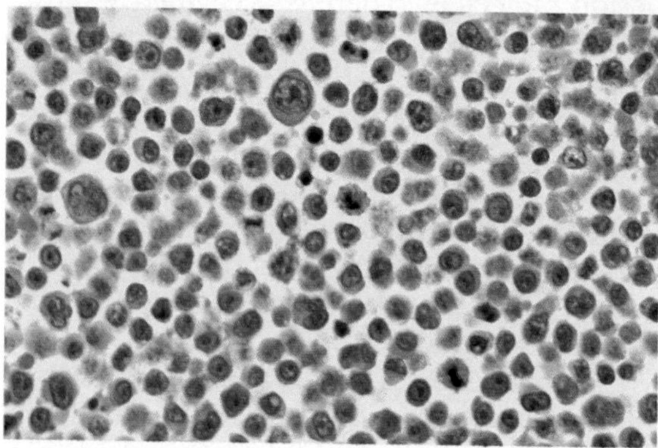

Figure 3-37

PRIMARY CENTRAL NERVOUS SYSTEM LYMPHOMA

Top: CT shows a well-demarcated intracranial mass.
Bottom: Biopsy of the mass reveals a large cell lymphoma of B-cell origin.

In 1999, Herrlinger et al. (89) reviewed the findings when PCNSL involves only the CNS (89). At initial presentation, patients have both general and focal signs and symptoms (90,91). Symptoms attributable to increased intracranial pressure have been reported in 15 to 60 percent of patients (92,93). Because many of the CNS lesions are in the periventricular region, the most frequent single symptom reported at time of admission, occurring in 24 to 73 percent of patients, is behavioral changes (92,94). The most common focal neurologic signs include hemiparesis in 40 to 50 percent and cerebellar signs (including ataxia) in 15 to 40 percent (92,94). At the time of the initial presentation, epileptic seizures are present in 2 to 33 percent and cranial nerve palsies in 5 to 31 percent of patients (95). Although only 1 to 2 percent of PCNSL cases arise in the spinal cord, seeding of lymphoma cells into the cerebrospinal fluid (CSF) has been reported in 42 percent of patients (88).

The diagnosis of PCNSL can be suspected clinically when the patient presents with typical retinal or sub-RPE infiltrates (fig. 3-36). A definitive diagnosis is only established by fluid or tissue specimens from the eye (vitreous and, rarely, chorioretinal biopsy) or the CNS (lumbar puncture or brain biopsy).

CT scans of immunocompetent patients with PCNSL show multiple, diffuse, periventricular lesions of high density before contrast injection. After contrast injection, dense periventricular enhancement appears (fig. 3-37) and may involve the corpus callosum. Systemic corticosteroid therapy may change this pattern, with resolution of the periventricular enhancement. When PCNSL recurs, it may appear different, with solid, ring-like enhancement foci away from the ventricle. MRI shows isointense lesions on T1-, and isointense to hyperintense lesions on T2-weighted imaging. Periventricular contrast enhancement is strong in 75 percent of cases (96).

Analysis of CSF from lumbar puncture may lead to a diagnosis of PCNSL and obviate the need for vitreous biopsies. A positive CSF aspirate has been reported in one third of patients with PCNSL, and multiple lumbar punctures may be needed to make the diagnosis (97). CSF specimens may contain less necrotic debris than vitreous aspirates; therefore, the lymphoma cells should be easier to recognize. On the other hand, there are fewer lymphoma cells, and these cells may not suffice for immunocytologic clonality studies. Because the potential morbidity of a vitreous biopsy is more significant than that of a lumbar puncture, the latter should be tried as the first step for tissue diagnosis.

Gross and Microscopic Findings. Enucleated eyes show a thickened retina with deposits of tumor cells under the RPE (figs. 3-38–3-40).

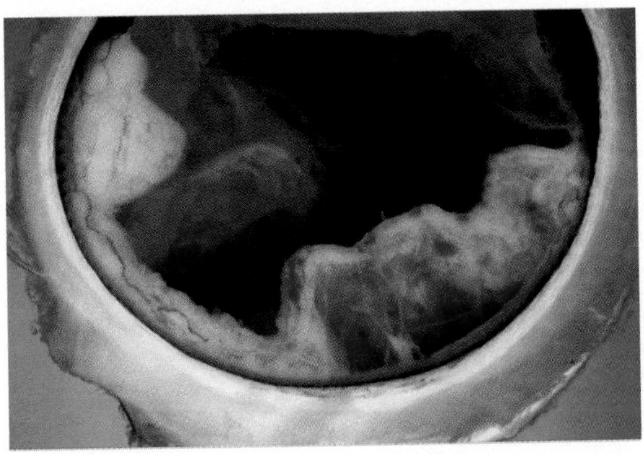

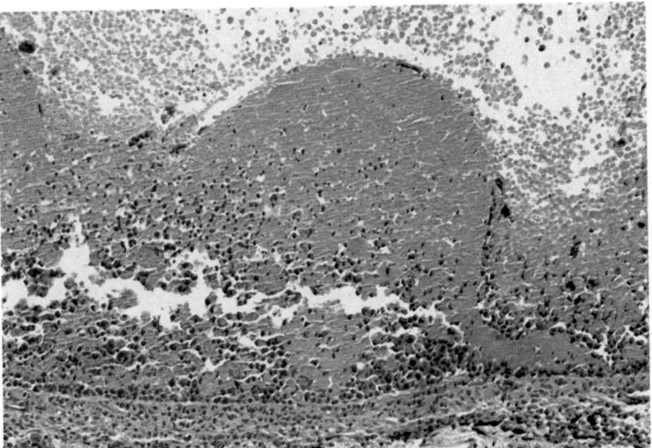

Figure 3-38

PRIMARY INTRAOCULAR B-CELL LYMPHOMA

Left: Diffuse thickening of the retina with deposits of tumor cells under the RPE.
Right: The sub-RPE deposits consist mostly of necrotic tumor cells.

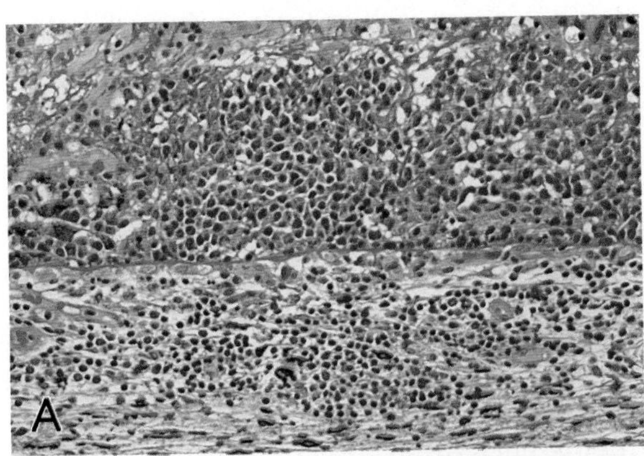

Figure 3-39

PRIMARY INTRAOCULAR B-CELL LYMPHOMA

A: Clusters of tumor cells are under the retina and the RPE. The choroid contains non-neoplastic reactive lymphocytes (PAS stain).

B: The tumor cells, which infiltrate the retina, subretinal space, and under the RPE, are positive for CD20 (B cells).

C: Higher magnification of the immunohistochemical preparation shows tumor cells expressing CD20.

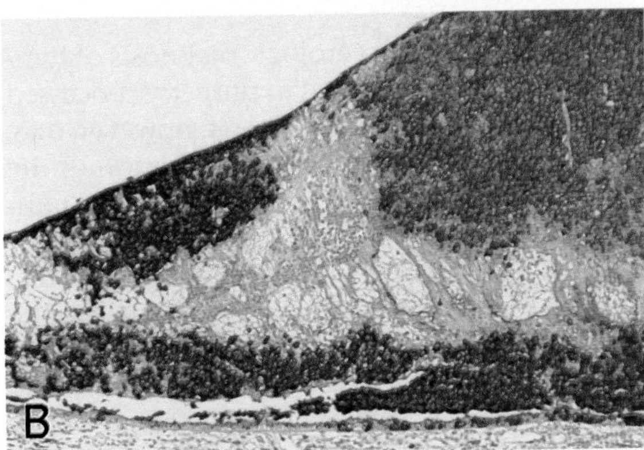

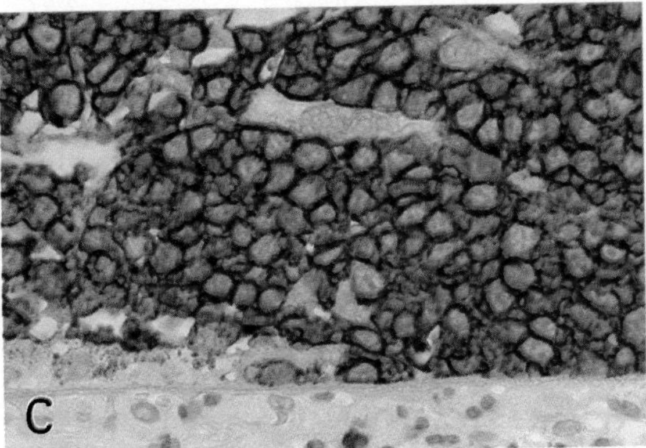

These sub-RPE deposits appear as mounds of white material on cross section. The vitreous body may show opacities from the tumor cell infiltration. Microscopically, the tumor cells are large, displaying hyperchromatic nuclei with single or multiple prominent nucleoli. Some neoplastic cells have indented nuclei with finger-like projections. Abnormal mitotic figures are common, and the neoplastic cells may be mixed with reactive T cells and macrophages. Necrosis of the tumor cells is a frequent finding. Although the tumor cells are seen in the retina,

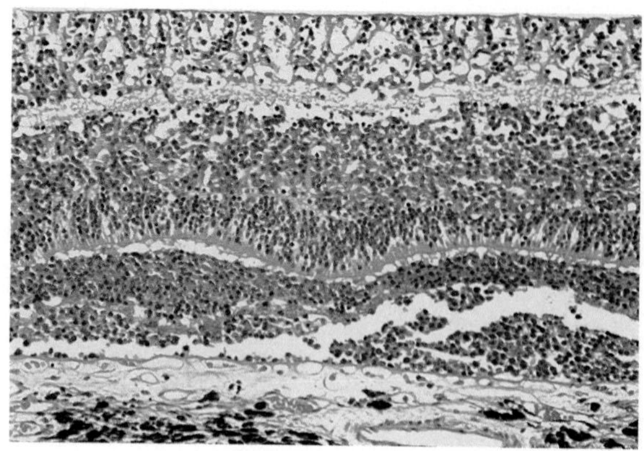
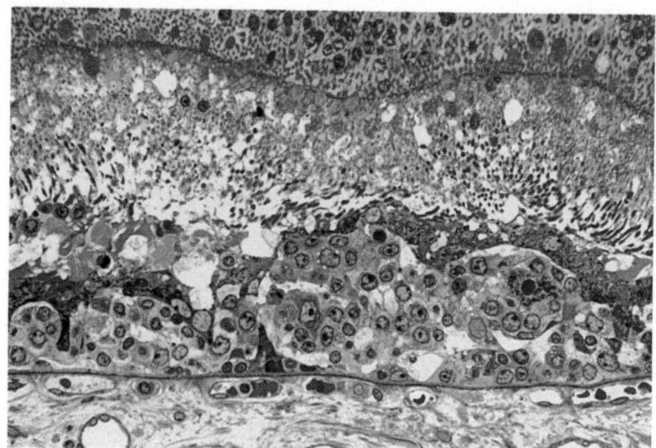

Figure 3-40

PRIMARY INTRAOCULAR B-CELL LYMPHOMA

Left: Subretinal and sub-RPE tumor infiltration. Reactive lymphocytes are absent in the choroid. Right: Higher magnification shows sub-RPE deposits of tumor cells (1-µm thin section).

primarily around the retinal vessels, a characteristic feature is deposits of tumor cells under the RPE and in the subretinal space (98). The choroid is usually thickened as a result of infiltration of non-neoplastic reactive mononuclear cells (fig. 3-39). These cells exhibit benign cytologic features and are significantly smaller than the neoplastic cells of the retinal or sub-RPE infiltrates.

Cytologic and Immunohistochemical Findings, and Molecular Studies. The diagnosis of intraocular lymphoma requires cytologic examination of a vitreous specimen, which is needle-aspirated or collected at the time of pars plana vitrectomy. The latter is preferred for lymphomas involving the retina and vitreous body because cellular yields are higher (99). Pars plana vitrectomy can also be used to obtain retinal, subretinal, or sub-RPE material, when such material is clinically evident as a subretinal or sub-RPE mound (100,101). Pars plana vitrectomy is used in cases where the clinical suspicion of lymphoma remains high despite negative needle-aspirated vitreous body biopsies. The vitreous body specimens are processed by various methods, such as filter technique, cytospin, and cell-block preparations.

The filter and cytospin methods are suitable for the fluid portion of the vitreous body sample; the settled portion can be used to prepare paraffin-embedded cell blocks. The two methods are complimentary. Paraffin-embedded cell blocks produce multiple sections that may be used for morphologic as well as immunohistochemical purposes. A useful method for improving cell-block quality is the celloidin bag technique (102,103).

When the above cytologic preparations are used, large cell lymphoma exhibits a characteristic cytologic appearance. Pleomorphic cells with hyperchromatic nuclei and an elevated nuclear to cytoplasmic ratio are typically seen (fig. 3-41). Nuclear membranes may show finger-like projections or folds and an irregular contour. Multiple nucleoli may be seen together with coarse nuclear chromatin. Also typical is the presence of necrotic cellular debris in the background (104).

In most cases, the cytologic diagnosis of lymphoma can be established in properly processed specimens. False-negative reports, however, may occur from improper or delayed fixation of the sample, which either damages or alters the staining properties of the neoplastic cells. Another factor that leads to diagnostic pitfalls is the distribution of variable proportions of neoplastic and inflammatory cells in the vitreous body (105). This variable distribution may mask the true pathology. Although some vitreous biopsies are clearly neoplastic or inflammatory by light microscopy, others are equivocal, posing a difficult diagnostic dilemma. Immunophenotypic and gene rearrangement studies may be helpful in some of these cases. To diagnose the lymphoma, the questions that have to be answered include whether the lesion is monoclonal or not and the lineage (i.e., B/T lymphocyte) of

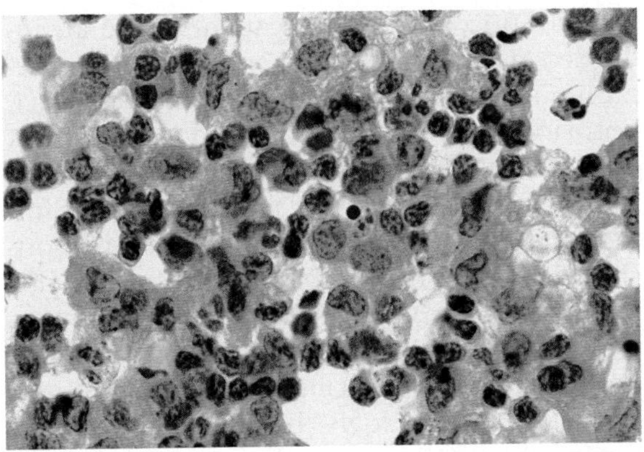

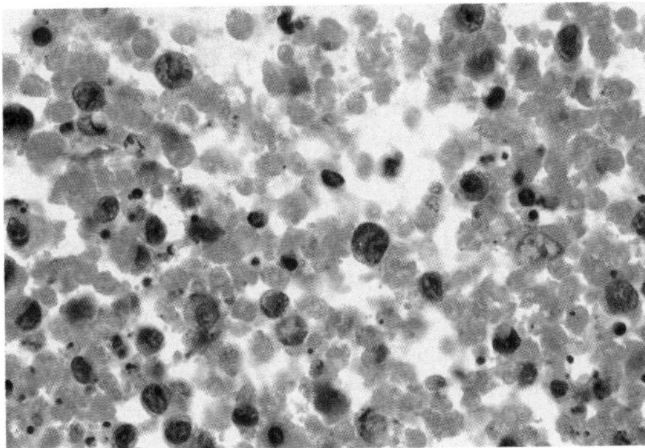

Figure 3-41

PRIMARY INTRAOCULAR LYMPHOMA

Left: Cytologic preparation of a vitrectomy specimen (cell block) reveals pleomorphic cells with hyperchromatic nuclei and a high nuclear to cytoplasmic ratio.

Right: Both viable and necrotic tumor cells are seen (thin prep technique).

the infiltrating cells. These questions may be answered either genotypically or phenotypically. Immunohistochemically, the tumor cells display markers for B cell lineage (fig. 3-42). In the vitreous body such neoplastic B cells may be mixed with reactive T cells and macrophages. In the enucleated globes, the retinal infiltrates are primarily made up of neoplastic B cells, whereas the choroidal infiltrates express the T-cell phenotype.

Flow cytometry analysis of the vitreous body material may be an adjunct to morphologic and immunohistochemical tests. It is not a primary, front-line diagnostic or prognostic tool, and cytology is still considered the gold standard (106). Flow cytometry, however, has several theoretical advantages over immunohistochemistry. It allows an objective cell count, as well as counts of cells simultaneously (positive or negative) for up to four different antigens. The number of cells in a tissue that can be evaluated simultaneously is greater with flow cytometry than with immunohistochemistry, and the results are therefore more quantitatively accurate. In addition, flow cytometry is far more sensitive than immunohistochemistry for the detection of immunoglobulin light chains. Cytopathology, however, remains essential for diagnosing this disease and cannot be replaced by immunohistochemistry or flow cytometry.

Gene rearrangement studies often enable determination of the clonality and lineage of lymphoid lesions, as well as the establishment of molecular fingerprint patterns of individual lymphoid neoplasms. This information is of prime importance for distinguishing lymphomas and reactive lymphoid processes. Some diagnostic difficulties encountered with immunohistochemical studies may be obviated by these newer molecular techniques. Moreover, these molecular studies are the only reliable methods for detecting clonality in T-cell neoplasms. Few studies have been published on the use of gene rearrangement analysis in intraocular lymphomas. Because the number of cells and, therefore, the DNA mass available from vitrectomy

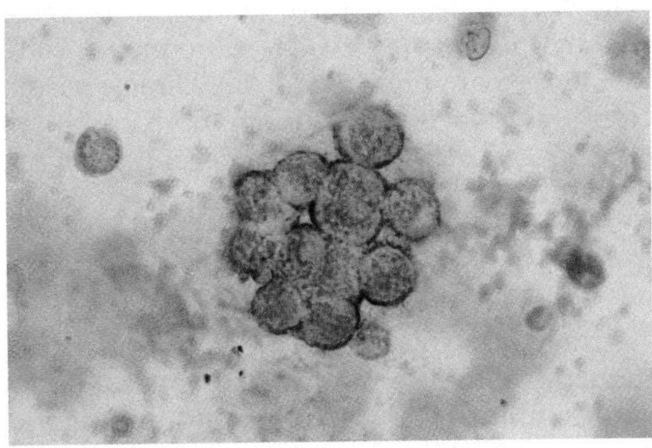

Figure 3-42

PRIMARY INTRAOCULAR LYMPHOMA

The neoplastic mononuclear cells in the vitreous body stain for L-26 (B cells).

specimens is usually limited, polymerase chain reaction (PCR) analysis is more applicable than Southern blot analysis. PCR combined with microdissection study of intraocular lymphoma cells may reveal clonal heavy chain immunoglobulin (IGH) gene rearrangement in the third framework of the VH region and *bcl-2*-associated translocation in tumor cells (107).

One theoretical problem that may reduce the sensitivity of clonality detection by PCR is the fact that small clones of tumor cells may be masked by a larger polyclonal background. In some cases of intraocular lymphoma, vitrectomy analysis is not diagnostic. Such patients show only a mixed population of inflammatory cells in vitreous body specimens obtained from repeated vitrectomies. The malignant cells may be sequestered only in the subretinal or sub-RPE space, where they give rise to the typical yellowish or cream-colored lesions, as appreciated by funduscopy. If such subretinal or sub-RPE lesions are present and the clinical suspicion of intraocular lymphoma remains high after a negative vitrectomy, a chorioretinal biopsy should be considered (108).

Treatment and Prognosis. The ideal therapeutic regimen for treating patients with PCNSL has yet to be identified. High-dose methotrexate therapy delivered intravenously, with intrathecal administration via an Ommaya reservoir, combined with radiotherapy and intravenous cytarabine has been used (109–111). Ocular disease is treated with radiotherapy at the time of CNS irradiation. With recurrence of ocular lymphoma, the patient requires lumbar puncture and MRI to determine whether the CNS disease is also recurrent. If so, therapy is directed at the entire CNS again. If CNS disease is absent, then intravitreal administration of methotrexate is considered (112).

Despite the various treatment modalities and regimens available, the long-term prognosis for patients with PCNSL remains poor, with the longest median survival reported to date being approximately 40 months. Multiple factors are of significance in predicting outcome and survival in patients with PCNSL, including age, Karnofsky performance status, neurological function classification level, single versus multiple lesions, and superficial cerebral/cerebellar hemisphere lesions versus deep periventricular region lesions.

Immunocompromised patients have an increased risk of malignancy, of which lymphoproliferative disease is an important type; in fact, non-Hodgkin's lymphoma is the second most common malignancy associated with AIDS (113). PCNSL in AIDS patients is similar to that of immunocompetent patients, in that both are non-Hodgkin's lymphomas; but in AIDS-related disease the underlying pathology is an uncontrolled proliferation of B cells brought about by Epstein-Barr virus infection. Unlike immunocompetent individuals, human immunodeficiency virus (HIV)-infected patients with lymphoma may not show choroidal inflammation.

AIDS patients with CNS lymphoma do not present with the characteristic radiographic appearances seen in immunocompetent patients. MRI may show diffuse disease involving the deep gray matter nuclei and white matter tracts, rather than a dominant mass. T2-weighted imaging shows extensive hyperintensities in the pons, cerebellum, white matter, and basal ganglia. In contrast to the usual periventricular and corpus callosum distribution in immunocompetent patients, an irregular, ring-like enhancement in the basal ganglia, with surrounding edema and mass effect, is a frequent CT finding in AIDS-related PCNSL (114).

Leukemia

Various leukemias can involve the retina, including *acute myeloblastic leukemia, acute lymphoblastic leukemia,* and *adult T-cell leukemia* (fig. 3-43). Funduscopic examination may reveal dilated retinal veins, vascular sheathing, and occlusions. Histologically, the infiltrates show immature neoplastic leukocytes in and around the retinal vessels. Perivascular accumulation of the leukemic cells is a common feature in the involved retina. The retinal infiltration is usually associated with choroidal and optic nerve involvement. In some cases, the neoplastic cells infiltrate the RPE layer and accumulate under it (115,116).

TUMORS OF THE RETINAL PIGMENT EPITHELIUM

Although reactive hyperplasia of the RPE is common, true neoplastic lesions of the RPE are rare (117). Clinically, the neoplasms are jet black, elevated masses that mimic melanomas or melanocytomas. They occur in eyes without any

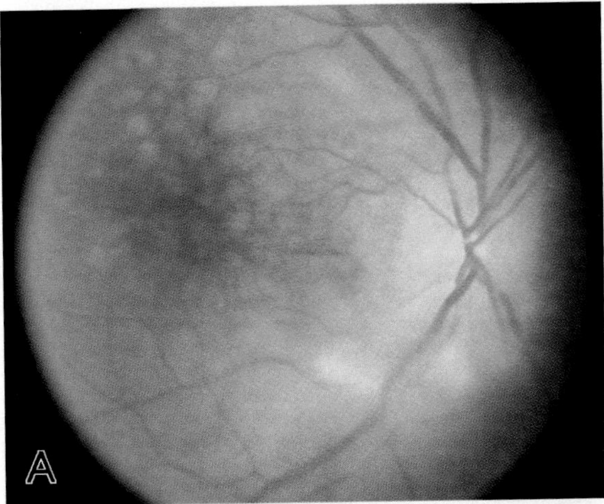

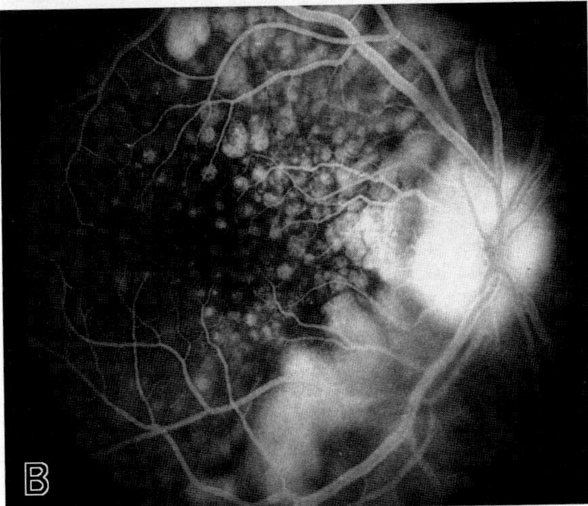

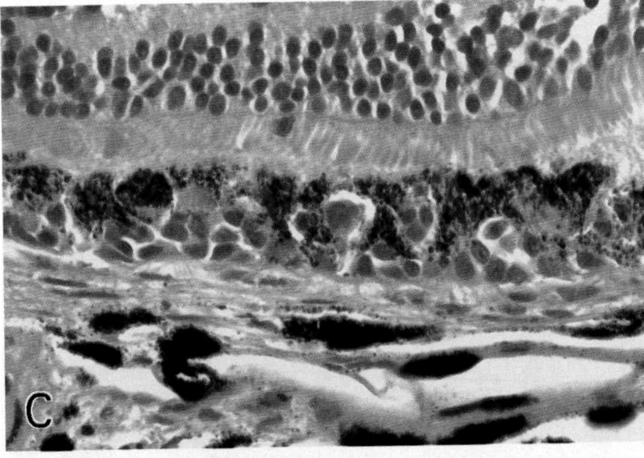

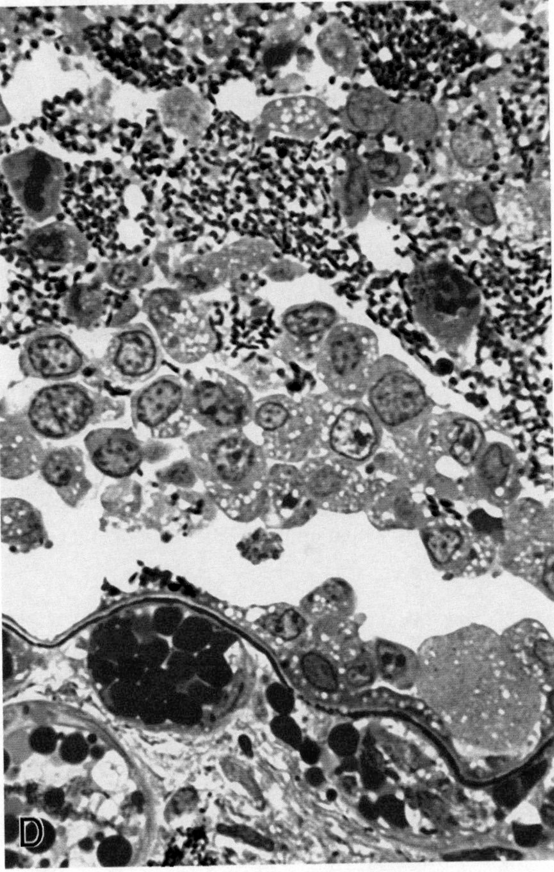

Figure 3-43

ADULT T-CELL LEUKEMIA

A: Ophthalmoscopic examination shows deep retinal infiltrates.

B: Fluorescein angiography reveals multiple RPE defects from the tumor cell infiltration.

C: The tumor cells are noted at the level of the RPE.

D: Several tumor cells are intermixed with the RPE cells (toluidine blue stain).

history or histopathologic evidence of trauma, inflammation, or other diseases. In a recently reported series of cases, the mean age at diagnosis was 53 years, and the age range was 28 to 79 years (118). RPE tumors may have benign cytologic features or anaplastic changes with mitotic activity. Tumors exhibiting the former cytologic features are considered adenomas, and the latter are diagnosed as carcinomas; however, no histologically verified cases of RPE carcinoma with distant metastasis have been documented. Moreover, scleral invasion is rare (119).

RPE adenomas have various histologic patterns: mosaic, tubular, papillary, and vacuolated (figs. 3-44, 3-45). These histologic patterns are often observed in different regions of the same tumor. The vacuoles have mucopolysaccharides containing sialic acid (using Alcian blue stain

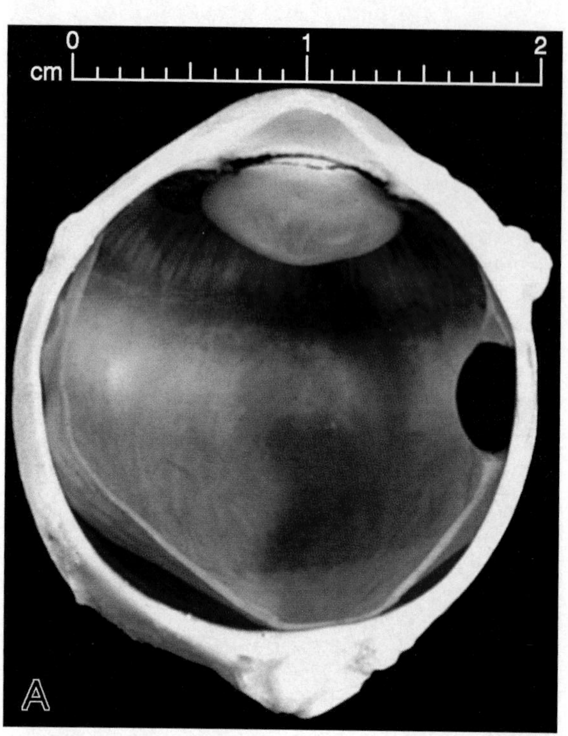

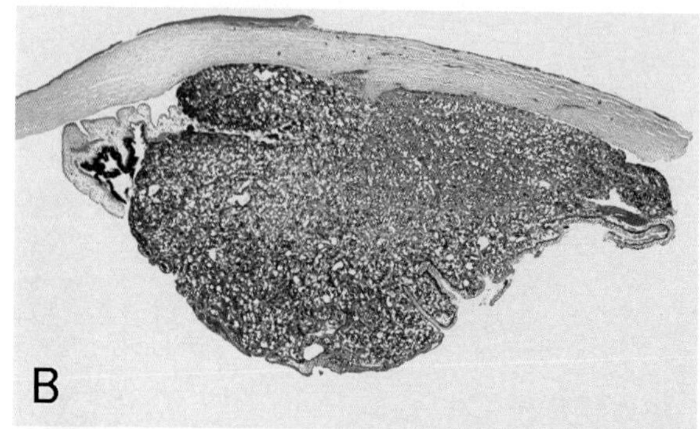

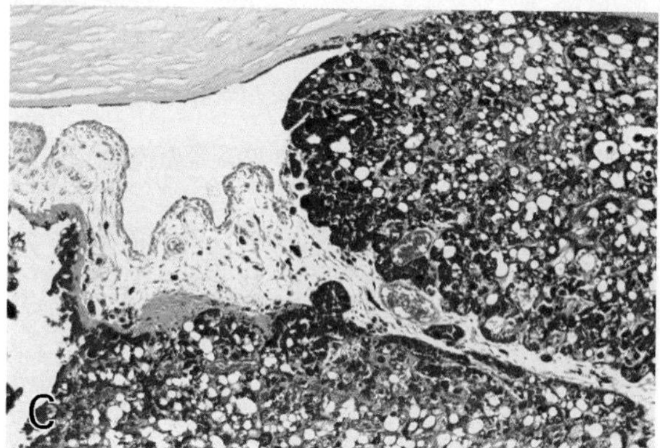

Figure 3-44

PIGMENT EPITHELIUM ADENOMA

A: A jet black adenoma is seen at the equator arising from the RPE.

B: Pigmented tumor arises from the ciliary epithelium and extends into the anterior chamber angle structures (iridocyclectomy specimen).

C: The tumor, which infiltrates the iris root and ciliary body, is composed of vacuolated cells.

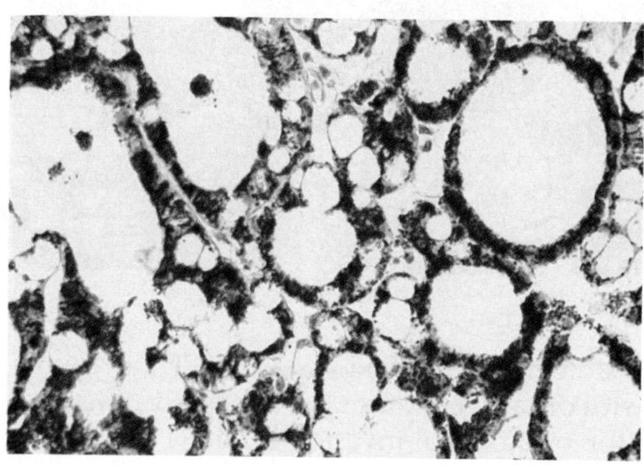

Figure 3-45

PIGMENT EPITHELIUM ADENOMA

Pigmented tumor of the ciliary epithelium has a mixed component of vacuolated cells and tubules.

before and after sialidase digestion). The tumor cells have large, oval pigment granules (fig. 3-46). Ultrastructurally, the neoplastic cells reveal basement membrane production, junctional complexes, and microvilli (fig. 3-47).

RPE adenocarcinomas show anaplastic changes and various histologic patterns, as seen in the adenomas. Nuclear pleomorphism, increased mitotic activity, and invasion of the choroid and optic nerve occur in tumors classified as adenocarcinomas.

Periodic observation for growth is suggested in the management of RPE adenomas and adenocarcinomas. Progressive tumors are treated mainly by enucleation (118).

METASTATIC NEOPLASMS

Isolated metastases to the retina are exceedingly rare. The metastases arise from breast,

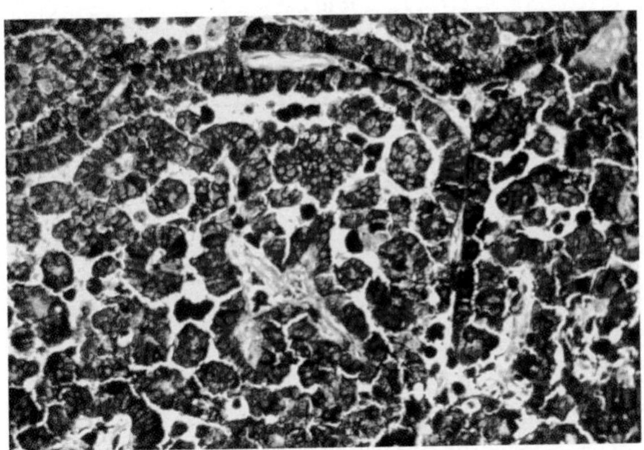

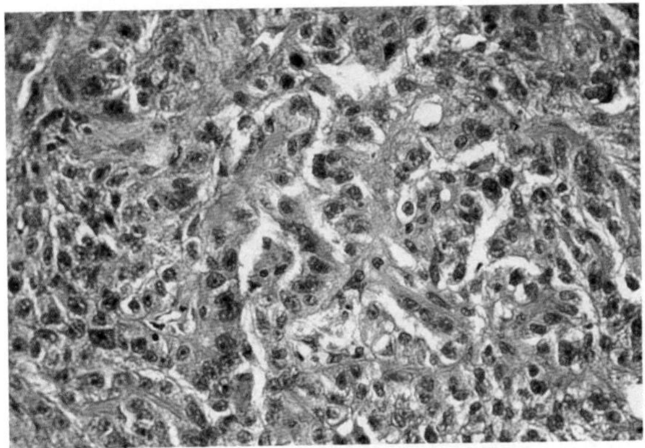

Figure 3-46

ADENOMA OF THE RETINAL PIGMENT EPITHELIUM

Left: Tubular and papillary structures are lined by heavily pigmented cuboidal cells. Right: Bleached section shows mild to moderate nuclear atypia with small nucleoli.

lung, gastrointestinal tract, and genitourinary system, and from cutaneous melanoma. Usually, the retinal metastases are noted in conjunction with optic nerve involvement and vitreous body seeding (120). Unlike metastases, direct invasion of the overlying retina is common in large primary choroidal melanomas.

NEUROEPITHELIAL TUMORS

Zimmerman (121) first suggested that primary neuroepithelial tumors of the ciliary body can be conveniently divided into two major groups: 1) those typically found in children, which are characterized histologically by their embryonic appearance and resemble primitive medullary epithelium (fig. 3-48), and 2) those observed mainly in adults, which are composed of histologic elements that resemble the fully differentiated ciliary epithelium. The former group is considered congenital, while the latter consists of acquired tumors. The congenital tumors include glioneuroma and medulloepithelioma. The acquired tumors can be benign or malignant. The former include pseudoadenomatous hyperplasia and adenomas of nonpigmented and pigmented ciliary epithelium; the latter, adenocarcinomas of nonpigmented and pigmented ciliary epithelium (Table 3-5).

Congenital Tumors of the Ciliary Epithelium

Glioneuroma. This tumor is an extremely rare choristomatous malformation in which brain-like tissue develops in association with a

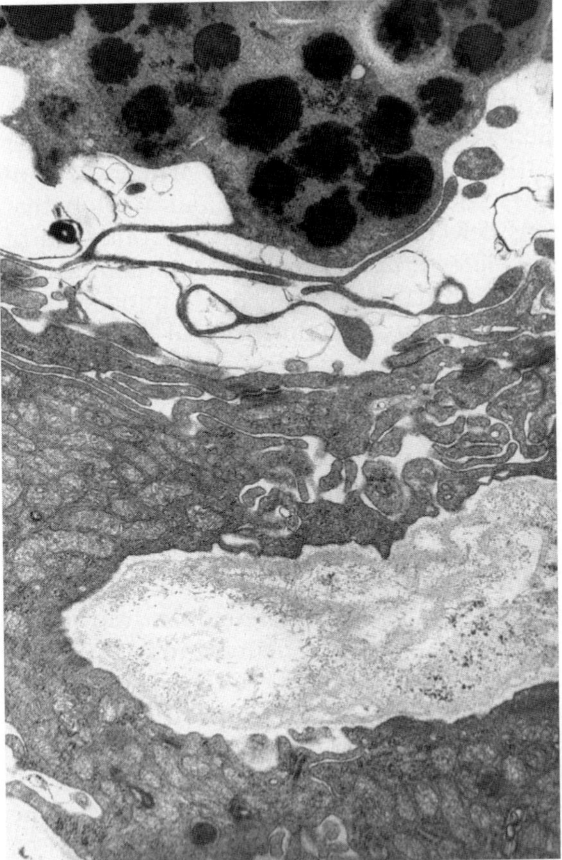

Figure 3-47

ADENOMA OF THE RETINAL PIGMENT EPITHELIUM

Transmission electron microscopy reveals pigmented cells that contain large melanosomes, clear cells with desmosomes, and a multilaminar basement membrane.

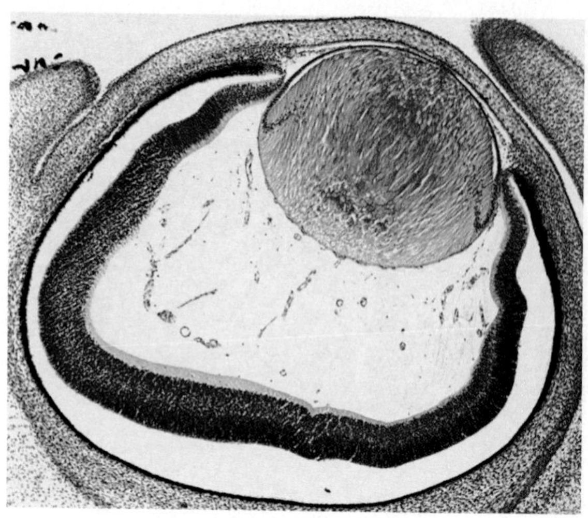

Figure 3-48

MEDULLARY EPITHELIUM

Ninth week (31 mm) embryonic eye shows the medullary epithelium at the edges (arrow) of the invaginated optic cup.

coloboma of the iris and ciliary body (122,123). Generally, these tumors are noted early after birth; however, they are observed rarely in teenagers and young adults without a colobomatous defect. The glioneuroma is composed of well-differentiated neural tissue containing glial and neuronal elements. These tumors express synaptophysin, neurofilament, GFAP, and S-100 protein (124).

Medulloepithelioma. Medulloepitheliomas are embryonic tumors that arise from the primitive medullary epithelium of the optic cup. The designation of *diktyoma* proposed by Fuchs (121) describes a particular arrangement of embryonic epithelial cords in a net-like arrangement. Verhoeff (125) preferred the term of *teratoneuroma* because of the resemblance of these tumors to immature neuroretinal tissue. In 1931, Grinker (126) proposed the name medulloepithelioma. Zimmerman, (121) who published a detailed histologic description of these tumors, preferred this term as well (121).

Medulloepitheliomas that contain heterotopic elements or tissues such as brain, cartilage, or rhabdomyoblasts are classified as *teratoid*, and those tumors lacking these elements are classified as *nonteratoid medulloepithelioma*. Both nonteratoid and teratoid medulloepitheliomas may be benign or malignant (Table 3-5). As a group these tumors are rarer than retinoblastoma.

Table 3-5

CLASSIFICATION OF NEUROEPITHELIAL TUMORS OF THE CILIARY BODY[a]

Classification
Congenital
Glioneuroma
Medulloepithelioma
Benign
Malignant
Teratoid medulloepithelioma
Benign
Malignant
Acquired
Nonpigmented
Benign
Pseudoadenomatous hyperplasia
Adenoma
Solid
Papillary
Pleomorphic
Malignant
Glandular and papillary
Pleomorphic, low grade
Anaplastic
Pigmented
Benign
Adenoma
Vacuolated
Malignant
Adenocarcinoma
Mixed pigmented and nonpigmented
Benign
Malignant

[a]Modified from reference 147.

Medulloepitheliomas arise commonly from the ciliary body and, rarely, from the retina (127) or optic disc or optic nerve (128,129). Although medulloepitheliomas are sporadic and nonfamilial tumors, they sometimes develop in patients following treatment for retinoblastoma or develop concurrently in patients with pinealoblastoma (130,131).

Benign Medulloepithelioma. Benign medulloepitheliomas occur in children averaging 5 years of age, with an interval of several months up to a few years between onset of signs and symptoms and recognition of the tumor (132,133). The most frequent signs are leukocoria, notching or subluxation of the lens, cataract, and a mass in the iris, ciliary body, or anterior chamber. Almost all tumors are unilateral. Ophthalmologic examination reveals a white, gray (fig. 3-49), or yellow mass of the posterior chamber, which may occasionally be pigmented. The ciliary body or iris may be involved. Free floating cystic

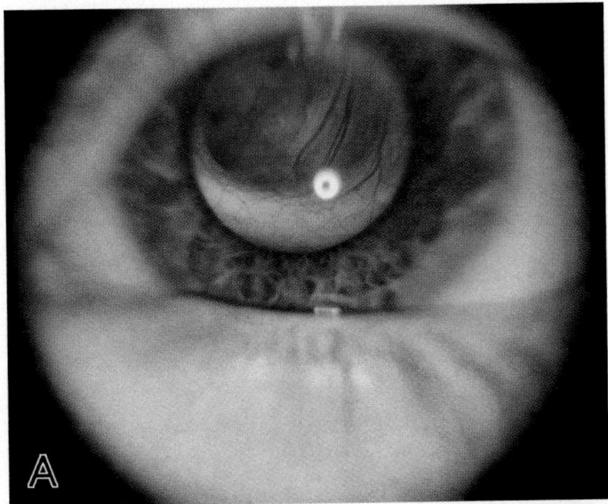

Figure 3-49

MEDULLOEPITHELIOMA

A: A gray-white vascularized mass is present behind the lens.

B: CT scan shows a ciliary body mass.

C: The enucleated eye reveals a mass arising from the ciliary body containing multiple small cysts.

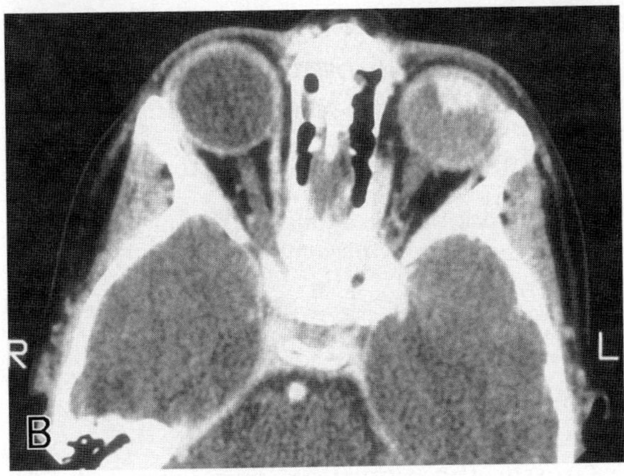

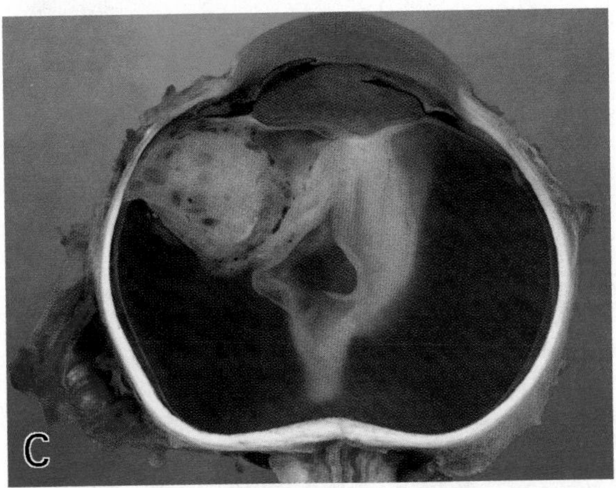

masses in the anterior chamber or vitreous body are seen in 60 percent of the patients (fig. 3-50).

The tumor is composed of sheets and cords of poorly differentiated neuroepithelial cells that resemble the embryonic ciliary epithelium and retina. These cords of tumor cells resemble fishnet, and, thus, the tumors were previously called diktyomas (fig. 3-51). The neuroepithelial tubules have polarized cells with one surface (internal) exhibiting fine fibrils of loose mesenchymal tissue rich in hyaluronic acid. Some tumors may be partially pigmented. Heteroplastic tissue, including rhabdomyoblasts and hyaline cartilage, may be observed (fig. 3-52).

Cytologic examination of anterior vitreous body aspirates may reveal partially pigmented neuroepithelial tubules (fig. 3-53). Electron microscopic examination may show lumens containing microvilli and bordered by numerous terminal bar complexes and gap junctions similar to those that are seen in the normal ciliary epithelium (134). Small, well-circumscribed tumors are managed by iridocyclectomy, while larger tumors may require enucleation of the globe.

Malignant Medulloepithelioma. Malignant medulloepithelioma has one or more of the following histologic features: 1) areas composed of poorly differentiated neuroblastic cells resembling those of retinoblastoma; 2) nuclear pleomorphism and marked abnormal mitotic activity; 3) areas resembling soft tissue sarcomas; and 4) invasion of the uvea, cornea, or sclera, with or without extraocular extension (132).

Most patients present during the first decade of life; the median age is 6 years at the time of diagnosis. In rare instances, malignant medulloepithelioma has been reported in adults aged of 28 to 79 years (135). Tumors are commonly located at the inferior, temporal (fig. 3-54), or inferotemporal meridians of the ciliary body. The signs and symptoms do not differ from those of benign tumors; however, malignant

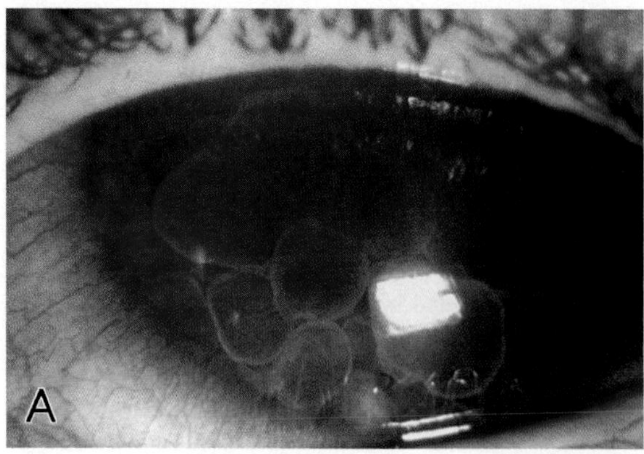

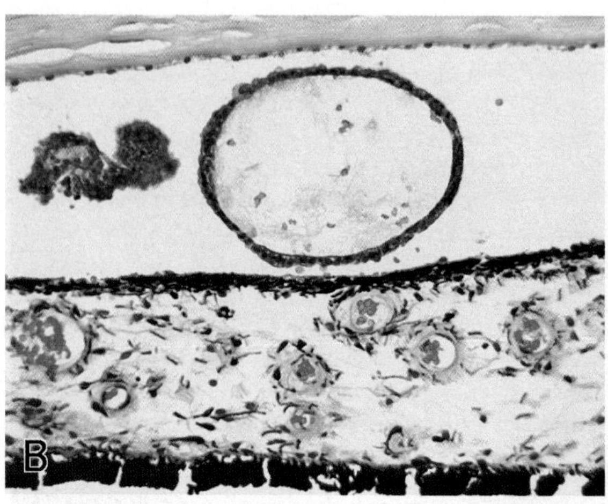

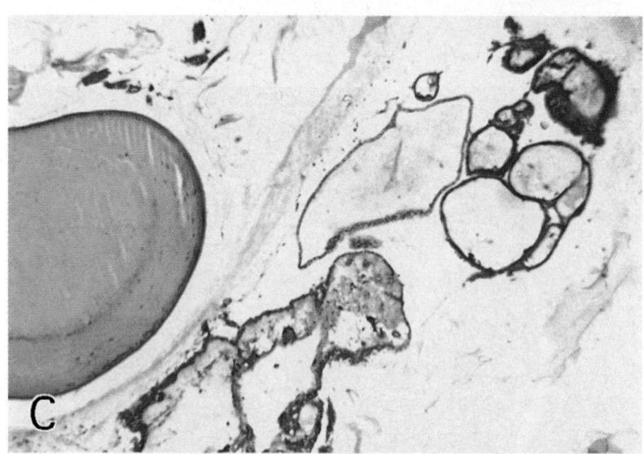

Figure 3-50

MEDULLOEPITHELIOMA

A: The tumor within the anterior chamber has multiple cysts.

B: A cyst of medulloepithelioma is seen in the anterior chamber.

C: The cystic masses of tumor in the anterior vitreous contain Alcian blue–positive mucopolysaccharides.

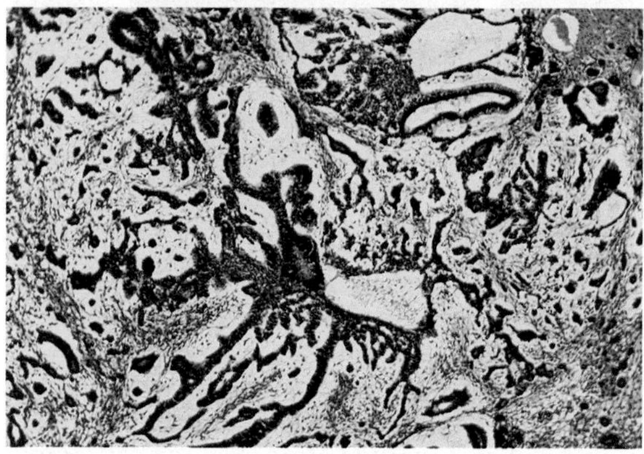

Figure 3-51

MEDULLOEPITHELIOMA

Pigmented cords of neoplastic cells resemble a fishnet.

medulloepithelioma is friable and frequently seeds the aqueous humor and anterior chamber. Proptosis and orbital involvement may be observed in some cases (fig. 3-55). Echographic findings of a highly reflective, irregularly structured tumor, with associated cystic changes involving the ciliary body region, are helpful in establishing a presumed diagnosis of medulloepithelioma.

Grossly, the tumors are nonpigmented and irregular in shape. They invade the anterior uvea, cornea, and sclera. An anterior fungating extraocular extension may be observed in neglected cases (fig. 3-56). The poorly differentiated neuroblastic component forms sheets or tubular structures lined by multilayered neuroblastic cells. In some tumors rosettes similar to those found in retinoblastoma and neuroblastoma are observed (fig. 3-57). The heterotopic elements include not only sarcomatous components but also benign-appearing hyaline cartilage. The malignant heteroplastic elements may appear as rhabdomyosarcoma (fig. 3-58) (136), spindle-cell sarcoma, and even chondrosarcoma. Minute foci of calcification may be found. These histologic components vary in different tumors.

Immunohistochemically, the neuroblastic cells are positive for NSE and synaptophysin, while intermixed cells stain for vimentin, GFAP, and S-100 protein (137). Heterotopic rhabdomyoblasts stain for desmin and muscle-specific actin. The cells lining the rosettes are positive for S-100

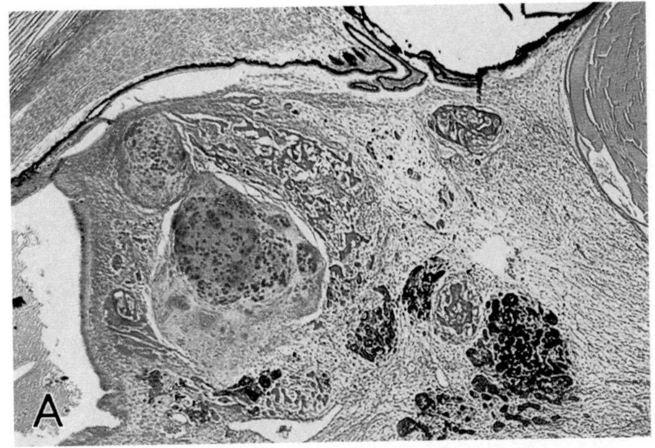

Figure 3-52

MEDULLOEPITHELIOMA

A: An island of hyaline cartilage in a teratoid medulloepithelioma (Alcian blue stain).

B: Benign teratoid medulloepithelioma exhibits heterotopic cartilage and myoblasts (hematoxylin and eosin [H&E] stain).

C: The myoblasts stain red with the trichrome method.

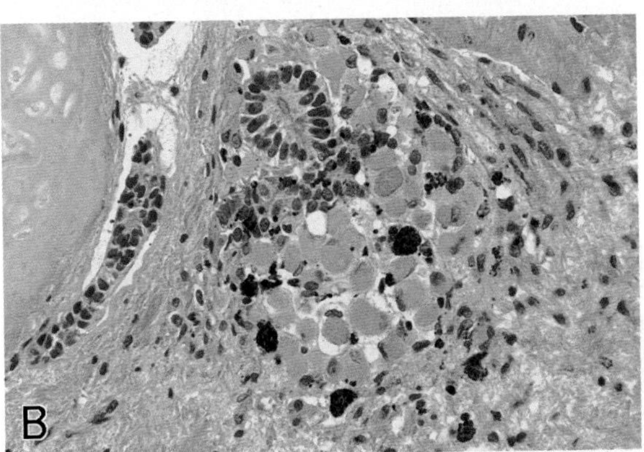

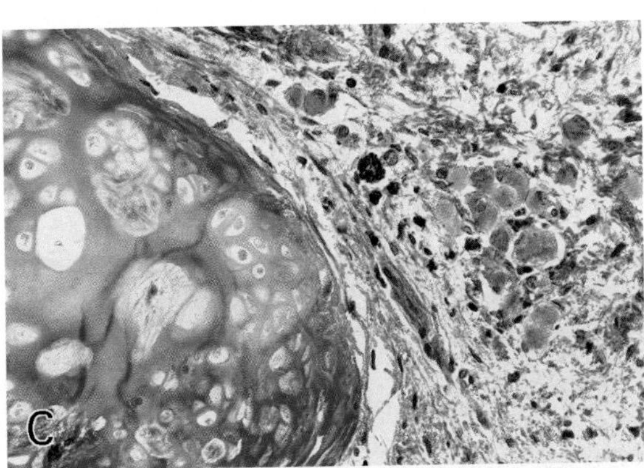

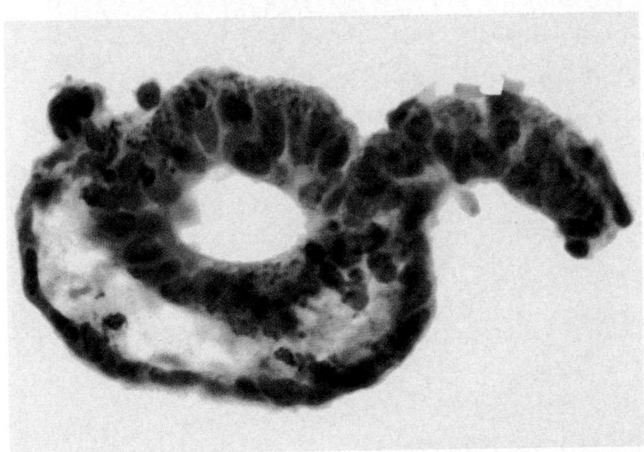

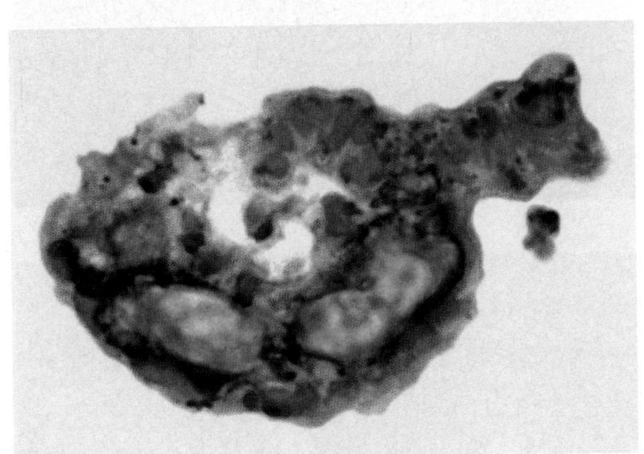

Figure 3-53

MEDULLOEPITHELIOMA

Left: Cytology of an anterior vitreous aspirate shows a neuroepithelial rosette with partially pigmented epithelial cells. Right: The tubule contains Alcian blue–positive mucopolysaccharides.

antigen and rhodopsin, suggesting photoreceptor differentiation (138). Cytologically, there are sheets and tubules of neuroblastic cells with scanty cytoplasm. Rosette-like structures resembling retinoblastoma may be observed.

Electron microscopy of the neural component shows zonulae adherents and well-developed junctional complexes with interdigitating cell processes. Betts et al. (139) reported that the primary cytogenetic abnormality in a case of

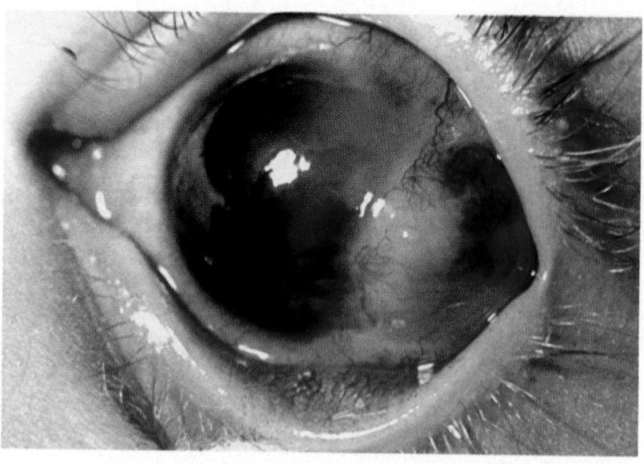

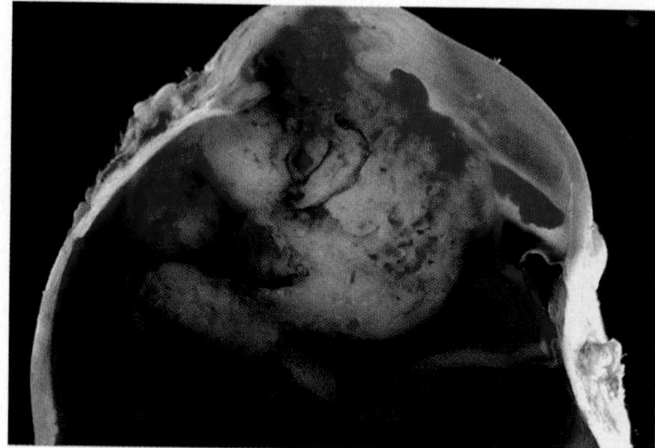

Figure 3-54

MALIGNANT MEDULLOEPITHELIOMA

Left: Recurrent malignant nonteratoid medulloepithelioma that developed in the ciliary body, temporally. Right: Gross examination shows a grayish white ciliary body mass with foci of hemorrhage.

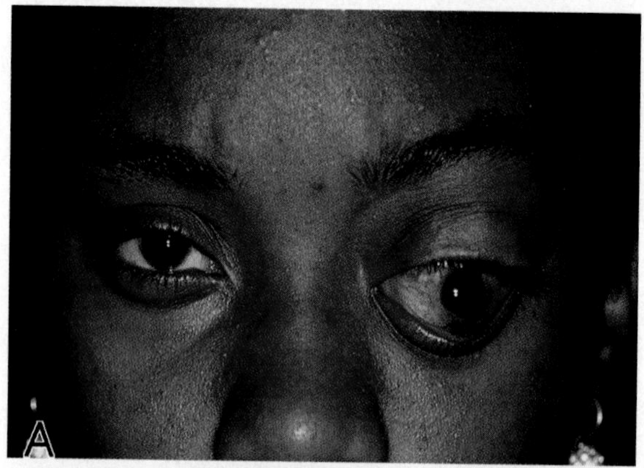

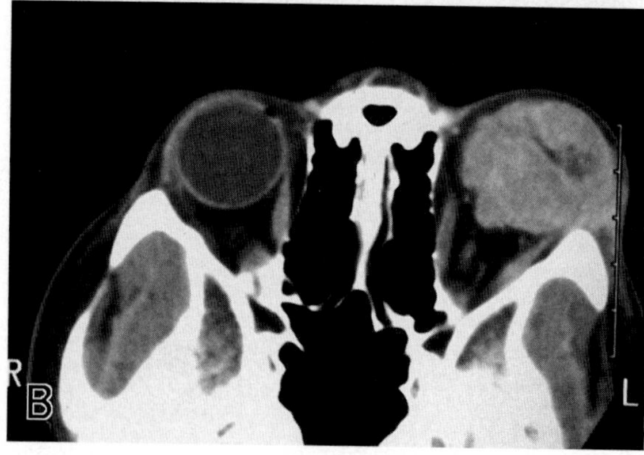

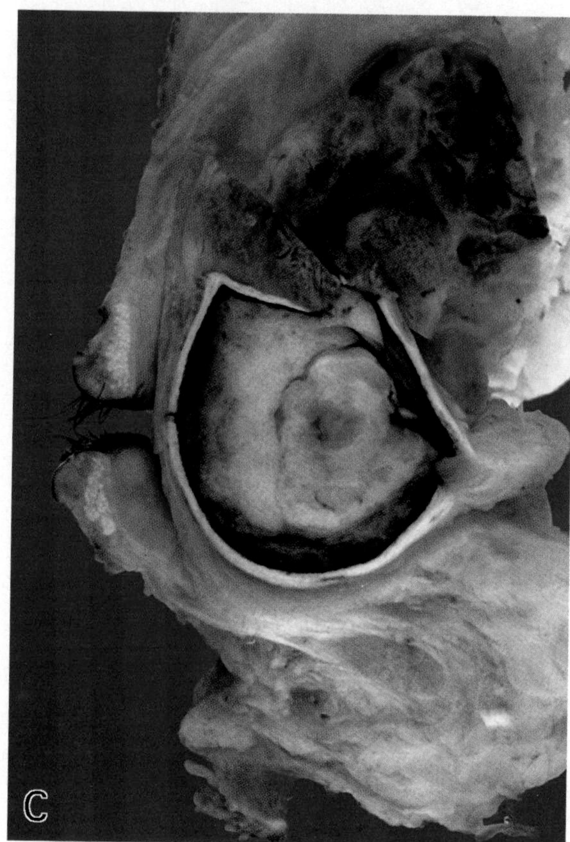

Figure 3-55

MALIGNANT TERATOID MEDULLOEPITHELIOMA

A: The patient developed massive proptosis of the left eye.
B: CT scan shows orbital invasion of the intraocular mass.
C: Orbital exenteration specimen shows massive orbital invasion superiorly.

intraocular medulloepithelioma was a der(16)t (1;16) chromosome, which has been found in a wide range of other tumor types. Additional abnormalities included del(6q) and monosomy 15.

Usually, the histologic diagnosis of medulloepithelioma of the ciliary body is not difficult. Solid cellular neuroblastic tumors disclosing prominent rosette-like structures arising from the retina, optic nerve, or disc could be confused with retinoblastoma; however, such tumors are extremely rare.

Although medulloepitheliomas have a high recurrence rate after local excision, only a few cases of regional metastatic disease have been published. Metastasis developed in 11 percent of histologically proven malignant cases, all of which had extraocular extension (132). In this series, metastases or direct extension of the tumor led to death in four patients: one from massive lymphatic spread to lung and mediastinum, and three from intracranial invasion. Rarely, patients develop parotid metastasis. Most medulloepitheliomas that are larger than 3 clock hours are best managed with enucleation. Local resection is usually associated with recurrences that later require enucleation. Adjunctive chemotherapy and radiotherapy have been used. The chemotherapy regimen is similar to that used in retinoblastoma.

Benign Acquired Tumors of the Ciliary Epithelium

Pseudoadenomatous Hyperplasia (Fuchs' Adenoma, Coronal Adenoma). These tumors are small (1 mm or less) and appear as white nodules in the pars plicata of the ciliary body (fig. 3-59). They represent localized hyperplasia of the nonpigmented ciliary epithelium and are found in 20 to 31 percent of eyes obtained at postmortem (140–142). Histologically, the lesions

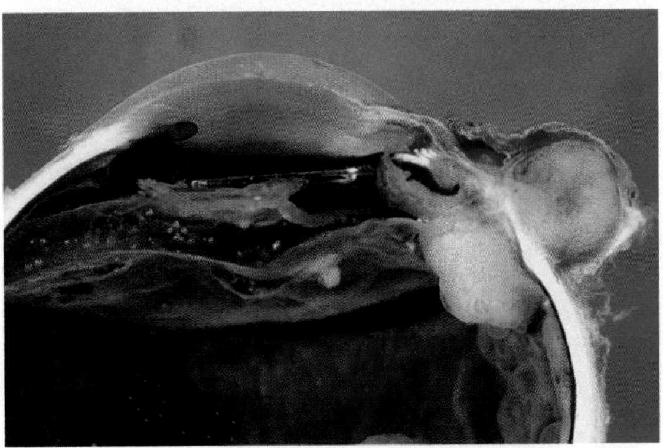

Figure 3-56

MALIGNANT MEDULLOEPITHELIOMA

Recurrent malignant nonteratoid medulloepithelioma of the ciliary body extends extraocularly. The tumor developed within a surgical coloboma of the ciliary body.

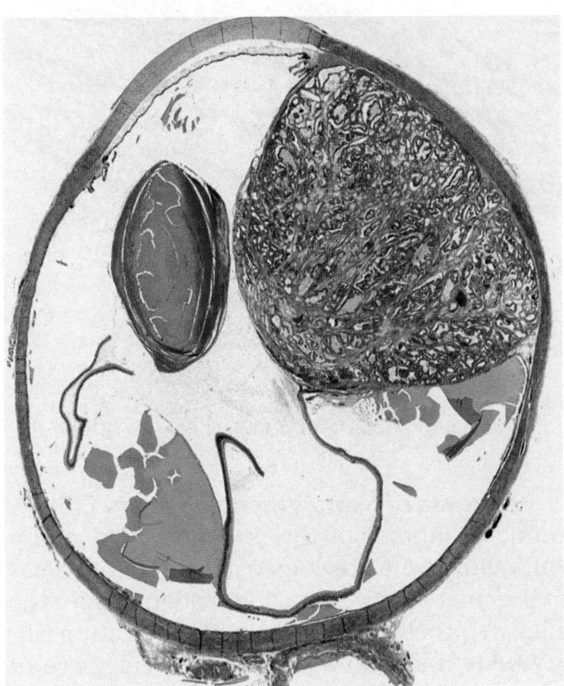

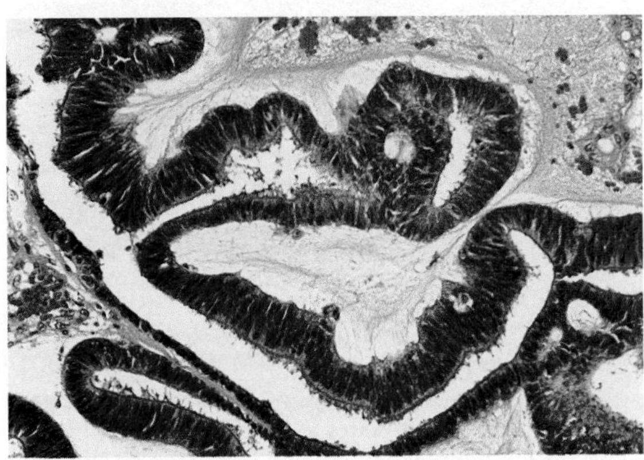

Figure 3-57

MALIGNANT NONTERATOID MEDULLOEPITHELIOMA IN AN ADULT PATIENT

Left: Large tumor of the ciliary epithelium displaces the lens.

Above: The tumor shows features of medullary epithelium with its inner surface forming primary vitreous and the outer surface displaying features of photoreceptor differentiation.

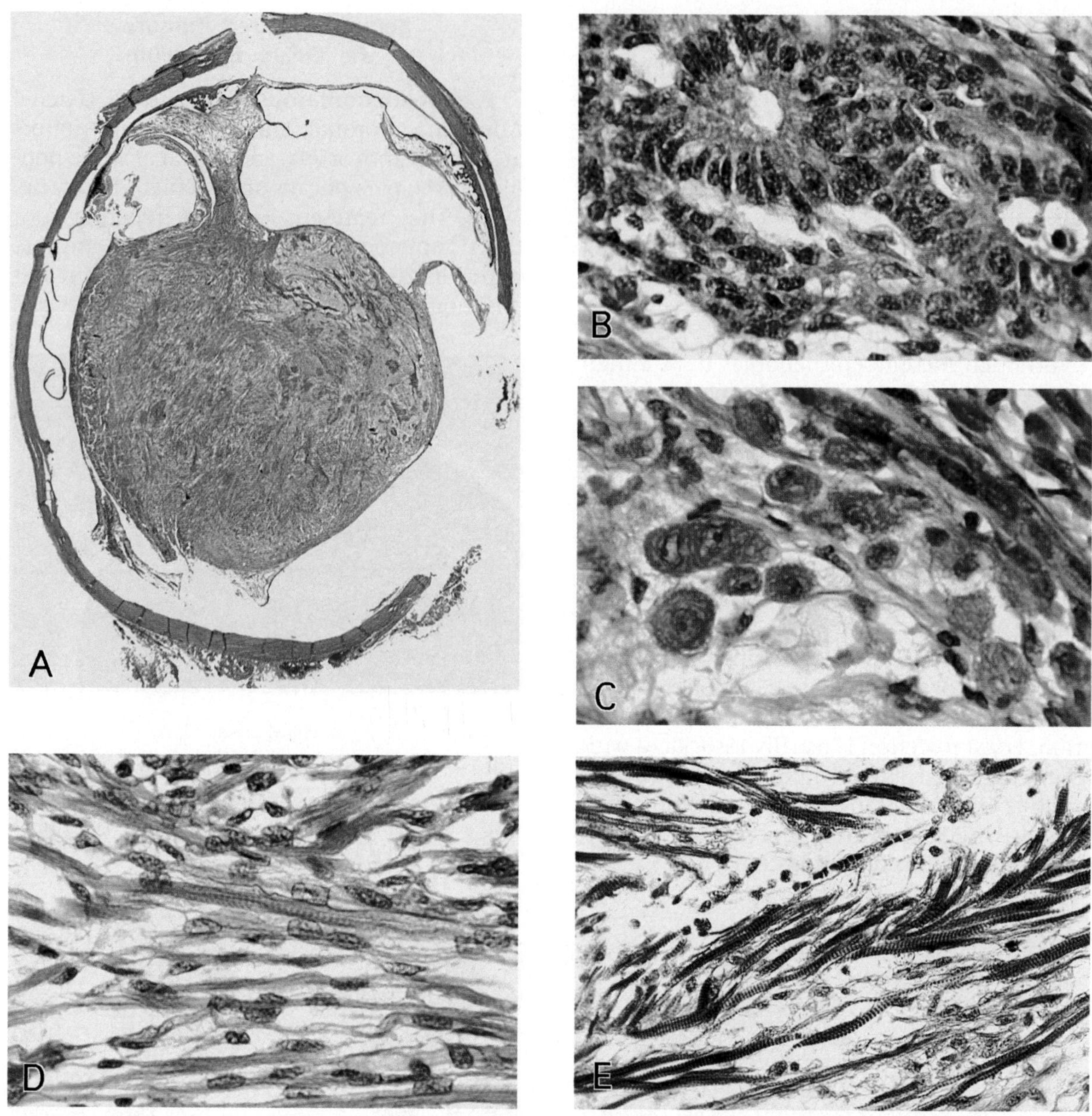

Figure 3-58

MALIGNANT TERATOID MEDULLOEPITHELIOMA

A: A large intraocular mass with a stalk attached to the ciliary epithelium.
B: Neuroepithelial rosettes are present.
C,D: The tumor contains globoid and spindle-shaped myoblasts.
E: The myoblasts display cross striations vividly outlined by staining with phosphotungstic acid hematoxylin (PTAH).

consist of solid cords or tubular proliferation of nonpigmented ciliary epithelium, with extracellular deposits of eosinophilic, PAS-positive basement membrane material (fig. 3-60) (143). They are associated with age and are not clinically significant.

Adenoma of Nonpigmented Ciliary Epithelium. Adenomas of the nonpigmented ciliary epithelium were previously called "epitheliomas of the ciliary epithelium." True adenomas of the ciliary epithelium may resemble clinically a ciliary body melanoma (144). The average age of

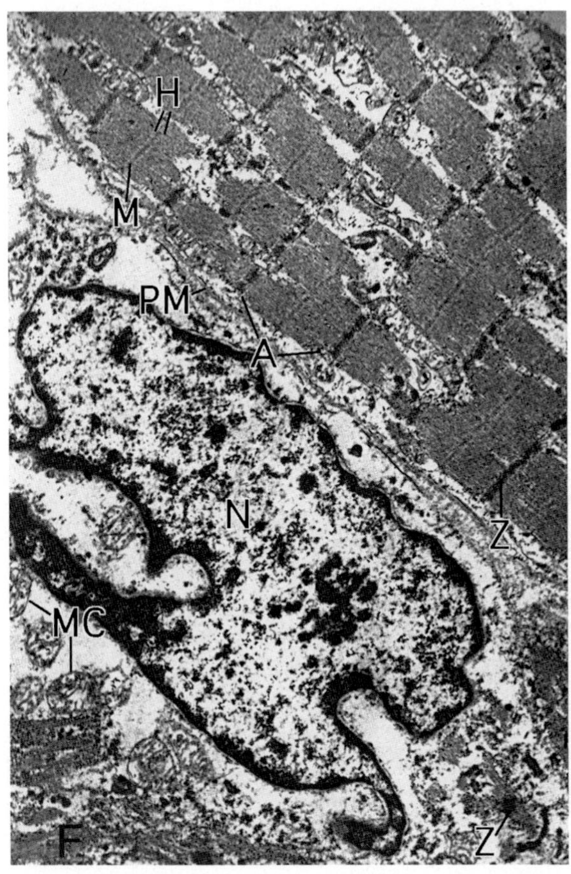

Figure 3-58F

Ultrastructure of the myoblasts reveals I bands with Z lines and A bands with M lines.

patients at the time of presentation of the tumor is about 40 years (145). The most frequent complaint is visual loss secondary to cataract, and the tumors may show evidence of sustained growth (146). A few tumors have been associated with an iris or ciliary body coloboma.

The adenomas are circumscribed, oval to round, solid, gray-white or flesh-colored tumors located in the inner aspect of the ciliary body,

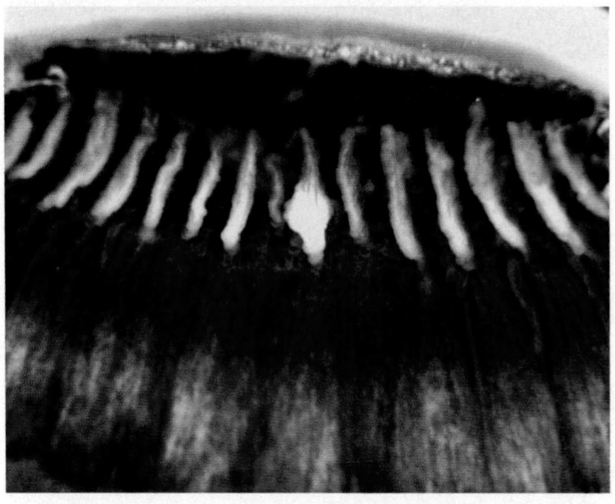

Figure 3-59

FUCHS' ADENOMA

Posterior view of the pars plicata shows a small, circumscribed, white nodule located at the tip of one ciliary process.

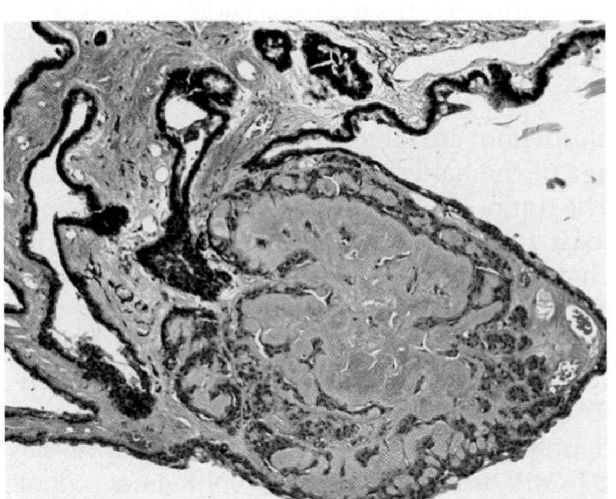

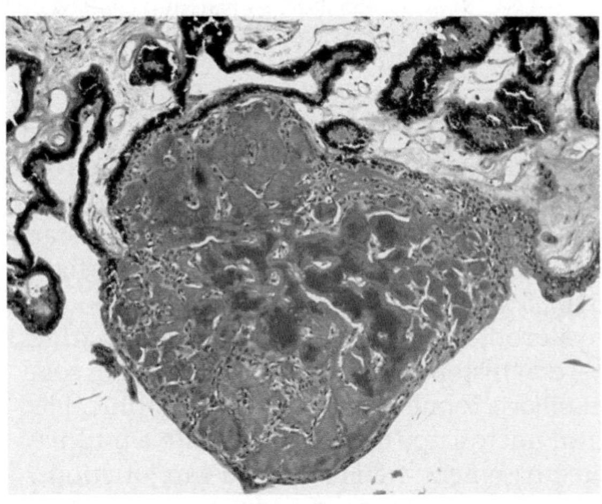

Figure 3-60

FUCHS' ADENOMA

Left: Nodular proliferation of nonpigmented ciliary epithelium with homogeneous eosinophilic deposits.
Right: Prominent PAS-positive basement membrane material is present.

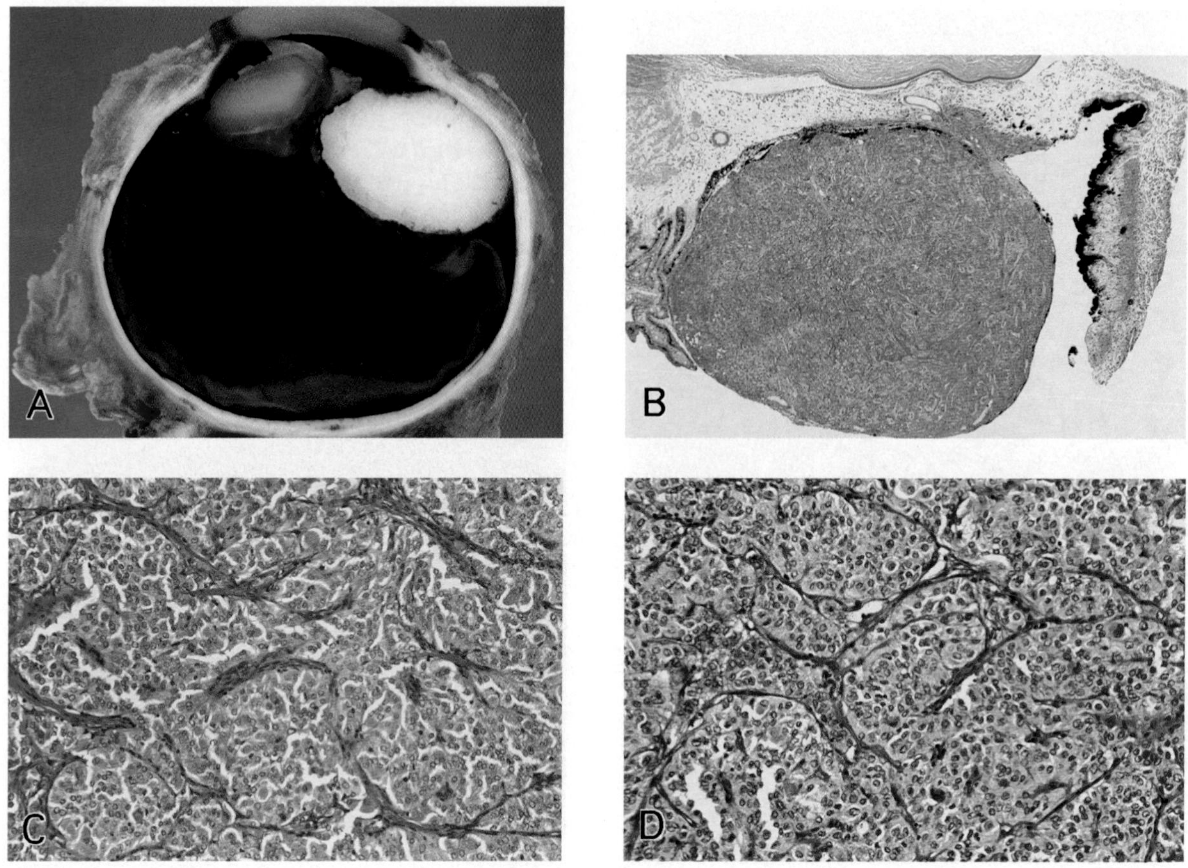

Figure 3-61

NONPIGMENTED ADENOMA

A: Globular grayish white tumor arises from the nonpigmented ciliary epithelium.
B: Low-power view of the ciliary body mass.
C: Tubuloacinar pattern is composed of regular cuboidal cells with small round nuclei.
D: The tumor lobules are demarcated by fibrovascular septa (PAS stain).

often indenting the lens (fig. 3-61A). They consist of cuboidal, columnar, or spindle-shaped cells arranged in cords or tubules that may be lined by a delicate PAS-positive basement membrane resembling the adult ciliary epithelium (fig. 3-61B). Some lesions contain extracellular pools of hyaluronidase-sensitive mucopolysaccharides. Several histopathologic patterns are seen: solid, papillary, tubuloacinar, and pleomorphic. Electron microscopy discloses cells with a multilayered basement membrane and gap junctions.

The management of suspected ciliary body adenomas is local resection. Following surgery, no recurrences are observed.

Adenoma of the Pigmented Ciliary Epithelium. Adenomas of the pigmented ciliary body epithelium are rarely encountered. The median age of the patients at presentation is 55 years. The tumor is a localized pigmented ciliary body mass that may be associated with cataractous changes and loss of vision. They are clinically indistinguishable from melanoma of the ciliary body; however, they are distinguished by their dark gray or jet black color and perpendicular edges without a mushroom-shaped configuration. Fine-needle aspiration biopsy reveals cells with features of pigment epithelium: cuboidal or columnar cells containing round to ovoid, fully melanized melanosomes measuring 0.6 to 1.0 µm; these findings help in the differential diagnosis. Histologically, the tumors develop from the pigment epithelium, usually without

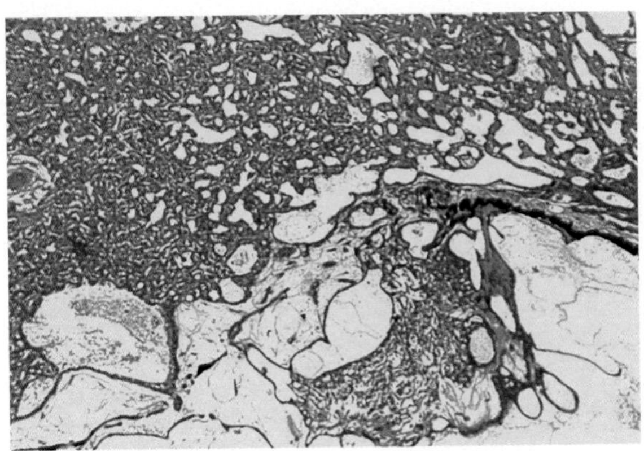

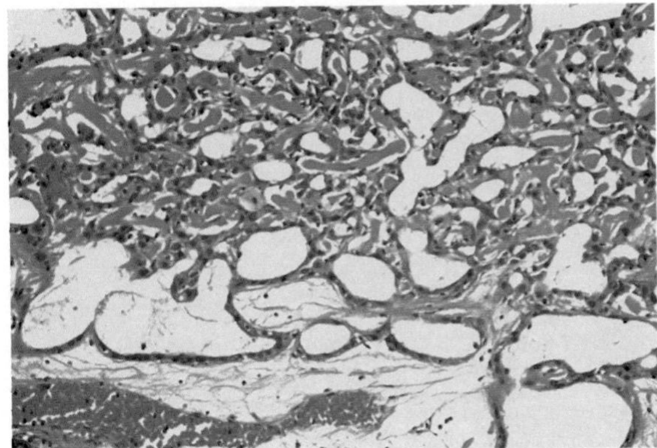

Figure 3-62

NONPIGMENTED ADENOCARCINOMA

Left: Low-grade well-differentiated epithelial tumor arises from the ciliary epithelium.
Right: The tumor is composed of cells resembling nonpigmented ciliary epithelium.

stromal involvement. Characteristically, numerous vacuoles contain hyaluronidase-resistant acid mucopolysaccharides. Nuclear atypia is mild, and mitotic figures are rare.

Adenocarcinoma of the Nonpigmented Ciliary Epithelium. Malignant acquired tumors of the nonpigmented ciliary epithelium (ANPCE) are exceedingly rare (147,148). Twenty-one cases reviewed from the files of the AFIP showed the mean age of patients to be 55 years (range, 23 to 87 years) (147). In all patients the tumor was unilateral. Many occurred in eyes with opaque media that had been blind for several years as result of trauma, ocular malformations, or other abnormalities. Patients present with proptosis or an epibulbar mass in a phthisical eye. The globe may show calcification as part of the phthisis, or in areas of tumor necrosis.

Histologically, the tumors span a spectrum from localized, low-grade, well-differentiated neoplasms that resemble the normal ciliary epithelium to poorly differentiated pleomorphic tumors (fig. 3-62). They are classified in the following categories: glandular or papillary, pleomorphic low-grade, pleomorphic with hyaline stroma, and anaplastic (figs. 3-63–3-65). Low-grade tumors show nuclear pleomorphism, increased mitotic activity, and areas of necrosis. The carcinomas usually invade the ciliary muscle, iris, anterior chamber angle structures, choroid, sclera, and optic nerve. The cells have pale cytoplasm and are often surrounded by a prominent PAS-positive basement membrane.

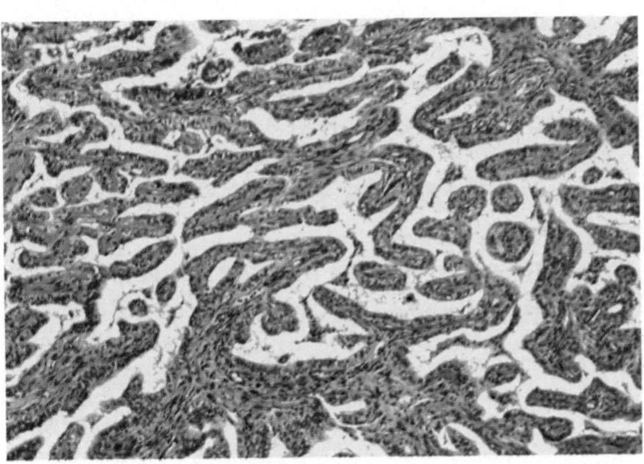

Figure 3-63

NONPIGMENTED ADENOCARCINOMA

Adenocarcinoma of the ciliary epithelium has a papillary pattern.

In some cases, the basement membrane is only demonstrated by electron microscopy. Immunohistochemically, the tumor cells often express different types of keratin (kermix, CAM5.2, and CK7) and are negative for HMB45 (149-151). Some tumors express NSE and vimentin. DNA analysis of a case with rapid growth showed a peridiploid DNA content (152).

The differential diagnosis includes metastatic clear cell and papillary carcinomas and amelanotic melanoma. Metastatic lesions and melanoma do not have a prominent basement membrane. Recurrences are frequent in pleomorphic and anaplastic tumors, and such

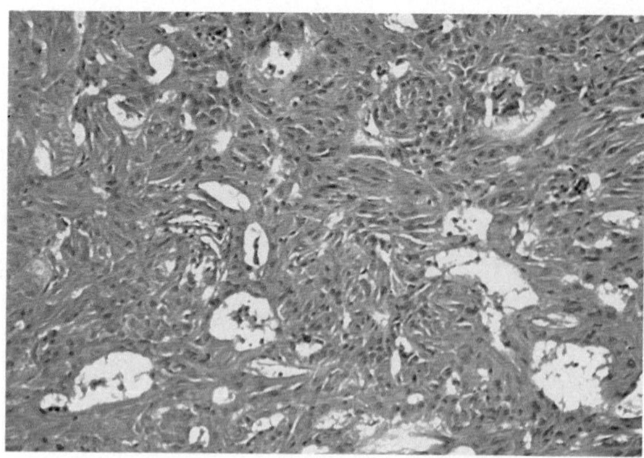

Figure 3-64

NONPIGMENTED ADENOCARCINOMA

This adenocarcinoma arising from the nonpigmented ciliary epithelium has a pleomorphic pattern with spindle-shaped cells.

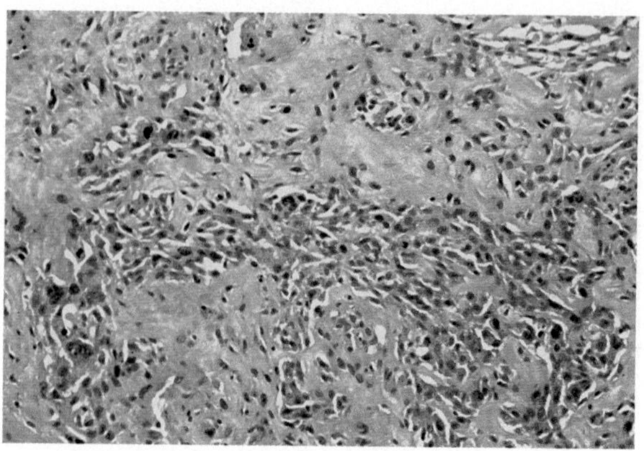

Figure 3-65

NONPIGMENTED ADENOCARCINOMA

Adenocarcinoma of the ciliary epithelium has a pleomorphic pattern and hyaline stroma.

recurrences usually develop in a few months. In a series of 16 cases compiled by the AFIP, five patients (31 percent) died as a result of tumor extension into the CNS or widespread disease. Tumors with epibulbar extension usually confer a bad prognosis.

Adenocarcinoma of the Pigmented Ciliary Epithelium. Adenocarcinomas arising from the pigment epithelium of the ciliary body are exceptionally rare. The criterion used for diagnosis and differentiation from adenoma of ciliary pigmented epithelium is local invasion including the iris, ciliary body stroma, anterior chamber angle, and sclera. The neoplastic cells may show moderate nuclear pleomorphism and rare mitotic figures.

REFERENCES

Anatomy and Histology

1. Fine BS, Yanoff M. Ocular histology. A text and atlas, 2nd ed. New York: Harper & Row; 1979:61–127.

Classification and Frequency

2. Green WR. Retina. In: Spencer WH, ed. Ophthalmic pathology: an atlas and textbook. Vol. 2. Philadelphia: WB Saunders; 1996:667–1332.
3. McLean IW. Retinoblastomas, retinocytomas and pseudoretinoblastomas. In: Spencer WH, ed. Ophthalmic pathology: an atlas and textbook. Vol. 2. Philadelphia: WB Saunders; 1996:1332–80.
4. McLean IW, Burnier MN, Zimmerman LE, Jakobiec FA. Tumors of the eye and ocular adnexa. Atlas of Tumor Pathology, 3rd Series, Fascicle 12. Washington, DC: Armed Forces Institute of Pathology; 1994:97–151.

Retinoblastoma

5. Gonzalez-Fernandez F, Lopes MB, Garcia-Fernandez JM, et al. Expression of developmentally defined retinal phenotypes in the histogenesis of retinoblastoma. Am J Pathol 1992;141:363–75.
6. Hurwitz RL, Bogenmann E, Font RL, Holcombe V, Clark D. Expression of the functional cone phosphotransduction cascade in retinoblastoma. J Clin Invest 1990;85:1872–8.
7. Devesa SS. The incidence of retinoblastoma. Am J Ophthalmol 1975;80:263–5.
8. Atchaneeyasakul L, Murphree AL. Retinoblastoma. In: Ryan SJ, ed. Retina, 3rd ed. St. Louis: Mosby; 2001:513–60.
9. Wiggs JL, Dryja TP. Predicting the risk of hereditary retinoblastoma. Am J Ophthalmol 1988; 106:346–51.

10. Usui Y, Rao NA. Pars plana ciliary epithelial proliferation in 13q deletion syndrome. Br J Ophthalmology 2003;87:1426.
11. Albert DM. Historic review of retinoblastoma. Ophthalmology 1987;94:654–62.
12. Ts'o MO, Fine BS, Zimmerman LE. The Flexner-Wintersteiner rosettes in retinoblastoma. Arch Pathol 1969;88:664–71.
13. Ts'o MO, Fine BS, Zimmerman LE, Vogel MH. Photoreceptor elements in retinoblastoma. A preliminary report. Arch Ophthalmol 1969;82: 57–9.
14. Ts'o MO, Fine BS, Zimmerman LE. The nature of retinoblastoma. II. Photoreceptor differentiation: an electron microscopic study. Am J Ophthalmol 1970;69:350–9.
15. Margo C, Hidayat A, Kopelman J, Zimmerman LE. Retinocytoma. A benign variant of retinoblastoma. Arch Ophthalmol 1983;101:1519–31.
16. Gallie BL, Phillips RA, Ellsworth RM, Abramson DH. Significance of retinoma and phthisis bulbi for retinoblastoma. Ophthalmology 1982;89: 1393–9.
17. Wiggs J, Nordenskjold M, Yandell D, et al. Prediction of the risk of hereditary retinoblastoma, using DNA polymorphism within the retinoblastoma gene. N Engl J Med 1988;318:151–7.
18. Herwig S, Strauss M. The retinoblastoma protein: a master regulator of cell cycle, differentiation and apoptosis. Eur J Biochem 1997;246:581–601.
19. Knudson AG Jr. Mutation and cancer: statistical study of retinoblastoma. Proc Natl Acad Sci U S A 1971;68:820–3.
20. Goodrich DW, Lee WH. Molecular characterization of the retinoblastoma susceptibility gene. Biochim Biophys Acta 1993;1155:43–61.
21. DerKinderen DJ, Koten JW, Tan KE, Beemer FA, Van Romunde LK, Den Otter W. Parental age in sporadic hereditary retinoblastoma. Am J Ophthalmol 1990;110:605–9.
22. Munier FL, Thonney F, Balmer A, et al. Prognostic factors associated with loss of heterozygosity at the RB1 locus in retinoblastoma. Ophthalmic Genet 1997;18:7–12.
23. Friend SH, Horowitz JM, Gerber MR, et al. Deletions of a DNA sequence in retinoblastomas and mesenchymal tumors: organization of the sequence and its encoded protein. Proc Natl Acad Sci U S A 1987;84:9059–63.
24. Lee EY, To H, Shew JY, Bookstein R, Scully P, Lee WH. Inactivation of the retinoblastoma susceptibility gene in human breast cancers. Science 1988;241:218–21.
25. Horowitz JM, Yandell DW, Park SH, et al. Point mutational inactivation of the retinoblastoma antioncogene. Science 1989;243:937–40.
26. Cairns P, Proctor AJ, Knowles MA. Loss of heterozygosity at the RB locus is frequent and correlates with muscle invasion in bladder carcinoma. Oncogene 1991;6:2305–9.
27. Bookstein R, Rio P, Madreperla SA, et al. Promoter deletion and loss of retinoblastoma gene expression in human prostate carcinoma. Proc Natl Acad Sci U S A 1990;87:7762–6.
28. Boynton RF, Huang Y, Blount PL, et al. Frequent loss of heterogeneity at the retinoblastoma locus in human esophageal cancers. Cancer Res 1991;51:5766–9.
29. Harbour JW, Lai SL, Whang-Peng J, Gazdar AF, Minna JD, Kaye FJ. Abnormalities in structure and expression of the human retinoblastoma gene in SCLC. Science 1988;241:353–7.
30. Murakami Y, Katahira M, Makino R, Hayashi K, Hirohashi S, Sekiya T. Inactivation of the retinoblastoma gene in a human lung carcinoma cell line detected by single-strand conformation polymorphism analysis of the polymerase chain reaction product of cDNA. Oncogene 1991;6:37–42.
31. Shields JA, Shields CL. Retinoblastoma. In: Shields JA, Shields CL, eds. Intraocular tumors. Philadelphia: Lippincott, Williams & Wilkins; 1999:208–31.
32. Mietz H, Hutton WL, Font RL. Unilateral retinoblastoma in an adult: report of a case and review of the literature. Ophthalmology 1997;104:43–7.
33. Grossniklaus HE, Dhaliwal RS, Martin DF. Diffuse anterior retinoblastoma. Retina 1998;18: 238–41.
34. Bunt AH, Tso MO. Feulgen-positive deposits in retinoblastoma. Incidence, composition and ultrastructure. Arch Ophthalmol 1981;99:144–50.
35. Tso MO, Zimmerman LE, Fine BS, Ellsworth RM. A cause of radioresistance in retinoblastoma: photoreceptor differentiation. Trans Am Acad Ophthalmol Otolaryngol 19780;74:959–69.
36. Rodrigues MM, Wiggert B, Shields J, et al. Retinoblastoma. Immunohistochemistry and cell differentiation. Ophthalmology 1987;94:378–87.
37. Gonzalez-Fernandez F, Lopes MB, Garcia-Fernandez JM, et al. Expression of developmentally defined retinal phenotypes in the histogenesis of retinoblastoma. Am J Pathol 1992; 141:363–75.
38. Messmer EP, Font RL, Kirkpatrick JB, Hopping W. Immunohistochemical demonstration of neuronal and astrocytic differentiation in retinoblastoma. Ophthalmology 1985;92:167–73.
39. Nork TM, Millecchia LL, Poulsen G. Immunolocalization of the retinoblastoma protein in the human eye and in retinoblastoma. Invest Ophthalmol Vis Sci 1994;35:2682–92.

40. Lin CC, Tso MO. An electron microscopic study of calcification of retinoblastoma. Am J Ophthalmol 1983;96:765–74.
41. Davila RM, Miranda MC, Smith ME. Role of cytopathology in the diagnosis of ocular malignancies. Acta Cytol 1998;42:362–6.
42. Messmer EP, Heinrich T, Hopping W, de Sutter E, Havers W, Sauerwein W. Risk factors for metastases in patients with retinoblastoma. Ophthalmology 1991;98:136–41.
43. Reese AB, Ellsworth RM. The evaluation and current concept of retinoblastoma therapy. Trans Am Acad Ophthalmol Otolryngol 1963;67:164–72.
44. Howarth C, Meyer D, Hustu HO, et al. Stage-related combined modality treatment of retinoblastoma. Results of a prospective study. Cancer 1980;45:851–8.
45. Pratt CB, Fontanesi J, Lu X, Parham DM, Elfervig J, Meyer. Proposal for a new staging scheme for intraocular and extraocular retinoblastoma based on an analysis of 103 globes. Oncologist 1997;2:1–5.
46. Rubin CM, Robison LL, Cameron JD, et al. Intraocular retinoblastoma group V: an analysis of prognostic factors. J Clin Oncol 1985;3:680–5.
47. Eng C, Li FP, Abramson DH, et al. Mortality from second tumors among long-term survivors of retinoblastoma. J Natl Cancer Inst 1993;85:1121–8.
48. Roarty JD, McLean IW, Zimmerman LE. Incidence of second neoplasms in patients with bilateral retinoblastoma. Ophthalmology 1988;95:1583–7.
49. Font RL, Jurco S 3rd, Brechner RJ. Postradiation leiomyosarcoma of the orbit complicating bilateral retinoblastoma. Arch Ophthalmol 1983;101:1557–61.
50. Abramson DH, Melson MR, Dunkel IJ, Frank CM. Third (fourth and fifth) nonocular tumors in survivors of retinoblastoma. Ophthalmology 2001;108:1868–76.
51. Eagle RC Jr, Shields JA, Donoso L, Milner RS. Malignant transformation of spontaneously regressed retinoblastoma, retinoma/retinocytoma variant. Ophthalmology 1989;96:1389–95.

Glial Tumors and Tumor-Like Conditions

52. Ulbright TM, Fulling KH, Helveston EM. Astrocytic tumors of the retina. Differentiation of sporadic tumors from phakomatosis-associated tumors. Arch Pathol Lab Med 1984;108:160–3.
53. Arnold AC, Helper RS, Yee RW, Maggiano J, Eng LF, Foos RY. Solitary retinal astrocytoma. Surv Ophthalmol 1985;30:173–81.
54. Jakobiec FA, Brodie SE, Haik B, Iwamoto T. Giant cell astrocytoma of the retina. A tumor of possible Mueller cell origin. Ophthalmology 1983;90:2565–76.
55. Bornfeld N, Messmer EP, Theodossiadis G, Meyer-Schwickerath G, Wessing A. Giant cell astrocytoma of the retina. Clinicopathologic report of a case not associated with Bourneville's disease. Retina 1987;7:183–9.
56. Margo CE, Barletta JP, Staman JA. Giant cell astrocytoma of the retina in tuberous sclerosis. Retina 1993;13:155–9.
57. Robertson DM. Ophthalmic manifestations of tuberous sclerosis. Ann N Y Acad Sci 1991;615:17–25.
58. de Juan E Jr, Green WR, Gupta PK, Baranano EC. Vitreous seeding by retinal astrocytic hamartoma in a patient with tuberous sclerosis. Retina 1984;4:100–2.
59. Yanoff M, Zimmerman LE, Davis RL. Massive gliosis of the retina. Int Ophthalmol Clin 1971;11:211–29.
60. Sahel JA, Frederick AR Jr, Pesavento R, Albert DM. Idiopathic retinal gliosis mimicking a choroidal melanoma. Retina 1988;8:282–7.
61. Berger B, Peyman GA, Juarez C, Mason G, Raichand M. Massive retinal gliosis simulating choroidal melanoma. Can J Ophthalmol 1979;14:285–90.
62. Nork TM, Ghobrial MW, Peyman GA, Tso MO. Massive retinal gliosis. A reactive proliferation of Muller cells. Arch Ophthalmol 1986;104:1383–9.

Vascular Tumors

63. Font RL, Ferry AP. The phakomatoses. Int Ophthalmol Clin 1972;12:1–50.
64. Horton WA, Wong V, Eldridge R. Von Hippel-Lindau disease: clinical and pathological manifestations in nine families with 50 affected members. Arch Intern Med 1976;136:769–77.
65. Ehlers N, Jensen OA. Juxtapapillary retinal hemangioblastoma (angiomatosis retinae) in an infant: light microscopical and ultrastructural examination. Ultrastruct Pathol 1982;3:325–33.
66. Jakobiec FA, Font RL, Johnson FB. Angiomatosis retinae. An ultrastructural study and lipid analysis. Cancer 1976;38:2042–56.
67. Prowse AH, Webster AR, Richards FM, et al. Somatic inactivation of the VHL gene in Von Hippel-Lindau disease tumors. Am J Hum Genet 1997;60:765–71.
68. Chan CC, Vortmeyer A, Chew EY, et al. VHL gene deletion and enhanced VEGF gene expression detected in the stromal cells of retinal angioma. Arch Ophthalmol 1999;117:625–30.
69. Goldberg RE, Pheasant TR, Shields JA. Cavernous hemangioma of the retina. A four-generation pedigree with neurocutaneous manifestations and an example of bilateral retinal involvement. Arch Ophthalmol 1979;97:2321–4.

70. Pancurak J, Goldberg MF, Frenkel M, Crowell RM. Cavernous hemangioma of the retina. Genetic and central nervous system involvement. Retina 1985;5:215–20.
71. Messmer E, Font RL, Laqua H, Hopping W, Naumann GO. Cavernous hemangioma of the retina. Immunohistochemical and ultrastructural observations. Arch Ophthalmol 1984;102:413–8.

Melanogenic Neuroectodermal Tumor of the Retina

72. Freitag SK, Eagle RC Jr, Shields JA, Duker JS, Font RL. Melanogenic neuroectodermal tumor of the retina (primary malignant melanoma of the retina). Arch Ophthalmol 1997;115:1581–4.

Lymphoid Malignancies

73. Paulus W. Classification, pathogenesis and molecular pathology of primary CNS lymphomas. J Neurooncol 1999;43:203–8.
74. Read RW, Zamir E, Rao NA. Neoplastic masquerade syndromes. Surv Ophthalmol 2002;47:81–124.
75. Char DH, Ljung BM, Deschenes J, Miller TR. Intraocular lymphoma: immunological and cytological analysis. Br J Ophthalmol 1988;72:905–11.
76. Davis JL, Solomon D, Nussenblatt RB, Palestine AG, Chan CC. Imunocytochemical staining of vitreous cells. Indications, techniques, and results. Ophthalmology 1992;99:250–6.
77. Kaplan HJ, Meredith TA, Aaberg TM, Keller RH. Reclassification of intraocular reticulum cell sarcoma (histiocytic lymphoma). Immunological characterization of vitreous cells. Arch Ophthalmol 1980;98:707–10.
78. Taylor CR, Russell R, Lukes RJ, Davis RL. An immunohistological study of immunoglobulin content of primary central nervous system lymphomas. Cancer 1978;41:2197–205.
79. Warnke R, Miller R, Grogan R, Pederson M, Dilley J, Levy R. Immunological phenotype in 30 patients with diffuse large-cell lymphoma. N Engl J Med 1980;303:293–300.
80. Eby NL, Grufferman S, Flannelly CM, Schold SC Jr, Vogel FS, Burger PC. Increasing incidence of primary brain lymphoma in the US. Cancer 1988;62:2461–5.
81. Corn BW, Donahue BR, Rosenstock JG, et al. Performance status and age as independent predictors of survival among AIDS patients with primary CNS lymphoma: a multivariate analysis of a multi-institutional experience. Cancer J Sci Am 1997;2:52–6.
82. Paulus W. Classification, pathogenesis and molecular pathology of primary CNS lymhomas. J Neurooncol 1999;43:203–8.
83. Paulus W, Jellinger K. Comparison of integrin adhesion molecules expressed by primary brain lymphomas and nodal lymphomas. Acta Neuropathol (Berl) 1993;86:360–4.
84. Walker J, Ober RR, Khan A, Yuen D, Rao NA. Intraocular lymphoma developing in a patient with Vogt-Koyanagi-Harada syndrome. Int Ophthalmol 1993;17:331–6.
85. DeAngelis LM, Yahalom J, Heinermann MH, Cirrincione C, Thaler HT, Krol G. Primary CNS lymphoma: combined treatment with chemotherapy and radiotherapy. Neurology 1990;40: 80–6.
86. Hochberg FH, Miller DC. Primary central nervous system lymphoma. J Neurosurg 1988;68: 835–53.
87. Peterson K, Gordon KB, Heinemann MH, DeAngelis LM. The clinical spectrum of ocular lymphoma. Cancer 1993;72:843–9.
88. Verbraeken HE, Hanssens M, Priem H, Lafaut BA, De Laey JJ. Ocular non-Hodgkin's lymphoma: a clinical study of nine cases. Br J Ophthalmol 1997;81:31–6.
89. Herrlinger U, Schabetg M, Bitzer M, Petersen D, Krauseneck P. Primary central nervous system lymphoma: from clinical presentation to diagnosis. J Neurooncol 1999;43:219–26.
90. Hobson DE, Anderson BA, Carr I, West M. Primary lymphoma of the central nervous system. Manitoba experience and literature review. Can J Neurol Sci 1986;13:55–61.
91. O'Neill BP, Illig J. Primary central nervous system lymphoma. Mayo Clin Proc 1989;64:1005–20.
92. Braus DF, Schwechheimer K, Muller-Hermelink HK, Schwarzkopf G, Volk B, Mundinger F. Primary cerebral malignant non-Hodgkins lymphomas: a retrospective clinical study. J Neurol 1992;239:117–24.
93. Parekh HC, Sharma RR, Lynch PG, Keogh AJ, Prabhu SS. Primary cerebral lymphoma: report of 24 patients and review of the literature. Br J Neurosurg 1992;6:563–73.
94. Grote TH, Grosh WW, List AF, Wiley R, Cousar JB, Johnson DH. Primary lymphoma of the central nervous system. A report of 20 cases and a review of the literature. Am J Clin Oncol 1989;12:93–100.
95. Balmaceda CM, Fetell MR, Selman JE, Seplowitz AJ. Diabetes insipidus as first manifestation of primary central nervous system lymphoma. Neurology 1994;44:358–9.
96. Rauschning W. Brain tumors and tumor-like masses: classification and differential diagnosis. In: Osborn AG, ed. Diagnostic neuroradiology. St Louis: Mosby; 1994:399–625.
97. Freilich RJ, DeAngelis LM. Primary central nervous system lymphoma. Neurol Clin 1995;13: 901–14.

98. Dean JM, Novak MA, Chan CC, Green WR. Tumor detachments of the retinal pigment epithelium in ocular/central nervous system lymphoma. Retina 1996;16:47–56.
99. Shields JA, Shields CL, Ehya H, Eagle RC Jr, De Potter P. Fine-needle aspiration of suspected intraocular tumors. The 1992 Urwick Lecture. Ophthalmology 1993;100:1677–84.
100. Ciulla TA, Pesavento RD, Yoo S. Subretinal aspiration biopsy of ocular lymphoma. Am J Ophthalmol 1997;123:420-2.
101. Pavan PR, Oteiza EE, Margo CE. Ocular lymphoma diagnosed by internal subretinal pigment epithelium biopsy. Arch Ophthalmol 1995;113:1233–4.
102. Engel HM, Green WR, Michels RG, Rice TA, Erozan YS. Diagnostic vitrectomy. Retina 1981;1:121–49.
103. Chess J, Sebag J, Tolentino FL, et al. Pathologic processing of vitrectomy specimens. A comparison of pathologic findings with celoidin bag and cytocentrifugation preparation of 102 vitrectomy specimens. Ophthalmology 1983;90:1560–4.
104. Scroggs MW, Johnston WW, Klintworth GK. Intraocular tumors. A cytopathologic study. Acta Cytol 1990;34:401–8.
105. Akpek EK, Ahmed I, Hochberg FH, et al. Intraocular-central nervous system lymphoma: clinical features, diagnosis, and outcomes. Ophthalmology 1999;106:1805–10.
106. Carey JL, Hanson CA. Flow cytometric analysis of leukemia and lymphoma. In: Keren DF, Hanson CA, Hurtubise PE, eds. Flow cytometry and clinical diagnosis. Chicago: American Society of Clinical Pathologists; 1994:197–308.
107. Shen DF, Zhuang Z, LeHoang P, et al. Utility of microdissection and polymerase chain reaction for the detection of immunoglobulin gene rearrangement and translocation in primary intraocular lymphoma. Ophthalmology 1998; 105:1664–9.
108. Kirmani MH, Thomas EL, Rao NA, Laborde RP. Intraocular reticulum cell sarcoma: diagnosis by choroidal biopsy. Br J Ophthalmol 1987;71:748–52.
109. Abrey LE, DeAngelis LM, Yahalom J. Long-term survival in primary CNS lymphoma. J Clin Oncol 1998;16:859–63.
110. Abrey LE, Yahalom J, DeAngelis LM. Treatment for primary CNS lymphoma: the next step. J Clin Oncol 2000;18:3144–50.
111. DeAngelis LM. Primary central nervous system lymphoma. Recent Results Cancer Res 1994;135:155–69.
112. Smith JR, Rosenbaum JT, Wilson DJ, et al. Role of intravitreal methotrexate in the management of primary central nervous system lymphoma with ocular involvement. Ophthalmology 2002;109:1709–16.
113. DeMario MD, Liebowitz DN. Lymphomas in the immunocompromised patient. Semin Oncol 1998;25:492–502.
114. Ramsey RG. Supratentorial brain tumors. In: Ramsey RG, ed. Neuroradiology, 3rd ed. Philadelphia: WB Saunders; 1994:250–330.
115. Kumar SR, Gill PS, Wagner DG, Dugel PU, Moudgil T, Rao NA. Human T-cell lymphotropic virus type I-associated retinal lymphoma. A clinicopathologic report. Arch Ophthalmol 1994;112:954–9.
116. Kohno T, Uchida H, Inomata H, Fukushima S, Takeshita M, Kikuchi M. Ocular manifestations of adult T-cell leukemia/lymphoma. A clinicopathologic study. Ophthalmology 1993;100:1794–9.

Tumors of the Retinal Pigment Epithelium

117. Tso MO, Albert DM. Pathological condition of the retinal pigment epithelium. Neoplasms and nodular non-neoplastic lesions. Arch Ophthalmol 1972;88:27–38.
118. Shields JA, Shields CL, Gunduz K, Eagle RC Jr. Neoplasms of the retinal pigment epithelium: the 1998 Albert Ruedemann, Sr, Memorial Lecture, Part 2. Arch Ophthalmol 1999;117:601–8.

Metastatic Neoplasms

119. Loeffler KU, Kivela T, Borgmann H, Witschel H. Malignant tumor of the retinal pigment epithelium with extraocular extension in a phthisical eye. Graefes Arch Clin Exp Ophthalmol 1996;234(Suppl 1):S70–5.
120. Mack HG, Jakobiec FA. Isolated metastases to the retina or optic nerve. Int Ophthalmol Clin 1997;37:251–60.

Neuroepithelial Tumors

121. Zimmerman LE. Verhoeff's "terato-neuroma." A critical reappraisal in light of new observations and current concepts of embryonic tumors. The fourth Frederick H. Verhoeff lecture. Am J Ophthalmol 1971;72:1039–57.
122. Spencer WH, Jesberg DO. Glioneuroma (choristomatous malformation of the optic cup margin): a report of two cases. Arch Ophthalmol 1973;89:387–91.
123. Addison DJ, Font RL. Glioneuroma of iris and ciliary body. Arch Ophthalmol 1984;102:419–21.
124. Kivela T, Kauniskangas L, Miettinen P, Tarkkanen A. Glioneuroma associated with colobomatous dysplasia of the anterior uvea and retina. A case simulating medulloepithelioma. Ophthalmology 1989;96:1799–808.

125. Verhoeff FH. A rare tumor arising from the pars ciliaris retinae (teratoneuroma), of a nature hitherto unrecognized and its relation to the so-called glioma retinae. Trans Am Ophthalmol Soc 1904;10:351–77.
126. Grinker RR. Gliomas of the retina, including the results of studies with silver impregnations. Arch Ophthalmol 1931;5:920–35.
127. Andersen SR. Medulloepithelioma of the retina. Int Ophthalmol Clin 1962;2:483–506.
128. O'Keefe M, Fulcher T, Kelly P, Lee W, Dudgeon J. Medulloepithelioma of the optic nerve head. Arch Ophthalmol 1997;115:1325–7.
129. Green WR, Iliff WJ, Trotter RR. Malignant teratoid medulloepithelioma of the optic nerve. Arch Ophthalmol 1974;91:451–4.
130. Minoda K, Hirose Y, Sugano I, Nagao K, Kitahara K. Occurrence of sequential intraocular tumors: malignant medulloepithelioma subsequent to retinoblastoma. Jpn J Ophthalmol 1993;37:293–300.
131. Mamalis N, Font RL, Anderson CW, Monson MC, Williams AT. Concurrent benign teratoid medulloepithelioma and pineoblastoma. Ophthalmic Surg 1992;23:403–8.
132. Broughton WL, Zimmerman LE. A clinicopathologic study of 56 cases of intraocular medulloepithelioma. Am J Ophthalmol 1978;85:407–18.
133. Shields JA, Eagle RC Jr, Shields CL, Potter PD. Congenital neoplasms of the nonpigmented ciliary epithelium (medulloepithelioma). Ophthalmology 1996;103:1998–2006.
134. Orellana J, Moura RA, Font RL, Boniuk M, Murphy D. Medulloepithelioma diagnosed by ultrasound and vitreous aspirate. Electron microscopic observations. Ophthalmology 1983;90:1531–9.
135. Husain SE, Husain N, Boniuk, M, Font RL. Malignant nonteratoid medulloepithelioma of the ciliary body in an adult. Ophthalmology 1998;105:596–9.
136. Zimmerman LE, Font RL, Andersen SR. Rhabdomyosarcomatous differentiation in malignant intraocular medulloepitheliomas. Cancer 1972;30:817–35.
137. Kivela T, Tarkkanen A. Recurrent medulloepithelioma of the ciliary body. Immunohistochemical characteristics. Ophthalmology 1988;95:1565–975.
138. Desai VN, Lieb WE, Donoso LA, Eagle RC Jr. Shields JA, Saunders R. Photoreceptor cell differentiation in intraocular medulloepithelioma: an immunohistopathologic study. Arch Ophthalmol 1990;108:481–2.
139. Betts DR, Leibundgut KE, Niggli FK. Cytogenetic analysis in a case of intraocular medulloepithelioma. Cancer Genet Cytogenet 1996;92:144–6.
140. Iliff WJ, Green WR. The incidence and histology of Fuchs's adenoma. Arch Ophthalmol 1972;88:249–54.
141. Hillemann J, Nagmann G. [Benign epithelioma (Fuchs) of the ciliary body.] Ophthalmologica 1972;164:321–35. (German.)
142. Bateman JB, Foos RY. Coronal adenomas. Arch Ophthalmol 1979;97:2379–84.
143. Brown HH, Glasgow BJ, Foos RY. Ultrastructural and immunohistochemical features of coronal adenomas. Am J Ophthalmol 1991;112:34–40.
144. Cursiefen C, Schlotzer-Schrehardt U, Holbach LM, Naumann GO. Adenoma of the nonpigmented ciliary epithelium mimicking a malignant melanoma of the iris. Arch Ophthalmol 1999;117:113–6.
145. Shields JA, Eagle RC Jr, Shields CL, De Potter P. Acquired neoplasms of the nonpigmented ciliary epithelium (adenoma and adenocarcinoma). Ophthalmology 1996;103:2007–16.
146. Shields JA, Eagle RC Jr, Shields CL, Singh AD, Torrisi PF. Clinicopathologic reports, case reports, and small case series: progressive growth of benign adenoma of the pigment epithelium of the ciliary body. Arch Ophthalmol 2001; 119:1859–61.
147. Spencer WH. Ophthalmic pathology: an atlas and textbook, 4th ed. Vol 2. Philadelphia: WB Saunders; 1996:1325–30.
148. Dryja TP, Albert DM, Horns D. Adenocarcinoma arising from the epithelium of the ciliary body. Ophthalmology 1981;88:1290–2.
149. Grossniklaus HE, Zimmerman LE, Kachmer ML. Pleomorphic adenocarcinoma of the ciliary body. Immunohistochemical and electron microscopic features. Ophthalmology 1990;97: 763–8.
150. Laver NM, Hidayat AA, Croxatto JO. Pleomorphic adenocarcinomas of the ciliary epithelium. Immunohistochemical and ultrastructural features of 12 cases. Ophthalmology 1999;106:103–10.
151. Terasaki H, Nagasaka T, Arai M, Harada T, Miyake Y. Adenocarcinoma of the nonpigmented ciliary epithelium: report of two cases with immunohistochemical findings. Graefes Arch Clin Exp Ophthalmol 2001;239:876–81.
152. Nicolo M, Nicolo G, Zingirian M. Pleomorphic adenocarcinoma of the ciliary epithelium: a clinicopathological, immunohistochemical, ultrastructural, DNA-ploidy and comparative genomic hybridization analysis of an unusual case. Eur J Ophthalmol 2002;12:319–23.

4 TUMORS OF THE OPTIC NERVE AND OPTIC NERVE HEAD

ANATOMY AND HISTOLOGY

The optic nerve, approximately 50 mm long, extends from the optic disc to the optic chiasm. For descriptive purposes, the nerve is divided into four portions: intraocular, intraorbital, intracanalicular, and intracranial. The intraocular portion, commonly known as the optic nerve head (fig. 4-1), is about 1.0 to 1.5 mm long and 1.5 mm in diameter. The intraocular portion traverses the sclera. The intraorbital portion, 30 to 40 mm long and 3 to 4 mm in diameter, follows a sinuous course, emerging from the back of the eye to enter the optic foramen at the apex of the orbit. The slack provided by this sinuous course allows for considerable eye movement. About 8 to 15 mm behind the globe, the central retinal artery, a branch of the ophthalmic artery, penetrates the dura and leptomeninges and reaches the center of the optic nerve. The intracanalicular portion, which is about 5 to 8 mm long, passes through the optic canal, where it is tightly fixed. The intracranial portion, approximately 10 mm long, joins with the contralateral nerve to form the optic chiasm. All of the central nervous system (CNS) sheaths, including the pia mater, arachnoid, and dura mater, surround the intraorbital portion of the optic nerve.

Histologically, the optic nerve head extends from the surface of the optic disc facing the vitreous cavity to the posterior scleral surface. The optic nerve head can be divided into the

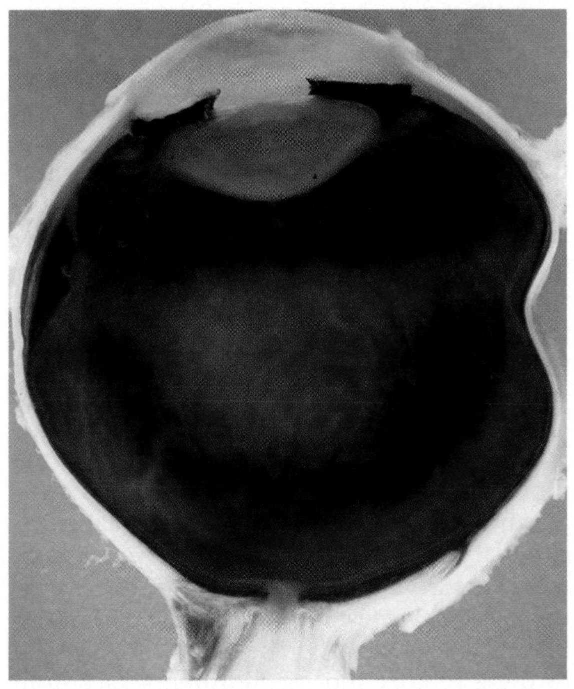

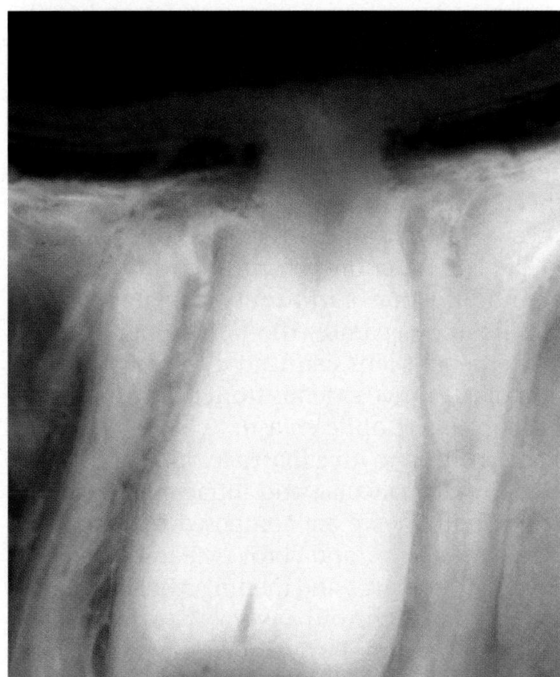

Figure 4-1

NORMAL OPTIC NERVE

Left: Sectioned specimen of globe and optic nerve. The nonmyelinated optic nerve head is seen.
Right: Higher magnification shows retina, choroid, sclera, and optic nerve. The retrobulbar nerve is myelinated.

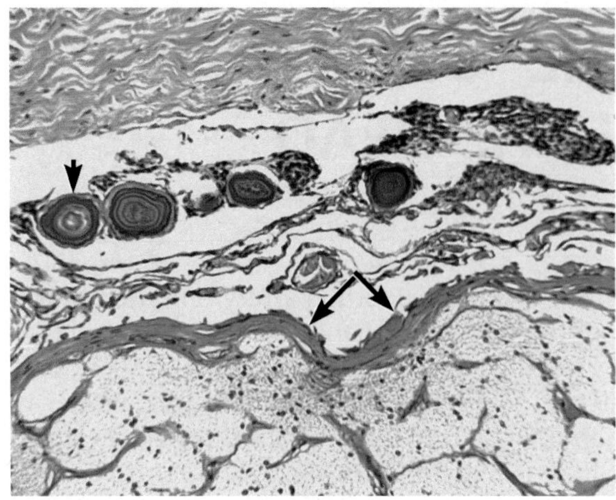

Figure 4-2

NORMAL OPTIC NERVE

Dura mater, arachnoid, and pia mater are seen. Psammoma bodies (short arrow) are present in the arachnoid layer and characteristic septa from the pia mater (long arrows) extend into the nerve.

prelaminar region and the lamina cribrosa region. The prelaminar region consists of nonmyelinated axons, arranged in bundles that are separated by columns of astrocytes and capillaries. The lamina cribrosa is a specialized, sieve-like region with many oval or round openings that permit the passage of the bundles of nerve fibers and the central retinal vessels. This region consists of dense, compact collagenous sheets of scleral trabeculae alternating with glial sheets. The astrocytes that line the openings in the lamina cribrosa form a continuous glial membrane that surrounds each nerve fiber bundle and separates the nerve fiber bundles from the adjacent connective tissue. Myelination of the nerve extends from the postlaminar portion to the optic chiasm.

In addition to myelinated axons, the intraorbital, intracanalicular, and intracranial portions of the optic nerve are composed of astrocytes, oligodendrocytes, and fibrovascular septa. Blood vessels, fibroblasts, and meningothelial cells are in the pia/archnoid layers. The axons are grouped into bundles by fibrovascular pial septa.

The intraorbital portion of the optic nerve is enclosed by three sheaths that are continuous with the meninges of the CNS: the dura mater, the arachnoid, and the pia mater. Anteriorly, the dura mater inserts into the sclera. Posteriorly, it divides into two layers. One of these layers fuses with the periosteum of the bony canal at the apex of the orbit; the remaining layer is tightly adherent to the bone of the canal harboring the optic nerve. When the optic nerve passes through the cranial foramen of the canal, the dura mater becomes the periosteum of the sphenoid bone without any other interposed tissues. Therefore, even small lesions that occur within the canal or at its openings will compress and damage the optic nerve.

The arachnoid, which is lined by meningothelia, contains numerous vessels, along with some fibroblasts and histiocytes. The meningothelia often proliferate in a concentric pattern to form onion-like structures, with or without foci of calcification, known as corpora arenacea (fig. 4-2).

The pia mater lies tightly on the surface of the nerve itself and consists of collagenous fibers, elastic fibers, and a fused glial layer. The pia mater invests the nerve and sends fibers into it to form the fibrovascular septa. The pia mater joins the sclera and choroid anteriorly; posteriorly, it continues through the optic foramen to form the single sheath around the intracranial portion of optic nerve.

The potential space between the dura mater and the arachnoid, known as the subdural space, does not communicate with the corresponding intracranial space and has little clinical significance. The subarachnoid space, between the arachnoid and the pia mater, is continuous with the corresponding intracranial space. It transmits cerebrospinal fluid, providing a pathway for the spread of tumor cells between the eye and the CNS.

CLASSIFICATION AND FREQUENCY

Tumors arising in the optic nerve head or the nerve are classified as benign or malignant neoplasms. In addition, there are other malignancies that secondarily involve the nerve; such tumors arise from anatomic structures adjacent to the nerve or metastasize to the nerve from distant organs (Table 4-1). The relative frequencies of these tumors and pseudotumors vary from one series to another. In one series reported by the Armed Forces Institute of Pathology (AFIP) the most common primary tumor was astrocytoma (Table 4-2). In contrast, the most common

Table 4-1

TUMORS OF THE OPTIC NERVE AND OPTIC NERVE HEAD

Primary Tumors and Pseudoneoplasms
- Benign
  - Meningioma
  - Juvenile pilocytic astrocytoma
  - Melanocytoma
  - Medulloepithelioma
  - Juvenile xanthogranuloma
  - Hemangioma/angiomatosis and hemangiopericytoma
  - Astrocytic hamartoma and giant calcified drusen
  - Juxtapapillary hamartoma
- Malignant
  - Malignant astrocytoma
  - Melanoma
  - Malignant teratoid medulloepithelioma

Secondary and Metastatic Tumors
- Retinoblastoma
- Melanoma
- Leukemia
- Leptomeningeal carcinomatosis
- Others

Table 4-2

TUMORS OF THE OPTIC NERVE AND OPTIC NERVE HEAD[a]

Type of Tumor	Number of Cases
Nerve	
Astrocytoma	17
Meningioma	8
Hemangiopericytoma	2
Melanoma	1
Lymphoma	1
Carcinoma, metastatic	1
Disc	
Melanocytoma	3
Astrocytoma	1

[a]Frequency distribution of 34 tumors from the Armed Forces Institute of Pathology (AFIP) Registry of Ophthalmic Pathology collected between 1984 and 1989.

Table 4-3

PRIMARY TUMORS OF THE OPTIC NERVE AND OPTIC NERVE HEAD[a]

Type of Tumor	Number of Cases
Nerve	
Meningioma	18
Astrocytoma	12
Melanoma	1
Optic Nerve Head	
Melanocytoma	1
Angiomatosis	1

[a]Frequency distribution of 33 tumors from the Doheny Eye Institute files collected between 1970 and 2000.

tumor in the series from the Doheny Eye Institute was meningioma, followed by astrocytoma (Table 4-3). Henderson (1) found that meningiomas were slightly more common than astrocytomas. Other tumors or pseudoneoplasms that are localized to the optic disc and seen only at this location are giant calcified drusen and juxtapapillary hamartoma. Although melanocytomas are observed in the uvea and conjunctiva, these tumors usually involve the optic nerve head and are unique to the eye.

MENINGIOMA

Definition. *Optic nerve meningioma* is a benign neoplasm that originates from the meningothelial cells present in the arachnoidal villi of the optic nerve sheath. This tumor, which is among the most common primary neoplasms of the optic nerve, is composed of nests of meningothelial cells along with vascular and fibrous tissues. Meningiomas can arise from any part of the optic nerve, but more than 80 percent are located at the orbital apex. Other sites of origin include the sphenoid ridge and ectopic meningothelial cells. A review of large series of meningiomas revealed that 90 percent arise intracranially and 10 percent in the orbit. Of the latter group, 96 percent arise from the optic sheath and 4 percent from a presumed ectopic site (Table 4-4).

Like CNS meningiomas, optic nerve meningiomas display a variety of morphologic features, including syncytial, fibroblastic, transitional with variable number of psammoma bodies, and angioblastic features. Most, however, show syncytial or transitional histologic features. Optic nerve meningiomas may not have the features associated with aggressive and malignant behavior seen in CNS meningiomas such as marked atypia and solid areas of tumor (known as "sheeting").

General Features. Cushing (4) coined the term meningioma to describe tumors originating from the CNS meninges. Although the histologic

Table 4-4

SITES OF ORIGIN FOR MENINGIOMAS INVOLVING THE ORBIT (5000 PATIENTS)[a]

Secondary tumors, intracranial origin: 4502 (90%)
Primary tumors, orbital origin: 498 (10%)
Ectopic: 21 (4%)
Optic sheath: 477 (96%)
Orbital optic nerve: 438 (92%)
Optic canal: 40 (8%)

[a]Modified from reference 3.

Table 4-5

CLINICAL CHARACTERISTICS OF OPTIC NERVE SHEATH MENINGIOMA[a]

Age:	40.8 yrs (range, 2.5–78 yrs) < 20 yrs: 11 (4 percent)	
Sex:	Women: 61%	Men: 39%
Laterality:	Unilateral: 95%	Bilateral: 5%

[a]Modified from reference 3.

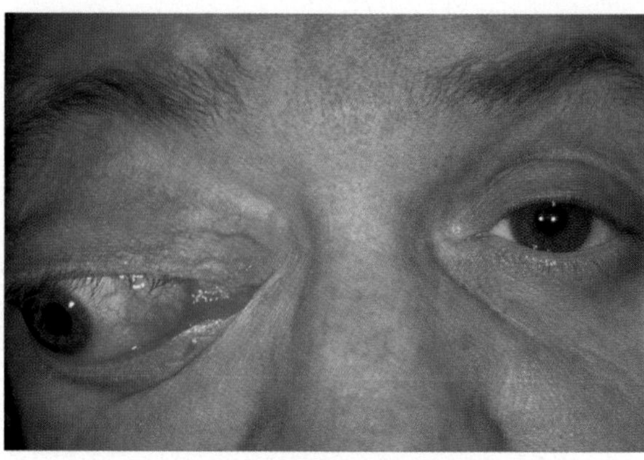

Figure 4-3

MENINGIOMA

Proptosis and inferior-lateral displacement of the right globe in optic nerve meningioma.

makeup of meningiomas led Cushing and Eisenhart to propose that they could arise from optic nerve sheath, the first unequivocal meningioma arising from the optic nerve was reported by Friedenwald (5). Primary optic nerve meningiomas constitute about 1.7 percent of orbital tumors.

There are contradictory reports about the age distribution of patients presenting with optic nerve meningioma. A few reports suggest that the tumor occurs primarily in young individuals; others report the occurrence of these tumors mainly in middle-aged individuals (3). In a review of reported series (3), the mean age at presentation is 40.8 years and the range varies from 2.5 to 78 years. The mean age is a little higher in women (42.5 years) than men (36.1 years) and the incidence is greater in women (ratio of 1.6 to 1.0). About 95 percent of tumors are unilateral; only 5 percent are bilateral (Table 4-5) (3). Patients with bilateral tumors tend to be younger, with a median age of 33.0 years. Bilateral meningiomas commonly occur in the optic canal (canalicular meningiomas) (6). Meningioma is more frequent in patients with neurofibromatosis, with an incidence of about 9 percent (3).

A number of factors may play a role in the development of intracranial meningioma: etiologic factors, such as ionizing radiation; hormonal disturbances involving estrogen and progesterone; viral infections with papova or adenoviruses; and chromosomal abnormalities, such as the loss of one copy of chromosome 22 or segments of DNA sequences from chromosome 22. Similar factors may play a role in the pathogenesis of optic nerve sheath meningioma. In addition to the chromosomal loss, intracranial meningiomas may express estrogen, progesterone, and androgen receptors. Progesterone receptors are expressed in two thirds of intracranial meningiomas, and estrogen receptors in one third (7).

Clinical Features. Visual loss is the most common finding, followed by proptosis (fig. 4-3) and chronic disc swelling (fig. 4-4) or optic atrophy. A clinical triad of visual loss, optic atrophy, and the presence of optociliary shunt vessels strongly suggests the diagnosis of optic nerve meningioma. The visual loss is gradual, and color vision is affected early. The neoplasm usually produces enlargement of the blind spot and/or visual field loss. Computerized tomography (CT) can detect optic nerve meningioma and such scans typically reveal a denser and thicker nerve sheath outlining the optic nerve as a central lucency (fig. 4-5). This radiographic sign is known as tram-tracking (3). Similar findings are noted on magnetic resonance imaging (MRI)

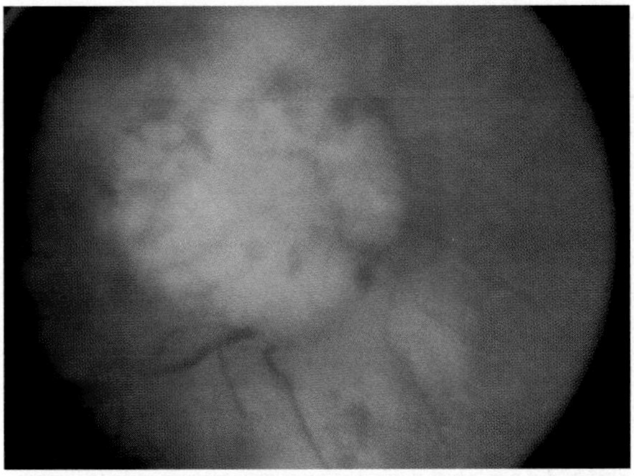

Figure 4-4

MENINGIOMA

Fundus photo of optic nerve meningioma shows a swollen optic disc with hemorrhages.

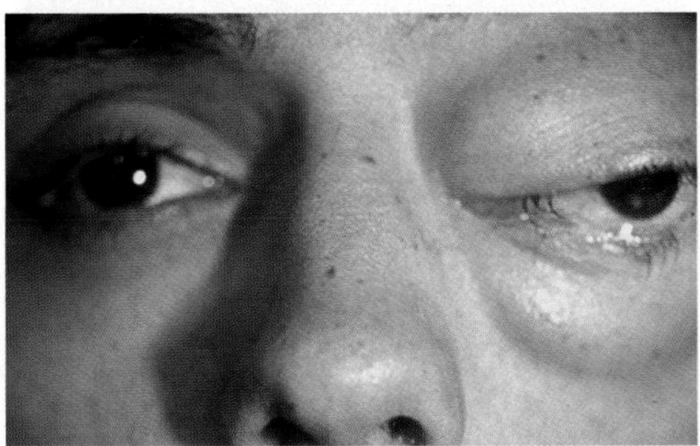

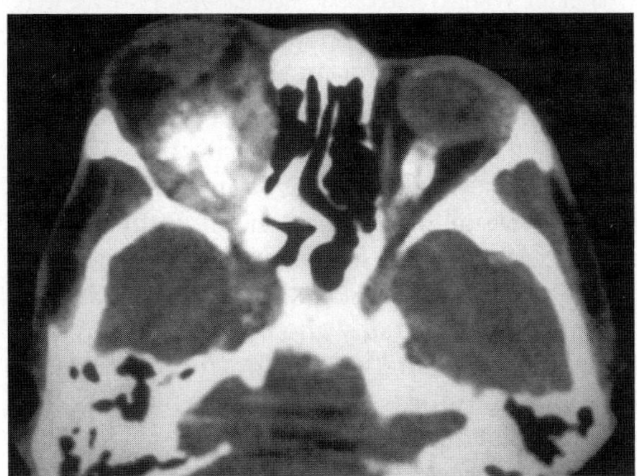

Figure 4-5

BILATERAL MENINGIOMAS

Top: The patient with neurofibromatosis 1 developed marked proptosis of the left eye.

Bottom: Computerized tomography (CT) shows bilateral meningiomas. The right optic nerve tumor exhibits a central lucency.

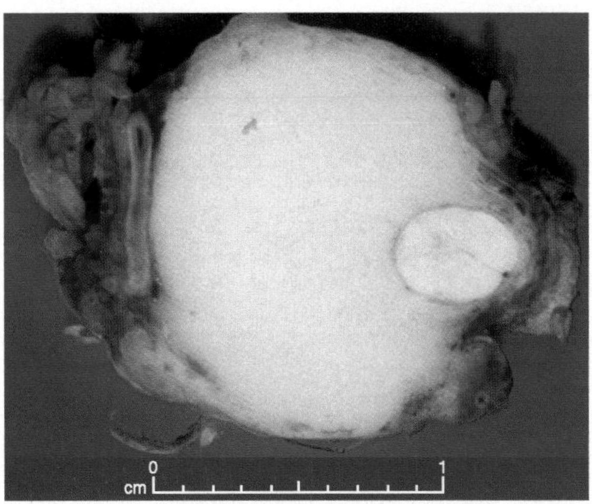

Figure 4-6

MENINGIOMA

The tumor partially encircles the optic nerve.

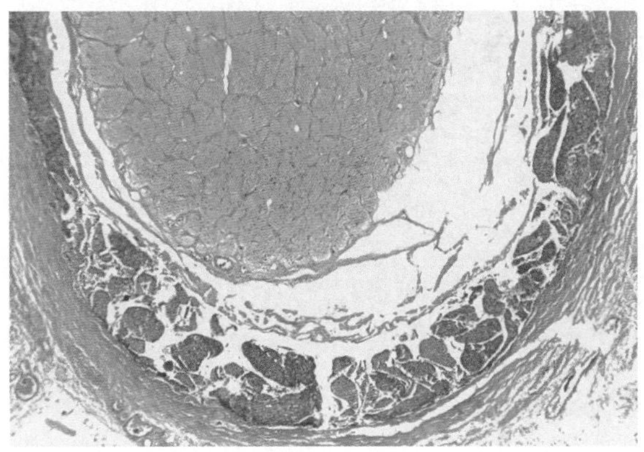

Figure 4-7

MENINGIOMA

The meningioma is localized to the arachnoid.

with fat suppression contrast administered T1-weighted imaging. In conjunction with the tram-tracking sign, T1-weighted MRI outlines the true anatomic borders of the optic nerve located in the optic canal and the orbit.

Gross and Microscopic Findings. Meningiomas emanating from the orbital part of the optic nerve may cause diffuse, plaque-like thickening of the meninges, or may be seen as a globular or fusiform mass replacing the orbital soft tissue (fig. 4-6). The tumor may be localized to the arachnoid (fig. 4-7); grow to compress the nerve, causing optic atrophy (fig. 4-8); or invade the dura and extend into the

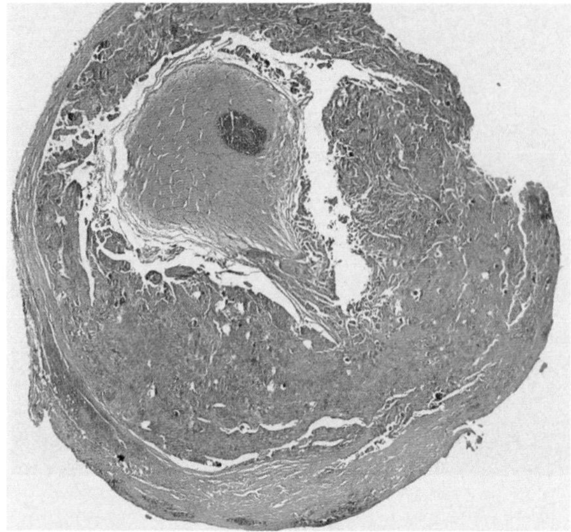

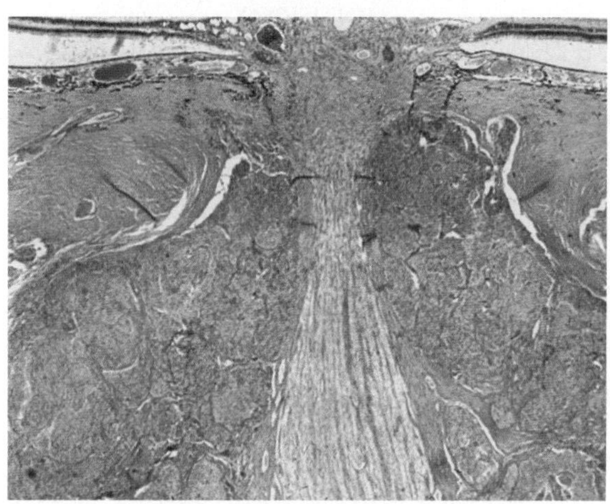

Figure 4-8

MENINGIOMA

Atrophic optic nerve is surrounded by meningioma.

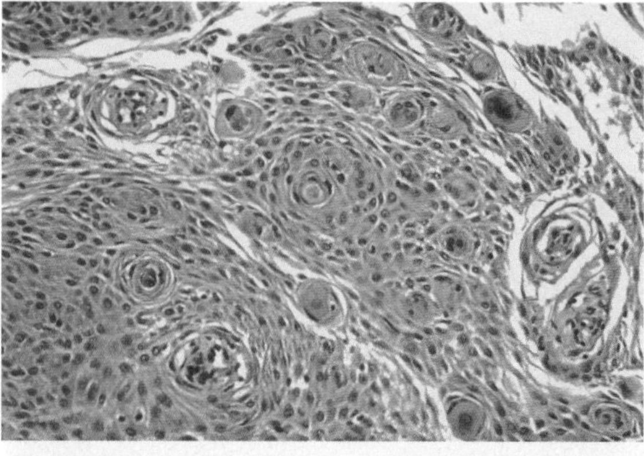

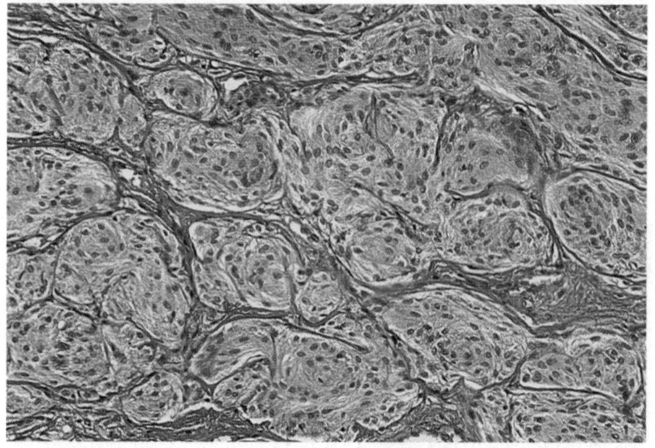

Figure 4-9

MENINGIOMA

Top: Syncytial meningioma with whorls of meningothelial cells.

Bottom: Whorls of neoplastic meningothelial cells are seen.

orbital soft tissue. Histologic analysis of *syncytial meningioma* reveals aggregates of lobules or whorls of meningothelial cells (fig. 4-9) with indistinct cell borders. The neoplastic cells have pale nuclei, some of which contain inclusion bodies. These inclusion bodies are cytoplasmic invaginations into the nuclei. Although inclusion bodies are occasionally seen in other histologic types of meningiomas, they are most typical of the syncytial type (8). Usually, the syncytial type also shows xanthoma cells and a small number of psammoma bodies.

Transitional meningioma consists of groups of meningothelial cells with syncytial features surrounded by elongated, fibroblast-like cells (fig. 4-10). There may be an abundance of meningiothelial whorls or psammoma bodies. Tumors containing a profusion of psammoma bodies largely exclude intervening meningothelial cells and are referred to as *psammomatous meningiomas*.

Fibroblastic and *angioblastic meningiomas* usually arise intracranially and secondarily involve the orbit; they rarely occur in the optic nerve. Fibroblastic tumors are composed of elongated cells arranged in sheets and fascicles. The typical whorled pattern and psammoma bodies may not be easily detected. Some fibroblastic meningiomas show a storiform pattern and resemble histiocytic tumors, with markedly elongated nuclei and dense chromatin, while others have plump nuclei with delicate chromatin. Ultrastructurally, fibroblastic meningiomas reveal occasional desmosomes and intermediate

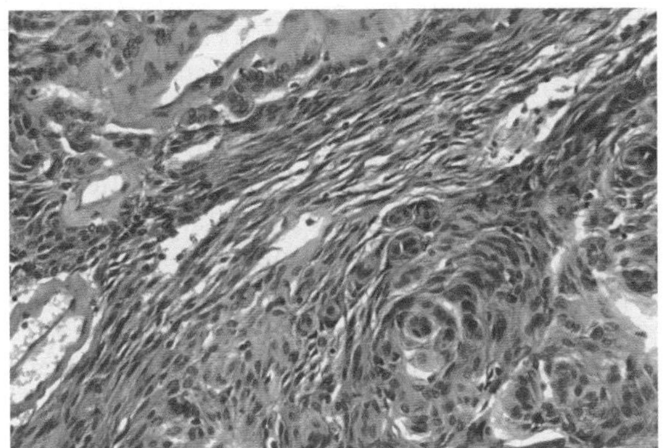

Figure 4-10

MENINGIOMA

Transitional meningioma shows features of syncytial and spindle-shaped meningothelial cells.

filaments (typical features of meningothelial cells), along with an abundance of extracellular basement membrane-like material. Like the fibroblastic type, angioblastic meningiomas (fig. 4-11) are extremely rare. The histogenesis of angioblastic meningioma is a subject of controversy; some reports show immunohistochemical evidence of a meningothelial origin, but such tumors may represent syncytial or transitional meningiomas containing a large number of blood vessels (3,8). Hemangiopericytomas and fibrous histiocytomas arise from the mesodermal component of the meninges, but these tumors more commonly arise from orbital soft tissue structures (9).

Immunohistochemical Findings. Neoplastic meningothelial cells are immunoreactive for epithelial membrane antigen (EMA). The positive reaction may occur in the cytoplasm or the membranes of the neoplastic cells (fig. 4-12). Membrane staining is considered useful for diagnosis. The tumors also react with antivimentin antibodies. Some meningiomas also react with antibodies directed against cytokeratin and S-100 protein.

Cytologic Findings. Rarely, a fine-needle aspiration biopsy is performed to confirm the diagnosis. Imprints or squash preparations are useful for recognizing meningiomas. Typically, meningiomas have wispy cytoplasm, delicate chromatin, small nucleoli, and intranuclear inclusions (fig. 4-13). They generally lack mitotic figures and areas of necrosis.

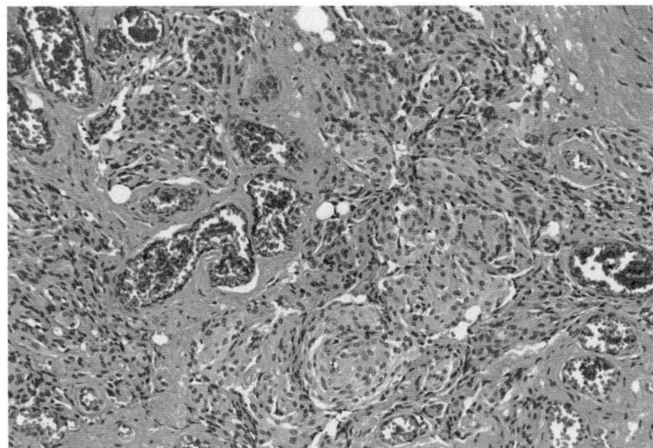

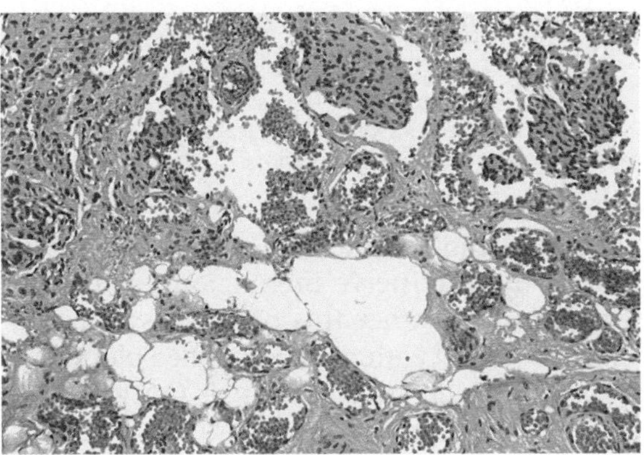

Figure 4-11

MENINGIOMA

Top: Prominent vascularity in an angioblastic meningioma.

Bottom: There are collections of meningothelial cells.

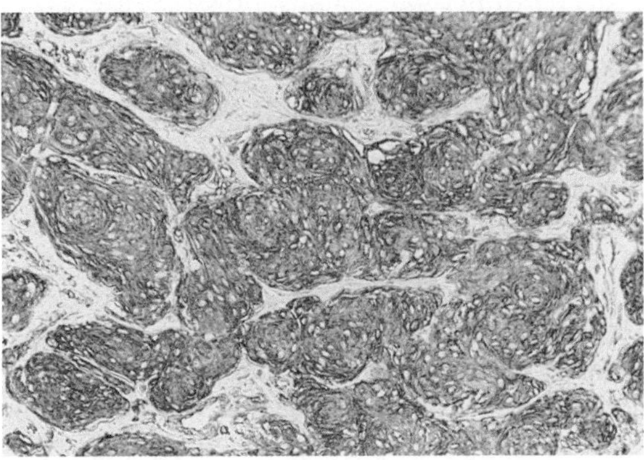

Figure 4-12

MENINGIOMA

Immunostaining is positive for epithelial membrane antigen.

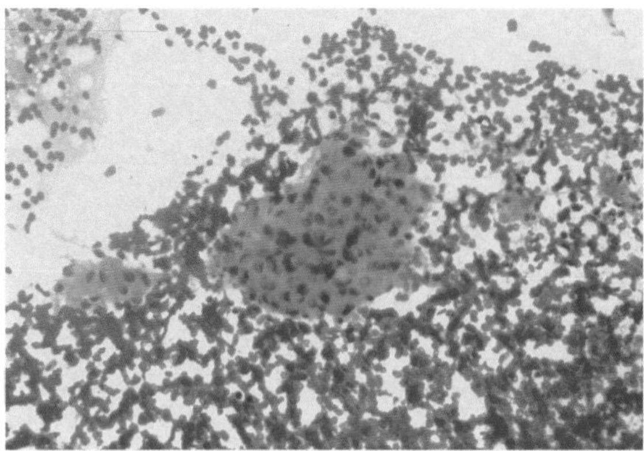

Figure 4-13

MENINGIOMA

Fine-needle aspiration biopsy preparation shows meningothelial cells displaying delicate chromatin, small nucleoli, and intranuclear inclusions.

Differential Diagnosis. The microscopic diagnosis of optic nerve meningioma is usually straightforward since this tumor has a characteristic whorled pattern, thick-walled blood vessels, and psammoma bodies. Optic nerve pilocytic astrocytoma may stimulate the proliferation of adjacent meningothelial cells and fibroblasts, resulting in an appearance that can be confused with a meningioma. This reactive process is contained within the dural sheet, in contrast to true meningiomas which usually invade the dura. Occasionally, leptomeningeal carcinomatosis resulting from metastatic lung or breast carcinoma may be mistaken for a syncytial meningioma. Usually, however, these carcinomas have hyperchromatic nuclei, abnormal mitotic figures, and foci of necrosis.

Special Studies. Researchers addressing the pathogenesis of meningioma and possible treatment options are attempting both to detect the estrogen and progesterone receptors on the tumor cells and to locate a chromosome 22 deletion that may play a role in tumor development. The significance of such studies in the management of optic nerve meningioma is not clear. Detecting a higher percentage of actively cycling tumor cells by labeling nuclear antigen with antibody Ki-67 may help identify aggressive meningiomas (8).

Treatment and Prognosis. Optic nerve meningioma produces a gradual loss of vision, disfiguring proptosis, and orbital pain; however, mortality from this tumor is rare among adults. Meningiomas in infants and young children, although infrequent, are much more aggressive than those in adults. Meningiomas occurring in children may require early surgical intervention (10). In general, adult patients with intraorbital optic nerve meningiomas who retain some vision are followed without surgical intervention. A recent report suggests that fractionated external beam radiation (5000–5500 cGy) may be considered as initial treatment in order to preserve visual function (11). Once vision is lost, surgical removal of the tumor may be offered to manage proptosis, orbital pain, and various intraocular complications. In contrast to the repeated MRI follow-up examinations used to track the spread of meningiomas localized to the orbital part of the nerve, meningiomas that extend toward the optic canal are usually managed surgically by a combined transorbital and transcranial approach, particularly in those patients with vision loss.

Occasional case reports suggest that optic canal meningiomas spread to the opposite side; however, there is no histologic confirmation of such spread. Bilateral canalicular meningiomas may originate from an intracranial meningeal focus, and then extend forward bilaterally into the canalicular optic nerve sheath (3). Rarely, malignant meningiomas are encountered, particularly in patients with multiple recurrences (figs. 4-14, 4-15). Histologically, such tumors show sheets of neoplastic cells with frequent mitoses.

JUVENILE PILOCYTIC ASTROCYTOMA

Definition. *Juvenile pilocytic astrocytoma* is a benign, primary optic nerve tumor that is mainly composed of fibrous astrocytes. Microscopically, these tumors display elongated spindle-shaped astrocytes with hair-like cytoplasmic processes. The tumor is also referred to as *optic nerve glioma*, but many prefer to use the term juvenile pilocytic astrocytoma, since most of these glial tumors occur in children. The typical clinical course is benign.

General Features. Although the clinical and histopathologic features of pilocytic astrocytoma have been well documented, controversies remain regarding the natural history, treatment, and hamartomatous versus neoplastic nature of

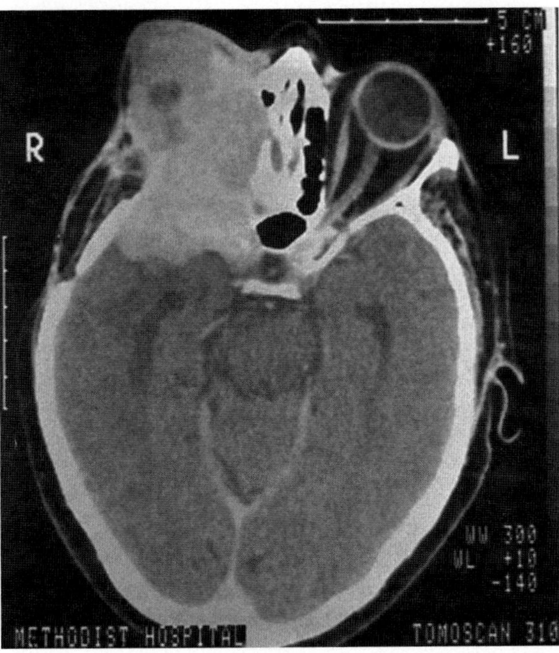

Figure 4-14

MENINGIOMA

CT scan of a recurrent orbital meningioma shows an infiltrative mass.

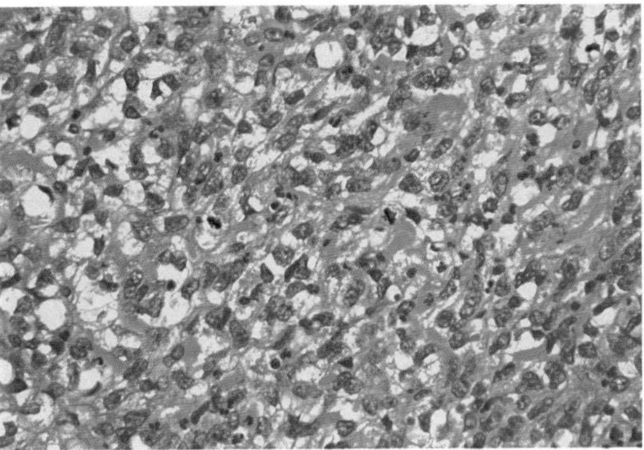

Figure 4-15

MALIGNANT MENINGIOMA AFTER RECURRENCE

Sheets of atypical cells have frequent abnormal mitoses.

these tumors. Regarding the latter, the propensity for optic nerve astrocytoma to invade the leptomeninges and to enlarge progressively implies that these masses are neoplastic in nature.

Pilocytic astrocytoma is mainly a tumor of childhood. Ninety percent of cases are diagnosed during the first two decades, with a median age of 5 years. The age at which the tumor becomes clinically apparent varies from 8 months to 38 years of age (12–14). The tumor is rarely present at birth (15). There is a female predominance (60 to 40 ratio). Optic nerve astrocytomas represent between 1 and 4 percent of all orbital tumors. About 48 percent involve the orbital portion of the nerve, 28 percent the intracranial portion, and 24 percent both the orbital and intracranial portions.

An association between optic nerve astrocytoma and neurofibromatosis type 1 is well established. It is estimated that as many as 30 percent of patients with juvenile pilocytic astrocytoma of the nerve have neurofibromatosis. The astrocytoma may be bilateral in these patients, but unilateral tumors are more common; multicentric tumors, rare in other patients, also occur in patients with neurofibromatosis. Astrocytomas tend to present at younger age (mean, 4.9 years) in patients with neurofibromatosis as compared to those without the disease (mean, 12 years) (12).

Clinical Features. The clinical presentation of optic nerve astrocytoma varies, depending on the location. Patients with orbital optic nerve astrocytoma have unilateral visual loss, proptosis (fig. 4-16, top), and disc swelling (fig. 4-16, bottom) or disc pallor. Visual loss is the initial and the most common symptom. The proptosis is usually axial (displacement of the globe anteriorly without horizontal or vertical displacement), often in the 3- to 8-mm range, but occasionally greater than 8 mm. The optic nerve mass is often fusiform and asymmetric. The tumor does not invade the surrounding orbital structures and is almost invariably confined by the dura mater.

Tumors located near the optic disc may compress adjacent tissue, resulting in rapid visual loss, disc swelling, and central retinal vein occlusion. In contrast, chiasmal astrocytomas may result in signs of hypothalamic and pituitary involvement. Such tumors also cause visual loss, strabismus, and nystagmus and may be associated with elevated intracranial pressure.

Neuroradiologic procedures, such as MRI or CT, help diagnose pilocytic astrocytoma. The tumor is seen as a fusiform enlargement (fig. 4-17), without signs of surrounding orbital soft tissue invasion (16).

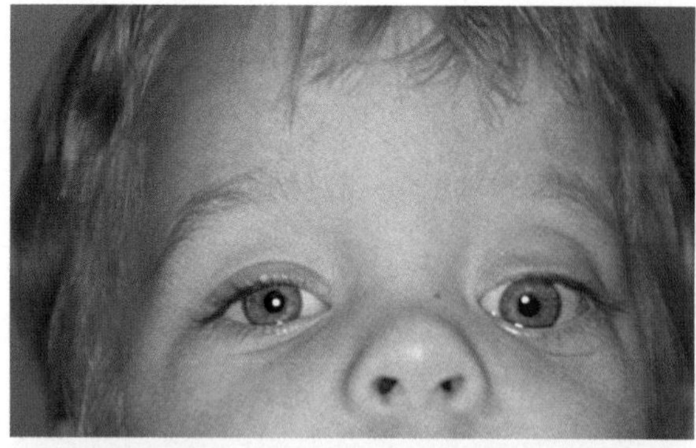

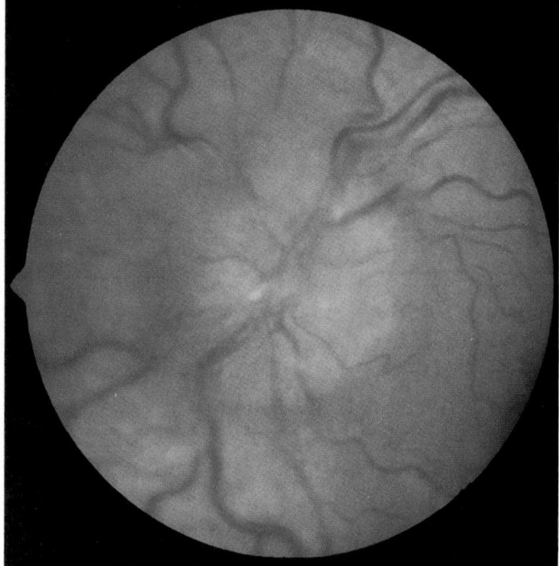

Figure 4-16

PILOCYTIC ASTROCYTOMA

A 2-year-old child with pilocytic astrocytoma of the orbital optic nerve presents clinically with proptosis (top) and optic disc swelling (bottom).

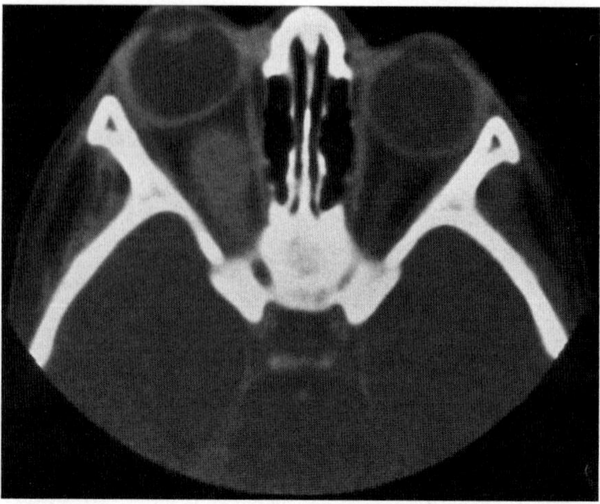

Figure 4-17

PILOCYTIC ASTROCYTOMA

CT reveals fusiform enlargement of the nerve without signs of surrounding orbital tissue invasion.

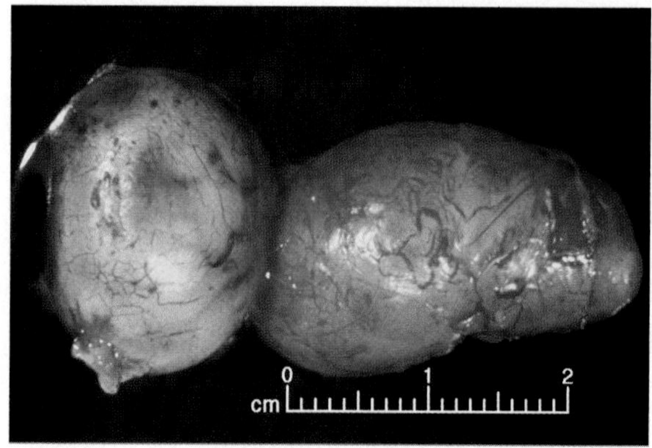

Figure 4-18

PILOCYTIC ASTROCYTOMA

Fusiform enlargement of a retrobulbar optic nerve astrocytoma.

Gross and Microscopic Findings. Grossly, astrocytomas arising from the intraorbital portion of the optic nerve have a fusiform appearance, with intact dura (fig. 4-18) that may be stretched and thin. Cross-section often reveals an enlarged, whitish or yellowish tan nerve surrounded by arachnoidal tissue of varying thickness. The latter is surrounded by dura, which although thin, is intact. Occasional tumors have a gelatinous or cystic appearance. Astrocytomas arising from the canalicular portion of the nerve may extend into the orbital and intracranial parts of the nerve; they may have a dumbbell shape. Near the tapering margins of the tumor the optic nerve may be of normal thickness. It is often difficult to distinguish the tumor margins from the uninvolved nerve; however, the tapered end of the tumor may be surrounded by variably thickened arachnoidal tissue.

Histologically, optic nerve astrocytomas are composed of spindle-shaped astrocytes with elongated, hair-like (pilocytic) processes (fig. 4-19). These astrocytes are relatively cohesive, with oval nuclei that are rarely hyperchromatic.

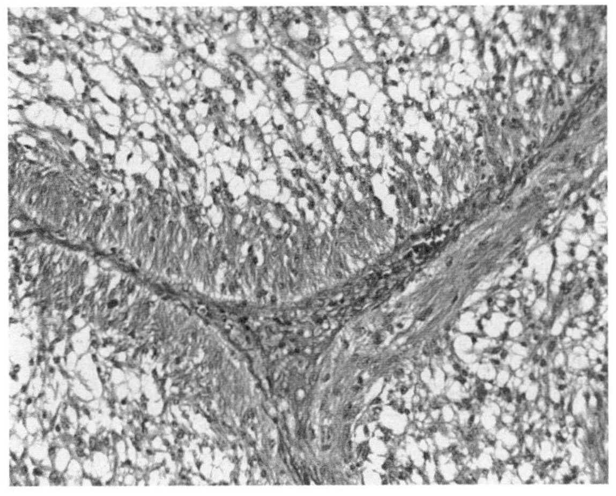

Figure 4-19

PILOCYTIC ASTROCYTOMA

Pilocytic cells are palisading around a blood vessel.

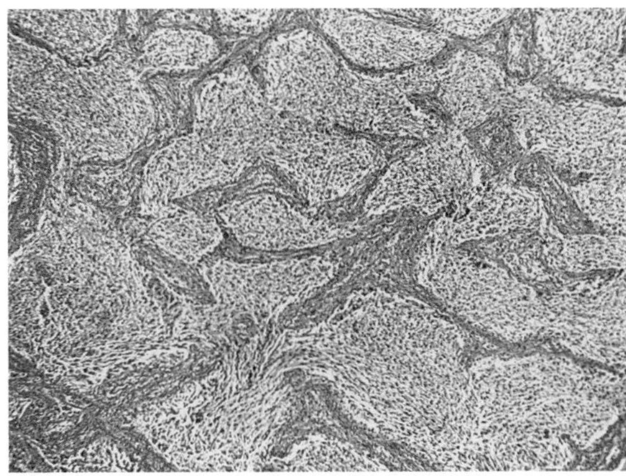

Figure 4-20

PILOCYTIC ASTROCYTOMA

Irregularly distended pial septa.

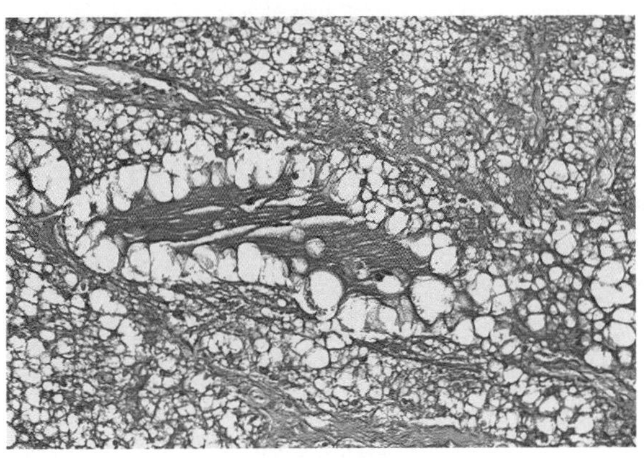

Figure 4-21

PILOCYTIC ASTROCYTOMA

Cystic changes with an accumulation of extracellular mucopolysaccharides (Alcian blue stain).

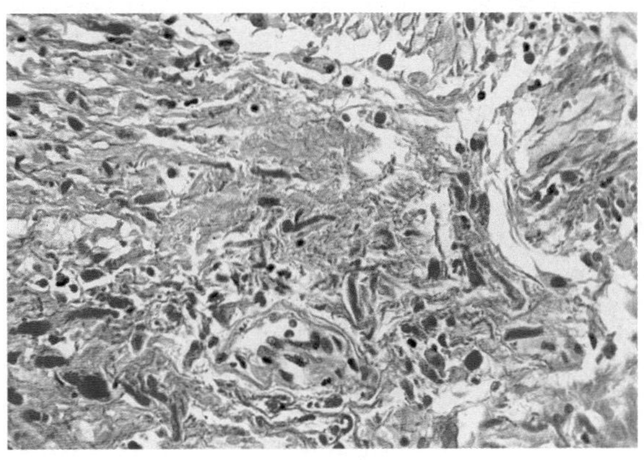

Figure 4-22

PILOCYTIC ASTROCYTOMA

Rosenthal fibers consist of eosinophilic, cylindric or carrot-shaped astrocytes with degenerative changes.

Mitotic figures are absent. The pilocytic cells form interlacing bundles that irregularly distend the pial septa of the optic nerve (fig. 4-20). The tumor may show thickened vessel walls and microcystic spaces that often contain extracellular acid mucopolysaccharides, which are believed to be produced by the astrocytes. Occasionally, such extracellular deposits are a prominent feature of the tumor, and these tumors are usually designated as *myxomatous glioma* (fig. 4-21). Along with the pilocytic astrocytes, some tumors contain a variable number of oligodendrocytes, which have small round nuclei and halo-like cytoplasm without glial fibrils.

Rosenthal fibers are a common histologic feature of optic nerve astrocytomas (fig. 4-22). These fibers, which represent degenerative changes of the astrocytes, usually display eosinophilic cylindric, spherical, or carrot-shaped swellings. Ultrastructurally, Rosenthal fibers are made up of electron-dense granular material and aggregates of glial filaments (fig. 4-23).

Other degenerative changes of astrocytoma include foci of calcification, aggregates of

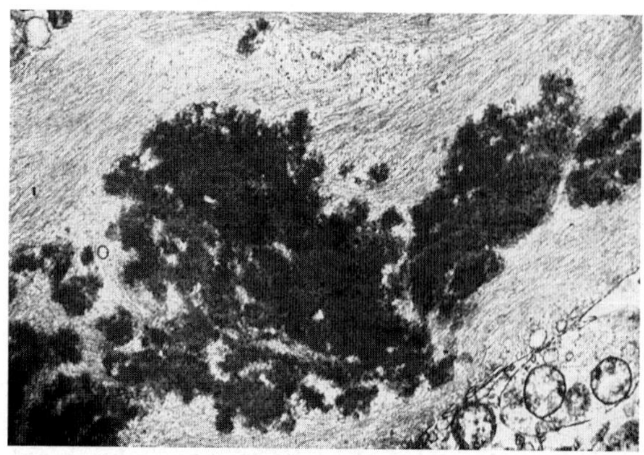

Figure 4-23

PILOCYTIC ASTROCYTOMA

Rosenthal fibers have glial filaments with electron-dense granular material.

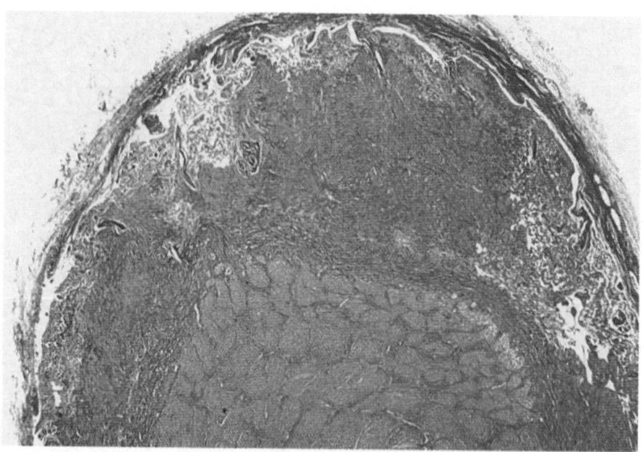

Figure 4-24

PILOCYTIC ASTROCYTOMA

Arachnoidal hyperplasia is admixed with neoplastic astrocytes in arachnoidal gliomatosis (Masson trichrome stain).

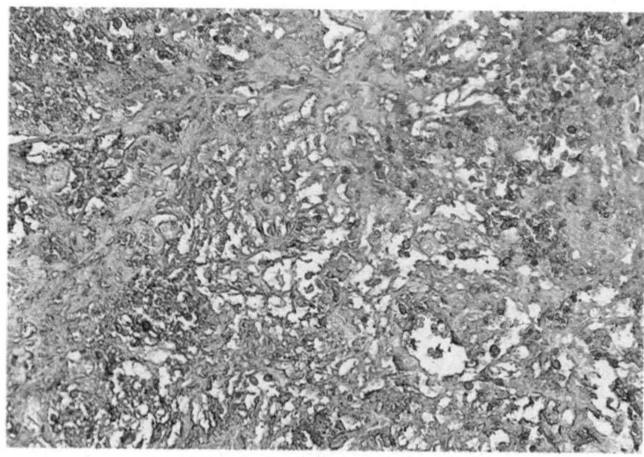

Figure 4-25

PILOCYTIC ASTROCYTOMA

Positive immunohistochemical staining with glial fibrillary acidic protein.

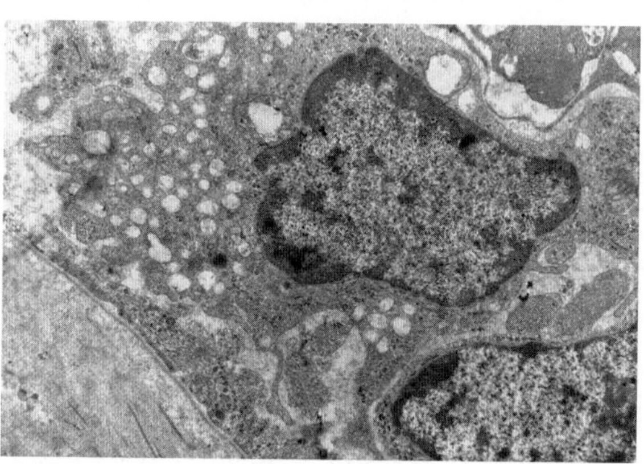

Figure 4-26

PILOCYTIC ASTROCYTOMA

Electron microscopic examination reveals neoplastic cells lined by basement membrane material.

lipoidal histiocytes, fibrosis, and the presence of dilated sinusoidal vascular channels. Tumors that display such prominent degenerative features have been labeled *ancient gliomas*.

Some pilocytic astrocytomas show thickened perineural tissue made up of arachnoidal hyperplasia admixed with neoplastic astrocytes (fig. 4-24). Such perineural thickening, known as *arachnoidal gliomatosis*, appears to be prominent in tumors associated with neurofibromatosis type 1 (12).

Immunohistochemical and Ultrastructural Findings. Pilocytic astrocytes are immunoreactive with the antibodies to glial fibrillary acidic protein (GFAP) (fig. 4-25). Ultrastructurally, the tumor cells show elongated cytoplasm containing glial filaments. The filaments measure 10 nm in diameter and are usually aggregated into bundles. The cytoplasm is surrounded by basement membrane (figs. 4-26, 4-27).

Differential Diagnosis. Fibroblastic meningiomas and peripheral nerve tumors are considered in the differential diagnosis of astrocytoma, although pilocytic features are characteristic of optic nerve astrocytoma. Immunohistochemical analysis with anti-GFAP antibody is often helpful for distinguishing pilocytic astrocytoma from these tumors. Moreover, astrocytomas

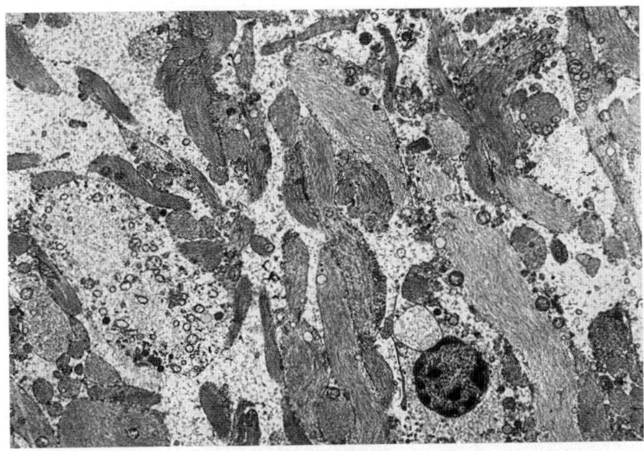

Figure 4-27

PILOCYTIC ASTROCYTOMA

The cytoplasm of the neoplastic cells contains bundles of glial filaments.

remain intradural, whereas transdural extension is often noted in meningiomas. Occasionally, the arachnoidal hyperplasia seen in astrocytomas may be confused with meningioma. In such cases, immunohistochemistry can help distinguish these two neoplasms.

It may be difficult to differentiate biopsy specimens of optic nerve astrocytomas obtained from the tumor margin from reactive gliosis of the nerve. In the former, the arrangement of the astrocytic nuclei is less orderly, and the nuclei appear more numerous. Moreover, the increase in glial cells may cause irregular enlargement of the affected nerve bundles, whereas in gliosis the nerve bundles are variably atrophic.

Special Studies. Neurofibromatosis type 1 (NF1) gene product, neurofibromin, is a protein that functions as a tumor suppressor. Loss of expression of this protein occurs in astrocytomas associated with NF1 (17). Although a significant number of nonpilocytic astrocytomas show *p53* gene mutations, the role of such a mutation in pilocytic astrocytoma is not clear. Pilocytic astrocytomas have chromosomal abnormalities involving chromosomes 7, 8, and 11 (18).

Treatment and Prognosis. Most juvenile pilocytic astrocytomas grow very slowly, with long periods of dormancy and some spontaneous regression. Regression has been noted in patients with and without neurofibromatosis (19). Rapid growth and malignant change are exceptional, and such features are rarely documented (14). Mortality from nonchiasmal optic nerve astrocytoma is rare, while chiasmal tumors may be associated with an unfavorable course because they involve cerebral structures. The morbidity and mortality of patients with such intracranial tumors is virtually the same, regardless of whether the patients have been treated, either surgically or by radiation, or have received no treatment (14).

MELANOCYTOMA

Definition. *Melanocytoma* is a deeply pigmented, benign tumor composed of tightly packed, ovoid to polyhedral melanocytes that are filled with melanin granules (20). They usually occur in the optic nerve head but also arise in the uveal tract and conjunctiva.

General Features. Melanocytomas were once considered either choroidal melanomas that invaded the disc or primary melanomas of the disc (20). Zimmerman and Garron (20) defined this entity in 1962, providing detailed the clinical and histopathologic characteristics as well as the natural history of these tumors. Since histologic analysis of this tumor reveals large, plump, polyhedral melanocytes, it is also known as a *magnocellular nevus*. Melanocytomas occur mainly in heavily pigmented individuals, including African-Americans and Caucasians of Mediterranean origin.

Clinical Features. The tumor is usually detected in an asymptomatic individual, or it may be associated with mild visual deterioration or a defect in the visual field (21). On ophthalmoscopic examination, the tumor is seen as an elevated gray to jet black mass, eccentrically located on the optic disc (fig. 4-28). The tumor usually extends into the juxtapapillary retina, and has fibrillated margins (22). Optic nerve head melanocytomas usually measure 3 mm in diameter and less than 2 mm in height. Bilateral occurrence is rare.

Gross and Microscopic Findings. Grossly, melanocytomas appear as a jet black mass with little or no variation in color (figs. 4-29, 4-30). The mass involves the disc and may extend posteriorly beyond the lamina cribrosa (fig. 4-31) and laterally to the adjacent retina and choroid. Microscopically, plump polyhedral cells packed with melanin are seen. The nuclear details are usually not discernible unless the

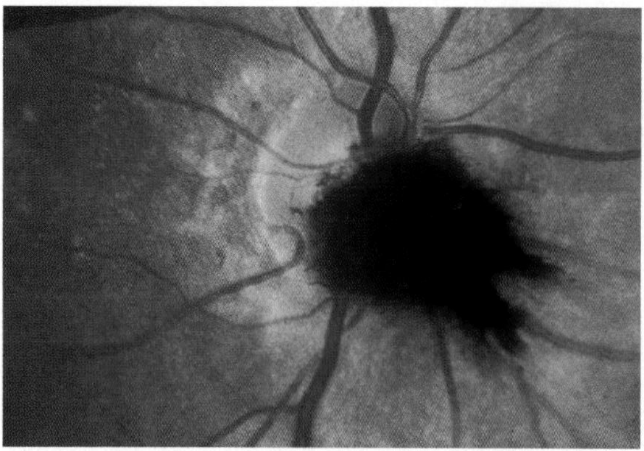

Figure 4-28

MELANOCYTOMA

An elevated jet black mass is eccentrically located on the optic disc. The margins of the tumor are feathery.

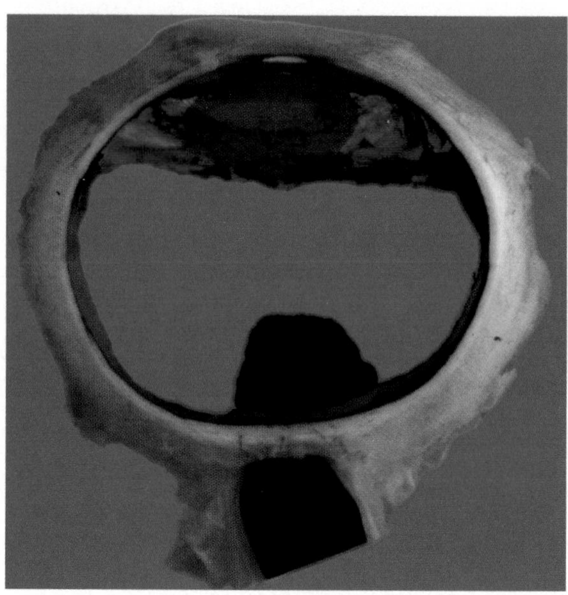

Figure 4-29

MELANOCYTOMA OF OPTIC DISC AND NERVE

The jet black mass covers the optic disc and extends into the retrobulbar nerve. Numerous melanin-laden macrophages surround the posterior lens surface.

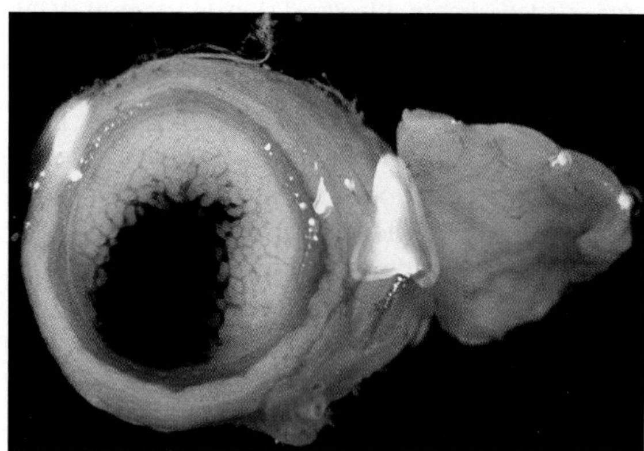

Figure 4-30

MELANOCYTOMA

A section of the retrobulbar optic nerve shows a jet black mass with feathery margins.

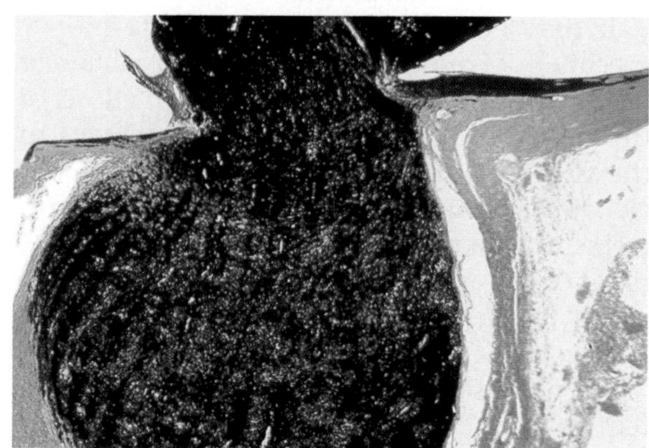

Figure 4-31

MELANOCYTOMA

The optic nerve head, juxtapapillary choroid, and postlaminar portion of the nerve are involved by tumor.

sections are bleached (fig. 4-32); such bleached sections show cells with small round nuclei and inconspicuous nucleoli (23).

Ultrastructural Findings. Ultrastructurally, two types of melanocytes are noted: one showing giant melanosomes and the other containing small round melanosomes that are characteristic of uveal melanocytes (fig. 4-33). The predominant cell type in most melanocytomas is the plump, polyhedral nevus cell packed with giant melanosomes (24).

Cytologic Findings. Fine-needle aspiration biopsy and cytologic preparations usually reveal uniformly heavily pigmented polyhedral cells with small round nuclei. The uniform cells may be associated with an admixture of spindle cells, but no epithelioid cells are observed.

Differential Diagnosis. Heavily pigmented choroidal melanomas or necrotic juxtapapillary choroidal melanomas that extend into the optic nerve require differentiation from melanocytoma. Bleached histologic sections are often

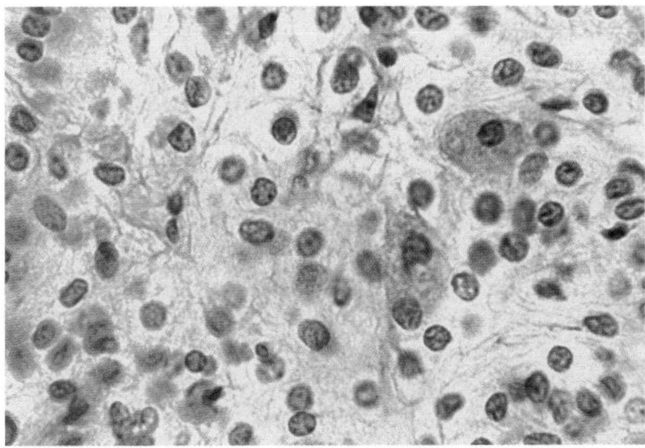

Figure 4-32

MELANOCYTOMA

Bleached preparation shows small round nuclei with inconspicuous nucleoli.

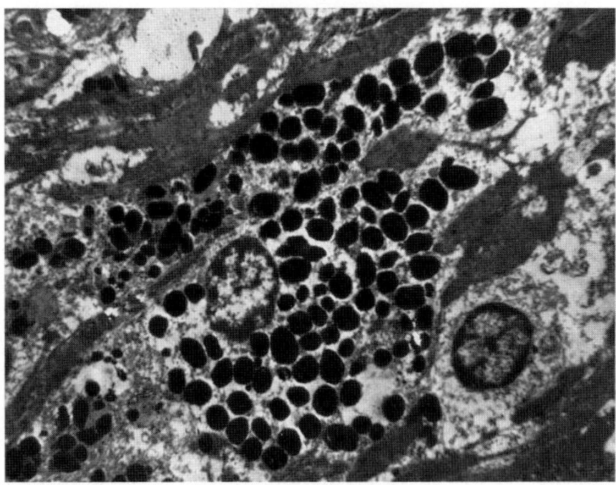

Figure 4-33

MELANOCYTOMA

Giant and small round melanosomes are present.

necessary to differentiate these tumors. Uveal melanomas usually exhibit an admixture of spindle and epithelioid cells, with large nuclei and prominent nucleoli. Necrotic melanomas usually have melanophages containing clumps of pigment granules. Juxtapapillary adenoma of retinal pigment epithelium may resemble melanocytoma, but the former exhibits pigmented cells displaying a vacuolated or a tubular pattern.

Treatment and Prognosis. Melanocytomas are benign tumors that require no surgical intervention. Malignant transformation is extremely rare (25,26). Patients with melanocytomas are usually followed periodically with fundus photography to document tumor growth and other abnormal morphologic changes.

ASTROCYTIC HAMARTOMA AND GIANT CALCIFIED DRUSEN

Astrocytic hamartoma and *giant calcified drusen* primarily occur in the optic disc, but they also arise from the adjacent retina. These tumors are seen in association with tuberous sclerosis or neurofibromatosis type 2 (NF2). They are slow-growing proliferations of plump, spindle-shaped astrocytes (figs. 4-34, 4-35). Clinically, hamartomas appear as flat, discoid masses protruding forward into the vitreous body. Cystic degeneration and calcification may occur. Lesions with extensive calcification are designated giant calcified drusen (fig. 4-36).

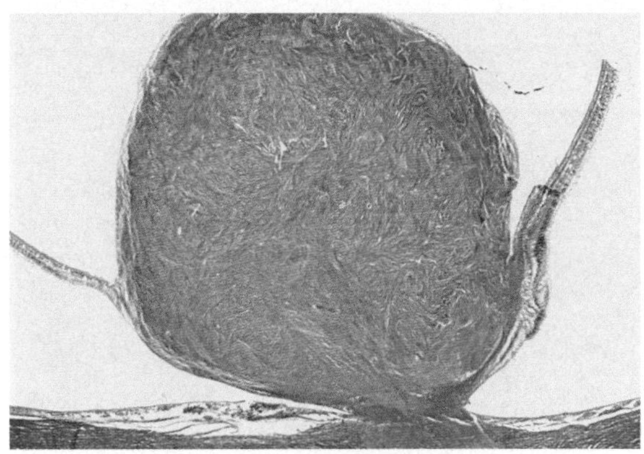

Figure 4-34

ASTROCYTIC HAMARTOMA

Astrocytic hamartoma arising from the optic disc (Masson trichrome stain).

HEMANGIOMA AND HEMANGIOPERICYTOMA

Capillary or *cavernous hemangiomas* arise from the optic disc (fig. 4-37) or along the optic nerve. Cavernous lesions are rare. Capillary hemangiomas vary in their presentation: they may be endophytic, extending into the vitreous body; exophytic, extending into the optic nerve head; or sessile. These capillary growths are often associated with von Hippel-Lindau disease. Histopathologically, the tumors have endothelium-lined capillaries that are interspersed with pale, vacuolated stromal cells (fig. 4-38). The latter cells are believed to be astrocytes that have

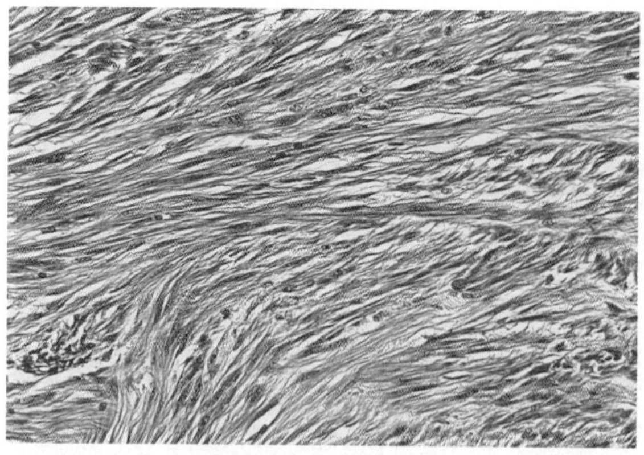

Figure 4-35

ASTROCYTIC HAMARTOMA

There are plump spindle-shaped astrocytes.

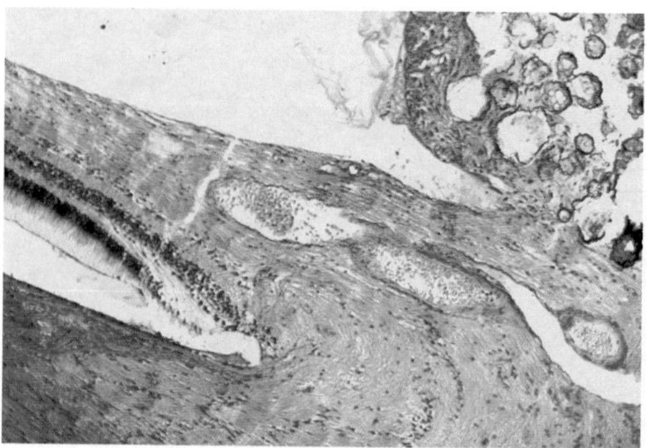

Figure 4-36

ASTROCYTIC HAMARTOMA

Giant drusen are characterized by extensive calcification of an astrocytic hamartoma.

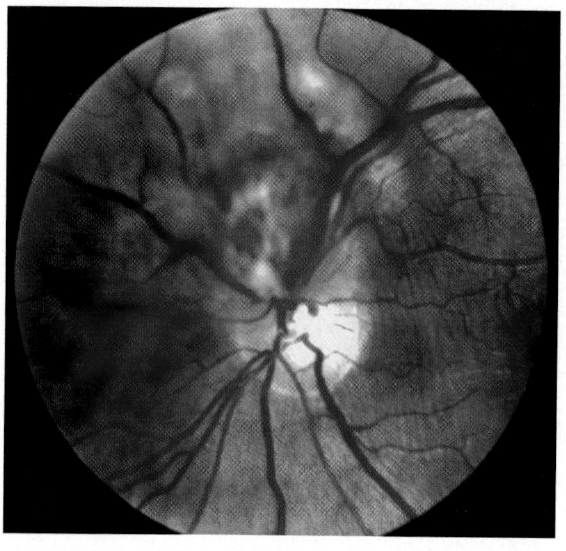

Figure 4-37

JUXTAPAPILLARY HEMANGIOMA

Juxtapapillary hemangioma arising at the optic disc in a patient with von Hippel-Lindau disease.

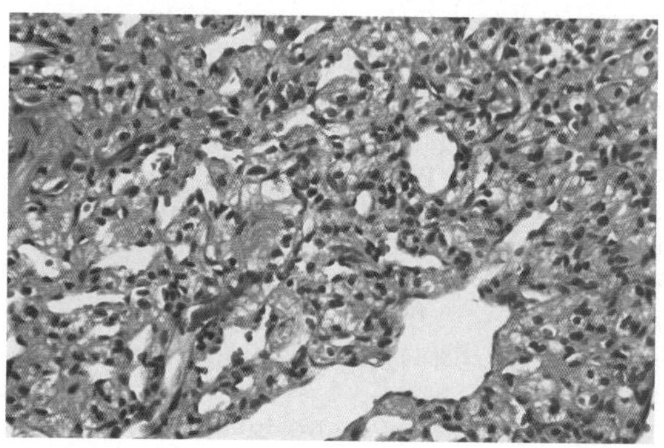

Figure 4-38

ANGIOMATOSIS

Endothelium-lined capillaries are interspersed with vacuolated stromal cells.

imbibed plasma lipids (27). A capillary hemangioma that displays lipidized stromal cells in association with von Hippel-Lindau disease is designated *angiomatosis retinae.*

Hemangiopericytomas rarely arise from the meninges of the optic nerve (28). Clinically, patients present with signs of optic atrophy, and CT scan may reveal a fusiform enlargement of the nerve (fig. 4-39A). Histopathologically, fascicles of spindle-shaped cells are interspersed among numerous irregular vascular channels (fig. 4-39B). The reticulum stain reveals a network of reticulin surrounding the tumor cells (fig. 4-39C).

MEDULLOEPITHELIOMA

Medulloepithelioma arises frequently from the ciliary body; this tumor only rarely originates in the optic disc or the nerve. Medulloepithelioma is believed to arise from embryonic neuroepithelium at any site along the course of the invaginated optic vesicle. The tumor is also known as *neuroepithelioma* or *diktyoma.*

Benign, malignant, teratoid, and nonteratoid medulloepitheliomas of the nerve display cords

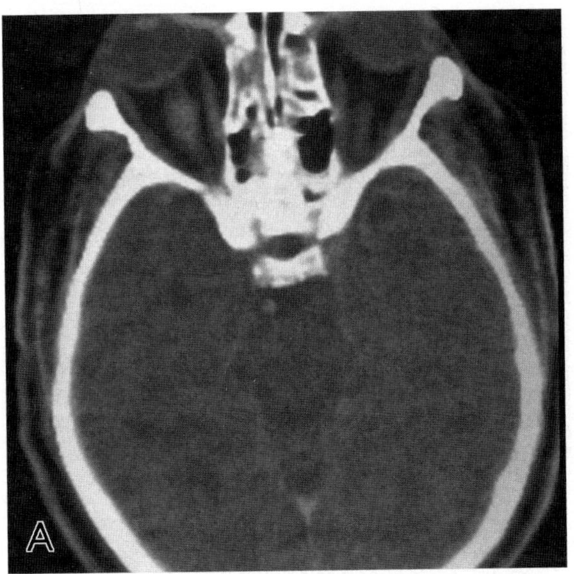

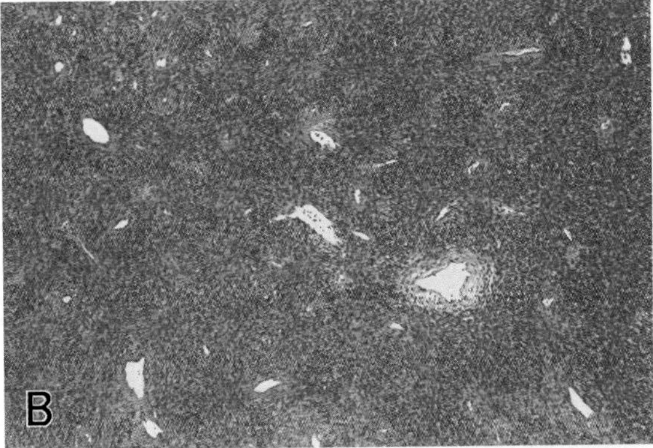

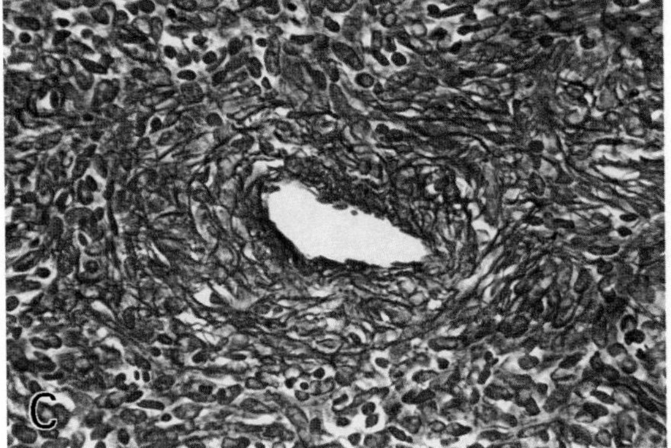

Figure 4-39

HEMANGIOPERICYTOMA

A: CT scan shows a fusiform mass involving the optic nerve.

B: Fascicles of spindle-shaped cells are interspersed among vascular channels.

C: A rich network of reticulin surrounds the neoplastic cells (reticulin stain).

and tubules of epithelium, resembling embryonal neuroepithelium (fig. 4-40). A hyaluronidase-sensitive mucopolysaccharide is present in the lumen of the tubules and between the sheets of tumor cells. If the tumor has heterologous elements, such as cartilage or rhabdomyoblasts, it is classified as a teratoid medulloepithelioma. Medulloepithelioma of the optic nerve occurs in children and adults, however, in children it is usually misdiagnosed as an astrocytoma preoperatively. Histologic features that distinguish benign from malignant medulloepithelioma are described in the chapter, Tumors of the Retina.

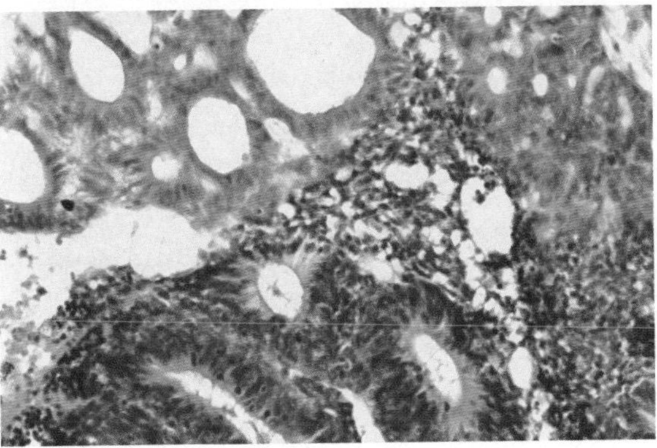

Figure 4-40

MEDULLOEPITHELIOMA

Cords and tubules of neoplastic epithelium in a nonteratoid medulloepithelioma.

JUVENILE XANTHOGRANULOMA

Rarely, the optic nerve is infiltrated by a xanthogranulomatous process in children. Optic nerve involvement in juvenile xanthogranuloma may be associated with uveal and retinal involvement and may occur in the absence of skin manifestations. Grossly, the infiltration is yellow (fig. 4-41A). Histologically, the nerve is infiltrated by mildly atypical histiocytes, some of which may have foamy cytoplasm mixed with occasional Touton giant cells (fig. 4-41B). These giant cells and the histiocytes reveal lipid droplets in frozen sections stained for fat (fig. 4-41C).

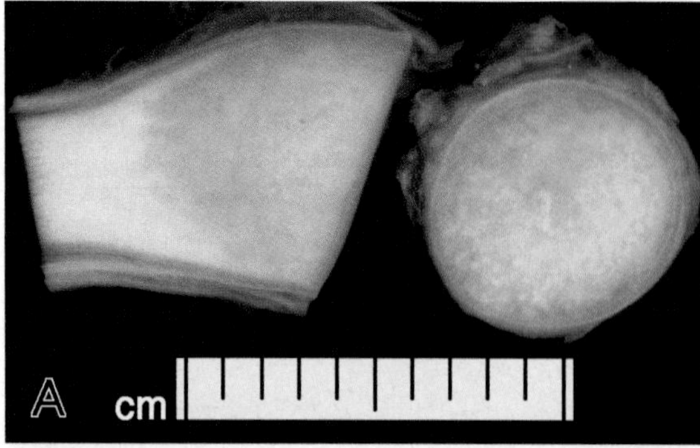

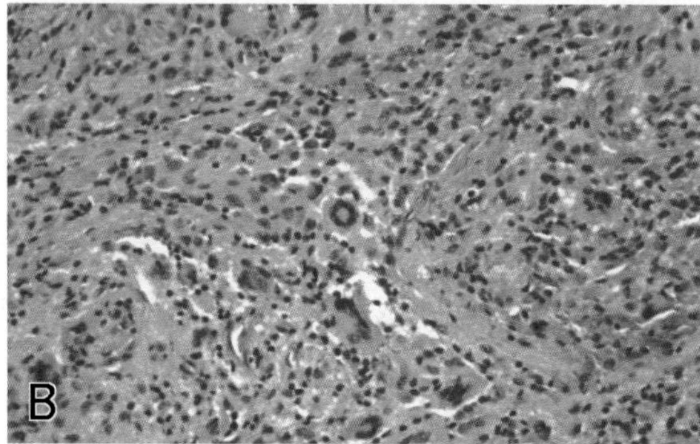

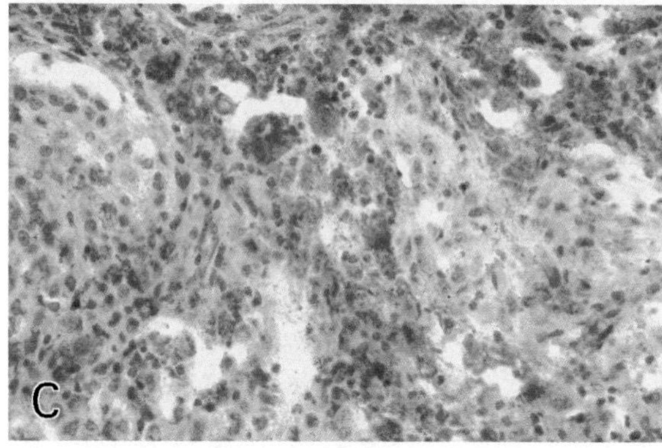

Figure 4-41

JUVENILE XANTHOGRANULOMA

A: Yellowish infiltration of the optic nerve in juvenile xanthogranuloma.

B: Histiocytic infiltration with some cells showing foamy cytoplasm.

C: Lipid deposits are present in the infiltrating histiocytes (oil red-O stain).

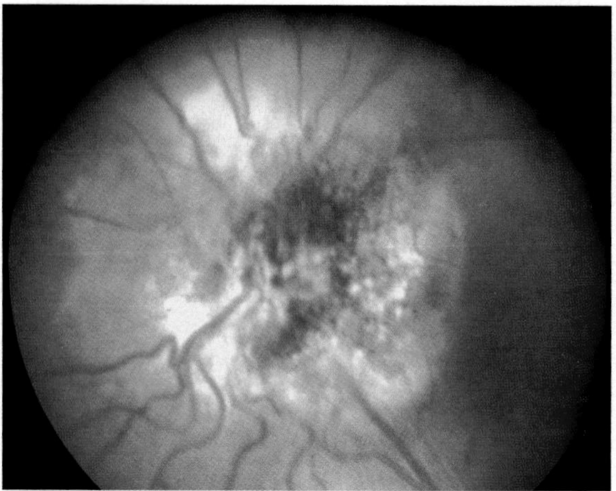

Figure 4-42

JUXTAPAPILLARY HAMARTOMA

Ophthalmoscopic view shows a mass obscuring the disc margins.

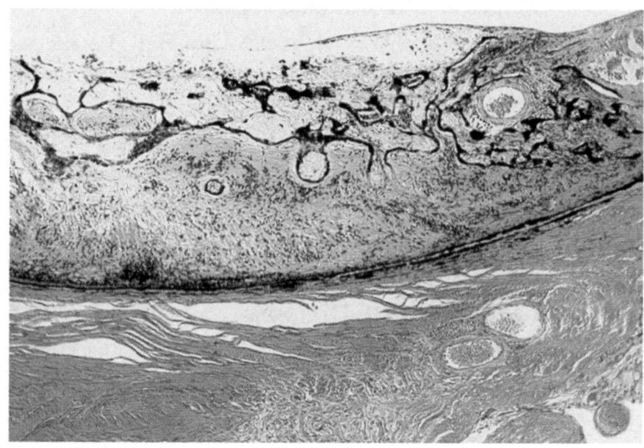

Figure 4-43

JUXTAPAPILLARY HAMARTOMA

Proliferated tubules of retinal pigment epithelium intermingle with glial cells.

JUXTAPAPILLARY HAMARTOMA

Juxtapapillary hamartoma, also known as *combined hamartoma of the retina and retinal pigment epithelium*, is a rare pseudoneoplasm that clinically simulates melanoma (29–31). Clinically, an irregular, ill-defined gray mass is seen obscuring the disc margins and surrounded by a gliotic retina containing tortuous retinal vessels (fig. 4-42). These lesions have prominent vascularity as seen with fluorescein angiography. Histologically, the mass is made up of proliferating juxtapapillary retinal pigment epithelium that involves the overlying retina and the optic disc (fig. 4-43). The proliferating retinal pigment epithelium is intermingled with glial cells; in some areas, the gliosis is prominent and surrounded by the proliferating retinal pigment epithelium. These lesions usually remain

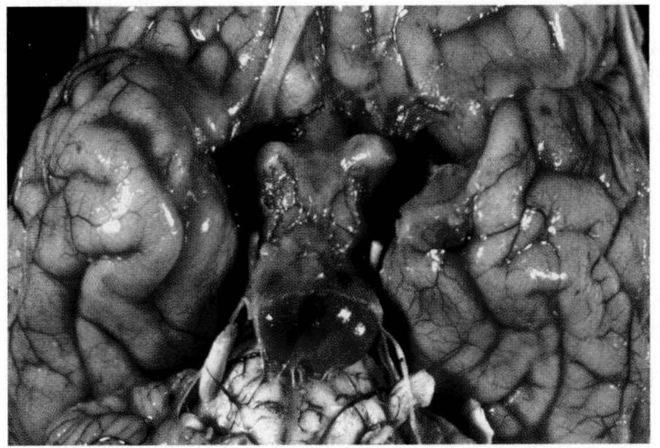

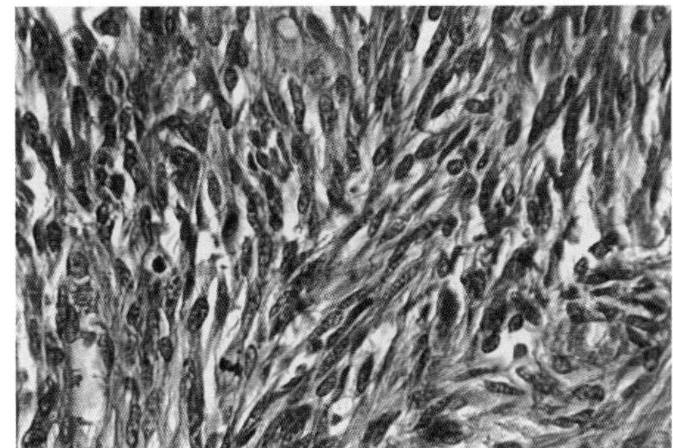

Figure 4-44

MALIGNANT ASTROCYTOMA

Left: Gross appearance of an optic chiasm astrocytoma.
Right: Atypical pleomorphic astrocytes and abnormal mitotic figures are seen.

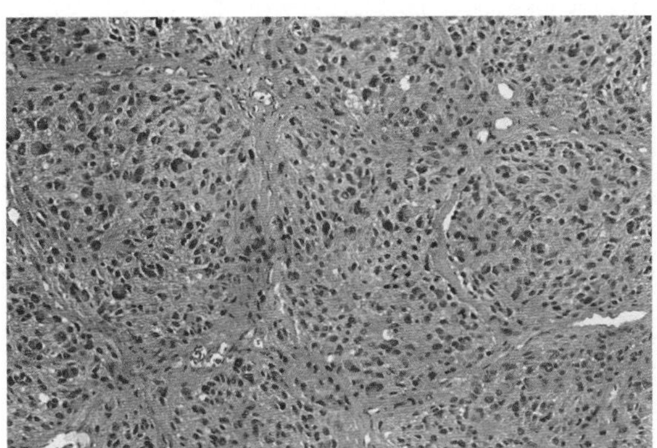

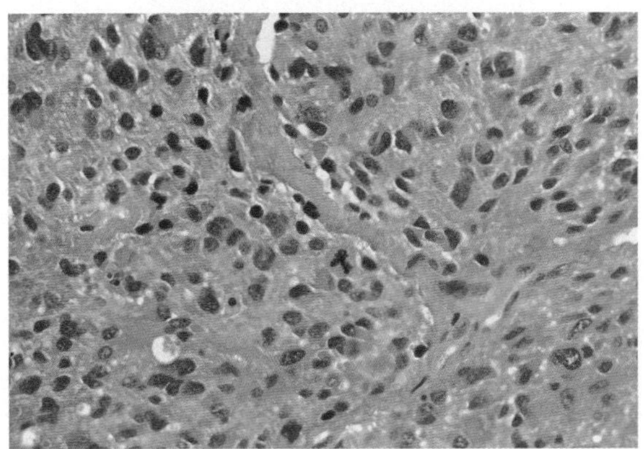

Figure 4-45

MALIGNANT ASTROCYTOMA

Malignant astrocytoma arising from optic nerve displays prominent hypercellularity (left) and pleomorphic cells (right).

stationary, but occasionally grow slowly. Familial occurrence of these hamartomas has been reported in association with NF2 and in a patient with Gorlin's syndrome (30,32).

MALIGNANT ASTROCYTOMA

Malignant astrocytic tumors rarely arise from the optic nerve and chiasm (fig. 4-44). These malignant neoplasms usually occur in adults between 22 and 79 years of age, with an average age of 52 years. There is no sex predilection. The tumors may present clinically with signs of visual field loss. Chiasmal tumors can extend bilaterally into the optic nerves, resulting in bilateral blindness.

Histopathologically, atypical, pleomorphic astrocytes (fig. 4-45); numerous mitoses; foci of necrosis; and invasion of the dura are seen. In some cases, the tumor extends through the dura to invade the surrounding orbital tissues. The tumors also show secondary vascular and endothelial cell proliferation. Malignant astrocytoma is associated with a bad prognosis, and death usually occurs in less than 1 year.

PRIMARY MALIGNANT MELANOMA

Primary melanomas of the optic disc and the nerve are rare. The tumors may arise from melanocytes of the optic nerve meninges, and they may develop in patients with congenital

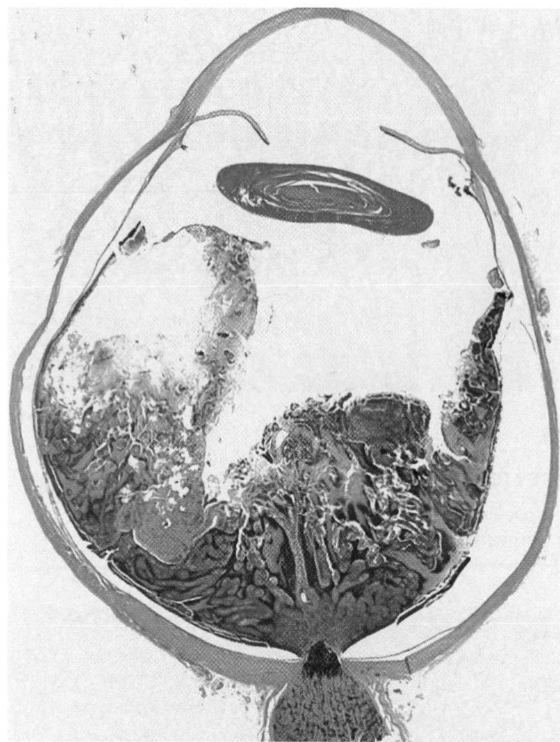

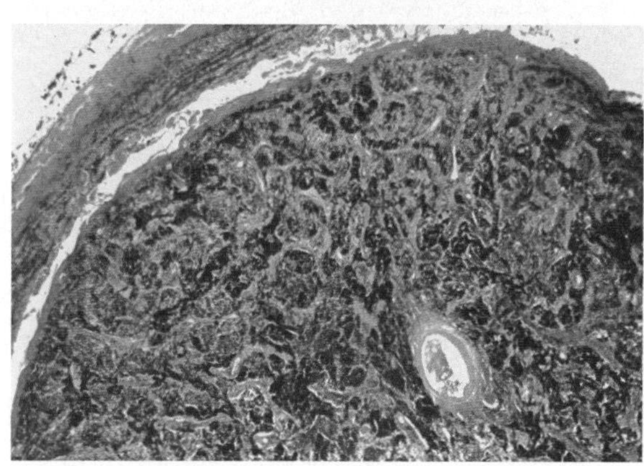

Figure 4-46

RETINOBLASTOMA WITH OPTIC NERVE INVASION

Top: Section of the globe shows retinoblastoma invading the nerve.

Bottom: Section of the optic nerve reveals retinoblastoma extending into the nerve.

melanosis oculi or the nevus of Ota. Most optic disc and nerve melanomas, however, are either a direct extension from a juxtapapillary choroidal melanoma or a cutaneous melanoma metastatic to the meninges of the nerve. Rarely, melanocytoma of the optic disc or optic nerve proper transforms into malignant melanoma.

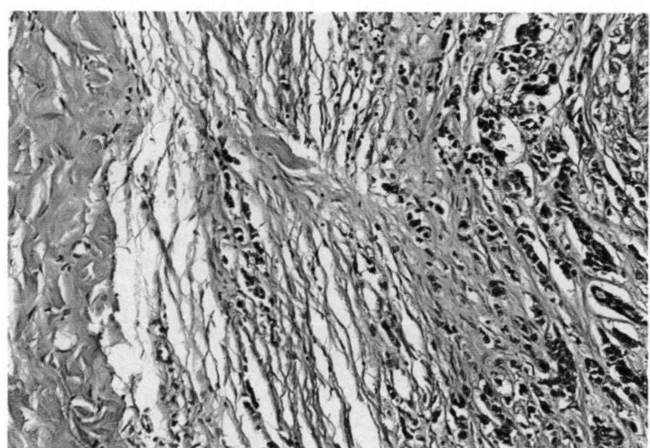

Figure 4-47

METASTATIC BRONCHOGENIC CARCINOMA

Metastatic bronchogenic carcinoma involves the optic nerve.

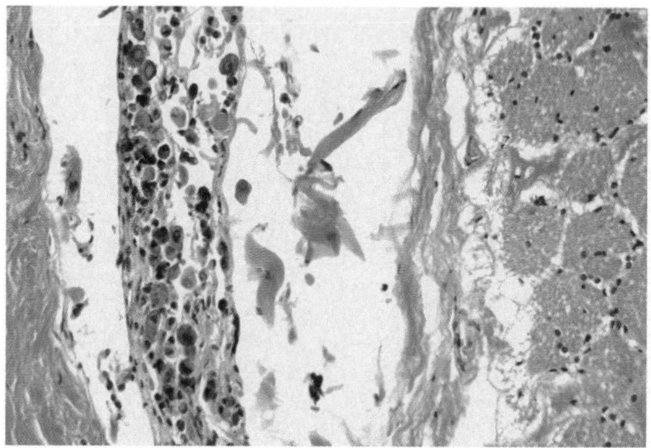

Figure 4-48

METASTATIC MELANOMA

Metastatic skin melanoma infiltrates optic nerve meninges.

SECONDARY AND METASTATIC TUMORS

The optic nerve head or the nerve may be involved through direct extension from either a juxtapapillary choroidal melanoma in adults or from a retinoblastoma in children (fig. 4-46). Secondary tumors of the nerve are more common than primary tumors (33). Although invasion of the optic nerve head and the nerve by a choroidal melanoma may not affect the overall prognosis, invasion of the optic nerve by retinoblastoma is associated with a worsened prognosis.

The optic nerve head or the nerve is frequently involved in both acute and chronic leukemia of various types. Primary lymphomas of the optic nerve head or the nerve are rare. Metastatic carcinomas (fig. 4-47) and cutaneous melanomas can involve either the optic nerve or its meninges (fig. 4-48). Common carcinomas that metastasize to the nerve include lung, breast, and stomach (34). Some of these present primarily as leptomeningeal carcinomatosis.

REFERENCES

Classification and Frequency

1. Henderson JW, Farrow GM. Orbital tumors, 2nd ed. New York: B.C. Decker; 1980.
2. McLean IW, Burnier MN, Zimmerman LE, Jakobiec FA. Tumors of the optic nerve and optic nerve head. In: McLean IW, Burnier MN, Zimmerman LE, Jakobiec FA. Tumors of the eye and ocular adnexa. Atlas of Tumor Pathology, 3rd Series, Fascicle 12. Washington DC: Armed Forces Institute of Pathology; 1994:299–316.

Meningiomas

3. Dutton JJ. Optic nerve sheath meningiomas. Surv Ophthalmol 1992;37:167–83.
4. Cushing H. The meningiomas (dural endotheliomas). Their source and favoured seats of origin (Cavendish lecture). Brain 1922:282–316.
5. Friedenwald JS. Cited in Cushing H, Eisenhardt L: Meningiomas—their classification, regional behavior, life history, and surgical end results. Springfield, Ill.: Charles C. Thomas; 1938:297.
6. Wilson WB. Meningiomas of the anterior visual system. Surv Ophthalmol 1981;26:109–27.
7. Bondy M, Ligon BL. Epidemiology and etiology of intracranial meningiomas: a review. J Neurooncology 1996;29:197–205.
8. Burger PC, Shibata T, Kleihues P. The use of monoclonal antibody Ki-67 in the identification of proliferating cells: application to surgical neuropathology. Am J Surg Pathol 1986;10:611–7.
9. Boniuk M, Messmer EP, Font RL. Hemangiopericytoma of the meninges of the optic nerve. A clinicopathologic report including electron microscopic observations. Ophthalmology 1985;92:1780–7.
10. Alper MG. Management of primary optic nerve meningiomas. Current status—therapy in controversy. J Clin Neuroophthalmol 1981;1:101–17.
11. Turbin RE, Thompson CR, Kennerdell JS, Cockerham KP, Kupersmith MJ. A long-term visual outcome comparison in patients with optic nerve sheath meningioma managed with observation, surgery, radiotherapy, or surgery and radiotherapy. Ophthalmology 2002;109:890–900.

Juvenile Pilocytic Astrocytoma

12. Stern J, Jakobiec FA, Housepian EM. The architecture of optic nerve gliomas with and without neurofibromatosis. Arch Ophthalmol 1980; 98:505–11.
13. Wright JE, McNab AA, McDonald WI. Optic nerve glioma and the management of optic nerve tumours in the young. Br J Ophthalmol 1989;73:967–74.
14. Borit A, Richardson EP Jr. The biological and clinical behaviour of pilocytic astrocytomas of the optic pathways. Brain 1982;105:161–87.
15. Yanoff M, Davis RL, Zimmerman LE. Juvenile pilocytic astrocytoma ("glioma") of the optic nerve: Clinico-pathologic study of sixty-three cases. In: Jakobiec FA, ed. Ocular and adnexal tumors. Birmingham, AL: Aesculapius Pub Co; 1978;685–707.
16. Jakobiec FA, Depot MJ, Kennerdell JS, et al. Combined clinical and computed tomographic diagnosis of orbital glioma and meningioma. Ophthalmology 1984;91:137–55.
17. Lau N, Feldkamp MM, Roncari L, et al. Loss of neurofibromin is associated with activation of RAS/MAPK and PI3-K/AKT signaling in a neurofibromatosis 1 astrocytoma. J Neuropathol Exp Neurol 2000;59:759–67.
18. Zattara-Cannoni H, Gambarelli D, Lena G, et al. Are juvenile pilocytic astrocytomas benign tumors? A cytogenetic study in 24 cases. Cancer Genet Cytogenet 1998;104:157–60.
19. Parsa CF, Hoyt CS, Lesser RL, et al. Spontaneous regression of optic glioma: thirteen cases documented by serial neuroimaging. Arch Ophthalmol 2001;119:516–29.

Melanocytoma

20. Zimmerman LE, Garron LK. Melanocytoma of the optic disc. Int Ophthalmol Clin 1962;2: 431–40.
21. Brown GC, Shields JA. Tumors of the optic nerve head. Surv Ophthalmol 1985;29:239-64.

22. Usui T, Shirakashi M, Kurosawa A, Abe H, Iwata K. Visual disturbance in patients with melanocytoma of the optic disk. Ophthalmologica 1990;201:92–8.
23. Rao NA, Spencer WH. Optic nerve. In: Spencer WH, ed. Ophthalmic pathology, 4th ed. Vol 1. Philadelphia: W.B. Saunders; 1996:584–87.
24. Juarez CP, Tso MO. An ultrastructural study of melanocytomas (magnocellular nevi) of the optic disk and uvea. Am J Ophthalmol 1980;90: 48–62.
25. Shields JA, Shields CL, Gunduz K, Eagle RC Jr. Neoplasms of the retinal pigment epithelium: the 1998 Albert Rurdemann Sr. memorial lecture, Part 2. Arch Ophthalmol 1999;117:601–8.
26. Meyer D, Ge J, Blinder KJ, Sinard J, Xu S. Malignant transformation of an optic disk melanocytoma. Am J Ophthalmol 1999;127:710–4.

Hemangioma and Hemangiopericytoma

27. Jakobiec FA, Font RL, Johnson FB. Angiomatosis retinae. An ultrastructural study and lipid analysis. Cancer 1976;38:2042–56.
28. Boniuk M, Messmer EP, Font RL. Hemangiopericytoma of the meninges of the optic nerve. A clinicopathologic report including electron microscopic observations. Ophthalmology 1985;92:1780–7.

Juxtapapillary Hamartoma

29. Gass JD. An unusual hamartoma of the pigment epithelium and retina simulating choroidal melanoma and retinoblastoma. Trans Am Ophthalmol Soc 1973;71:171–83.
30. De Potter P, Stanescu D, Caspers-Velu L, Hofmans A. Photo essay: combined hamartoma of the retina and retinal pigment epithelium in Gorlin syndrome. Arch Ophthalmol 2000;118: 1004–5.
31. Font RL, Moura RA, Shetler DJ, Martinez JA, McPherson AR. Combined hamartoma of sensory retina and retinal pigment epithelium. Retina 1989;9:302–11.
32. Bouzas EA, Parry DM, Eldridge R, Kaiser-Kupfer MI. Familial occurrence of combined pigment epithelial and retinal hamartomas associated with neurofibromatosis 2. Retina 1992;12:103–7.

Secondary and Metastatic Tumors

33. Christmas NJ, Mead MD, Richardson EP, Albert DM. Secondary optic nerve tumors. Surv Ophthalmol 1991;36:196–206.
34. Ferry AP, Font RL. Carcinoma metastatic to the eye and orbit. I. A clinicopathologic study of 227 cases. Arch Ophthalmol 1974;92:276–86.

5 TUMORS OF THE EYELIDS

ANATOMY AND HISTOLOGY

Each eyelid is composed of six layers. The epidermal surface of the skin of the eyelids forms the outermost layer, and the epithelium covering the palpebral conjunctiva is the innermost layer. Between these lie the dermis, the loose subcutaneous layer, the orbicularis muscle, and the tarsal plate (fig. 5-1). The anatomic structures of the eyelids and their relation to the anterior orbit and globe are depicted in figure 5-2. The mucocutaneous junction of the lid is located at the eyelid margin, just posterior to the openings of the meibomian gland ducts. Between the meibomian ducts and the lashes is the gray line, which is a sulcus extending over most of the length of the lid margin.

The epidermis is composed of two cell types: keratinocytes and dendritic cells. The keratinocytes are arranged in four layers: the deepest is the basal cell layer, the squamous cell layer (stratum spinosum) and granular layer are intermediate, and the non-nucleated horny layer is superficial. The basal keratinocytes form a single row of cells resting on a basement membrane that is attached to the dermis. The cells are columnar and their long axes are perpendicular to the skin surface. They are connected to each other by intercellular bridges and may contain

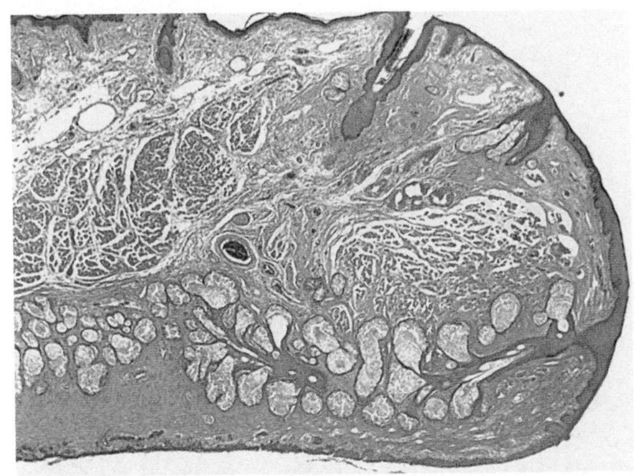

Figure 5-1

MUCOCUTANEOUS JUNCTION OF THE EYELID

In cross section, the layers of the mucocutaneous junction are: epidermis, dermis, orbicularis muscle fibers, submuscular plane, the tarsus housing the meibomian glands, and the palpebral (tarsal) conjunctiva. The opening of the meibomian duct is located in front of the mucocutaneous junction of the eyelid.

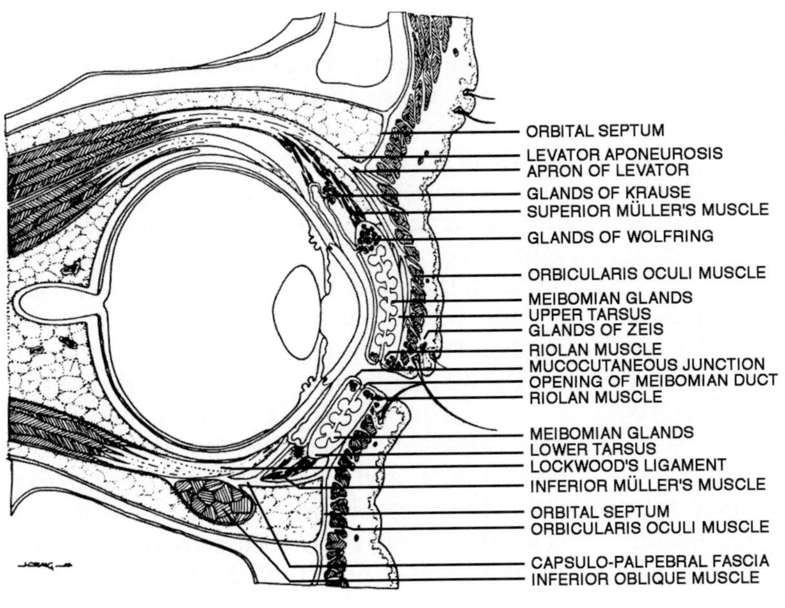

Figure 5-2

EYELID STRUCTURES

Schematic drawing outlining the important eyelid structures.

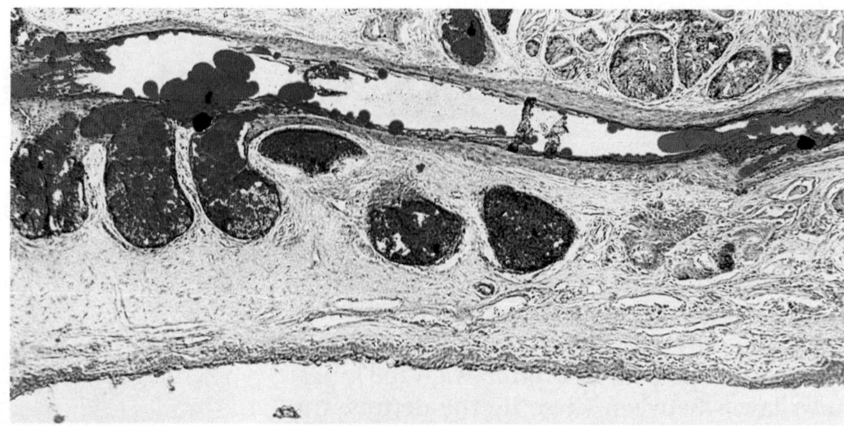

Figure 5-3

MEIBOMIAN GLANDS

The meibomian glands are holocrine glands that open into the lumen of the meibomian duct (oil red-O stain).

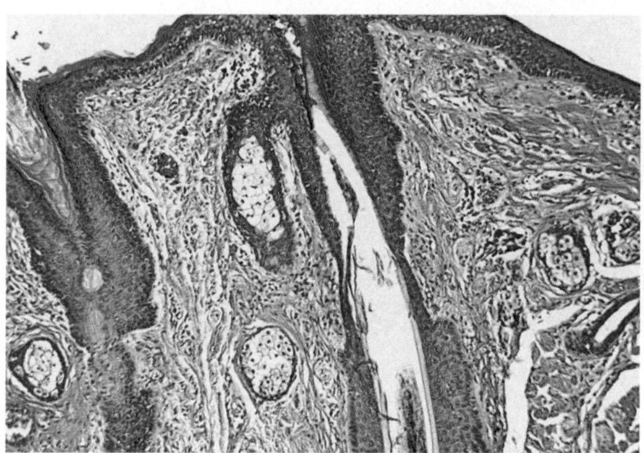

Figure 5-4

GLANDS OF ZEIS

The sebaceous glands of Zeis open laterally into the infundibular portion of the hair follicle.

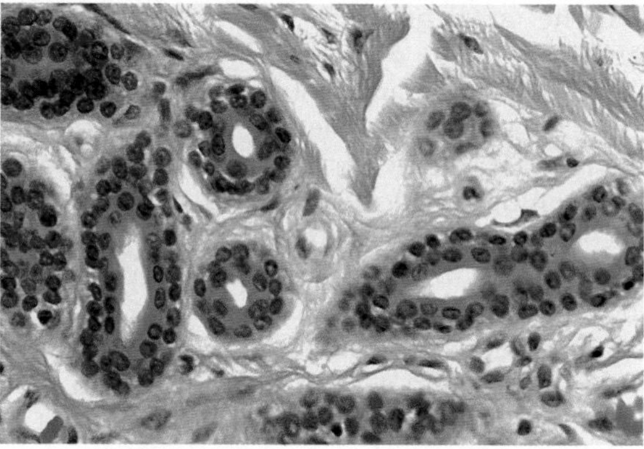

Figure 5-5

ECCRINE SWEAT GLAND DUCTS

Eccrine sweat ducts in the dermis are lined by a double layer of cells (an inner secretory and an outer myoepithelial layer).

variable amounts of melanin pigment derived, in part, from adjacent dendritic melanocytes. The squamous cell layer is composed of a mosaic of polygonal keratinocytes that flatten superficially where they run parallel to the surface. The granular layer forms a row of elongated flat cells containing coarse basophilic keratohyaline granules. The external horny layer consists of flat keratinized cells devoid of nuclei.

A variety of epidermal appendages (glands and cilia) are present in the eyelids. The sebaceous glands are holocrine (figs. 5-3, 5-4). Their acini possess no lumens and extrude their secretory products by decomposition of their cells. They are composed of several lobules that lead into a common excretory duct which opens into the pilosebaceous follicle. The sebaceous glands of the lashes (glands of Zeis) empty their products into the follicles of the cilia (fig. 5-4). Their cells have foamy cytoplasm and empty into a duct that is lined by stratified squamous epithelium and is continuous with the outer root sheath of the hair follicle. The meibomian glands are situated within the tarsal plates (fig. 5-3) where they are arranged vertically and parallel to each other; they are larger in the upper tarsus. There are 25 in the upper lid and 20 in the lower. They secrete sebum, which is extruded into the meibomian ducts, the orifices of which open on the lid margin just behind the gray line.

The eccrine sweat glands are composed of three segments: a secretory portion, an intradermal duct, and an intraepidermal duct (fig. 5-5). The secretory portion is composed of three cell types: clear cells, dark cells that contain periodic acid–Schiff (PAS)-positive diastase-re-

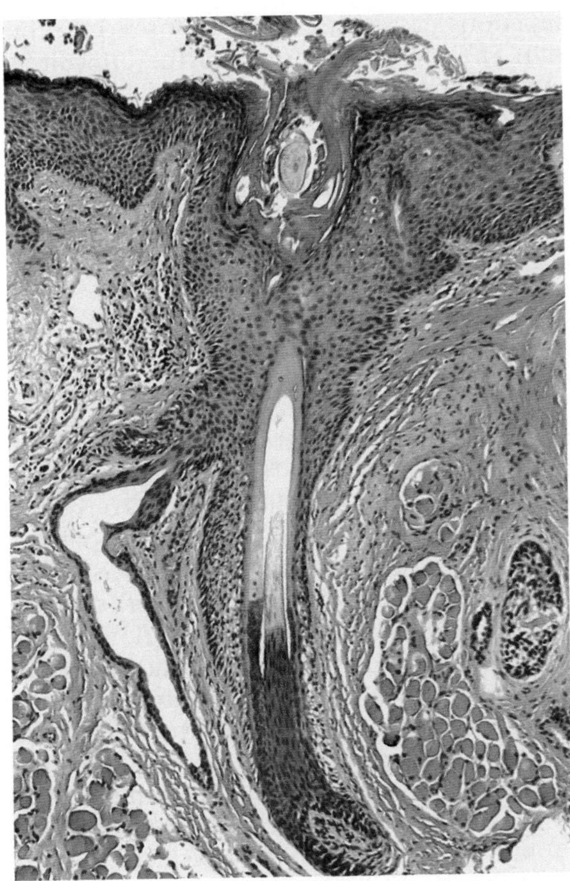

Figure 5-6

GLANDS OF MOLL

The glands of Moll terminate in the infundibular portion of the hair follicle.

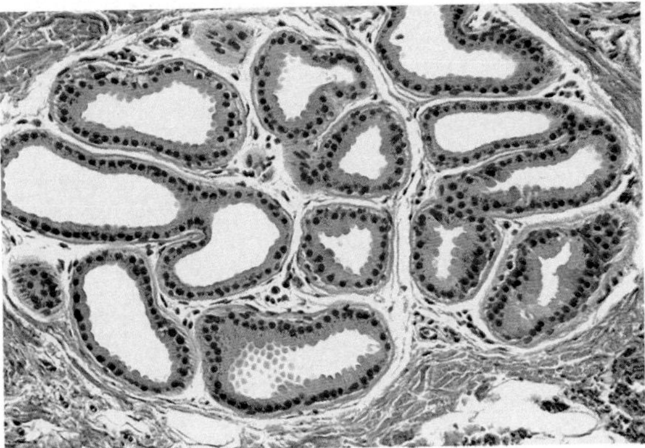

Figure 5-7

GLANDS OF MOLL

Apocrine glands of Moll show areas of decapitation secretion.

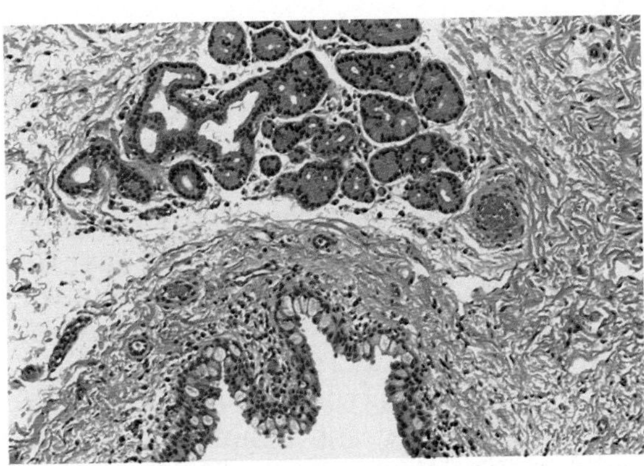

Figure 5-8

GLANDS OF KRAUSE

Glands of Krause (accessory lacrimal glands) are in the upper fornix.

sistant neutral mucopolysaccharides, and myoepithelial cells. The intradermal eccrine duct is composed of two layers of small, cuboidal, deeply basophilic epithelial cells. The lumen of the intradermal duct is lined by a PAS-positive eosinophilic cuticle that is readily visible with the light microscope. The intraepidermal eccrine duct is also referred to as the eccrine pore or acrosyringium. It pursues a spiral course as it penetrates the epidermis.

The apocrine glands of Moll lie near the eyelid margin and empty their secretions into the follicles of the lashes (fig. 5-6). The cells lining the apocrine glands have secretory apical granules and areas of decapitation (fig. 5-7).

Accessory lacrimal glands with histologic features identical to those seen in the main lacrimal gland are often found in the substantia propria of the conjunctiva. The glands, which are located deep in the subconjunctival tissues at the fornices, are known as Krause's glands (fig. 5-8). These number approximately 42 in the upper fornix and 6 to 8 in the lower. The glands of Wolfring (or Ciaccio) (fig. 5-9) are larger than the glands of Krause. In the upper lid, two to five glands are situated at the upper border of the tarsus and two at the inferior edge of the lower tarsus.

The hair of the skin of the eyelid is scanty and fine. The two or three rows of cilia are unusually long and strong, and do not possess arrector pili muscles.

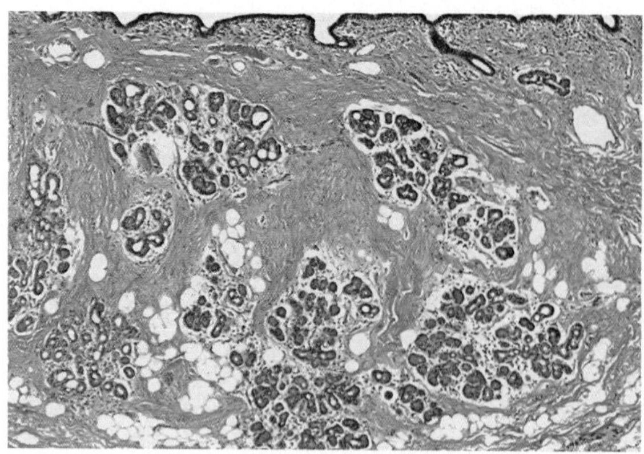

Figure 5-9

GLANDS OF WOLFRING

Accessory lacrimal glands of Wolfring are located at the upper edge of the tarsus.

The dermis is loose and delicate. It is composed of a papillary layer and a reticular layer. The papillary dermis forms numerous cone-shaped dermal papillae which extend upward into the epidermis. The ridges of epidermis separating the papillae are called the rete ridges. The reticular dermis contains thick bundles of collagen and variable amounts of elastic and reticulin fibers, as well as a ground substance containing mucopolysaccharides. Small nerve fibers, blood vessels, and lymphatics are also found in the reticular dermis. The subcutaneous layer of the eyelids contains a small amount of adipose tissue. It is very loosely adherent to the underlying orbicularis muscle.

The lymphatics of the eyelids are arranged in pre- and post-tarsal plexuses that communicate by cross-channels. The pretarsal group drains the dermis, pretarsal orbicularis muscle, and adjacent structures, and the post-tarsal group drains the palpebral conjunctiva and meibomian glands. The lymphatics of the outer two thirds of the upper lid and the outer one third of the lower lid drain into the preauricular nodes. The lymphatics of the inner two thirds of the lower lid and the inner one third of the upper lid drain into the submandibular nodes.

The orbicularis oculi muscle forms an elliptic sheet of concentrically arranged, striated muscle fibers within the eyelids. In the upper lid, the tendon of the levator palpebrae superioris passes through it to insert into the skin and tarsus. A portion of the orbicularis muscle, known as the muscle of Riolan, consists of striated muscle fibers that lie adjacent to the tarsal plate near the eyelid margin. Portions of this muscle are located superficial to the meibomian glands and the remainder (subtarsal portion) lies deep to them.

In the upper lid, the striated fibers of the palpebral portion of the levator palpebrae superioris merge anteriorly into a dense fibrous membrane, the levator aponeurosis, which divides into three or more collagenous sheets that insert like an apron into the deeper aspect of the orbicularis muscle. The smooth muscle of Müller in the upper lid lies adjacent to the orbital septum under the levator palpebrae superioris. It originates among the fibers of the levator in the upper lid and the inferior rectus in the lower. The fibers of the superior and inferior Müller muscle insert, in part, into the margins of the tarsal plates and also insert into collagenous tissue attached to the deep fibers of the orbicularis muscle.

The orbital septum is a thin membrane of fibrous and elastic connective tissue which has multiple attachments to the orbicularis muscle, the levator palpebrae superioris, and the tarsal plates. All pathologic processes located behind the orbital septum are considered to be intraorbital.

The tarsi are flat, semilunar plates which contribute to the rigidity of the eyelids. They are composed of collagenous tissue and elastic fibers, and contain the meibomian glands.

The epithelium of the tarsal conjunctiva is stratified columnar and contains goblet cells. It becomes stratified squamous near the mucocutaneous junction of the eyelid. The underlying conjunctival stroma is thin and closely adherent to the tarsus.

TUMORS

The eyelid is the site of several tumors that also occur elsewhere in the skin. Sebaceous carcinomas develop frequently from the meibomian glands of the upper eyelid, while basal cell carcinomas mostly develop in the lower eyelid. Since basal cell carcinomas are covered in the Fascicle on nonmelanocytic tumors of the skin, this tumor is only briefly discussed.

Table 5-1

CLASSIFICATION OF TUMORS OF THE EYELID

Tumors of Epidermis
- Benign
  - Squamous cell papilloma
  - Seborrheic keratosis
  - Keratoacanthoma
  - Benign lichenoid keratosis
  - Large cell acanthoma
  - Others
- Precancerous
  - Dysplasia
  - Actinic keratosis
  - Bowen's disease
  - Radiation dermatosis
  - Large cell acanthoma
  - Others
- Malignant
  - Basal cell carcinoma
  - Squamous cell carcinoma
  - Others

Melanocytic Tumors
- Benign
  - Nevocellular nevi (junctional, compound, and dermal)
  - Blue nevi and cellular blue nevi
  - Epidermal pigmented lesions (freckle, lentigo simplex, solar lentigo)
- Malignant
  - Melanoma (lentigo maligna, superficial spreading melanoma, nodular melanoma)

Tumors of Eccrine Glands
- Benign
  - Syringoma
  - Eccrine poroma
  - Nodular hydradenoma (eccrine acrospiroma, clear cell hydradenoma)
  - Eccrine spiradenoma
  - Chondroid syringoma
- Malignant
  - Mucinous eccrine carcinoma
  - Adenocarcinoma of eccrine sweat glands
  - Primary adenoid cystic carcinoma

Apocrine Gland Tumors
- Benign
  - Apocrine cystadenoma (Moll gland cyst)
  - Apocrine hydradenoma papilliferum
  - Syringocystadenoma papilliferum
- Malignant
  - Apocrine adenocarcinoma

Sebaceous Gland Tumors
- Benign
  - Sebaceous gland adenoma
- Malignant
  - Sebaceous gland carcinoma (meibomian gland ca, Zeiss gland ca)

Tumors of Hair Follicles
- Inverted follicular keratosis
- Trichoepithelioma
- Trichofolliculoma
- Trichillemoma
- Pilomatrixoma
- Others

Vascular Tumors
- Benign
  - Hemangioma
  - Lymphangioma
  - Glomus tumor
  - Intravascular papillary endothelial hyperplasia
- Malignant
  - Angiosarcoma (malignant hemangioendothelioma)
  - Kaposi's sarcoma

Histocytic and Fibrohistiocytic Tumors
- Xanthoma
- Langerhans cell histiocytosis
- Xanthogranulomas
- Fibrous histiocytoma

Lymphoid Tumors
- Benign
  - Reactive lymphoid hyperplasia
  - Atypical lymphoid hyperplasia
- Malignant
  - Lymphomas
  - Mycosis fungoides (cutaneous T-cell lymphoma)
  - Lymphomatoid granulomatosis

Miscellaneous Tumors
- Phakomatous choristoma
- Merkel cell carcinoma
- Nodular fasciitis
- Juvenile fibromatosis
- Granular cell tumor
- Myxoma

Secondary and Metastatic Tumors

BENIGN EPITHELIAL TUMORS

Tumors of the surface epithelium are divided according to their clinical behavior and histologic features into three main groups: benign, precancerous, and malignant (Table 5-1). Although the tendency is for benign lesions to grow more slowly and to ulcerate less frequently than malignant ones, the clinical features of lesions in each group often overlap. The important benign lesions originating from the surface epithelium are squamous cell papilloma, pseudocarcinomatous hyperplasia, keratoacanthoma, seborrheic keratosis, and inverted follicular keratosis (Table 5-2).

Table 5-2

EPIDERMAL TUMORS OF THE EYELID[a]

Type of Tumor	Number of Cases
Benign	
Squamous cell papilloma	237
Seborrheic keratosis	120
Keratoacanthoma	20
Clear cell acanthoma	1
Premalignant	
Dysplasia	31
Malignant	
Basal cell carcinoma	410
Squamous cell carcinoma	28
Miscellaneous	
Pseudoepitheliomatous hyperplasia	15

[a]Frequency distribution of 862 tumors from the Doheny Eye Institute files collected between 1970 and 2000.

Squamous Cell Papilloma

Squamous cell papilloma is the most common benign lesion of the eyelid. The lesion is usually sessile or pedunculated, and has a color similar to that of the adjacent lid skin. Papillomas are often multiple and tend to involve the lid margin. A small keratin crust can often be palpated on their surface (*keratotic papilloma*). Squamous cell papilloma is composed of finger-like projections of vascularized connective tissue covered by hyperplastic epithelium. The epidermis is usually acanthotic, with elongation of the rete ridges, and shows areas of hyperkeratosis and focal parakeratosis.

Seborrheic Keratosis

Seborrheic keratosis, also known as *basal cell papilloma, seborrheic wart,* and *senile verruca*, is one of the most frequently observed benign skin lesions involving the eyelids and face of middle-aged and older individuals. In whites, the lesions are tan to dark brown and appear as well-demarcated, lobulated (occasionally papillary), cerebriform excrescences, with a verrucous, slightly raised, friable surface. They vary in size from a few millimeters to several centimeters.

According to the predominant histologic features, the lesions are classified into three histologic types: hyperkeratotic, acanthotic, and adenoid. All share variable proportions of hyperkeratosis, acanthosis, and papillomatosis. "Pure" lesions of each type are uncommon, and frequently one or more types are seen in different areas of the same lesion. The acanthotic epidermis often contains keratin-filled cystic inclusions, referred to as horn cysts when they are formed within the mass and pseudohorn cysts when they represent invaginations of surface keratin. Hyperkeratotic lesions have a greater tendency for papillomatosis than do those of the acanthotic type. In the latter, the epidermis is notably thickened, and hyperkeratosis is relatively reduced. The adenoid type of seborrheic keratosis exhibits even less evidence of keratinization and shows elongated, branching, epithelial strands composed of a double row of basaloid cells.

An increased amount of melanin pigment is almost invariably present within keratinocytes and is observed especially in the adenoid and acanthotic types. Thus, seborrheic keratosis may be clinically confused with a pigmented basal cell carcinoma or even with a malignant melanoma. Seborrheic keratosis is not a premalignant lesion, however, and does not evolve into squamous or basal cell carcinoma. Irritated seborrheic keratosis often exhibits infiltration of the dermis by chronic inflammatory cells, accompanied by squamous cell proliferation. In some cases the histopathologic appearance may resemble a squamous cell carcinoma.

Inverted Follicular Keratosis

This benign lesion usually presents as a nodular or wart-like keratotic mass that may be pigmented, simulating a melanocytic lesion (1). *Inverted follicular keratosis* has a tendency to recur if incompletely excised. This may result in the erroneous clinical impression that the lesion is a squamous cell carcinoma.

Histologically, the epithelium exhibits lobular acanthosis, with proliferation of both basaloid and squamoid elements interspersed with areas of acantholysis. Squamoid eddies are frequently observed. Inverted follicular keratosis is believed to be a form of irritated seborrheic keratosis.

Benign Lichenoid Keratosis

Benign lichenoid keratosis, also known as *lichen planus-like keratosis*, usually appears as a solitary, indurated nodule or plaque measuring from 5 to 20 mm in diameter. Its surface is smooth or slightly verrucous; it may occur in areas that have been exposed to the sun as well as in nonexposed areas.

Histopathologically, the lesion bears a striking resemblance to lichen planus. The epidermis, which frequently exhibits increased eosinophilia, shows irregular acanthosis with areas of parakeratosis. The dermis contains a band-like mononuclear cell infiltrate that embraces the epidermis. In addition, colloid bodies (Civatte bodies) are commonly observed (2). Direct immunofluorescence shows that the colloid bodies contain immunoglobulin (Ig)M and fibrinogen (3). Benign lichenoid keratosis can be distinguished from lichen planus by the absence of hypergranulosis and the presence of parakeratosis. Benign lichenoid keratosis has been reported to involute spontaneously (4).

Large Cell Acanthoma

Large cell acanthoma is a slightly keratotic, solitary lesion, usually smaller than 10 mm, whose histologic appearance resembles actinic keratosis, seborrheic keratosis, or Bowen's disease. Large cell acanthoma is a pale, thick, waxy, hyperkeratotic, avascular plaque; although usually solitary, multiple lesions also have been reported (5). The lesion occurs in the sun-exposed areas of middle-aged patients, with a slight predominance in women.

The histologic features are those of a benign epidermal proliferation and are characterized by a sharply circumscribed population of uniformly hyperplastic polygonal keratinocytes that are twice their normal size, with proportional enlargement of their nuclei and cytoplasm. Scattered dyskeratotic cells with an increased number of colloid bodies are observed. The epidermal rete ridges may bud downward or elongate in a club-shaped manner. The dermis frequently contains focal lymphocytic infiltrates that may hug the basal layer of the epidermis, mimicking the histologic features observed in lichen planus-like keratosis.

Pseudocarcinomatous Hyperplasia

Pseudocarcinomatous hyperplasia, also known as *pseudoepitheliomatous hyperplasia,* may be clinically and histopathologically confused with carcinoma. The lesion is usually elevated and has an irregular surface that may be ulcerated or crusted, mimicking either a squamous cell or basal cell carcinoma. The lesion can occur anywhere in the eyelid and typically is of short duration (a few weeks to several months). Pseudocarcinomatous hyperplasia is characteristically associated with a chronic inflammatory process and may be caused by some mycotic infections (blastomycosis, chromomycosis), insect bites, drugs (bromoderma, iododerma), burns, or radiation therapy. In addition, certain tumors, such as granular cell myoblastoma or malignant lymphoma, may evoke pseudoepitheliomatous hyperplasia of the overlying epidermis. For many lesions, the cause is undetermined.

Pseudocarcinomatous hyperplasia is characterized by invasive acanthosis with interconnected islands of well-differentiated squamous epithelium, often containing multiple small microabscesses. Disturbing cytologic features such as nuclear hyperchromatism and atypical mitoses are usually absent. A moderate inflammatory reaction consisting of occasional multinucleated giant cells and eosinophils may be seen at the base of the lesion. The inflammation usually extends to the level of the sweat glands. Despite the benign features, occasional lesions exhibit epithelial hyperplastic changes that may be difficult to differentiate from those of low-grade squamous cell carcinoma. Detailed clinical information and repeated biopsies may be necessary to establish an unequivocal diagnosis.

Keratoacanthoma

Keratoacanthoma is a specialized variant of pseudocarcinomatous hyperplasia that occurs mainly in exposed areas of the skin and usually develops in a period of weeks or a few months. In a series of 44 cases of keratoacanthoma of the eyelid, 36 lesions had been present for 2 months or less (6). A typical keratoacanthoma is a dome-shaped nodule with a central, keratin-filled crater and elevated, rolled margins. Keratoacanthoma of the eyelid is one of the tumors that occurs in immunosuppressed individuals (7).

Microscopic examination of a typical eyelid keratoacanthoma discloses a cup-shaped nodular elevation and thickened epidermis containing islands of well-differentiated squamous epithelium surrounding a central mass of keratin. Frequently, the base of the lesion is uniform and well demarcated from the adjacent dermis by a moderate inflammatory reaction. Collections of neutrophils that form microabscesses are usually present within some of the islands of squamous epithelium. The islands of proliferating squamous epithelium may reach the orbicularis muscle, which in the eyelid normally lies close to the epidermis.

The ostensible epithelial infiltration of striated muscle, as well as its occasional apparent extension around cutaneous nerves, without clear-cut perineural or lymphatic invasion, has contributed to misdiagnosis as squamous cell carcinoma. Other lesions in the differential diagnosis are actinic keratosis, inverted follicular keratosis, and other epithelial lesions with a cup-shaped configuration such as isolated dyskeratosis follicularis, syringocystadenoma papilliferum, and adenoid squamous cell carcinoma.

PRECANCEROUS EPITHELIAL LESIONS

Actinic Keratosis

Actinic keratosis is the most common precancerous cutaneous lesion. It is also known as *solar keratosis* since it occurs in sun-exposed areas of the body of fair-skinned, middle-aged individuals. Prolonged exposure to sunlight with inadequate protection is a predisposing factor. Actinic keratosis is a single, or more often multiple, scaly, keratotic, flat-topped lesion sometimes showing a nodular, horny, or warty configuration. The lesions usually measure only a few millimeters. Early lesions appear as erythematous scales with little or no infiltration. Patients with actinic keratosis often have other cutaneous premalignant and malignant lesions, including squamous cell, basal cell, and adnexal carcinomas and malignant melanoma. If untreated, 12 to 13 percent of lesions become squamous cell carcinoma (8).

The prognosis of patients with squamous cell carcinoma that arose from actinic keratosis is excellent, and metastases are rare (9). Squamous cell carcinoma arising from actinic keratosis should be regarded as a separate, nonaggressive entity distinct from squamous cell carcinoma arising de novo, which is capable of metastasis.

The lesions of actinic keratosis consist of atypical keratinocytes that often form irregular buds which extend into the papillary dermis and underlie focal areas of parakeratosis. The lesions typically spare the orthokeratotic epithelium of the follicular ostia, but atypical keratinocytes may extend along the outer sheath of the pilosebaceous follicles. Clefts form as a result of dysplastic keratinocytic proliferation, dyskeratosis, and loss of intercellular bridges.

According to the predominant histologic features, three types of actinic keratosis are recognized: hypertrophic, atrophic, and bowenoid. In all three the upper dermis shows moderate to severe basophilic collagen degeneration and a moderate lymphoplasmacytic infiltrate. A fourth type of actinic keratosis has been recognized and is referred to as solitary lichen planus-like keratosis.

Bowen's Disease

The cutaneous lesions of *Bowen's disease* appear as erythematous, pigmented, crusty, scaly, fissured, keratotic plaques. The plaques are round and sharply demarcated, with occasional heaped-up margins. The disease involves both sexes but occurs predominantly in whites who have a fair complexion and are sun-sensitive. The disease predominantly strikes middle-aged to older individuals of an average age of 55 years at the time of diagnosis. Two thirds of the patients with Bowen's disease have single lesions.

Treatment is necessary because at least 5 percent of these lesions have clinical and microscopic evidence of an invasive carcinoma. Forty-two percent of patients develop other cutaneous and mucocutaneous premalignant and malignant lesions, including actinic keratosis, basal cell carcinoma of different types, squamous cell carcinoma, actinic keratosis with squamous cell carcinoma, adenoid squamous cell carcinoma, and adenoid cystic (mucinous) carcinoma. At least 25 percent of all patients with Bowen's disease have primary internal or extracutaneous cancers.

It appears that early, adequate excision of the cutaneous lesion does not prevent the subsequent development of systemic premalignant and malignant lesions. The locations of the primary systemic cancers, in order of frequency of involvement, are respiratory system, gastrointestinal tract, genital and urinary organs, reticuloendothelial system, oral cavity, breast, endocrine system, soft tissues, and mucous membranes of the conjunctiva and lip (8,10). Both cutaneous and internal malignancies are most apt to develop 6 to 7 years after Bowen's disease is diagnosed, but they may coexist at any time. If thorough studies are carried out from the time of diagnosis of Bowen's disease to the death of the patient, at least 75 percent of affected individuals will show evidence of primary systemic cancer (8).

Microscopically, typical lesions show hyperkeratosis, parakeratosis, plaque-like acanthosis, and hypogranulosis. The epidermis exhibits a striking loss of normal polarity as well as abnormal keratinocytic maturation. The loss of normal epidermal architecture is characterized by an atypical epithelial proliferation with hyperchromatic nuclei, multinucleated cells, vacuolated cells, malignant dyskeratotic cells, and abnormal mitotic figures. These changes occur at all levels of the epidermis and are confined by an intact dermoepidermal basement membrane. They closely resemble features of actinic keratosis. Examination of serial sections of Bowen's lesions shows involvement of the ducts of the hair follicles and sebaceous glands. The lesions tend to affect the outer sheaths of the hair follicles and replace the sebaceous gland cells. The acrosyringium (intraepidermal eccrine duct) generally is uninvolved. Because of the presence of atypical vacuolated cells, the lesion may be confused with sebaceous gland carcinoma. Sometimes, extensive skip areas of uninvolved epidermis are present.

Strong evidence suggests that ingestion of arsenic is a cause of Bowen's disease. In addition, hereditary predisposition, exposure to petroleum byproducts, trauma, and cutaneous injury from ionizing radiation have been suggested as etiologic factors (8).

Radiation Dermatosis

Cells in active division, such as the basal keratinocytes of the skin of the eyelid, are more susceptible to irradiation damage than are nondividing cells. Early *radiation dermatosis* is characterized by erythema that develops in the first 2 days after radiation exposure and becomes increasingly apparent during the next several days. The erythema is associated with intracellular and extracellular edema of the epidermal cells and of the papillary layer of the dermis. In severe cases, the intraepidermal edema may progress to form vesicles or bullae. In subsequent weeks, desquamation of keratin, with areas of parakeratosis and increased pigmentation, occurs, owing to stimulation of dendritic melanocytes. In the late stage, areas of atrophy, telangiectasis, and irregular hyperpigmentation develop.

The principal eyelid changes following therapeutic irradiation include epilation; acute and chronic dermatitis; pigment changes; atrophy and telangiectasis of the skin; ectropion; entropion; loss of sebaceous, Krause, and Wolfring glands; and postradiation tumors.

Histopathologically, early radiation changes include intracellular edema of the epidermal cells with pyknosis of the nuclei. The epithelial cells of the hair follicles, sebaceous glands, and sweat glands develop degenerative changes. In late radiation dermatosis, the epidermal cells show nuclear atypia, with individual cell keratinization and atypical keratinocytes. These changes are similar to those observed in actinic keratosis. Additional changes include hyperpigmentation and atrophy of the epidermis, with scattered melanophages in the papillary dermis; fibrosis and homogenization of the dermis; and atrophy of adnexal structures. The most striking and characteristic changes are observed in the blood vessels, which initially become dilated and may show endothelial cell swelling and edema of their walls. Later, the capillaries in the upper dermis become telangiectatic, and the vessels in the deeper portions of the dermis show thrombosis and recanalization of their lumens. In severe cases of late radiation dermatosis, ulceration may occur. Epithelial neoplasms, including basal cell carcinoma and squamous cell carcinoma, may develop. Squamous cell carcinomas arising in areas of radiation dermatosis are often of the spindle cell type, exhibit a high degree of malignancy, and have a tendency to metastasize. The dermis often displays large, plump fibroblasts with fusiform or stellate outlines and basophilic cytoplasm. These cells are usually isolated and should not be confused with tumor cells, which are often grouped in small islands.

Xeroderma Pigmentosum

Xeroderma pigmentosum is a progressive disorder that begins in early childhood and affects sun-exposed areas of the skin. It is inherited in

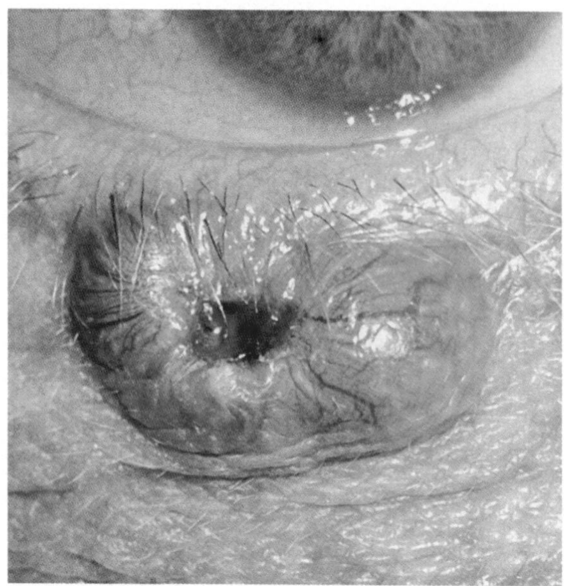

Figure 5-10

BASAL CELL CARCINOMA

Basal cell carcinoma, noduloulcerative type, involves the right lower lid.

an autosomal recessive fashion, and affected patients often have a history of family inbreeding. Some patients have neurologic abnormalities, retarded growth, or delayed sexual development. Xeroderma pigmentosum has a worldwide distribution and affects all races. Defective DNA repair processes are etiologically involved in the clinical manifestations of the disease. The skin and conjunctival tissues share the same defective repair of DNA after ultraviolet light–induced damage. Involvement of the eyelids and conjunctiva by multiple epithelial neoplasms in some cases leads to bilateral orbital exenteration.

The skin manifestations of xeroderma pigmentosum pass through three stages. In the first stage, the exposed skin shows slight erythema associated with scaling and numerous freckles. In the second stage, mottled pigmentation with telangiectases resembles the changes observed in chronic radiation dermatosis. In the third stage, various types of malignant neoplasms develop, including squamous cell carcinoma, basal cell carcinoma, malignant melanoma, and different types of sarcoma. The incidence of malignant melanoma has been estimated to be approximately 3 percent (11).

The first stage of the disease is nonspecific histologically and reveals hyperkeratosis with thinning of the epithelial layer and irregular hyperpigmentation throughout the basal cell layer. Focal lymphocytic infiltrates are usually present in the upper dermis. In the second stage, the irregular patches of hyperpigmentation with acanthosis and the atypical downward cellular proliferation resemble the features of actinic keratosis. The third stage is characterized by the development of multiple neoplasms, as mentioned above (12). Electron microscopic examination of the involved epidermis reveals an increased number of normal-sized melanosomes, as well as giant melanosomes (macromelanosomes), within melanocytes and keratinocytes.

MALIGNANT EPITHELIAL TUMORS

Basal Cell Carcinoma

Basal cell carcinoma accounts for 85 to 95 percent of all malignant epithelial tumors of the eyelid (13). It primarily affects the lower lid and inner canthus of fair-skinned adults; the upper eyelid and outer canthus are less commonly affected. Prolonged exposure to sunlight seems to be an important predisposing factor. Several clinical types of basal cell carcinoma have been described: noduloulcerative, pigmented, morphea or sclerosing, and superficial basal cell carcinoma; fibroepithelioma; nevoid basal cell carcinoma syndrome; linear basal cell nevus; and generalized follicular basal cell nevus. The last two types are extremely rare; most eyelid lesions belong in the first category.

The *noduloulcerative type of basal cell carcinoma* appears clinically as a raised, firm, pearly nodule, often exhibiting small telangiectatic vessels on its surface. As the nodule slowly increases in size, it may undergo central ulceration (figs. 5-10, 5-11); eventually the lesion appears as a slowly enlarging ulcer surrounded by a prominent rolled border ("rodent ulcer") (fig. 5-12).

Pigmented basal cell carcinoma is similar to the nodular or noduloulcerative type except for the presence of melanotic pigmentation (fig. 5-13). There are no significant differences between pigmented and nonpigmented basal cell carcinomas with respect to the age and sex of the patient or to the location, duration, and rate of

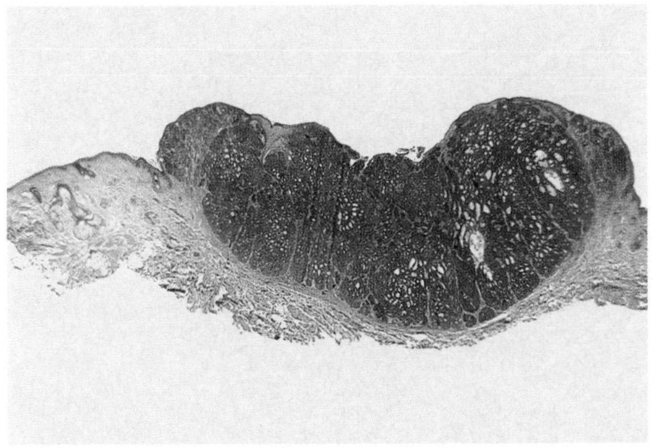

Figure 5-11

BASAL CELL CARCINOMA

Low-power view of basal cell carcinoma, noduloulcerative type.

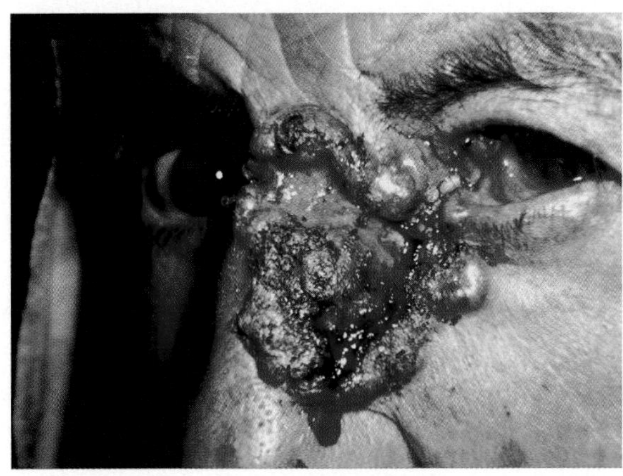

Figure 5-12

BASAL CELL CARCINOMA

Extensive basal cell carcinoma, noduloulcerative type, of the left inner canthus and nose.

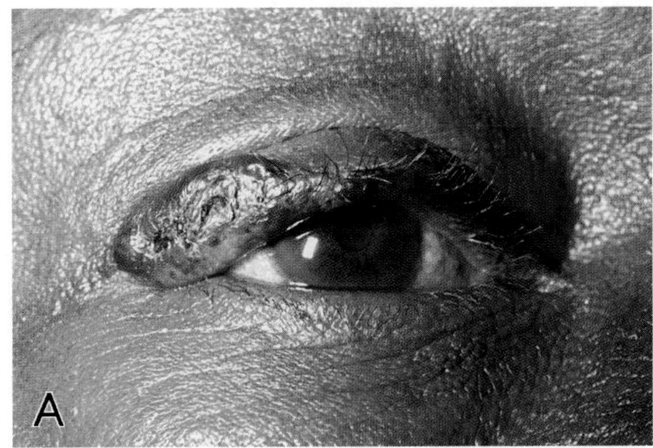

Figure 5-13

PIGMENTED BASAL CELL CARCINOMA

A: Pigmented basal cell carcinoma of the lateral portion of right upper lid.

B: Pigmented basal cell carcinoma.

C: Lobule of basal cell carcinoma with foci of melanin pigment.

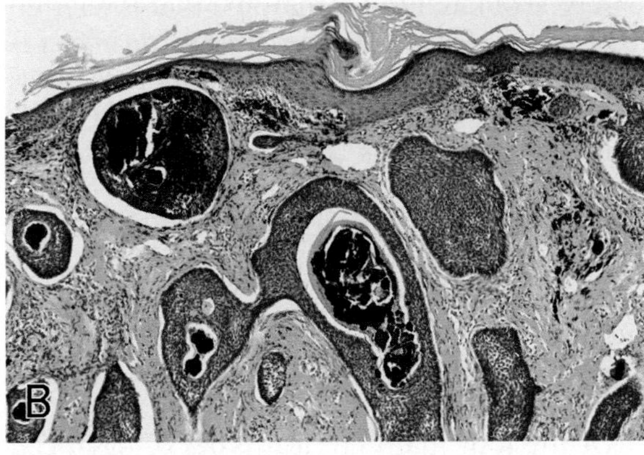

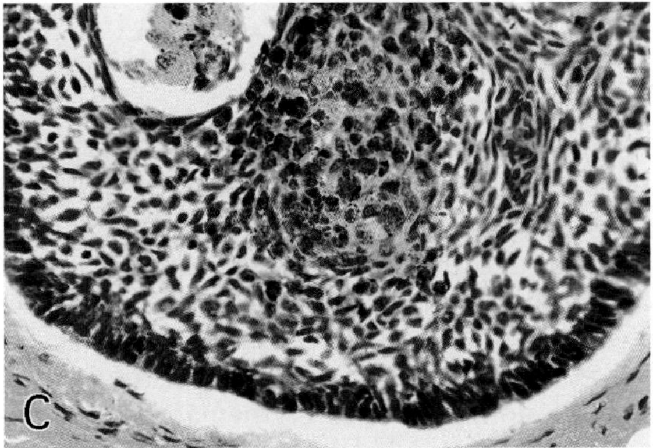

recurrence of the tumor. The pigmented lesion can be clinically misdiagnosed as malignant melanoma. The pigmentation is caused by the presence of melanocytes with slender cytoplasmic processes that contain melanin granules and are interspersed between the epithelial tumor cells. In some lesions, the pigmentation is also due to melanin pigment within the tumor cells or to collections of melanophages within the epithelial lobules.

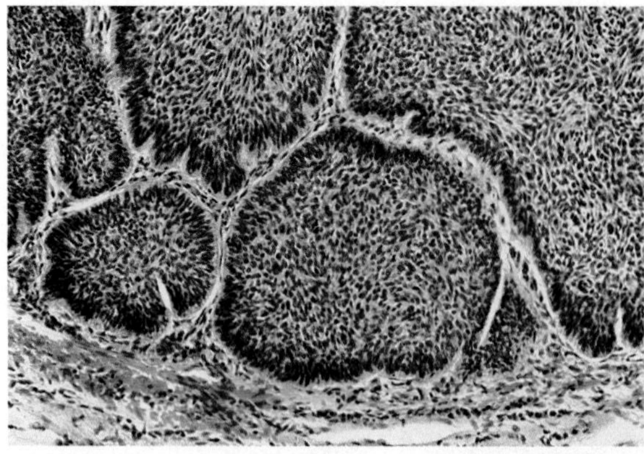

Figure 5-14

BASAL CELL CARCINOMA

Solid type of basal cell carcinoma with peripheral palisading of nuclei.

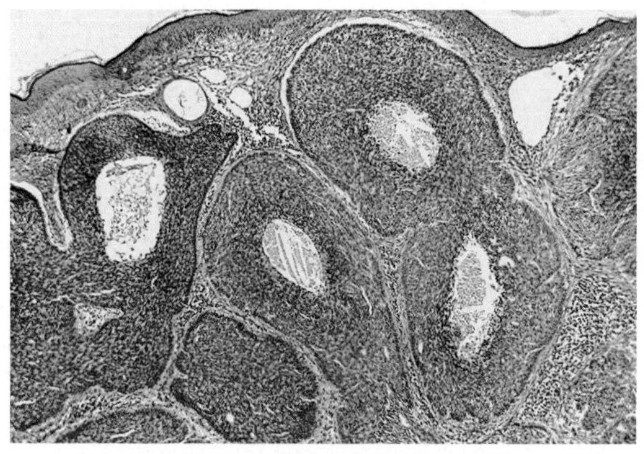

Figure 5-15

CYSTIC BASAL CELL CARCINOMA

Each tumor lobule has a central focus of necrosis.

The *morphea or sclerosing type of basal cell carcinoma* appears as a pale, indurated plaque with an ill-defined border. Noduloulcerative, pigmented, and morphea or sclerosing basal cell carcinomas have a predilection to involve the face. *Superficial basal cell carcinoma* may arise in the eyelid but usually is found on the trunk. These lesions appear as erythematous, scaling patches that extend peripherally and often have a pearly border. Frequently, they exhibit superficial ulceration and crusting.

Basal cell carcinomas arise from the pluripotential primary epithelial germ cells of the basal cell layer of the epidermis. Undifferentiated tumors (*solid basal cell carcinomas*) are composed of solid epithelial lobules with prominent peripheral palisading of the nuclei (fig. 5-14). The differentiated type may show features characteristic of several cutaneous appendages: tumors with differentiation toward hair structures are called *keratotic*, those with features resembling sebaceous glands are called *cystic* (fig. 5-15), and those differentiating toward apocrine and eccrine structures are referred to as *adenoid basal cell carcinomas* (fig. 5-16). Some of these tumors differentiate toward more than one of these cutaneous appendages.

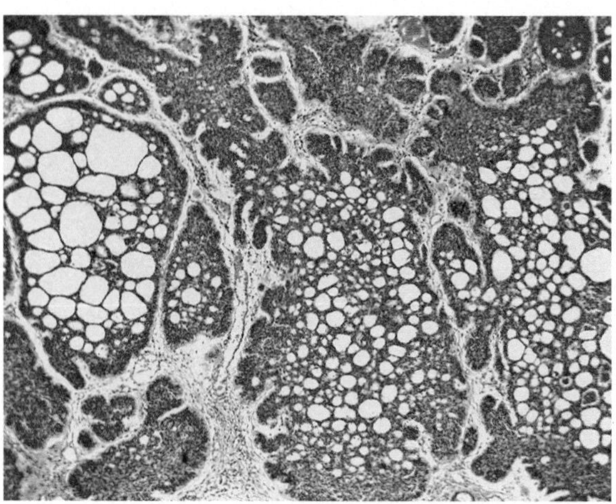

Figure 5-16

BASAL CELL CARCINOMA

Basal cell carcinoma with adenoid cystic pattern.

A type of basal cell carcinoma that is referred to as *metatypical*, or *basosquamous, carcinoma* is of special interest. It has morphologic features intermediate between those of basal cell carcinoma and squamous cell carcinoma; hence, it is often referred to as "intermediate" basosquamous and metatypical basal cell carcinoma (fig. 5-17). This type of basal cell carcinoma pursues a more aggressive course, infiltrates deeply, and may metastasize. Wide local excision is recommended to avoid recurrences and possible metastatic disease.

Of the four main clinical types of basal cell carcinoma that involve the face and eyelid, the noduloulcerative type is most capable of exhibiting areas of adenoid, cystic, or keratotic differentiation. The pigmented, morphea, and superficial types usually display few or no differentiating features.

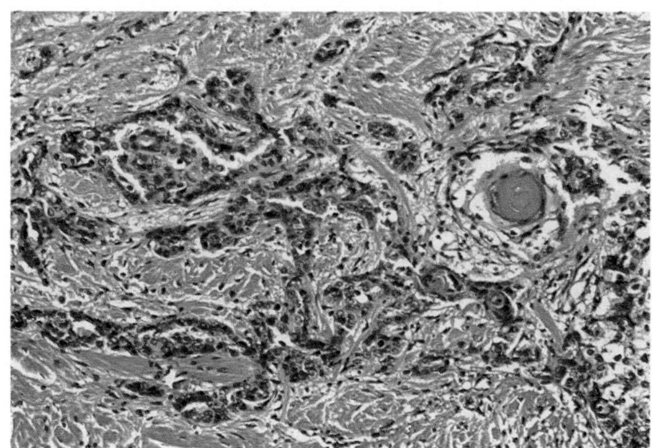

Figure 5-17

BASAL CELL CARCINOMA

Metatypical (basosquamous) basal cell carcinoma.

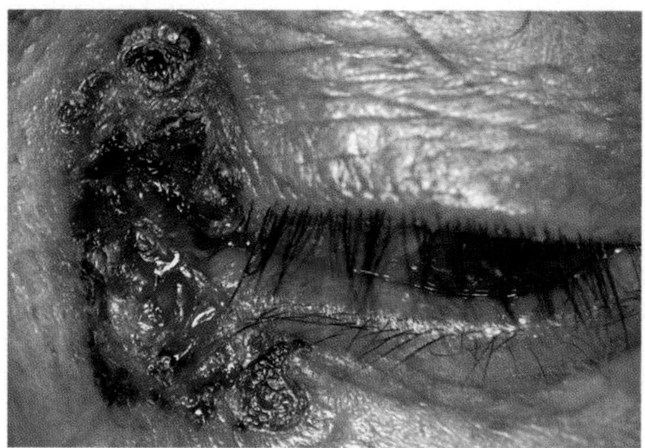

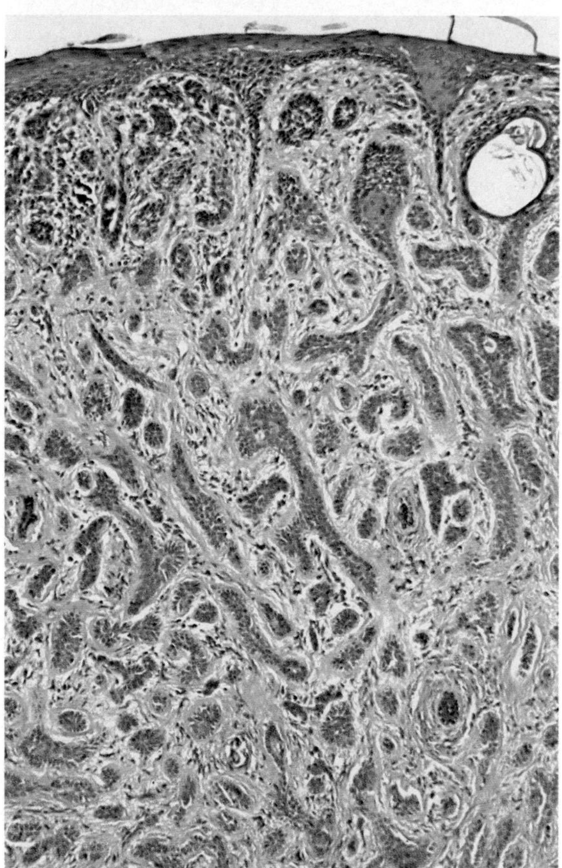

Figure 5-18

BASAL CELL CARCINOMA

Clinical appearance (top) and histologic features (bottom) of morphea type variant of basal cell carcinoma.

The growth pattern of basal cell carcinoma is quite variable, and four basic morphologic patterns have been described: nodular, ulcerative, morphea (sclerosing), and multicentric. Doxanas et al. (14) describe the nodular pattern as a localized, pearly nodule with superficial telangiectatic vessels on its surface. A pseudocapsule is formed as the tumor enlarges and compresses adjacent dermal structures. This type of basal cell carcinoma may have variable histologic features, ranging from solid proliferation of basaloid cells to areas exhibiting adenoid or cystic differentiation.

The ulcerative pattern shows a central ulcer crater with a raised, pearly epithelial margin. A pseudocapsule is not usually observed in this type. Because of surface ulceration, a chronic dermal inflammatory infiltrate is commonly present.

The morphea (sclerosing) pattern appears clinically as a pale, indurated plaque (fig. 5-18, top). Histologically, it is characterized by elongated strands of basaloid cells embedded in a dense fibrous stroma (fig. 5-18, bottom). The narrow epithelial strands, one to two cell layers in thickness, resemble those seen in metastatic scirrhous carcinoma of the breast. This type of basal cell carcinoma is aggressive and deeply infiltrates into the adjacent dermis and subcutis. Eyelid tumors of this type may erode into the paranasal sinuses and invade orbital structures.

The multicentric pattern exhibits an irregular nodular surface with telangiectatic vessels. It may involve the epidermis in a diffuse, multicentric manner and extend into the superficial dermis.

The ulcerative, morphea, and multicentric types of basal cell carcinoma often extend beyond the margins of apparent clinical involvement.

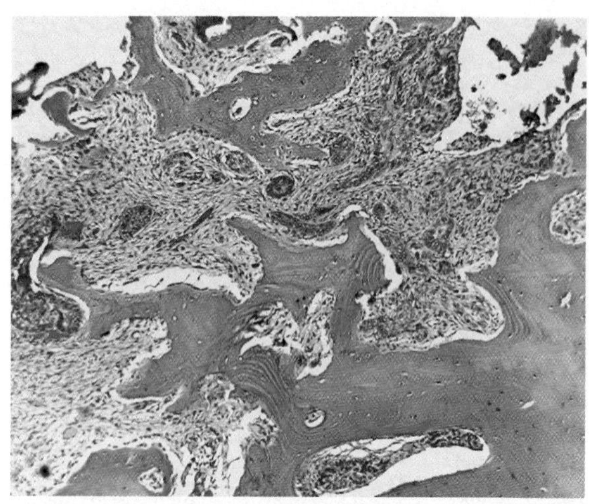

Figure 5-19

BASAL CELL CARCINOMA

Infiltrating basal cell carcinoma invades orbital bones.

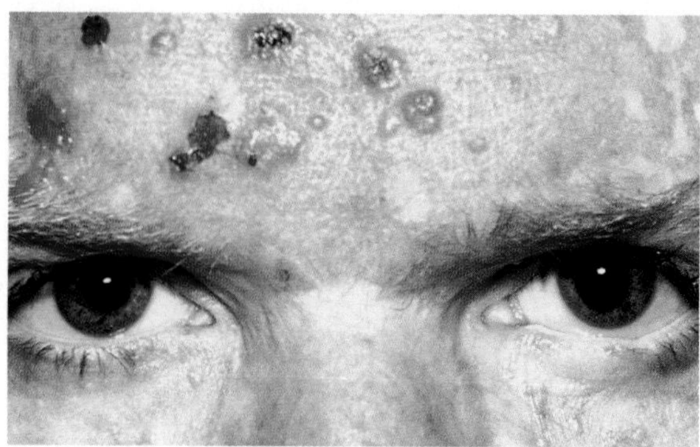

Figure 5-20

NEVOID BASAL CELL CARCINOMA SYNDROME

Multiple basal cell carcinomas of the forehead in a young male.

For this reason, frozen sections are mandatory to monitor the margins of surgically excised specimens to be certain that the tumor has been completely removed. This technique enables the surgeon to remove the entire lesion in a single excision while sacrificing the least amount of normal tissue and thus facilitating reconstruction of the eyelid.

Although radiotherapy has been successful for most types of basal cell carcinoma, it is less efficacious with tumors of the morphea type (15). Extensive lesions of this type that have invaded the orbital bones (fig. 5-19) are usually managed by orbital exenteration.

Basal cell carcinoma rarely metastasizes, and death from tumor is unusual (16). The incidence of metastasis has been estimated to range from 0.028 percent to 0.55 percent, depending upon the population surveyed (17). The most common metastatic sites are lung, bone, lymph nodes, liver, spleen, and adrenal gland. The mean survival time after metastasis is 1.6 years. Frequently, primary and recurring tumors have histologic features of metatypical (basosquamous) carcinoma, whereas the metastatic lesions generally have metatypical or adenoid patterns.

Nevoid Basal Cell Carcinoma Syndrome

Nevoid basal cell carcinoma syndrome, which is also known as *nevoid basal cell epithelioma syndrome* and *Gorlin-Goltz syndrome,* is inherited as an autosomal dominant disorder with high penetrance, variable degrees of expressivity, and equal involvement among men and women (17–19). It is characterized by multiple basal cell carcinomas (figs. 5-20, 5-21) involving the nose, eyelids, cheek, trunk, neck, and arm, associated with cysts of the jaw (odontogenic keratocysts), skeletal anomalies (most commonly bifid ribs), neurologic abnormalities (ectopic calcification, mental retardation), and endocrine disorders (ovarian cysts, testicular disorders). The incidence of this syndrome among individuals with basal cell carcinoma is 0.7 percent (18). In about half the patients with this syndrome, numerous, 1- to 3-mm, palmar and plantar pits develop around the second decade of life. Other clinical findings include scoliosis, short fourth metacarpals (brachymetacarpalism), calcification of the dura mater and, in some patients, cerebellar medulloblastoma.

The variety of ocular and periocular findings include prominence of the supraorbital ridges, hypertelorism, dystopia canthorum, internal strabismus, congenital blindness, glaucoma, congenital cataract, and colobomas of the choroid and optic nerve (20). Chromosomal studies of several patients with this syndrome have revealed a normal karyotype (21).

The skin lesions, which appear in childhood and around puberty, are multiple, grayish white, pearly nodules, some of which are umbilicated (fig. 5-20). They increase in size and number, and are haphazardly distributed over the face and

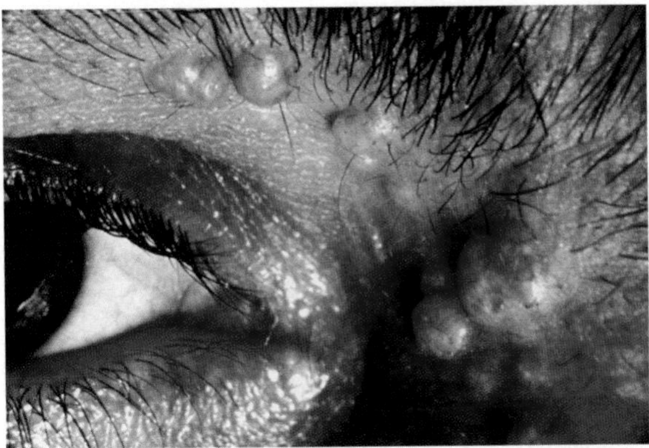

Figure 5-21

NEVOID BASAL CELL CARCINOMA SYNDROME

Multiple, grayish white, pearly nodules are observed in the right inner canthus and upper eyelid.

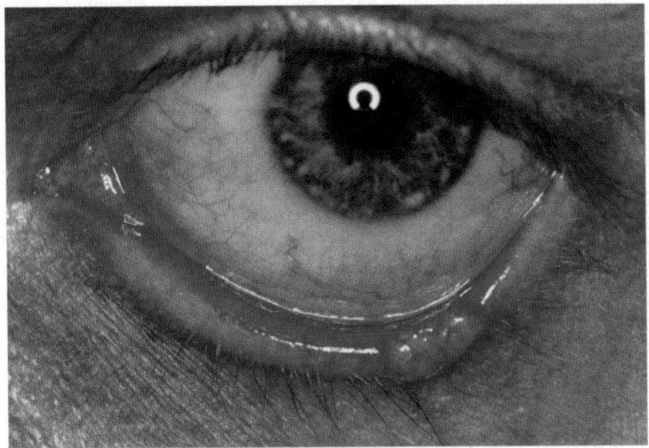

Figure 5-22

SQUAMOUS CELL CARCINOMA

The lower eyelid is involved.

body. When the face is involved, almost invariably the upper eyelids are affected. Zackheim and coworkers (22) found the eyelids to be affected in 21.6 percent of cases. Microscopically, the lesions show different variants of basal cell carcinoma (solid, adenoid, and keratotic), and the lesions of nevoid basal cell carcinoma syndrome cannot be distinguished histologically from those of conventional basal cell carcinoma. The possibility of this syndrome, however, should be considered when a basal cell carcinoma is associated with the following findings: a young patient, usually between the ages of 10 and 30 years; the presence of multiple tumors; a histologic pattern showing superficial multicentric tumors; and foci of osteoid within the tumor (23).

Clinically, the facial and eyelid lesions of the nevoid basal cell carcinoma syndrome resemble those seen in patients with multiple trichoepitheliomas (Brooke's tumor). The lesions in trichoepithelioma, however, tend to affect the nasolabial folds, remain small, and hardly ever ulcerate. In contrast, the lesions of the nevoid basal cell carcinoma syndrome are haphazardly distributed and may enlarge, ulcerate deeply, and display an invasive character. Histochemical studies may help distinguish these two entities. There is an abundance of sulfated acid mucopolysaccharides in lesions of nevoid basal cell carcinoma (especially of the adenoid type), compared with the lesions of multiple trichoepitheliomas, which contain mainly hyaluronic acid.

Squamous Cell Carcinoma

Squamous cell carcinoma typically involves the margin of the lower eyelid, but it may be located elsewhere in the eyelid (fig. 5-22). In the upper eyelid and outer canthus, squamous cell carcinoma is more common than basal cell carcinoma (24). Less than 5 percent of epithelial neoplasms of the eyelid, however, are squamous cell carcinomas. The overall ratio of squamous cell to basal cell carcinoma in the eyelid is about 1 to 39 (25). The tumor may arise de novo or from preexisting lesions, such as intraepithelial carcinoma or actinic keratosis. Squamous cell carcinoma may also develop following radiation therapy and in patients with xeroderma pigmentosum.

The lesion usually is an elevated, indurated plaque or nodule that tends to ulcerate and has irregular borders. In well-differentiated tumors, the masses of keratin may give the lesion a grayish white, granular appearance. Early lesions of squamous cell carcinoma of the eyelid rarely metastasize and patients have an excellent prognosis. Wide local excision is usually curative. Advanced or neglected cases are often associated with metastases to the preauricular and submandibular lymph nodes.

In well-differentiated tumors, the cells are polygonal with abundant acidophilic cytoplasm. Characteristic dyskeratotic cells with formation of keratin pearls are observed (fig. 5-23). The nuclei are prominent and hyperchromatic, and vary in size and staining properties

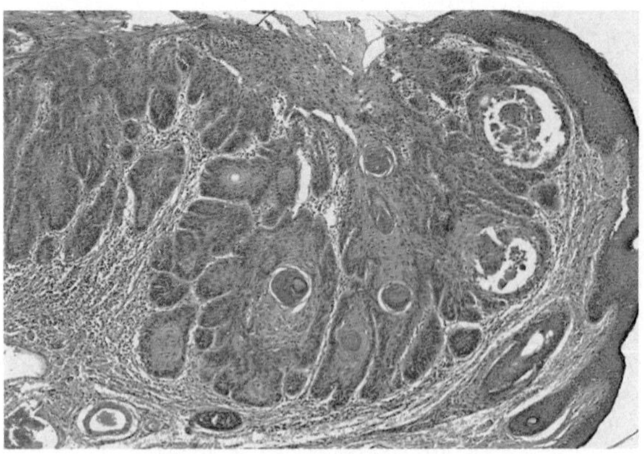

Figure 5-23

SQUAMOUS CELL CARCINOMA

Moderately well-differentiated squamous cell carcinoma with keratin pearls.

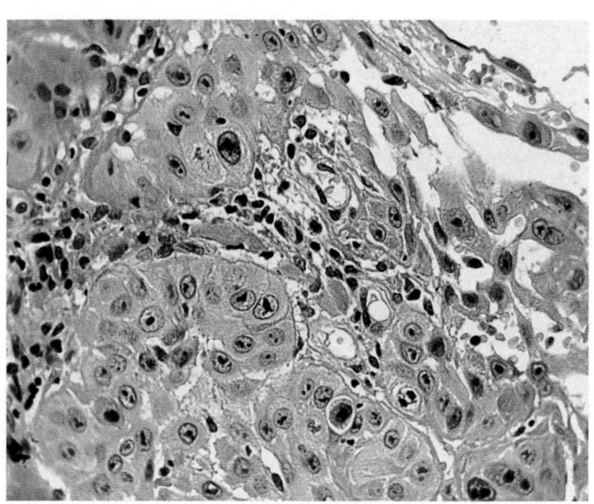

Figure 5-24

SQUAMOUS CELL CARCINOMA

High-power view shows large polyhedral cells with eosinophilic cytoplasm.

(fig. 5-24). Intercellular bridges can be easily found in well-differentiated tumors, but they may be difficult to demonstrate in poorly differentiated lesions that may show little or no evidence of keratinization.

Spindle Cell Squamous Carcinoma

A *spindle cell variant of squamous cell carcinoma* occasionally involves the skin of the eyelid. This lesion may be confused with fibrous histiocytoma, fibromatosis, or fibrosarcoma. Careful review of multiple sections, however, usually shows dysplastic keratinocytes, focal areas of intraepithelial carcinoma of the overlying epidermis, areas displaying intercellular bridges, or small foci of keratinization. In some cases, immunohistochemical or electron microscopic examination may be required to establish the definitive diagnosis.

Adenoid Squamous Cell Carcinoma

Adenoid squamous cell carcinoma, a variant of squamous cell carcinoma, is also known as *adenoacanthoma* and *pseudoglandular squamous cell carcinoma*. It tends to involve the sun-exposed areas of the head and neck of elderly individuals. Eyelid involvement is uncommon. Patients have a good prognosis. Local excision is usually curative.

The lesion appears as a slightly elevated nodule with central ulceration and elevated margins (fig. 5-25), sometimes resembling a keratoacanthoma. Histologically, the tumor often exhibits a cup-shaped configuration, with cords of infiltrating, atypical epithelial cells extending into the upper dermis. Toward the center of the tumor lobules are areas of acantholysis (fig. 5-26), with formation of lumens containing dyskeratotic cells; the peripheral portions of the lobules are lined by a single cohesive layer of cuboidal epithelial cells that form adenoid (pseudoglandular) structures.

The most frequent precursor lesion of adenoid squamous cell carcinoma is actinic keratosis with acantholysis. Often the lesion appears to originate from the pilar outer root sheaths, but in some instances it arises from the epidermis. Histochemical studies have demonstrated the presence of hyaluronic acid within the adenoid structures, in contrast to other apocrine and eccrine sweat gland tumors in which the mucopolysaccharide is a nonsulfated, hyaluronidase-resistant mucosubstance of the sialomucin type. Additionally, the desquamated acantholytic cells usually contain moderate amounts of glycogen (26).

MELANOCYTIC TUMORS

Melanocytic lesions of the skin arise from three sources: nevus cells, melanocytes of the epidermis, and melanocytes of the dermis. All are derived embryologically from neural crest cells. The morphologic characteristics of nevus

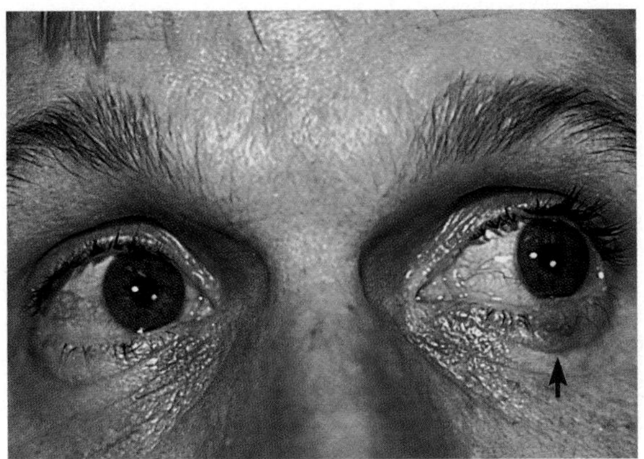

Figure 5-25

ADENOID SQUAMOUS CELL CARCINOMA

Lesion of the left lower eyelid (arrow).

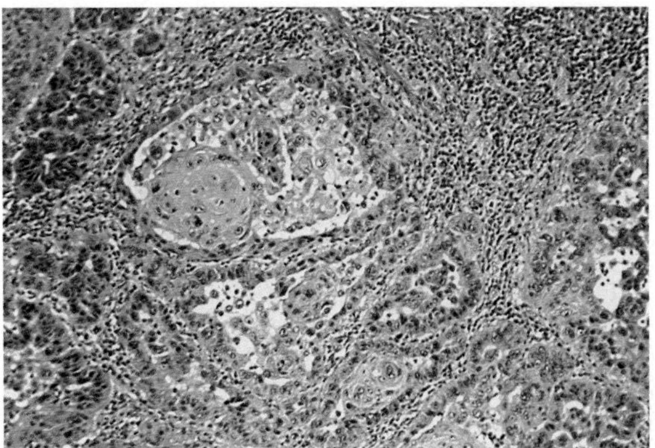

Figure 5-26

ADENOID SQUAMOUS CELL CARCINOMA

The tumor contains numerous acantholytic cells that have a pseudoglandular pattern.

cells and melanocytes are similar; however, nevus cells show a characteristic arrangement in nests and lack dendritic processes. Because these processes are short and stubby in epidermal melanocytes, they are not easily identified by light microscopy. Lesions arising within the epidermis are either melanocytic or nevocytic in origin, whereas those located entirely within the dermis (blue and cellular blue nevi) are believed to be melanocytic. The frequency distribution of melanocytic tumors accessioned at the Doheny Eye Institute over a 30-year period is summarized in Table 5-3.

Table 5-3

TUMORS OF MELANOCYTIC ORIGIN OF THE EYELID[a]

Type of Tumor	Number of Cases
Benign	
Dermal nevus	147
Compound nevus	12
Spindle and epithelioid cell nevus	2
Blue nevus	2
Malignant	
Melanoma	9

[a]Frequency distribution of 172 tumors from the Doheny Eye Institute files collected between 1970 and 2000.

Nevocellular Nevus

Nevocellular nevi are benign melanocytic lesions that frequently occur on the surface of the eyelid or on the lid margin. Histologically, nevi are divided into three types: junctional, compound, and intradermal. Stages intermediate between a junctional and a compound nevus may be encountered, as well as between a compound and an intradermal nevus. Based on the clinical features and the degree of pigmentation of the lesion, the histology of the nevi can be predicted. Hormonal factors associated with puberty or pregnancy may cause increased pigmentation and enlargement of nevi. Nevus cells in the upper, middle, and lower dermis have been referred to as types A, B, and C, respectively (27). Type A nevus cells exhibit large, round to oval nuclei and well-outlined cytoplasm and resemble epithelioid cells. Type B nevus cells are usually smaller, resemble lymphoid cells, and rarely contain melanin. Type C nevus cells resemble fibroblasts since they exhibit elongated spindle-shaped nuclei and contain little or no melanin.

Junctional nevi arise from the deeper layers of the epidermis ("junctional region") and do not involve the underlying dermis. They are flat, pigmented lesions. This type of nevus, like the compound nevus, has the capacity to evolve into a malignant melanoma. Although connected to the epidermis, nevus cells are able to "drop off" into the dermis, and many nevi that appear to be purely junctional in one area are found to be compound in other areas.

Compound nevi possess features of junctional and intradermal nevi. In an appreciable portion of these lesions, nests of intradermal nevus cells

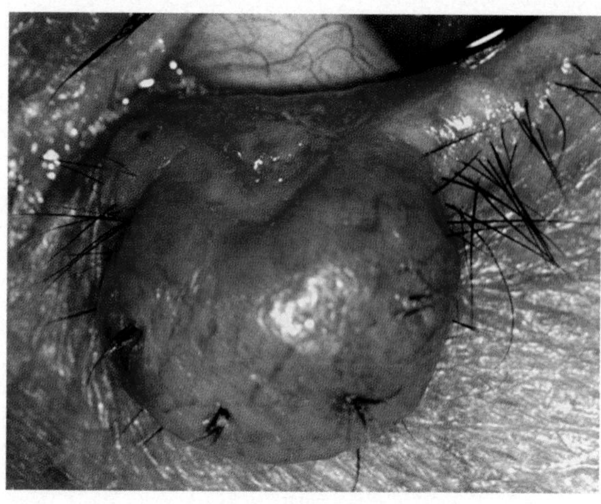

Figure 5-27

INTRADERMAL NEVUS

Pedunculated intradermal nevus is attached to the eyelid margin.

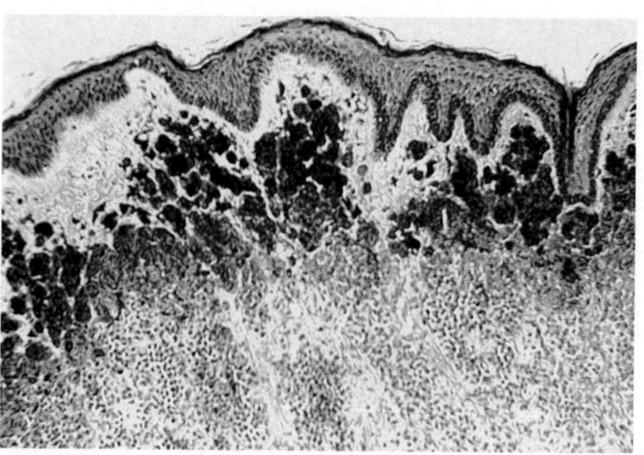

Figure 5-28

INTRADERMAL NEVUS

Heavily pigmented nevus cells in the upper dermis.

appear to have "dropped off" the epidermis into the dermis. This type of nevus is more common than the purely junctional nevus and may also undergo malignant change. In some instances, compound nevi involve an equal portion (mirror image) of the upper and lower eyelid margins ("kissing nevus"). This type of congenital nevus occurs when the developing lid folds, containing embryonic nests of nevus cells, meet during the 8th week and remain fused until the end of the 5th month, when separation occurs.

Intradermal nevi are the most common and the most benign of the three types of nevocellular nevi (fig. 5-27). Malignant change in a purely intradermal nevus is extremely rare. The surface of an intradermal nevus may have a papillomatous, domed, or pedunculated configuration. The presence of hairs in an elevated pigmented nodule usually indicates that the lesion is intradermal.

On microscopic examination, the nests of nevus cells in the dermis are separated from the overlying epidermis by an intact collagenous layer of upper dermis (Grenz zone) (fig. 5-28). In the eyelid, nevus cells may extend into the deeper dermis and reach the fibers of the orbicularis muscle. Often, nests of large, multinucleated nevus cells are present. These giant nevus cells occur only in mature intradermal nevi, and they are considered to indicate the benign nature of the lesion. In some instances, an intradermal nevus does not form nests in the upper dermis and is composed of spindle-shaped nevus cells embedded in a loosely arranged, collagenous stroma. These lesions resemble a solitary neurofibroma and are referred to as *neural nevi*. Occasionally, intradermal nevi contain large foci of fat cells intermixed with the nevus cells—a combination of an intradermal nevus with a nevus lipomatosus.

Four variants of nevocellular nevi have been described: *balloon cell nevi, spindle* or *epithelioid nevi ("juvenile melanoma"), halo nevi,* and *congenital giant pigmented nevi.*

Balloon cells may comprise only a small portion of an intradermal or compound nevus, or they may be the major component of the nevus. Transitions between typical nevus cells and balloon cells are occasionally observed. The balloon cells are larger than conventional nevus cells, measuring 20 to 40 µm in diameter. Their nuclei are small and pyknotic, and are located either paracentrally or eccentrically at one pole of the cell. The cytoplasm has a finely granular or vacuolated appearance, with well-demarcated boundaries. Scattered multinucleated balloon cells are frequently seen.

Electron microscopic studies have shown that the balloon cells contain numerous nonmelanized melanosomes that tend to coalesce and are located within large vacuoles (28). In contrast, melanosomes of intradermal and junctional nevus cells are smaller, spindle-shaped

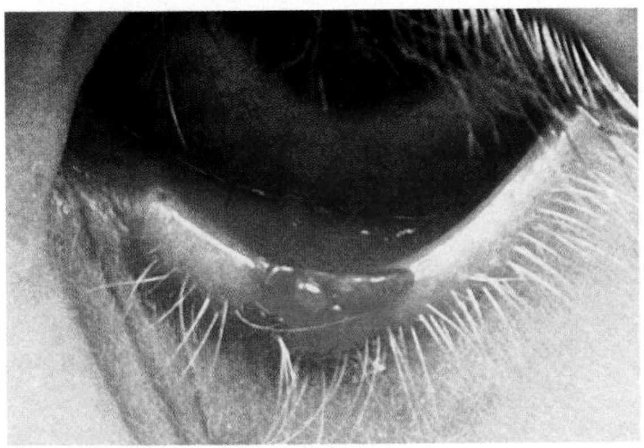

Figure 5-29

NEVUS OF THE EYELID

Spindle/epithelioid nevus of the eyelid in a blonde Caucasian child.

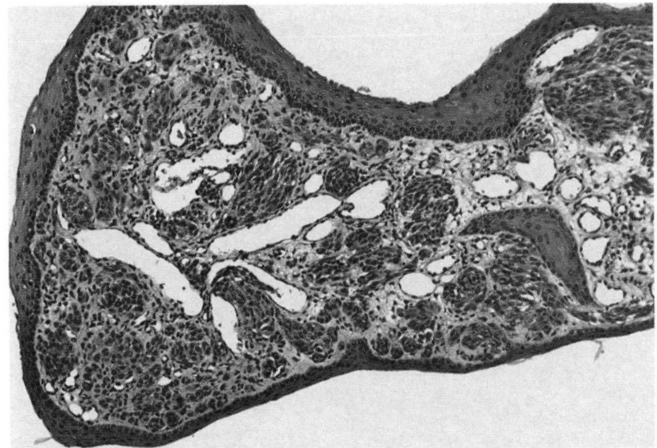

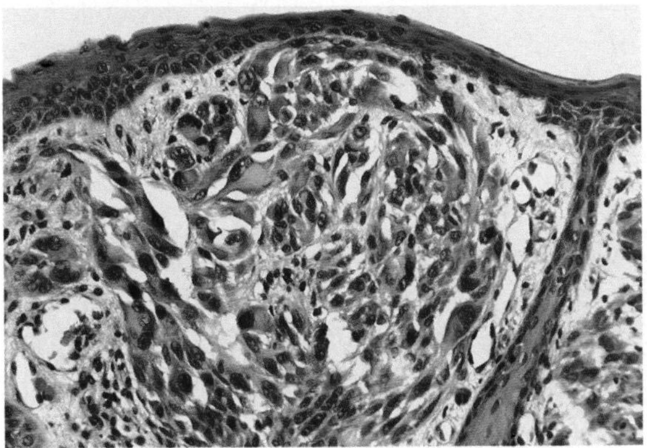

Figure 5-30

NEVUS OF THE EYELID

Top: Spindle/epithelioid cell nevus of eyelid in a child. Bottom: High-power view shows the admixture of large epithelioid cells and spindle cells.

rather than round, usually do not coalesce, and are fully melanized.

Spindle or epithelioid nevus (juvenile melanoma) is a form of compound nevus that mainly affects children and young adults (figs. 5-29, 5-30). The lesion appears as a dome-shaped nodule involving the face or the extremities. Because of the scarcity of melanin, the lesion is reddish pink rather than brown. Histologically, the lesion is a variant of a compound nevus, containing fascicles of spindle-shaped cells showing a "windblown" appearance, intermixed with larger epithelioid cells with polyhedral outlines (fig. 5-30). Despite disturbing cytologic features (an "active" junctional zone, scattered mitotic figures, and the presence of secondary inflammation), the lesion usually pursues a benign clinical course. Electron microscopic examination discloses lysosomal degradation of melanosomal complexes within the nevus cells and incomplete melanization (29).

Giant Congenital Melanocytic Nevus

Giant congenital melanocytic nevus (CMN) is a rare, large, congenital, melanocytic lesion that affects the eyelids and periorbital skin (fig. 5-31). The nevus presents a dramatic clinical appearance, causing considerable emotional distress for patients and their families. Although the term "giant" has been applied to these extensive periorbital lesions, they are usually considerably smaller than histologically identical nevi that affect the skin of other portions of the body, where the appellation is reserved for CMN measuring more than 10 cm in greatest diameter. Patients with giant CMNs that affect the head and neck may clinically manifest epilepsy and mental retardation associated with leptomeningeal melanocytosis, or even a primary malignant melanoma of the meninges and brain. The incidence of cutaneous melanoma with high mortality in patients with giant CMN has been reported to vary from 6.3 to 12.0 percent (30). The malignant melanoma may be present at birth, or it may arise in infancy or later in life.

Three histologic patterns can be observed in giant CMN: a compound nevus (fig. 5-32), an intradermal nevus, and a blue nevus. In addition, nevus cells are observed around pilosebaceous units (fig. 5-33), sweat ducts, vessel walls, and dermal nerves.

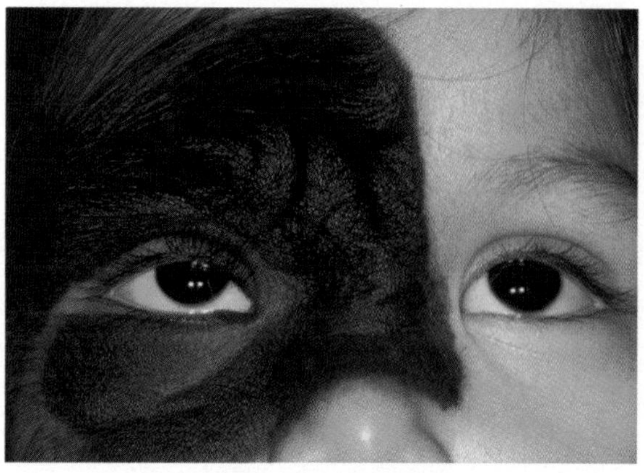

Figure 5-31

LARGE CONGENITAL NEVUS

Large congenital hairy nevus involves the eyelids and brow region, cheeks, and bridge of nose.

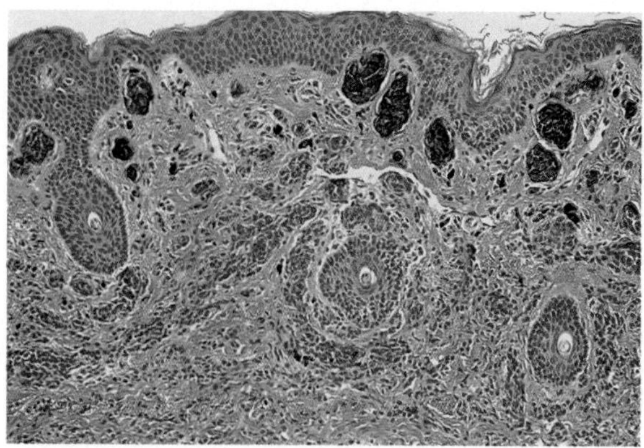

Figure 5-32

CONGENITAL NEVUS

Histologic features of the compound pattern from the congenital hairy nevus shown in figure 5-31.

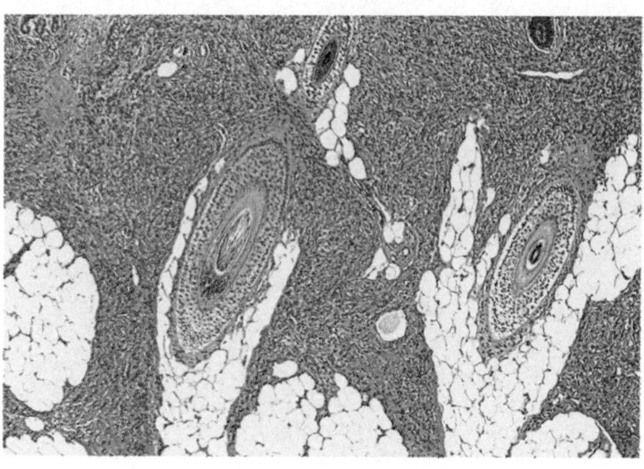

Figure 5-33

CONGENITAL NEVUS

Congenital hairy nevus surrounds large hair follicles in the subcutis. The nevus cells are spindle shaped and form an Indian-file pattern.

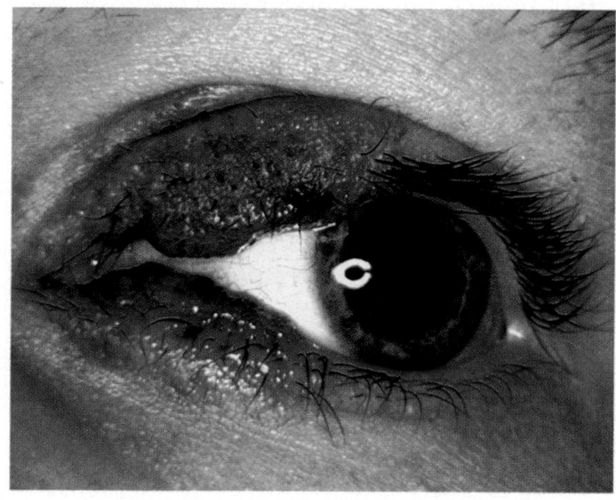

Figure 5-34

KISSING NEVUS

Kissing nevus of eyelid in a young child.

Kissing nevus of the eyelids in young children (figs. 5-34, 5-35) is a variant of CMN. It involves both upper and lower eyelids and histologically displays nevus cells in the dermis that extend into the tarsus (fig. 5-35). The clinical appearance of the nevus is due to the development of the lesion prior to the fourth month of fetal development when the eyelids are fused (fig. 5-36).

Unlike the development of most cutaneous melanomas, which originate from intraepidermal melanocytes at the dermoepidermal junction, the development of a malignant melanoma from a giant CMN usually takes place deep in the dermis. There is formation of sheets of undifferentiated cells containing little or no melanin pigment.

Blue Nevus, Cellular Blue Nevus, and Nevus of Ota

These lesions arise from deeply located melanocytes that have been arrested in the dermis before reaching the epidermis. Two types are recognized: the *blue nevus* and the *cellular blue nevus* (fig. 5-37). Blue nevus is a dome-shaped,

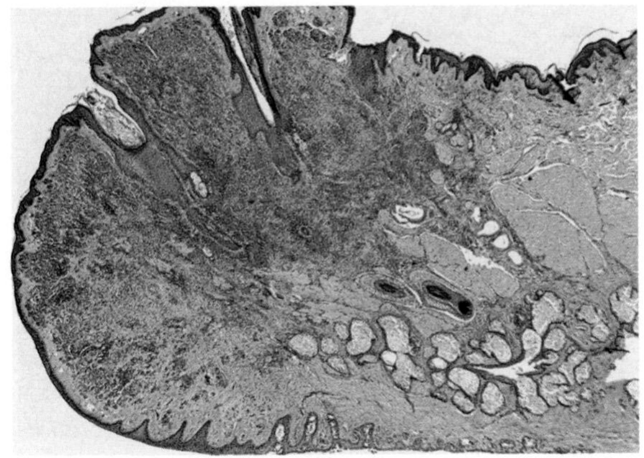

Figure 5-35

KISSING NEVUS

Low-power microscopy shows involvement of the dermis and early extension into the tarsus.

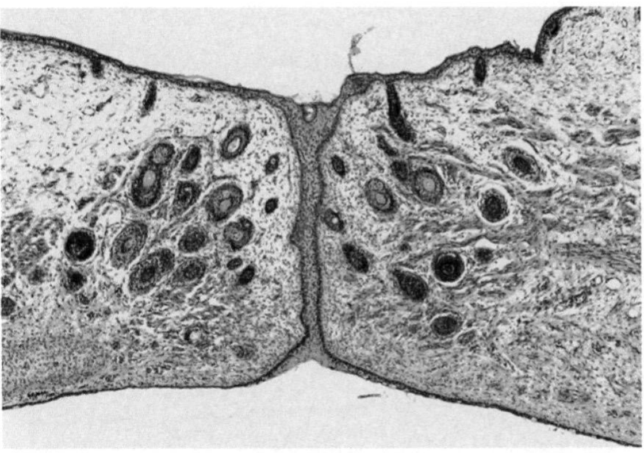

Figure 5-36

EYELIDS OF A FETUS

The eyelids are fused until the end of the fourth month of fetal development, which explains the clinical appearance of kissing nevus.

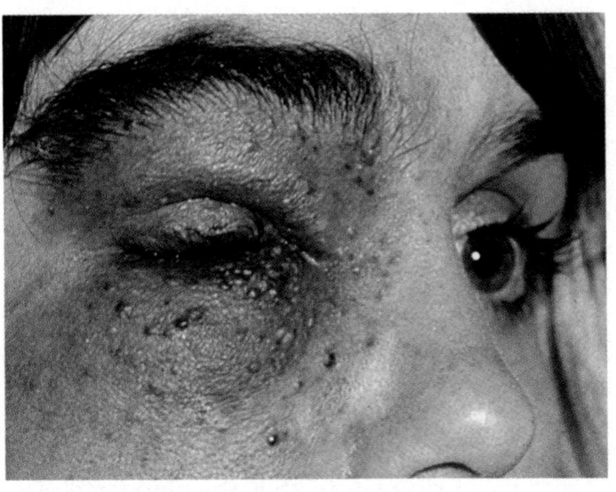

Figure 5-37

CELLULAR BLUE NEVUS

Cellular blue nevus involves the skin of eyelids and cheek.

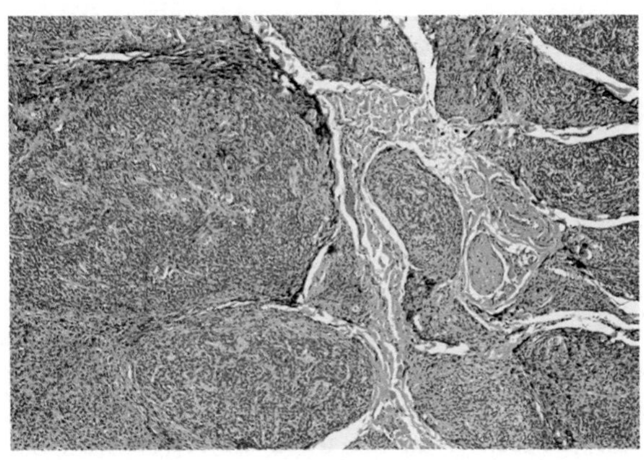

Figure 5-38

CELLULAR BLUE NEVUS

Hypercellular lobules are composed of spindle-shaped cells surrounded by heavily pigmented melanocytes.

small lesion, the blue color of which results from the scattering of light by melanin particles within deeply located dermal melanocytes. When a compound nevus is present over a conventional blue nevus, the lesion is called a *combined nevus*. Malignant degeneration does not occur in conventional blue nevi. Histologically, the lesions are composed of elongated, slender, slightly wavy, heavily pigmented melanocytes with numerous dendritic processes that primarily involve the lower dermis and the subcutaneous fat. Melanophages are frequently intermixed with the bundles of melanocytes.

Cellular blue nevi are composed of islands of deeply pigmented, dendritic melanocytes interspersed with bundles of nonpigmented cells that have a "neuroid" appearance (fig. 5-38). Frequently, the islands of nevus cells extend into the subcutaneous tissue. The buttock and sacrococcygeal regions are sites of predilection, with a female to male incidence of 2.2 to 1 (31). Cellular blue nevi may give rise to malignant melanomas. On occasion, it is difficult to be certain whether this change has occurred, since a benign cellular blue nevus may exhibit cells with pleomorphic nuclei. The

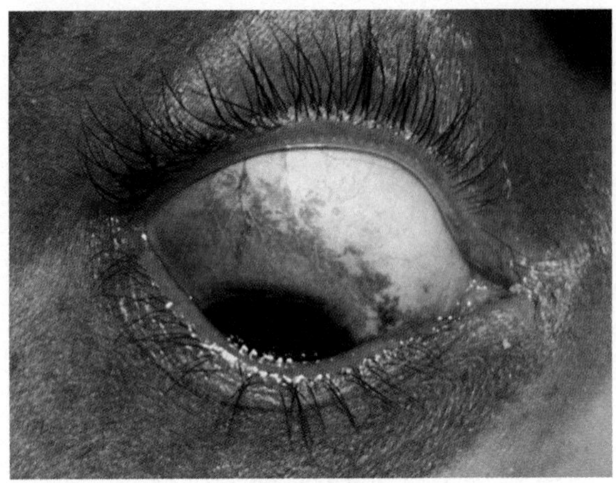

Figure 5-39

NEVUS OF OTA

The patient had an ipsilateral choroidal melanoma.

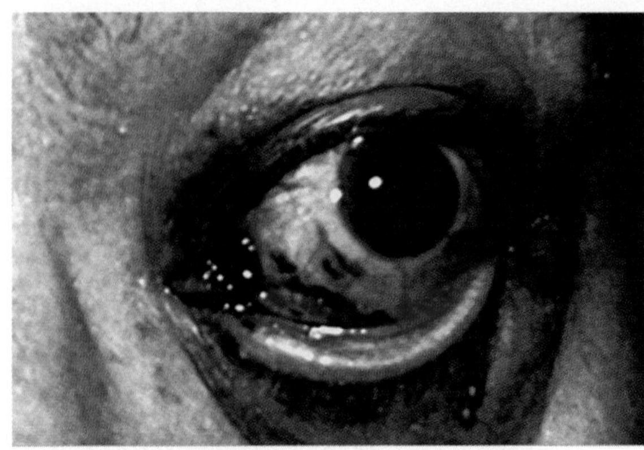

Figure 5-40

NEVUS OF OTA

Malignant melanoma of the conjunctiva with orbital invasion in a patient with a nevus of Ota.

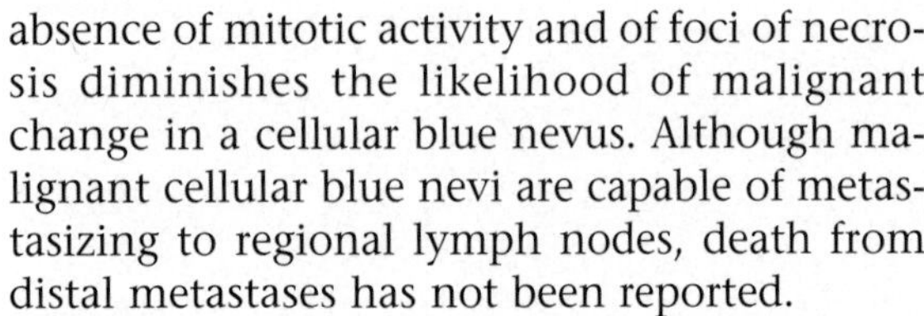

absence of mitotic activity and of foci of necrosis diminishes the likelihood of malignant change in a cellular blue nevus. Although malignant cellular blue nevi are capable of metastasizing to regional lymph nodes, death from distal metastases has not been reported.

Nevus of Ota, also known as *oculodermal melanocytosis*, is a variant of the blue nevus, with the distribution of melanocytes in the deep dermis of the eyelid and surrounding adnexa, sclera, and orbital and uveal tissue. Melanomas can develop from the uveal melanocytes (fig. 5-39) and the deep melanocytes of the conjunctiva (fig. 5-40).

Freckle

This pigmented lesion, also known as *ephelis*, appears as a small, brown macule scattered over the sun-exposed areas of the skin, including the eyelids. In contrast to lentigo simplex, sunlight exposure deepens the pigmentation of freckles. Histopathologically, there is hyperpigmentation of the basal cell layer but no elongation of the rete ridges. The basal layer of the epidermis contains large, dopa-positive melanocytes, but their number is not increased.

Lentigo Simplex

The lesions of *lentigo simplex* are flat and brown to black, and measure approximately 1 to 2 mm in diameter. They are clinically indistinguishable from junctional nevi. They are not affected by exposure to sunlight. There is an increased number of basal melanocytes, with elongation of the rete ridges and scattered melanophages in the upper dermis. Occasionally, nests of nevus cells are present at the dermoepidermal junction *(nevoid lentigo)*.

Solar Lentigo

Solar lentigo occurs in elderly whites; it is also known as *senile lentigo*. The lesions are multiple and appear as dark-brown macules with irregular outlines. They may resemble the lesions of seborrheic keratosis, which histologically differs from lentigo simplex in that the elongated rete ridges are club-shaped and exhibit irregular tortuosity. There is considerable hyperpigmentation and increased numbers of melanocytes throughout the basal cell layer. In addition, the synthesis of melanin is increased and there is a delay in lysosomal destruction of melanosomes.

MALIGNANT MELANOMA

Malignant melanoma constitutes approximately 1 percent of all malignant neoplasms of the eyelid. The clinical features, histopathologic findings, biologic behavior, and prognosis of primary eyelid melanomas parallel those of other cutaneous malignant melanomas. Four different types of primary cutaneous melanoma are recognized: lentigo maligna melanoma, superficial spreading melanoma, nodular melanoma, and acral lentiginous melanoma.

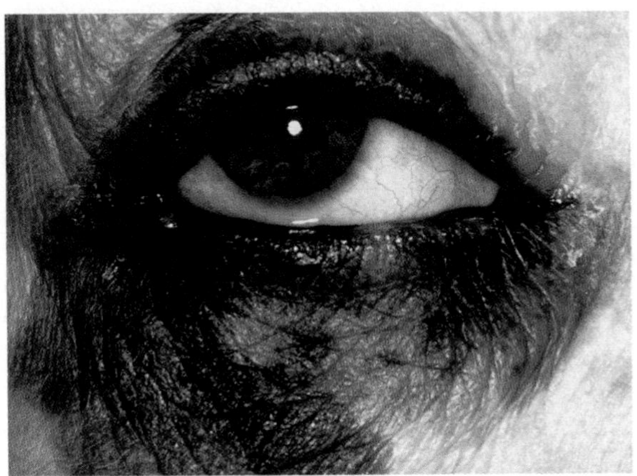

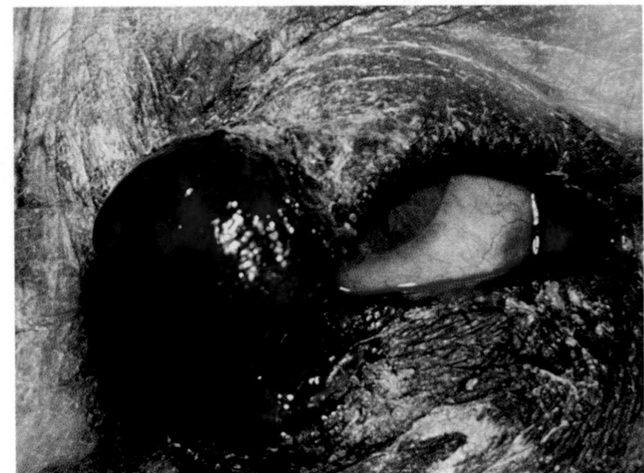

Figure 5-41

LENTIGO MALIGNA

Left: Lentigo maligna, also known as Hutchinson's melanotic freckle.
Right: Seven years later the patient developed an invasive malignant melanoma.

Virtually all cutaneous malignant melanomas initially develop from the neoplastic transformation of intraepidermal melanocytes, with the initial melanocytic proliferation extending horizontally (noninvasive horizontal growth phase). This stage is followed by an invasive (vertical growth) phase. The duration of the atypical, melanocytic intraepidermal migration is shortest for nodular melanoma and longest for lentigo maligna melanoma.

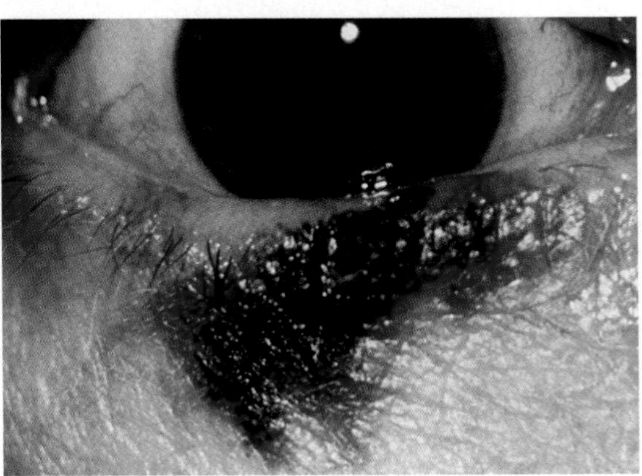

Figure 5-42

LENTIGO MALIGNA

Lentigo maligna with biopsy-proven early malignant melanoma.

Lentigo Maligna and Lentigo Maligna Melanoma

Lentigo maligna, also known as *Hutchinson's melanotic freckle,* is the precursor lesion of *lentigo maligna melanoma* (fig. 5-41). It appears as a flat, nonpalpable macule with irregular borders and a variable degree of pigmentation (tan to brown). It occurs mainly in the sun-exposed areas of elderly individuals (fig. 5-42). Peripheral extension occurs slowly, with waxing and waning of the lesion. Involvement of the lower lid and canthal regions is common. Areas of depigmentation may occur at sites of regression. The size of the lesion increases gradually and may reach 6 to 7 cm in diameter (horizontal growth phase). This preinvasive phase may last 10 to 15 years.

Histopathologically, there is diffuse hyperplasia of atypical, pleomorphic melanocytes throughout the basal cell layer of the epidermis, extending into the outer sheaths of the pilosebaceous structures (fig. 5-43). When dermal invasion occurs (vertical growth phase), the lesion becomes elevated, forming a dark-brown to black nodule (lentigo maligna melanoma). The invading malignant melanoma cells often are composed of fascicles of spindle-shaped cells. The estimated incidence of malignant transformation of lentigo maligna is 25 to 30 percent (32).

Superficial Spreading Melanoma

Superficial spreading melanoma, also referred to as *pagetoid melanoma,* differs from lentigo maligna melanoma in several respects. It occurs

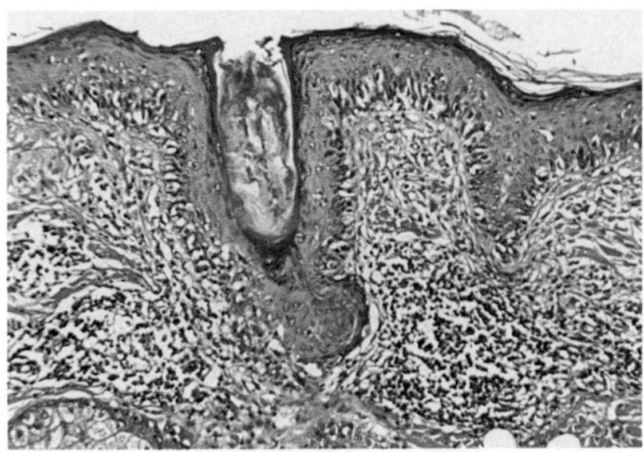

Figure 5-43

LENTIGO MALIGNA

There is a spindle-shaped melanocytic proliferation of the basal cell layer of the epidermis and outer sheaths of the hair follicle.

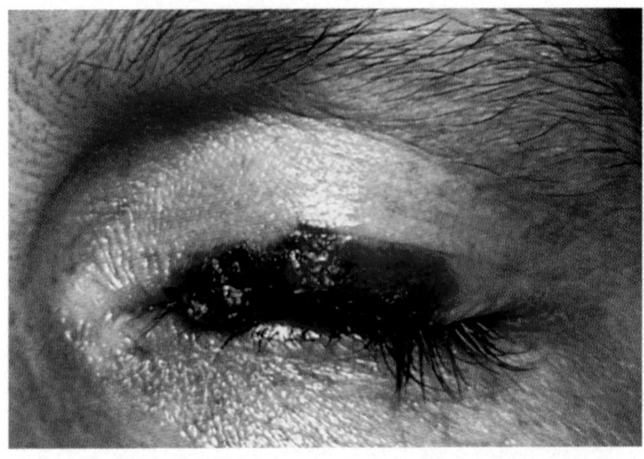

Figure 5-44

SUPERFICIAL SPREADING MELANOMA

Lesion of the left upper eyelid.

in younger individuals (median age, fifth decade), is smaller (average size, 2.5 cm) (fig. 5-44), and primarily involves nonexposed cutaneous surfaces.

The epidermal component consists of atypical melanocytes that exhibit pagetoid features (fig. 5-45). In contrast to lentigo maligna, the cells do not preferentially line up along the basal layer of the epidermis but instead are found singly and in nests at all levels of the epidermis. The atypical melanocytic cells tend to be uniform in size and shape, and often have epithelioid features. In the invasive vertical growth phase, the malignant melanoma cells vary in size and shape, and may take on the configuration of epithelioid, spindle, or nevus-like cells, or of a mixture of cell types.

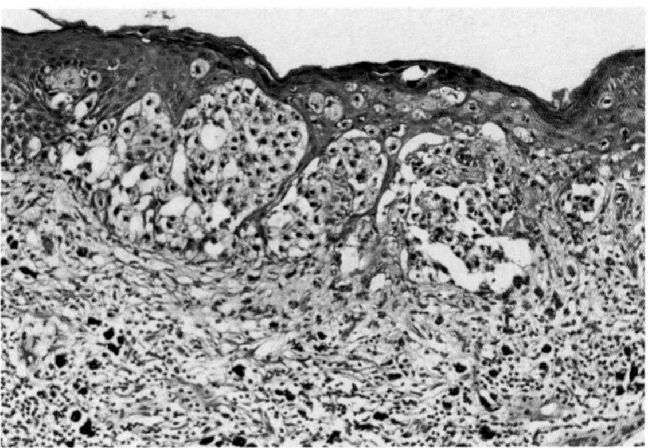

Figure 5-45

SUPERFICIAL SPREADING MELANOMA ("PAGETOID MELANOMA")

The epidermis contains nests of atypical melanocytes that exhibit pagetoid features and extend upward into the more superficial epidermal layers.

Nodular Melanoma

Nodular melanoma is a small, blue-black (fig. 5-46) or amelanotic, pedunculated nodule that is almost always palpable when first noted and rapidly increases in size to 1 to 3 cm (fig. 5-47). It usually occurs in the 40- to 50-year age group and is twice as common in men as in women. It involves exposed and unexposed areas of the skin, including the mucous membranes (buccal mucosa, genitalia, and anal canal).

This invasive melanoma has adenoid structures predominantly composed of large anaplastic epithelioid cells. Dermal invasion is always present at the onset (fig. 5-46, right). Some authorities believe that no horizontal growth phase is present in nodular melanoma; however, others are of the opinion that a transient horizontal phase occurs and that the lesion then rapidly undergoes a vertical growth phase with prominent dermal invasion. Nodular melanoma exhibits a more rapid growth and a more extensive depth of invasion than do other types of cutaneous malignant melanoma.

Acral Lentiginous Melanoma

Acral lentiginous melanoma occurs on the palms and soles, the distal phalanges (especially

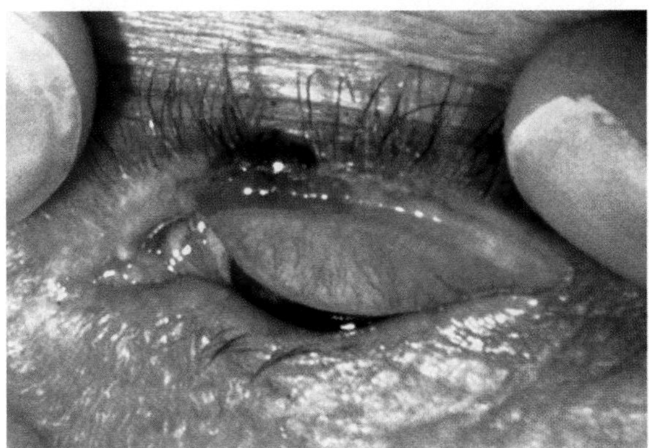
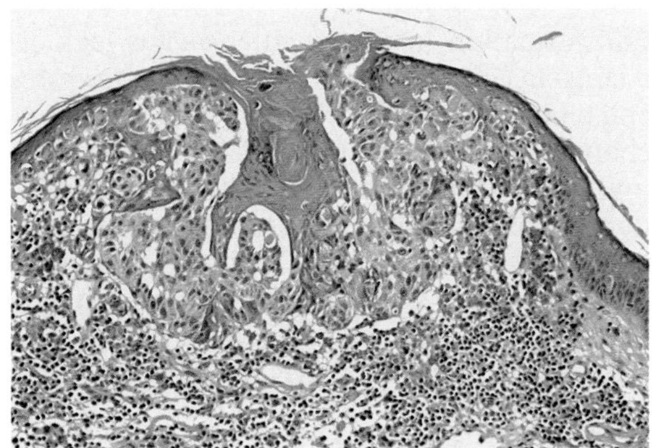

Figure 5-46

NODULAR MELANOMA

Left: Incipient nodular melanoma of the left upper lid.
Right: Histologic features of invasive malignant melanoma.

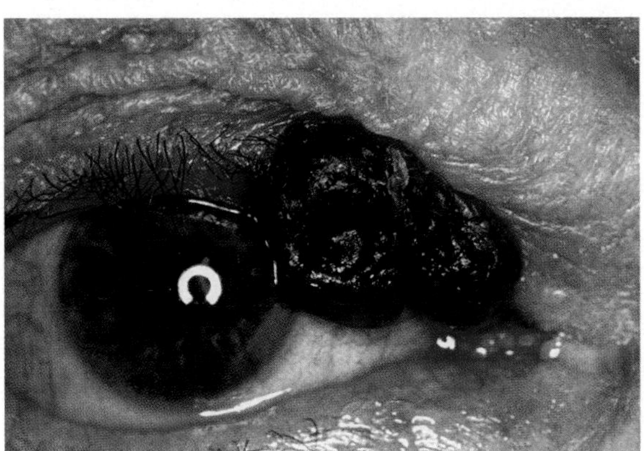
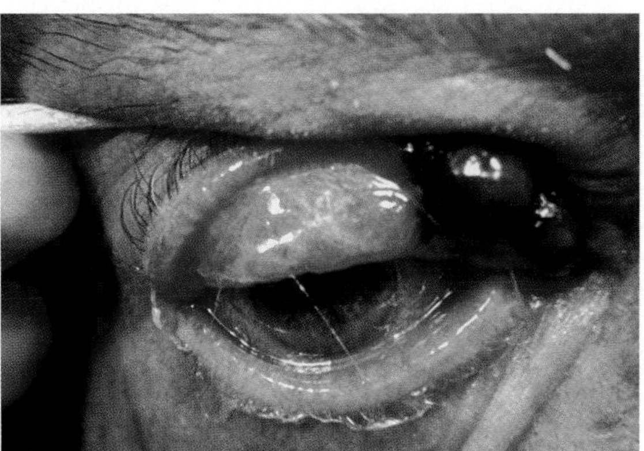

Figure 5-47

NODULAR MELANOMA

Nodular malignant melanoma of the right upper lid involving the tarsal conjunctiva. This patient died 2 years later with metastases.

the periungual and subungual regions), and the mucous membranes that are lined by stratified squamous epithelium. The lesions resemble those of lentigo maligna melanoma and appear as macules of varying pigmentation, ranging from tan brown to black. In the early, preinvasive, intraepidermal phase the lesions appear histologically benign in some areas, whereas other portions exhibit clear-cut malignancy. Histologically, the atypical melanocytes appear dendritic and are confined to the dermal/epidermal junction. Once the vertical phase is established, the invasive component is frequently of the spindle cell type. The prognosis is intermediate between that of a superficial spreading and a nodular melanoma.

Melanoma Arising from a Nevus

Malignant melanomas of all types arise in association with preexisting nevi, especially nevi that are totally intraepidermal. About 50 percent of superficial spreading melanomas studied with step sections show nevus cells at the base of the lesion; in other types of malignant melanoma, the percentage of nevus cells is considerably less. Approximately 20 percent of nodular melanomas are associated with a nevus. Ominous signs suggestive of malignant transformation in a pigmented nevus include change in color (especially shades of red, white, and blue and sudden darkening); change in size; change in surface characteristics (crusting, oozing, bleeding, or ulceration); change in consistency (especially softening or friability); changes in symptomatology (pain, itching, or tenderness); change in shape (rapid elevation in a previously flat lesion); and changes in the surrounding skin (redness, swelling, or the appearance of satellite lesions).

Clark and associates (33) proposed a prognostic classification system based upon levels of invasion of cutaneous malignant melanoma. Five levels of invasion were defined: level 1, the tumor is entirely confined to the epidermis with an intact epithelial basement membrane; level 2, the tumor extends beyond the epithelial basement membrane, with early invasion of the papillary dermis, without abutting the reticular dermis; level 3, the tumor fills the entire papillary dermis and reaches the interface between papillary and reticular dermis; level 4, the tumor penetrates the reticular dermis; and level 5, the tumor invades the subcutaneous tissues. The 5-year survival rate after treatment (listed by tumor type and by level of invasion) is given in Table 5-4.

Breslow (34) introduced the concept of tumor thickness as an important parameter in evaluating the prognosis of primary cutaneous melanomas. The maximal tumor thickness in histologic sections is measured by drawing a straight line from the uppermost part of the granular layer of the epidermis to the deepest point of penetration of the tumor. Breslow reported that patients with lesions less than 0.76 mm in thickness have a 100 percent 5-year survival rate, whereas those with lesions thicker than 1.5 mm have a less than 50 percent 5-year survival rate. Those with tumors with a thickness between 0.76 and 1.5 mm were found to have an intermediate 5-year survival rate. Clark's level of invasion system and Breslow's measurement of tumor thickness can be used as complementary factors in estimating the prognosis of patients with malignant melanoma (35).

The histologic type of malignant melanoma is regarded by most authorities to have prognostic value. Overall, patients with nodular malignant melanoma are considered to have the worst prognosis, whereas those with lentigo maligna melanoma have the best prognosis. The superficial spreading malignant melanoma carries an intermediate prognosis. The denser the inflammatory infiltrate, the better the prognosis, whereas absence of an inflammatory infiltrate is associated with a high index of mortality. The sex of the patient and the location of the melanoma are significant. Men have a worse prognosis than women; lesions situated in the extremities and the head and neck confer a better prognosis than do lesions involving the trunk and mucous membranes. Involvement of the draining lymph nodes as well as widespread tumor dissemination are ominous signs.

Table 5-4

FIVE-YEAR SURVIVAL RATE OF PATIENTS WITH CUTANEOUS MALIGNANT MELANOMA (AFTER THERAPY)[a]

	5-Year Survival (%)	Level of Invasion	5-Year Survival After Therapy (%)
Lentigo maligna melanoma	90	1-2	100
Superficial spreading melanoma	69	3	80
Nodular melanoma	44	4	65
Nodular melanoma		5	15

[a]Data from Kopf AW, Bart RS, Rodriguez-Sains RS, Ackerman AB, eds. Malignant melanoma. New York: Masson; 1979.

Malignant Melanoma

Grossniklaus and McLean (36), in a clinicopathologic study of 32 patients with cutaneous malignant melanoma of the eyelid, found that the lower eyelid was more frequently affected (21 patients, 66 percent of cases) than the upper eyelid. The melanomas were classified as nodular in 19 patients (59 percent), superficial spreading in 7 patients (22 percent), and lentigo malignant melanoma in 6 patients (19 percent). Associated histopathologic findings included solar elastosis in 13 tumors (41 percent), nevus cells in 18 lesions (38 percent), and basal cell carcinoma in 4 tumors (13 percent). Only 1 of 18 patients who had follow-up data available died of metastatic melanoma. Melanomas that occur in the lid margin may be associated with a worse prognosis than melanomas of the eyelid that spare the margin (37).

Dysplastic Nevus Syndrome

Dysplastic nevus syndrome is also known as *B-K mole syndrome* (named after two patients [Beth and Kruger] in whom the condition was first observed). It is characterized by multiple, large, atypical cutaneous nevi, frequently 5 to 10 mm in size, that have irregular outlines and a haphazard mixture of tan, brown, black, and pink coloration. The lesions mainly involve the upper part of the trunk and extremities. The term dysplastic has been applied because of the atypical clinical and histologic features of these lesions.

The nevi are usually noticeable in children and adolescents, and continue to grow throughout adult life. The condition is inherited as an autosomal dominant trait. Family members of involved patients are at high risk for developing cutaneous melanomas (some of which are multicentric), which may be detected early in life by careful and periodic dermatologic evaluation. The large moles of the dysplastic nevus syndrome may be precursors of malignant melanoma (38).

Histologically, the dysplastic nevi have areas of atypical melanocytic hyperplasia (often referred to as "melanocytic dysplasia"), patchy lymphocytic dermal infiltrates, delicate fibroplasia, and neovascularization of the papillary dermis. These histologic features are virtually identical to those observed in the areas of regression that are frequent in superficial spreading melanoma and in the halos of halo nevi.

BENIGN SEBACEOUS GLAND TUMORS

The eyelid contains a large number of sebaceous, sweat, and apocrine glands as well as hair follicles. It is therefore prone to the development of a wide variety of benign and malignant neoplasms arising in these structures (Table 5-5).

Table 5-5

TUMORS OF SEBACEOUS GLANDS OF THE EYELID[a]

Type of Tumor	Number of Cases
Benign	
Sebaceous hyperplasia	7
Sebaceous adenoma	4
Malignant	
Sebaceous gland carcinoma	82

[a]Frequency distribution of 93 tumors in the Doheny Eye Institute collected between 1970 and 2000.

Adenomatoid Sebaceous Hyperplasia. Also referred to as *senile sebaceous nevus*, this lesion occurs predominantly on the skin of the face and scalp of older individuals. The skin of the eyelids, the meibomian glands, and the sebaceous glands of the caruncle may be affected. The lesions are small (2 to 3 mm), elevated, soft, yellowish nodules, some of which are umbilicated. They are composed of well-demarcated lobules of fully mature sebaceous glands, usually grouped around a centrally located, dilated sebaceous duct. The localized dermal nodule usually compresses the adjacent adnexal structures. *Sebaceous gland adenomas* display clinical and histologic features similar to those observed in adenomatoid sebaceous gland hyperplasia.

Multiple Hamartoma Syndrome (Cowden's Disease). This is an autosomal dominant condition characterized by multiple dome-shaped, flesh-colored papules and verrucoid lesions that affect the face and eyelids, oral mucosa, and acral portions of the upper extremities (punctate keratoses of the palms). The syndrome is associated with lesions of the thyroid gland (goiter, adenoma, and carcinoma) and breast (fibrocystic disease and carcinoma) (39). It is important to recognize this syndrome because of the high incidence of associated malignancies, especially of the thyroid gland and breast. About half the biopsy specimens from the facial papules of patients with this syndrome display the histologic features of trichilemmoma (40). Some cutaneous facial papules show nonspecific hyperkeratosis and acanthosis (41).

Muir-Torre Syndrome. The association of sebaceous gland tumors of skin and visceral malignancy is known as Muir-Torre syndrome. Approximately 70 percent of patients with this condition have a positive family history of malignancy with an apparent autosomal dominant mode of transmission (42,43). The most common internal carcinomas are colorectal (47 percent), genitourinary (21 percent), breast (12 percent), hematologic (9 percent), and head and neck (4 percent) (43). Histologically, the sebaceous lesions are mostly sebaceous adenomas, whereas the other lesions are either adenomatoid sebaceous hyperplasia or basal cell carcinoma with foci of sebaceous differentiation.

The Muir-Torre syndrome differs from two other syndromes in which multiple cutaneous

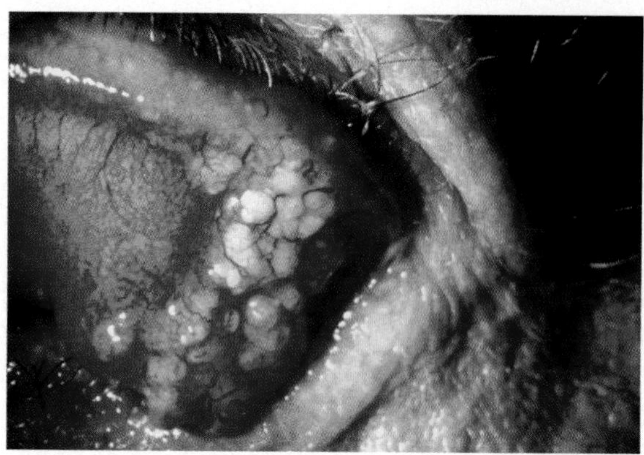

Figure 5-48

MEIBOMIAN GLAND CARCINOMA

The lobular pattern is striking.

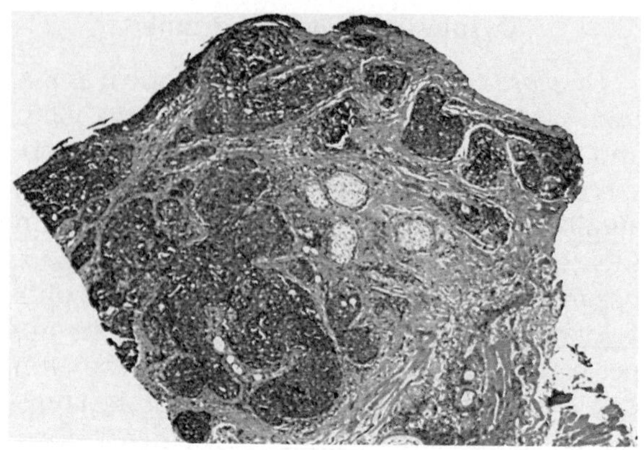

Figure 5-49

MEIBOMIAN GLAND CARCINOMA

Low-power microscopic view shows tumor lobules filling the meibomian glands.

tumors and visceral lesions develop: *Gardner's syndrome* and *Oldfield's syndrome*. Gardner's syndrome is characterized by intestinal polyposis, multiple osteomas of facial bones, fibromas and epithelial inclusion cysts of the skin, and fibromatosis (desmoid tumors) of the abdominal wall, mesentery, and breast (44). Oldfield's syndrome is typified by familial polyposis of the colon associated with multiple sebaceous cysts (45).

SEBACEOUS GLAND CARCINOMA

Definition. The malignant tumors arising from various sebaceous glands of ocular adnexa include *meibomian gland carcinoma, Zeis gland carcinoma,* and *carcinomas arising from sebaceous glands of the skin of the eyelid and caruncle.* These tumors reveal varying degrees of sebaceous differentiation. They can invade the orbit, metastasize to regional lymph nodes, and disseminate hematogenously to various visceral organs.

Epidemiology and General Features. Sebaceous gland carcinoma comprises 1 to 3 percent of all malignant eyelid tumors (46,47). The disease affects elderly patients (sixth to seventh decade); the rare cases reported before age 40 usually have followed prior radiation therapy either for retinoblastoma or cavernous hemangioma of the face (48). There appears to be a female predominance. In a series of 88 patients in the United States, 57 percent were female; about two thirds of 156 cases reported from Shanghai were female (48,49). Although all races have been reported to be affected, Ni and coworkers (49,50) reported that sebaceous gland carcinoma is encountered with greater frequency in China than in the United States and Western Europe. More recently this tumor was ranked second in frequency (32.7 percent) among 525 malignant eyelid tumors in Shanghai; the most common malignant eyelid tumor in this series was basal cell carcinoma (51).

Sebaceous gland carcinoma arises almost exclusively in the eyelid and only with extreme rarity elsewhere in the skin of the body (52). The most common sites of origin in the eyelid are the meibomian glands (figs. 5-48–5-50) and the sebaceous glands of the lashes (glands of Zeis) (figs. 5-51, 5-52). Less frequently, sebaceous gland carcinoma may originate from the sebaceous glands in the caruncle or the skin of the eyebrow. The upper lid is involved in about two thirds of the cases, probably because the meibomian glands are more numerous in the upper tarsus than the lower. Lesions originating from the glands of Zeis appear as small, yellowish nodules located at the lid margin just in front of the gray line. Some tumors appear to originate from both the meibomian glands and the glands of Zeis, whereas the exact site of origin cannot be determined in others. Rarely, the carcinoma arises from the four eyelids following radiation (53). Tumor arising from the sebaceous glands of the caruncle appears as a subconjunctival, multilobulated, grayish yellow mass, usually covered by an intact epithelium.

Clinical Features. A broad spectrum of clinical features are associated with sebaceous gland

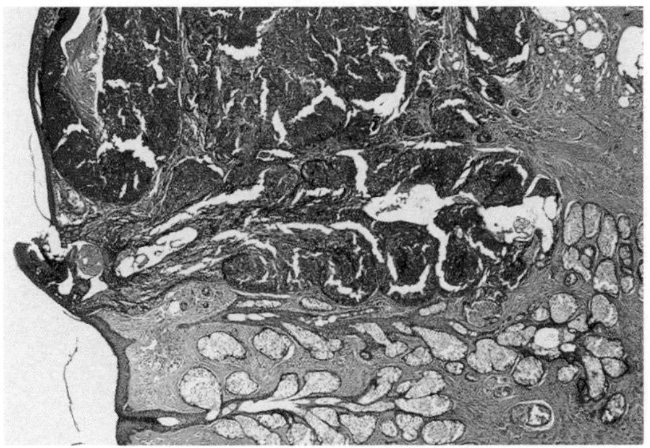

Figure 5-50

MEIBOMIAN GLAND CARCINOMA

Section through the opening of the meibomian ducts shows that tumor lobules have replaced the meibomian glands. Uninvolved normal meibomian glands are seen below.

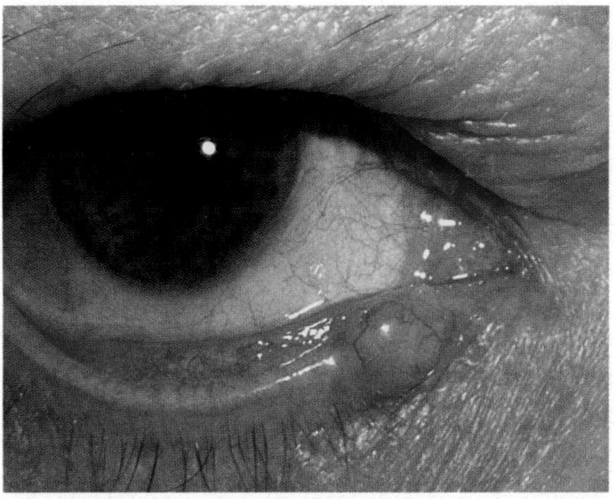

Figure 5-51

ZEIS GLAND CARCINOMA

Sebaceous gland carcinoma of the eyelid margin arising from Zeis gland causes ectropion.

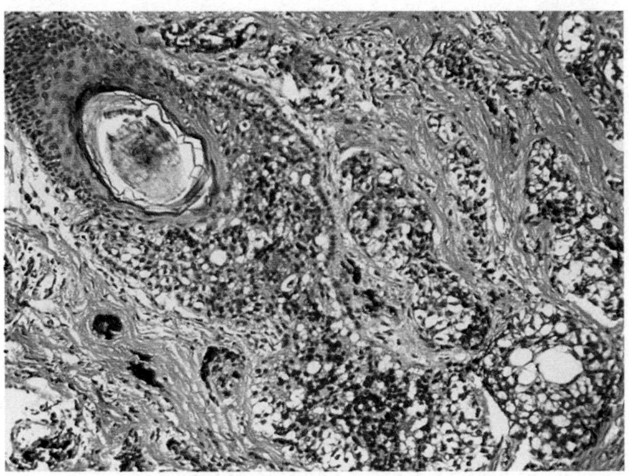

Figure 5-52

ZEIS GLAND CARCINOMA

Sebaceous gland carcinoma arising from Zeis gland. Tumor cells involve the walls of an eyelash follicle.

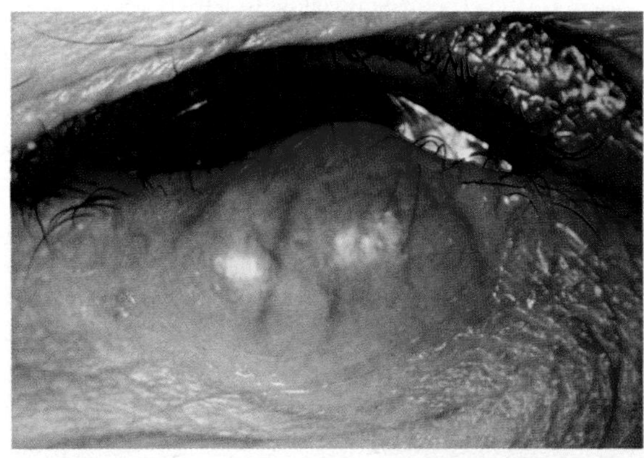

Figure 5-53

SEBACEOUS GLAND CARCINOMA

Sebaceous gland carcinoma of the eyelid masquerading as a chalazion.

carcinoma (figs. 5-53–5-60). Most commonly, it is a small, firm nodule resembling a chalazion (fig. 5-53). Frequently it appears as an atypical or recurring chalazion, showing a rubbery consistency. Some patients with a meibomian gland carcinoma have diffuse, plaque-like thickening of the tarsus (fig. 5-57) or a fungating or papillomatous lesion resembling a squamous cell papilloma or a papillary squamous cell carcinoma. The diagnosis is confirmed by the histologic demonstration of tumor originating from the meibomian glands. Other lesions appear as a localized, yellowish mass in the lid margin or as a diffuse or nodular thickening of the eyelids associated with loss of lashes. The latter finding is caused by neoplastic involvement of the follicles of the lashes.

A distinctive clinical feature of some sebaceous gland carcinomas, which may not be fully appreciated when the patient is examined initially, is persistent unilateral keratoconjunctivitis, blepharitis, meibomitis, or blepharoconjunctivitis that does not totally respond to antibiotic therapy ("masquerade syndrome") (figs.

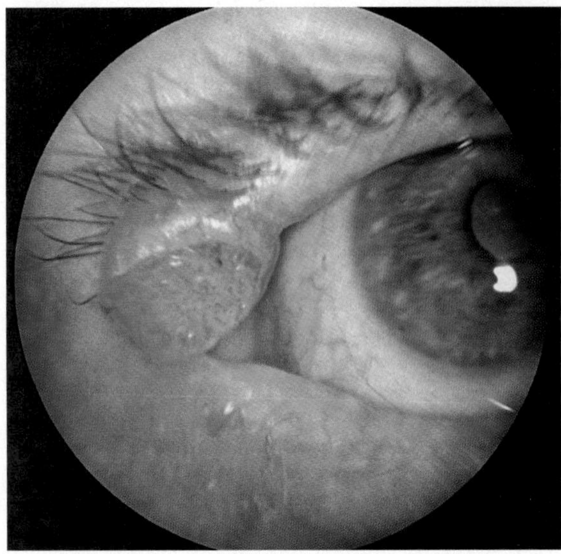

Figure 5-54

SEBACEOUS GLAND CARCINOMA

The mass is yellowish tan.

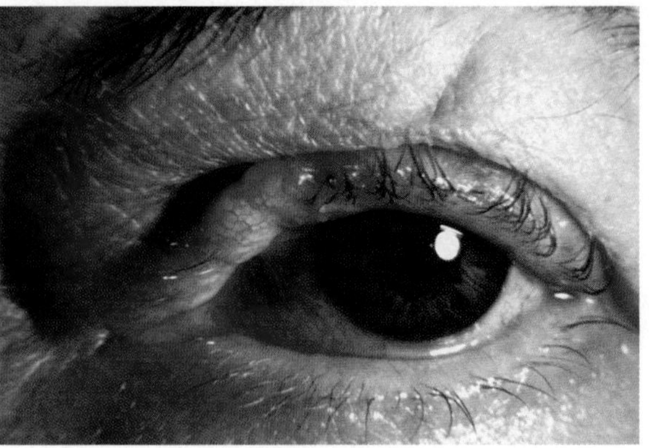

Figure 5-55

SEBACEOUS GLAND CARCINOMA

Nodular thickening of the left upper eyelid and loss of lashes.

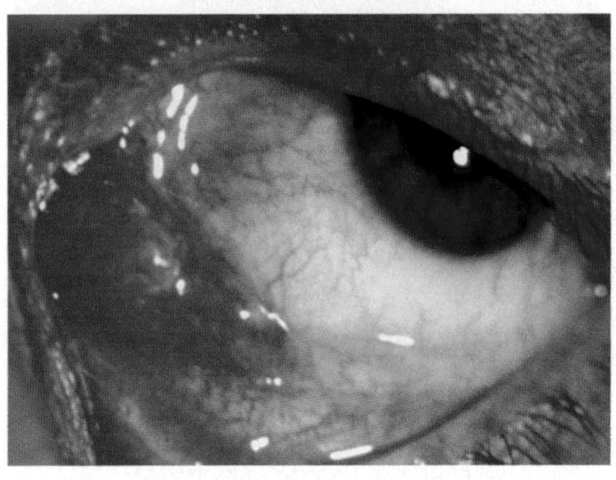

Figure 5-56

SEBACEOUS GLAND CARCINOMA OF THE CARUNCLE

The mass involves the caruncle.

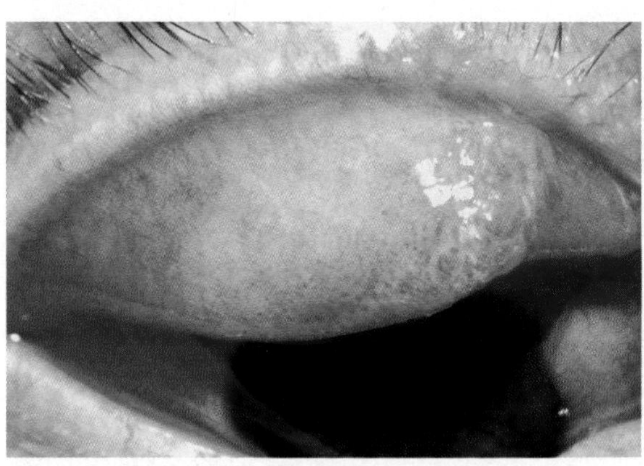

Figure 5-57

MEIBOMIAN GLAND CARCINOMA

Diffuse involvement of the right upper tarsus.

5-58–5-60). This appearance is, in part, caused by the tendency of sebaceous gland carcinoma cells to invade the overlying epithelium, forming single or several small nests of cells (pagetoid invasion), or to completely replace the entire thickness of the epithelium (intraepithelial sebaceous carcinoma). Independent, multicentric foci of intraepithelial neoplastic cells may invade both lids, the conjunctiva, and occasionally, the corneal epithelium, where they may cause a superficial keratitis with areas of scarring and vascularization. The accompanying diffuse eczematoid blepharoconjunctivitis may be associated with crusting and ulceration of the lid margin for many months or even years before the underlying sebaceous gland carcinoma becomes clinically evident. In such patients, it is often necessary to obtain multiple biopsy specimens from the lid margin as well as the palpebral and bulbar conjunctivae to determine the extent of pagetoid involvement. Many patients with diffuse pagetoid or intraepithelial carcinoma involving the skin of the eyelids, the conjunctiva, and/or the cornea are best managed by orbital exenteration.

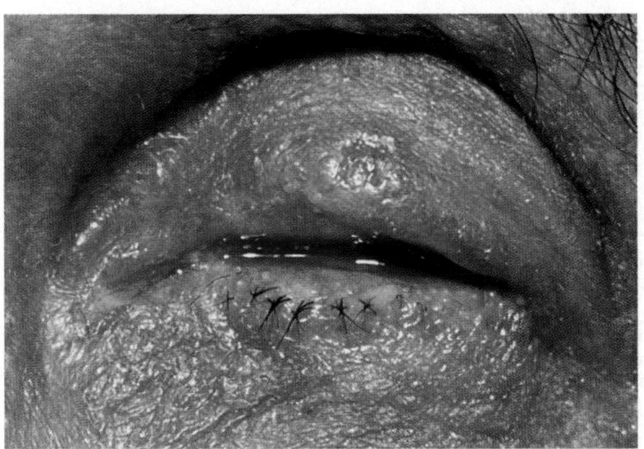

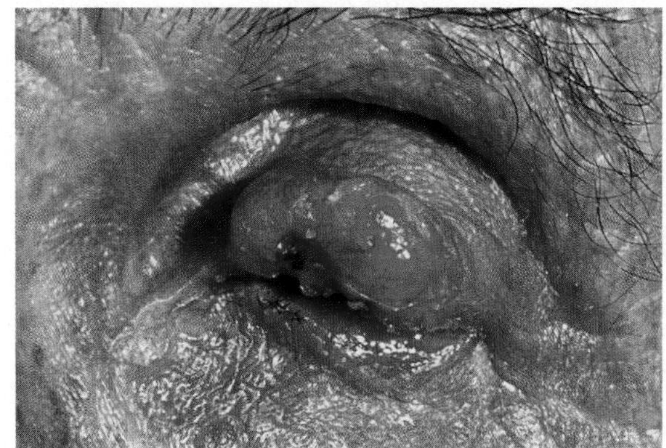

Figure 5-58

SEBACEOUS GLAND CARCINOMA

Left: Sebaceous gland carcinoma was initially treated as chronic ulcerative blepharitis with loss of lashes ("masquerade syndrome").

Right: Two years later, a mass developed in the left upper eyelid.

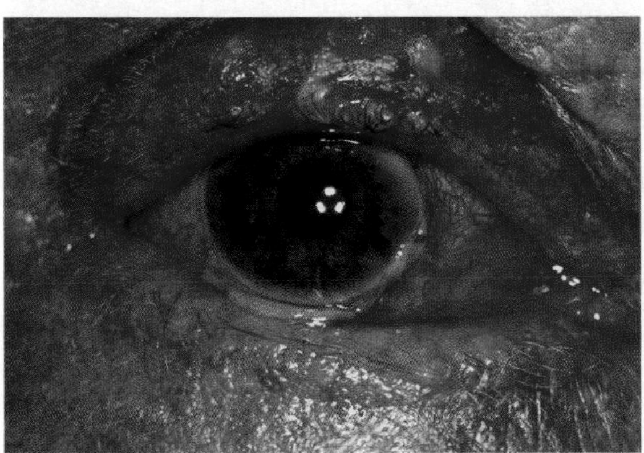

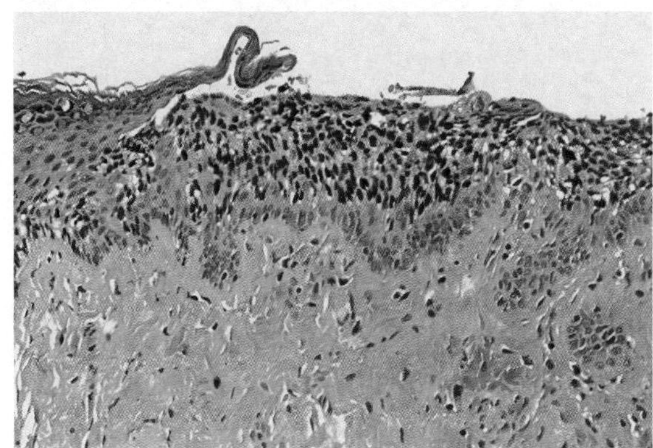

Figure 5-59

SEBACEOUS GLAND CARCINOMA

Left: Chronic blepharoconjunctivitis of the right upper eyelid.

Right: Biopsy of upper eyelid disclosed sebaceous gland carcinoma in situ.

Rarely, sebaceous gland carcinoma appears as a small, umbilicated, grayish white nodule at the lid margin resembling a basal cell carcinoma, or it may have the clinical appearance of a large cutaneous horn. Rarely, a meibomian gland carcinoma presents initially as a mass in the fossa of the lacrimal gland, simulating a malignant lacrimal gland tumor.

Microscopic Features. Sebaceous gland carcinoma is classified by degree of differentiation into three groups: well-differentiated, moderately differentiated, and poorly differentiated tumors (54). Well-differentiated tumors contain many neoplastic cells that exhibit sebaceous differentiation. These cells have an abundant, finely vacuolated cytoplasm that often appears foamy or frothy (fig. 5-61). The vacuoles often cause notching of the nuclear membrane. The nuclei are centrally placed or slightly displaced toward the periphery of the cells. Areas of sebaceous differentiation are frequently observed toward the center of the tumor lobules. Moderately differentiated tumors have only a few areas of highly differentiated sebaceous cells. The majority of the tumor is composed of neoplastic cells with hyperchromatic nuclei and prominent

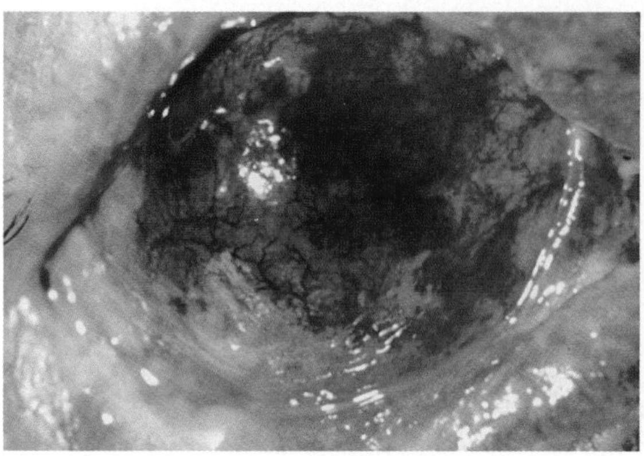

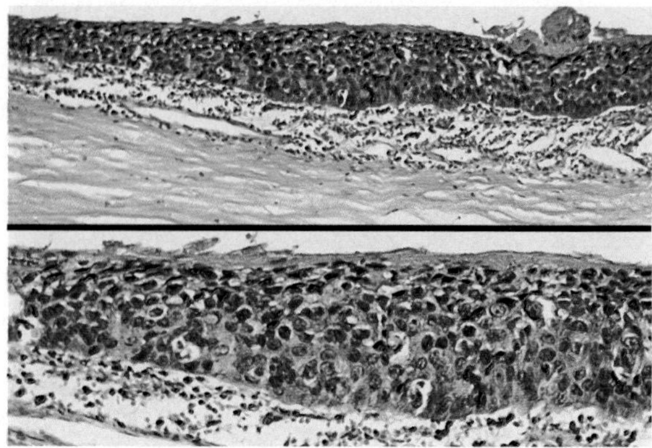

Figure 5-60

SEBACEOUS GLAND CARCINOMA

Left: Sebaceous gland carcinoma masquerading as chronic blepharitis with keratoconjunctivitis.
Right: Sebaceous gland carcinoma in situ replacing the corneal epithelium, with loss of the Bowman layer.

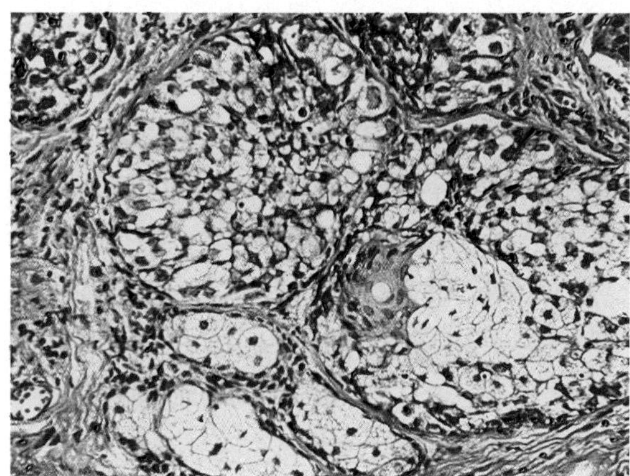

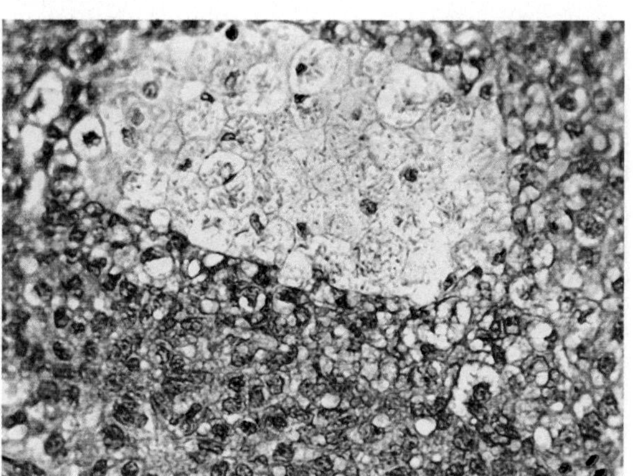

Figure 5-61

SEBACEOUS GLAND CARCINOMA

Well-differentiated sebaceous gland carcinoma with a lobular pattern.

nucleoli and abundant basophilic cytoplasm. The poorly differentiated, or anaplastic, variant of the tumor displays the features of an anaplastic carcinoma (53). The majority of the cells exhibit pleomorphic nuclei, with prominent nucleoli and scanty cytoplasm, which may show variable staining properties. Often, mitotic activity is moderately increased, and the mitoses are frequently atypical and bizarre (aneuploidy) (fig. 5-62). Frozen section and oil red-0 stains for lipid help establish an unequivocal diagnosis.

Four histologic patterns have been recognized: lobular, comedocarcinoma (fig. 5-63), papillary (fig. 5-64), and mixed (54). In the lobular pattern, the neoplastic cells form well-demarcated lobules of variable size. The lobules exhibit basaloid features, with a peripheral arrangement of the basophilic cells, which have hyperchromatic nuclei and scanty cytoplasm. In some areas, the cells have a vacuolated or foamy appearance that is highly characteristic of sebaceous differentiation. The comedocarcinoma pattern is characterized by large lobules with prominent central foci of necrosis (fig. 5-63). The viable cells in the lobules and the central necrotic tumor cells often stain intensely

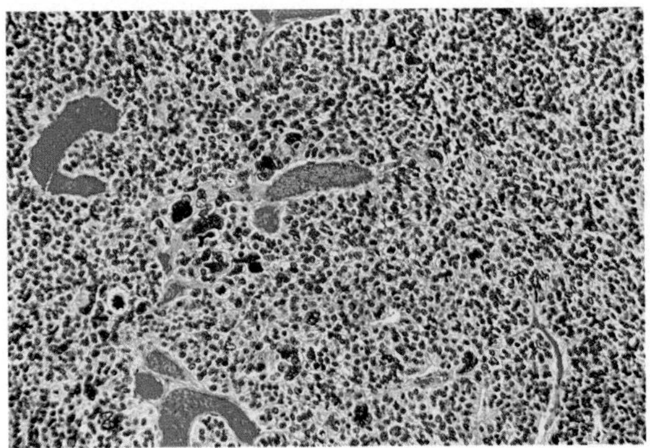
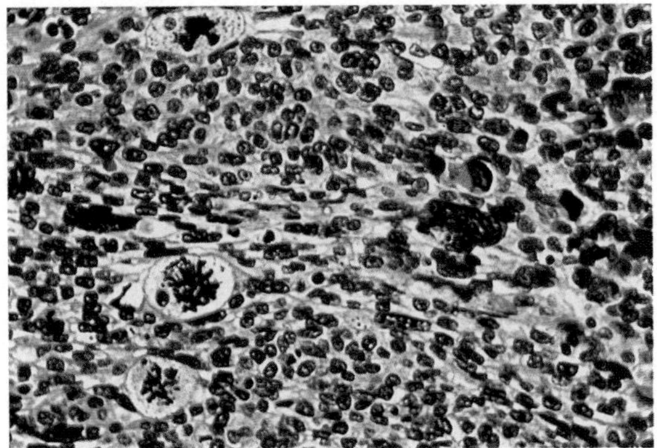

Figure 5-62

SEBACEOUS GLAND CARCINOMA

Anaplastic variant of sebaceous gland carcinoma with bizarre atypical mitoses. Prominent aneuploidy is seen.

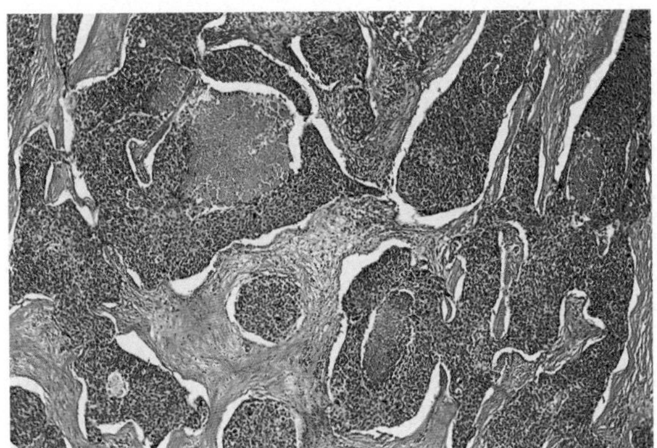
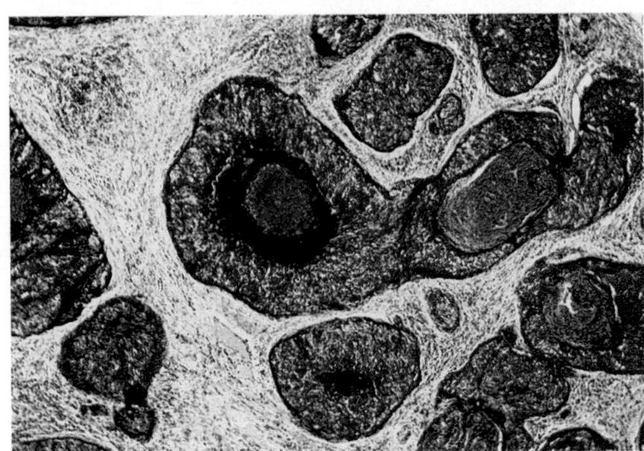

Figure 5-63

SEBACEOUS GLAND CARCINOMA

The lobules have central necrosis (comedocarcinoma pattern) (hematoxylin and eosin [H&E] and oil red-O stains).

for lipid. Tumors with the papillary pattern are composed of papillary fronds of neoplastic cells (fig. 5-64). They may resemble a squamous cell papilloma or carcinoma and tend to occur on the conjunctival surface. Careful histologic examination usually reveals foci of sebaceous differentiation. Tumors with a mixed pattern often show an admixture of lobular and comedocarcinoma-like areas; other tumors may show a combination of papillary areas with either comedocarcinoma or a lobular pattern.

Tumors are also classified according to their extent of infiltration (54). Minimally infiltrative neoplasms are made up of compact lobules; the neoplastic cells extend to a minor degree into the adjacent stroma from the periphery of the lobules. At the other extreme, highly infiltrative tumors are composed of infiltrating cords of epithelial cells that have only a few areas with a lobular pattern (fig. 5-65). Occasionally, the infiltrating cords of tumor cells are arranged in single rows of cells (Indian-file appearance).

Modes of Spread. *Intraepithelial Spread.* Sebaceous gland carcinoma spreads into the epithelium of the conjunctiva, cornea, and/or skin of the eyelids in two ways. Intraepithelial spread is mainly observed in moderately to highly infiltrative carcinomas. Pagetoid spread resembles the intraepithelial spread of a ductal carcinoma of the breast onto the skin of the nipple and surrounding areola (Paget's disease of the breast) (figs. 5-66–5-68). The neoplastic cells invade the

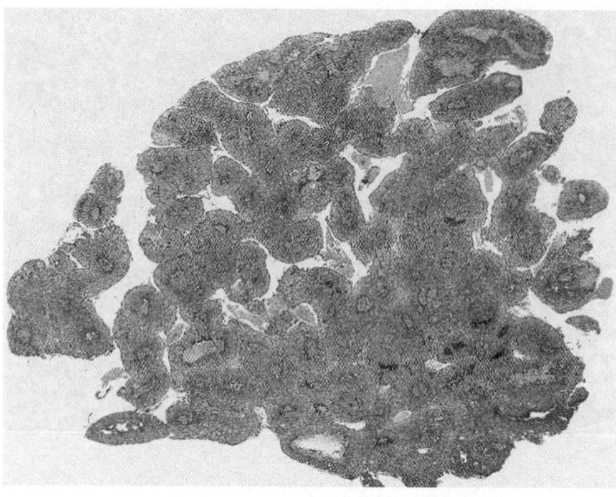

Figure 5-64

SEBACEOUS GLAND CARCINOMA

The papillary variant of sebaceous gland carcinoma mimics papilloma.

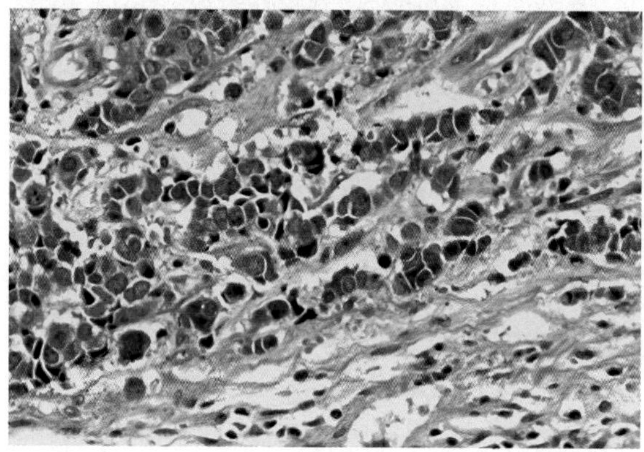

Figure 5-65

SEBACEOUS GLAND CARCINOMA

Sebaceous carcinoma with an infiltrating pattern (Indian-file pattern) mimics metastatic mammary carcinoma.

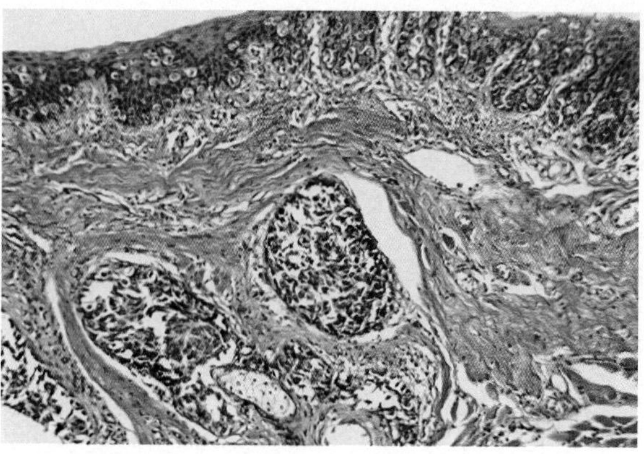

Figure 5-66

MEIBOMIAN GLAND CARCINOMA

There is pagetoid involvement of the overlying tarsal conjunctiva.

overlying epithelium as single cells or as small nests of cells that typically are devoid of intercellular bridges and often compress the adjacent epithelial cells. Pagetoid cells exhibit hyperchromatic nuclei and abundant vacuolated cytoplasm that contains variable amounts of lipid (fig. 5-69).

The second type of intraepithelial spread is a more diffuse process, with full-thickness replacement of surface epithelium by neoplastic cells (fig. 5-60, right). The changes resemble those observed in intraepithelial (in situ) squamous cell carcinoma or in Bowen's disease of the skin. They are characterized by a diffuse proliferation of large, pleomorphic neoplastic cells that exhibit increased mitotic activity. Involvement of the epithelium of the conjunctiva, cornea, or epidermis of the eyelids is often multifocal, with skip areas of unaffected epithelium. Occasionally, intraepithelial clefts containing desquamated acantholytic cells are formed. Such clefts may cause sloughing of the friable, involved epithelium, leaving behind only a single row of neoplastic cells that replaces the basal epithelial layer like "a row of tombstones" (fig. 5-68).

Most investigators agree that the histologic demonstration of intracytoplasmic lipid in the tumor cells is crucial in establishing an unequivocal diagnosis of sebaceous gland carcinoma, especially in poorly differentiated tumors (48,54). Even with pagetoid involvement or carcinoma in situ changes, lipid has been demonstrated in the areas of intraepithelial involvement (fig. 5-69).

Another feature of sebaceous gland carcinoma that is important in planning appropriate surgical management is the tendency for the tumors to be of multicentric origin. Independent foci with upper and lower lid involvement have been observed in 6 to 10 percent of cases (55). The presence of multicentricity suggests that an unknown carcinogen, possibly related to prolonged contact of unsaturated fatty acids

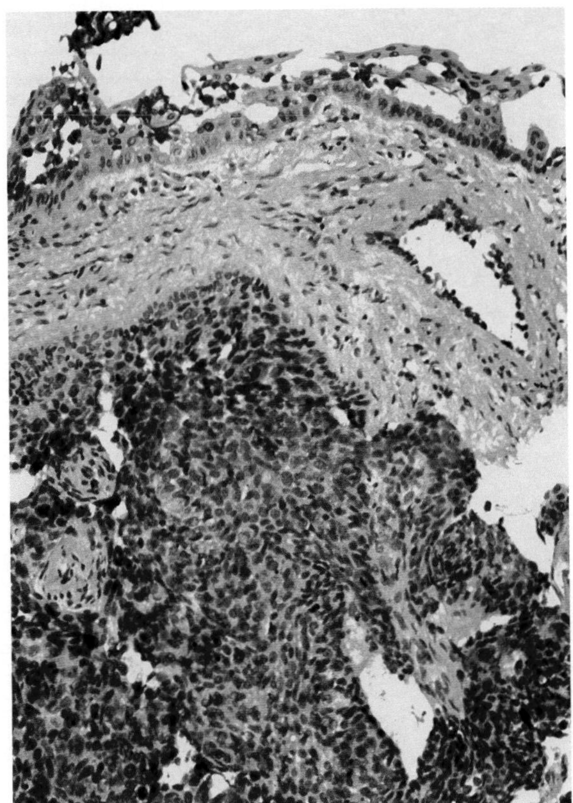

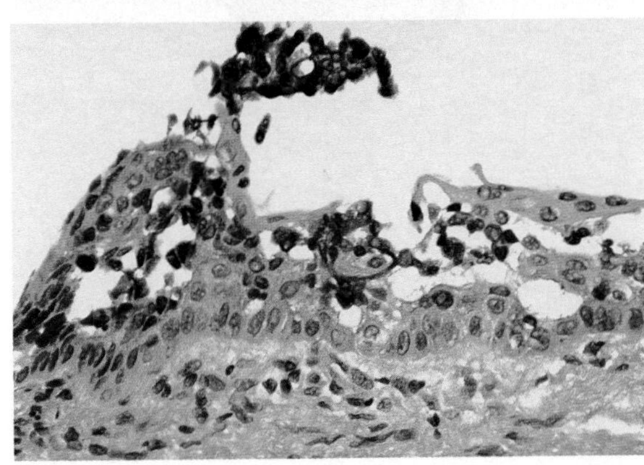

Figure 5-67

MEIBOMIAN GLAND CARCINOMA

There is pagetoid involvement of the conjunctival epithelium. Acantholytic clefts are seen in the involved epithelium. Low-power (top) and high-power (bottom) views.

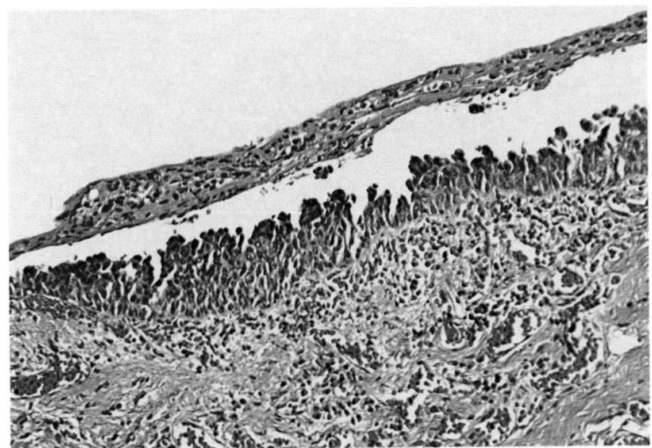

Figure 5-68

SEBACEOUS GLAND CARCINOMA

There is a necrotic sheet of epithelial cells with a "tombstone" pattern of viable tumor cells at its base.

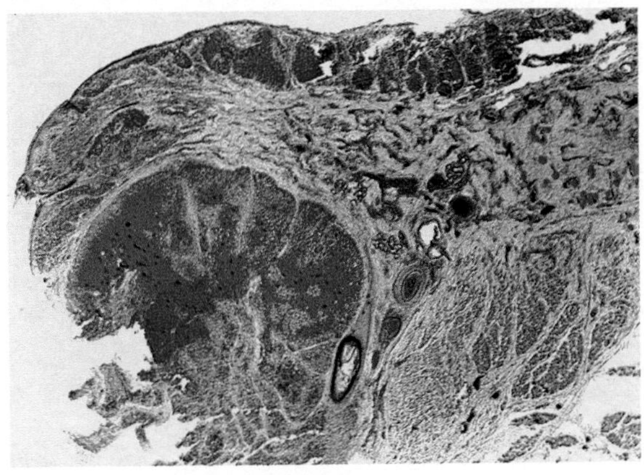

Figure 5-69

SEBACEOUS GLAND CARCINOMA

Sebaceous gland carcinoma with pagetoid spread to overlying epithelium (oil red-O stain).

with the glandular elements of the lid, may play a role in the pathogenesis of sebaceous gland carcinoma. Other environmental or genetic factors that may play a role have not been evaluated for this neoplasm.

Spread by Direct Extension. Sebaceous gland carcinoma may spread by direct extension into the adjacent structures (orbit, paranasal sinuses, intracranial cavity). Moderately to poorly differentiated tumors with infiltrating properties are often associated with areas of perineural infiltration and with invasion into the lumen of lymphatic vessels (figs. 5-70, 5-71). Among the 95 patients studied by Rao, McLean, and Zimmerman (54), 22 developed metastases to the preauricular (figs. 5-72, 5-73) and cervical lymph nodes. The primary eyelid tumor may be relatively small and associated with a huge preau-

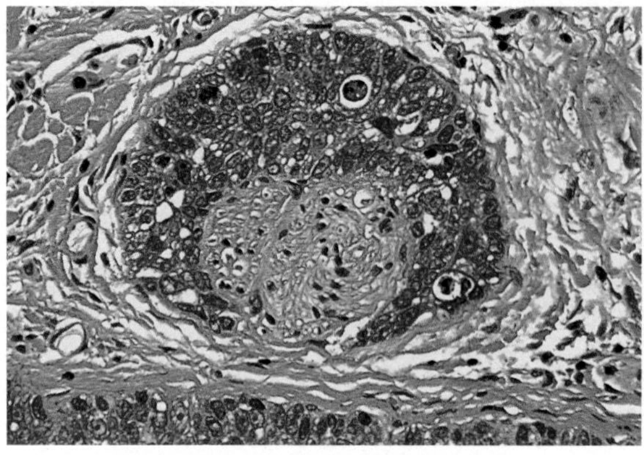

Figure 5-70

SEBACEOUS GLAND CARCINOMA

Perineural invasion.

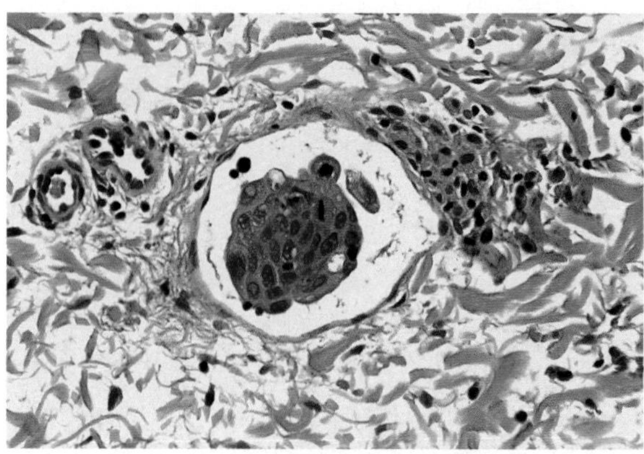

Figure 5-71

SEBACEOUS GLAND CARCINOMA

Lymphatic invasion.

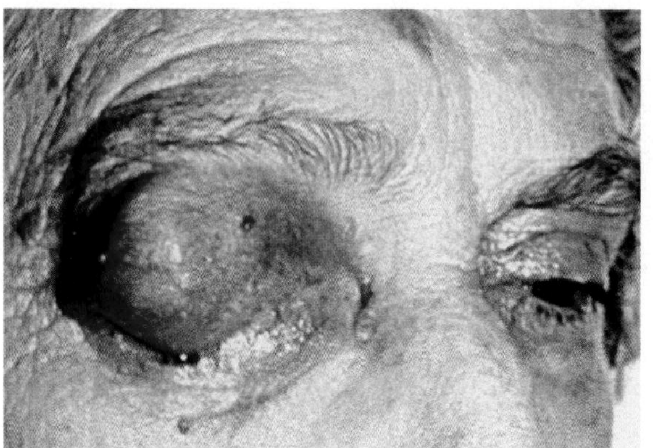

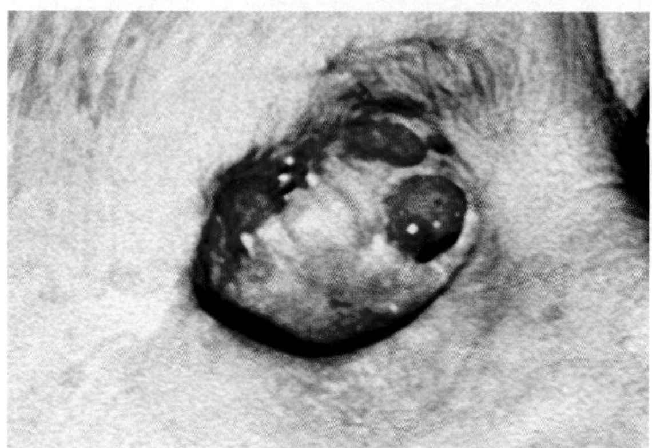

Figure 5-72

SEBACEOUS GLAND CARCINOMA

Sebaceous gland carcinoma (before and after exenteration) with preauricular lymph node metastasis.

ricular mass. In the series of cases reported by Rao et al., the recurrence rate was 33 percent. Direct orbital invasion occurred in 19 percent of cases, and metastases to periauricular, cervical lymph nodes, or both, in 23 percent of cases; 22 patients died as a result of the tumor. Vascular invasion with distant metastases involving the lungs, liver, brain, and skull often were associated with previous or simultaneous regional lymph node metastases.

Immunohistochemical Findings. Immunohistochemical preparations help differentiate sebaceous gland carcinoma from basal cell and squamous cell carcinomas. Sebaceous gland carcinoma stains with epithelial membrane antigen (EMA) while basal cell carcinoma does not. Unlike most sebaceous gland carcinomas, squamous cell tumors are negative for CAM5.2. Breast cancer antigen-1 (BRST-1) may be positive in sebaceous tumors but not in the squamous cell carcinomas (57). Immunohistochemical detection of human milk fat globule subclasses 1 and 2 are also useful for diagnosing sebaceous gland carcinomas (58).

Ultrastructural Findings. Electron microscopic examination of the neoplastic cells utilizing glycol methacrylate-glutaraldehyde-urea reveals myelin-like structures at the periphery of the cells and a homogenous interior structure (56). The myelin-like structures may be

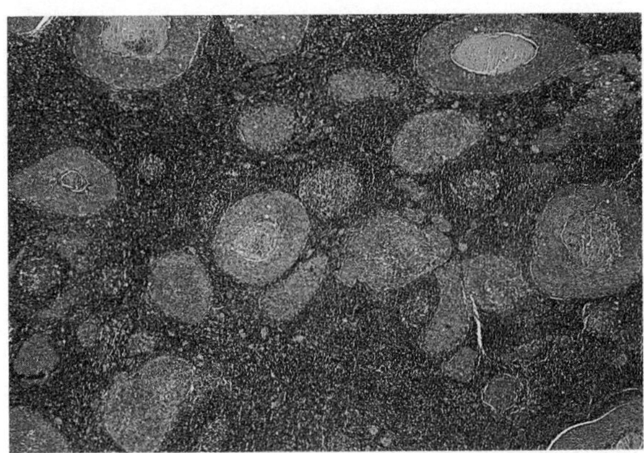

Figure 5-73

SEBACEOUS GLAND CARCINOMA

Preauricular lymph nodes are involved.

derived from smooth surface endoplastic reticulum. A true membrane enclosing the lipid droplet is not seen (56).

Molecular Studies. Sebaceous carcinomas of the ocular adnexa express the tumor suppressor gene, *p16*, in over 50 percent of cases. These tumors do not express *bcl-2*, however, and *p53* is mutationally inactive (59,60). The tumors may express estrogen and progesterone receptors and overexpress *c-erbB-2* (61).

Treatment and Prognosis. Rao and colleagues (54,55) analyzed the prognostic significance of the location, size, and site of origin of sebaceous gland tumors; the duration of symptoms prior to excision; and the histologic pattern and degree of cellular differentiation. They concluded that a poor prognosis results from location of the tumor in the upper eyelid, size of 10 mm or more in maximal diameter, origin from the meibomian glands, duration of symptoms for more than 6 months, an infiltrative growth pattern, and moderate to poor sebaceous differentiation. Additional findings indicating a poor prognosis include multicentric origin; intraepithelial carcinomatous changes (pagetoid involvement or bowenoid changes) of the conjunctiva, cornea, or epidermis of the eyelid; and invasion of lymphatic channels, vascular structures, and the orbit.

It appears that early diagnosis and adequate treatment with primary, wide surgical excision can significantly improve the prognosis (54,55). Because of the relatively high recurrence rate of incompletely excised sebaceous gland carcinomas, most investigators agree that frozen section control is required to ensure complete excision of the tumor. Radiation may be used for palliation in elderly patients with large tumors who are unable to tolerate radical surgery, or in patients who refuse surgical excision of the tumor (62).

Table 5-6

TUMORS OF THE ECCRINE AND APOCRINE GLANDS OF THE EYELID[a]

Type of Tumor	Number of Cases
Benign	
Syringoma	8
Chondroid syringoma	8
Apocrine hidrocystoma	5
Eccrine hidrocystoma	4
Eccrine acrospiroma	4
Hidradenoma papilliferum	4
Eccrine poroma	2
Eccrine spiradenoma	2
Apocrine cystadenoma	2
Malignant	
Mucinous sweat gland carcinoma	14
Syringomatous sweat gland carcinoma	1
Apocrine sweat gland carcinoma	1
Papillary apocrine hidradenoma with malignant change	1
Primary signet ring carcinoma	1
Miscellaneous	
Sudoriferous cyst	119

[a]Frequency distribution of 176 tumors from the Doheny Eye Institute files collected between 1970 and 2000.

TUMORS OF THE ECCRINE AND APOCRINE GLANDS OF THE EYELID

Several types of eccrine and apocrine tumors are observed in the eyelids. The frequency distribution of these tumors, as assessed at a single institution, is summarized in Table 5-6.

Syringoma

Syringoma is a common, benign sweat gland tumor of the eyelid. It occurs predominantly in young women near puberty or in early adulthood. The lesions are usually multiple and appear as yellowish, waxy nodules averaging 1 to 2 mm in size (fig. 5-74A).

Each nodule is composed of small ductal elements embedded in a dense fibrous stroma

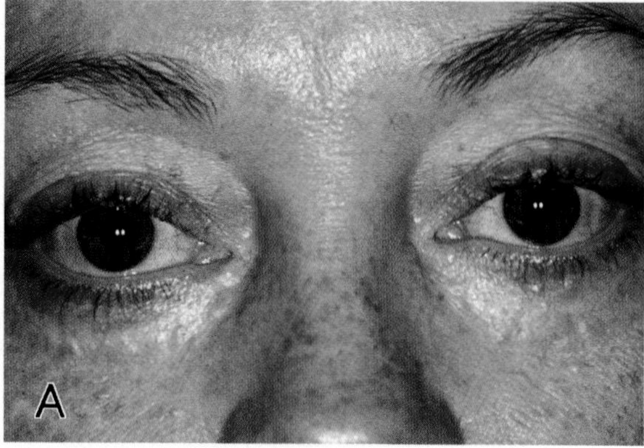

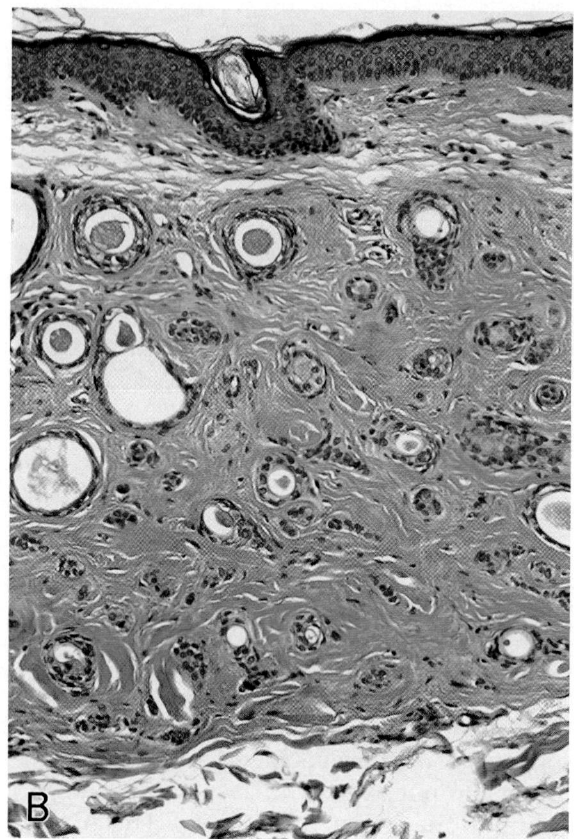

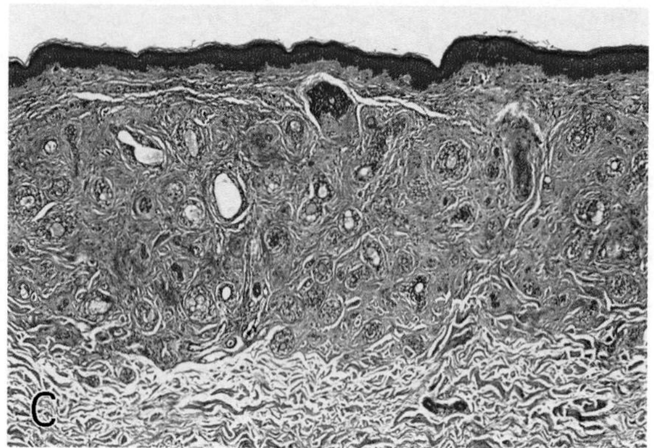

Figure 5-74

ECCRINE SYRINGOMA

A: Syringomas involving skin of cheeks and lower eyelids.
B: Eccrine syringoma (H&E stain).
C: Dense collagen fibers demarcate the dermal nodule (Masson trichrome stain).

(fig. 5-74B,C). The walls of the ducts are usually lined by two rows of epithelial cells. Frequently, the inner cells are flat and vacuolated. Myoepithelial cells are absent. Typically, some of the ducts exhibit comma-shaped tails (resembling tadpoles) intermixed with solid strands of basaloid cells. The lumens of the ducts usually contain basophilic mucoid material. Rarely, some of the ductal elements are lined by several layers of glycogen-rich clear cells. Some ducts show cystic dilatation filled with keratin. These keratin-filled cysts may rupture and elicit a secondary granulomatous reaction. They may also undergo calcification.

Enzyme histochemical and electron microscopic studies have established that syringoma is a tumor with differentiation toward epidermal eccrine sweat ducts (63). The tumor contains eccrine enzymes, such as succinic dehydrogenase, phosphorylase, and leucine aminopeptidase. The presence of keratin-filled cystic ducts is an additional finding supporting the histogenesis of this tumor from intraepidermal eccrine sweat ducts (64).

Pleomorphic Adenoma

Pleomorphic adenoma is also known as *mixed tumor of the skin* and *chondroid syringoma*. The tumor is commonly located on the head and neck and may involve the face and the eyelid (65). It is believed to arise from the sweat glands of the skin.

Pleomorphic adenoma appears as an intradermal, multilobulated mass, usually ranging from 0.5 to 3.0 cm in diameter. Histologically, it is identical to the pleomorphic adenoma that

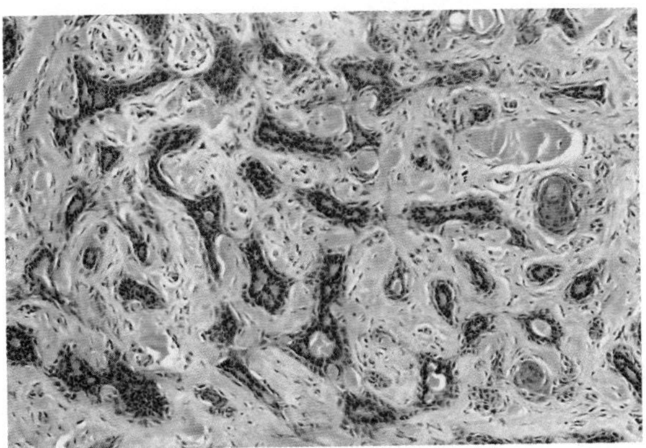
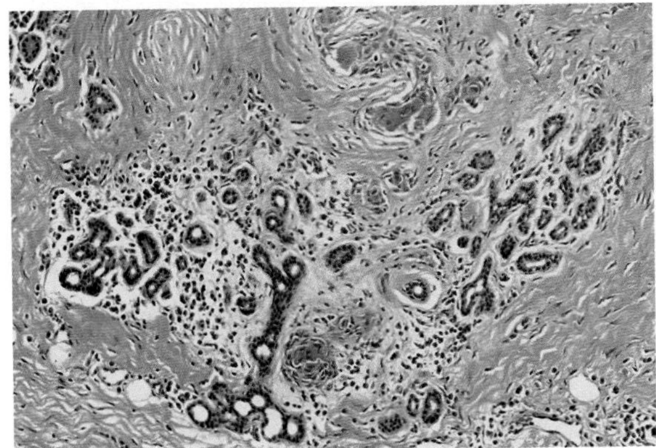

Figure 5-75

BENIGN MIXED TUMOR OF GLANDS OF WOLFRING

Left: Tumor arising from the glands of Wolfring in the upper eyelid.
Right: View adjacent to tumor depicts accessory glands of Wolfring.

arises in the lacrimal gland or in the accessory eyelid glands of Wolfring (fig. 5-75). It is composed of tubular structures lined by a double layer of epithelial cells that are in a mucoid stroma; the stroma often exhibits areas of chondroid metaplasia. The inner cells lining the ducts are secretory and produce a mucopolysaccharide; the outer cells are myoepithelial. It is believed that the stroma is derived from the outer myoepithelial cells, which are capable of undergoing fibrous, myxoid, or chondroid metaplastic changes.

When pleomorphic adenoma enlarges, it compresses surrounding structures of the eyelid. Recurrences from an incompletely removed tumor are usually histologically identical to the initial lesion; however, the initial lesion or recurrence may display malignant change.

Eccrine Acrospiroma

Eccrine acrospiroma is also referred to as *clear cell hidradenoma*, *clear cell myoepithelioma*, and *porosyringoma*. Eccrine acrospiroma appears clinically as a single, nodular, solid or cystic mass. The skin overlying the dermal nodule is flesh-colored to reddish blue (occasionally hemorrhagic) and is sometimes thickened and verrucous (66,67).

The lesion is a well-circumscribed, solid dermal nodule composed of lobulated masses of epithelial cells; however, some lesions are cystic and contain serous, gelatinous, or hemorrhagic fluid. In some instances the dermal tumor merges with the overlying acanthotic epidermis at the periphery of the mass. Enzyme histochemical and electron microscopic studies have established the eccrine origin of these lesions (68).

Two cell types are present in different areas of the tumor. One cell type is round to polyhedral in configuration, with moderate to large amounts of eosinophilic cytoplasm surrounding a round to oval nucleus with a distinct nucleolus. The second type is as a glycogen-rich clear cell with distinct boundaries (fig. 5-76). The nucleus is small and eccentric. In many areas, a transition from eosinophilic cells to clear cells is observed. Mitotic figures are infrequent or absent. Some tumors are almost entirely composed of clear cells, hence the name clear cell hidradenoma.

A characteristic feature of the tumor is the presence of small ductal lumens that are lined by a prominent eosinophilic cuticle, resembling that observed in eccrine sweat ducts. Occasional mucin-containing cells may be present within the lobules of clear cells (66). Some tumors have foci of squamous metaplasia with the formation of keratin pearls.

Mucinous Sweat Gland Adenocarcinoma

Mucinous sweat gland adenocarcinoma, also known as *mucinous adenocarcinoma, colloid carcinoma, gelatinous carcinoma,* and *"adenocystic" carcinoma,* is a rare primary adnexal neoplasm of the skin. The tumors range in size from 0.4 to 2.5 cm, occur predominantly in middle-aged adults

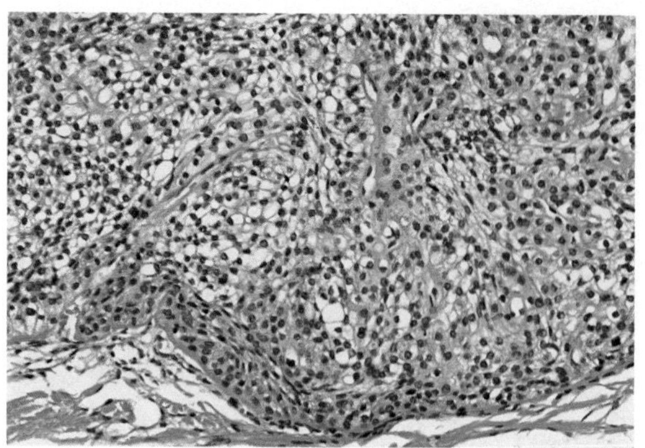

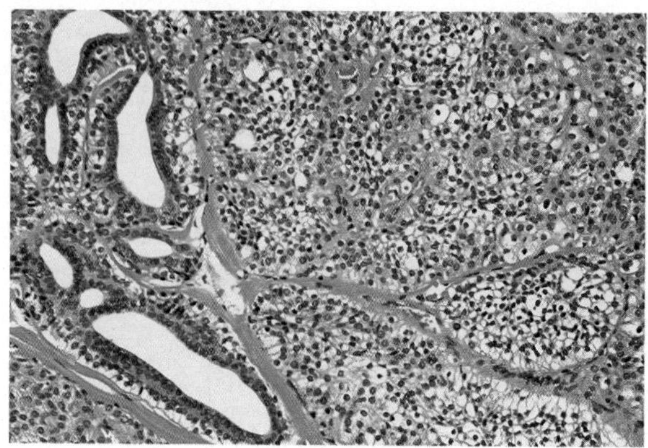

Figure 5-76

ECCRINE ACROSPIROMA

Left: Glycogen-rich clear cells are seen.
Right: Large eccrine ducts are intermixed within the lobules of clear cells.

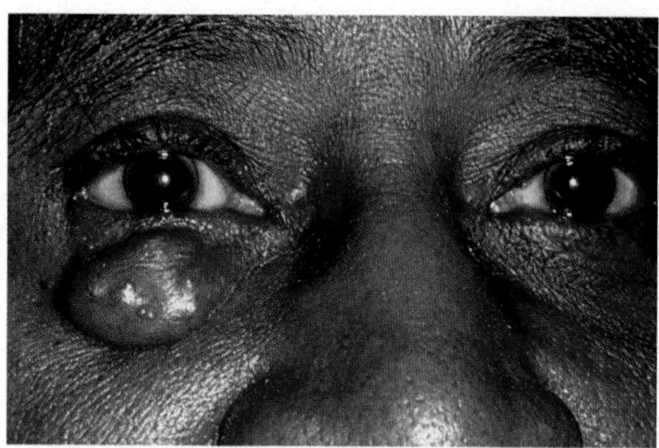

Figure 5-77

MUCINOUS SWEAT GLAND ADENOCARCINOMA

A:. A multilobulated, nonulcerated mass of the right lower eyelid is mucinous sweat gland adenocarcinoma of eccrine origin.

B: Tumor lobules are surrounded by pools of mucin.

C: High-power view shows dark cells located mostly at the periphery of the lobules.

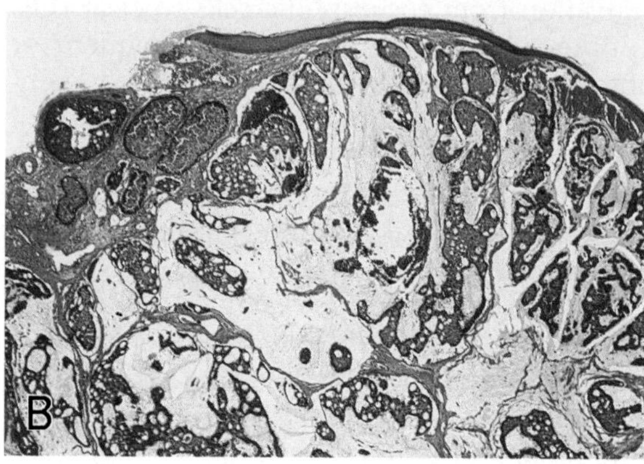

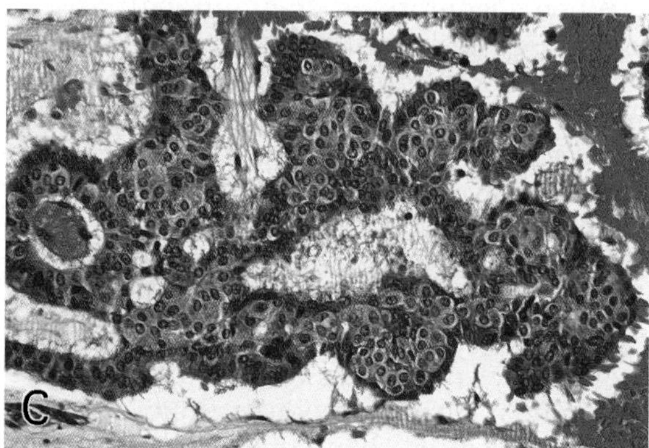

(median age, 60 years), and have a predilection for men (69). The lesion is often described as an elevated nodule or a lobulated mass that may appear firm, indurated, or cystic (fig. 5-77A). The color varies from bluish to pink to red.

Microscopically, elongated cords and lobules of epithelial cells float in large pools of mucin, which are separated by thin, fibrovascular septa (fig. 5-77B,C). Small ductal structures or gland-like lumens are often observed within the epithelial islands, producing the characteristic "adenocystic" pattern seen in most of the tumors. Some tumors also have large, solid epithelial lobules. Nuclear pleomorphism is usually slight or absent. Most tumors invade the reticular dermis, and some extend into the subcutis.

The tumor lobules are composed of a dual population of light and dark cells. The dark cells are located at the periphery of the lobules; the light cells are more central. The dark cells are believed to secrete the surrounding mucin, which is a form of nonsulfated mucopolysaccharide containing sialic acid (sialomucin). With electron microscopy, the dark cells are seen to have bulbous expansions and to contain bundles of thin filaments, membrane-bound dense granules, and numerous secretory vacuoles that tend to coalesce and form large subplasmalemmal vacuoles (69).

Patients with mucinous adenocarcinoma have a better prognosis than do those with other forms of sweat gland adenocarcinoma (69); 11 percent of the tumors metastasize to regional lymph nodes, and 31 percent recur locally. The best management of mucinous adenocarcinomas of low malignant potential is wide, en bloc excisional biopsy. The mucinous sweat gland carcinoma may invade the orbit and adjacent bony structures.

Primary Cutaneous Adenoid Cystic Carcinoma

Primary cutaneous adenoid cystic carcinoma is the rarest eccrine sweat gland tumor of the eyelid. The tumor is microscopically indistinguishable from adenoid cystic carcinoma of the major salivary and lacrimal glands. The main entity in the differential diagnosis is the adenoid cystic type of basal cell carcinoma, from which it can be easily differentiated by the lack of continuity with the epidermis or hair sheaths and the absence of peripheral palisading of the nuclei. Primary adenoid cystic carcinoma is immunoreactive to antibodies against carcinoembryonic antigen, amylase, and S-100 protein (70); the adenoid cystic type of basal cell carcinoma does not immunoreact with these three monoclonal antibodies. When adenoid cystic carcinoma affects the eyelid, the differential diagnosis should include origin from the superficial lobe of the lacrimal gland with secondary lid involvement, as well as a primary neoplastic process originating from the accessory lacrimal glands of Wolfring or from ectopic lacrimal gland tissue. Metastatic disease to the eyelid from a tumor arising from the major or minor salivary glands should be excluded.

Adenocarcinoma of Eccrine Sweat Glands

Adenocarcinoma of eccrine sweat glands is also known as *infiltrating signet ring carcinoma*. This tumor is one of a variety of adnexal tumors involving the skin of the eyelid (71–73). Clinically, the lesion appears as a nodular, indurated mass with diffuse, infiltrating margins. The overlying skin may be red. The clinical course is usually prolonged (5 to 10 years), with one or more recurrences after excision and a tendency for orbital invasion.

The tumor is composed of compact cords of atypical epithelial cells diffusely infiltrating the collagen fibers of the reticular dermis and extending into striated muscle and subcutaneous tissue. In many areas, a pattern of atypical histiocytoid cells arranged in single rows is evident (Indian-file pattern). The nuclei of the atypical cells are round to oval and contain a single inconspicuous nucleolus. Mitotic figures are usually scarce. The cytoplasm is abundant, and has a foamy or vacuolated appearance. Some cells contain single vacuoles that give them a characteristic signet ring appearance. These highly characteristic intracytoplasmic vacuoles stain with the Alcian blue, mucicarmine, and PAS techniques. Ultrastructural examination shows highly characteristic, intracytoplasmic lumens and abundant endoplasmic reticulum with smooth and rough surfaces, lipid droplets, and many membrane-bound cytoplasmic inclusions, some which have a filamentous substructure (74).

Adenocarcinoma of eccrine sweat gland closely resembles histiocytoid mammary carcinoma, infiltrating lobular carcinoma, and signet ring carcinoma of the breast (74). The possibility of metastatic carcinoma from the breast in female patients should be considered. If the eyelid lesion occurs in a man, the possibility of a primary neoplasm elsewhere must be ruled out. If the results are negative, the possibility of a primary eccrine sweat gland carcinoma of the eyelid should be considered.

Adenoma and Adenocarcinoma of the Glands of Moll

Apocrine adenoma arising from the glands of Moll is an extremely unusual neoplasm of the eyelid. For a given lesion to be accepted as an apocrine adenoma derived from the glands of

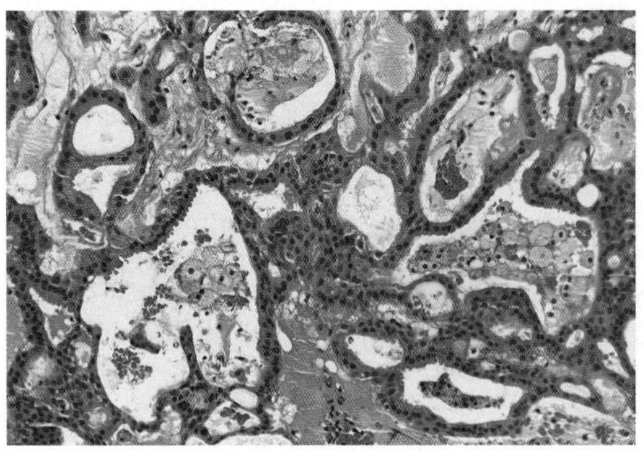

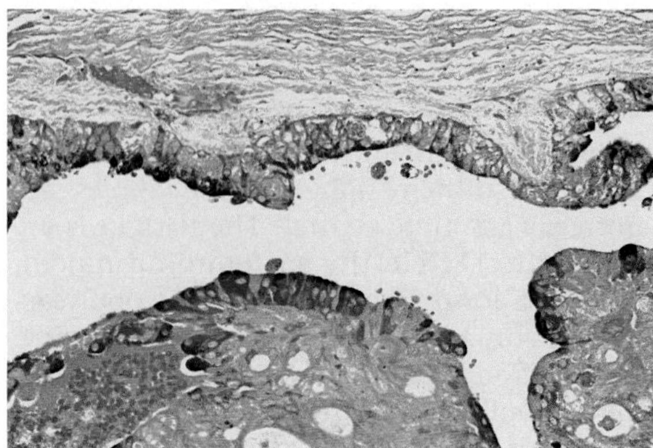

Figure 5-78

MOLL GLAND ADENOMA

Left: Prominent cytoplasmic acidophilia and foci of decapitation secretion are seen.
Right: Iron-positive granules are located mostly in apical snouts.

Table 5-7

TUMORS OF THE PILAR STRUCTURES OF THE EYELID[a]

Type of Tumor	Number of Cases
Benign	
Inverted follicular keratosis	18
Pilomatrixoma	14
Adnexal tumor	14
Trichoepithelioma	4
Trichofolliculoma	3
Trichilemmoma	1
Hamartomatous hair follicle tumor	1
Proliferating trichilemmal tumor	1
Malignant	
Malignant adnexal tumor	3

[a]Frequency distribution of 59 tumors from the Doheny Eye Institute files collected between 1970 and 2000.

Moll, it must be located at the lid margin, and the cuboidal tumor cells should display a strongly eosinophilic cytoplasm with areas of decapitation secretion (fig. 5-78, left). The cells also may show iron-positive intracellular granules (present in only one third of the tumors) (fig. 5-78, right), as well as diastase-resistant, PAS-positive granules located in the apical portions.

Examples of *adenocarcinoma arising from glands of Moll* have been recorded (fig. 5-79A) (75,76,77). These tumors are characterized by a glandular arrangement of large cells with abundant eosinophilic cytoplasm and evidence of decapitated secretion (fig. 5-79B,C). Other sweat gland tumors, sebaceous carcinoma with pagetoid invasion, and metastatic carcinomas should be considered in the differential diagnosis. Apocrine adenocarcinomas of the eyelid may invade surrounding structures and can metastasize (78).

TUMORS OF THE PILAR STRUCTURES OF THE EYELID

Benign tumors arising from hair follicles include trichoepithelioma (solitary and multiple), trichofolliculoma, trichilemmoma, and pilomatrixoma (benign calcifying epithelioma of Malherbe). Most tumors arising from hair follicles are benign (Table 5-7), based on a series collected from the Doheny Eye Institute over a 30-year period.

Trichoepithelioma

Trichoepithelioma, also known as *epithelioma adenoides cysticum, multiple benign cystic epithelioma,* and *Brooke's tumor,* is a firm, elevated, skin-colored nodule. It tends to involve the face but can occur anywhere on the body. It has no pattern of inheritance and characteristically appears late in life. Multiple trichoepitheliomas are inherited in an autosomal dominant manner with incomplete penetrance (79). The lesions typically arise in adolescence and tend to increase in size and number. They appear as multiple, round, firm nodules ranging from 2 to 8 mm in diameter, and mainly involve the face, including the forehead and lids; occasionally, the scalp, neck, and upper trunk are also involved. In contrast to basal cell carcinoma and

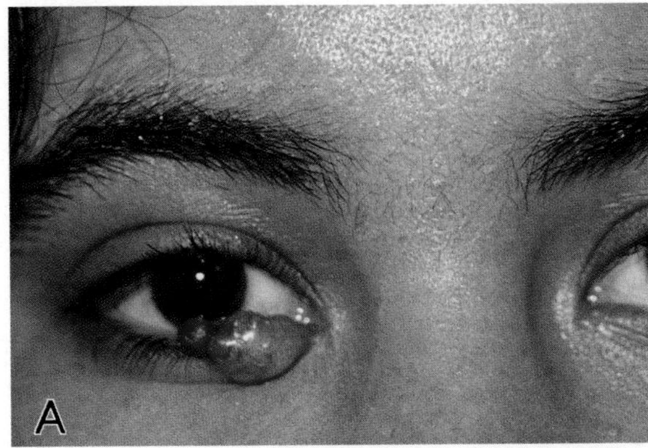

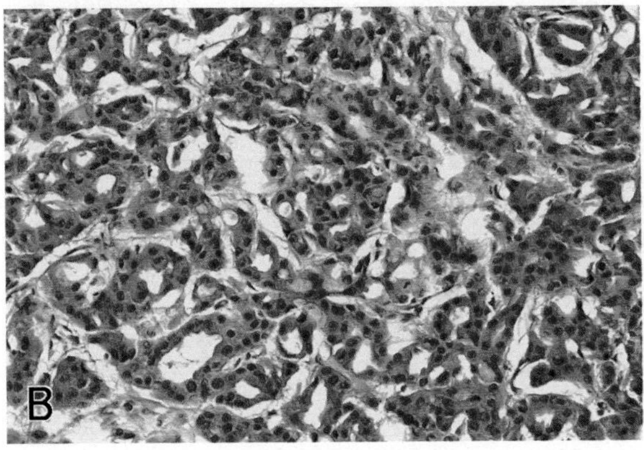

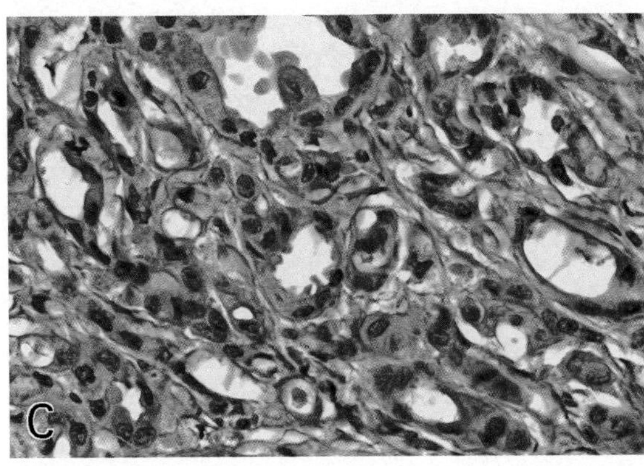

Figure 5-79

MOLL GLAND ADENOCARCINOMA

A: Clinical appearance of Moll gland adenocarcinoma. B,C: Histologic appearance shows prominent cytoplasmic acidophilia with areas of decapitation secretion.

the lesions of the nevoid basal cell carcinoma syndrome, ulceration is rare. Transformation of trichoepithelioma into a basal cell carcinoma occurs rarely (79).

Microscopic examination discloses multiple horny cysts with a fully keratinized center surrounded by islands of proliferating basaloid cells. The stroma of the tumor is abundant and well demarcated from the surrounding dermis (fig. 5-80). Some lesions have a high degree of differentiation, with abortive formation of hair papillae and hair shafts. The horn cysts in trichoepithelioma, which represent immature hair structures, allow this tumor to resemble keratotic basal cell carcinoma. It is therefore sometimes difficult to distinguish multiple trichoepitheliomas from this and other keratinizing neoplasms on histologic grounds alone. In trichoepithelioma the keratinization is typically abrupt and complete, differing from the gradual and incomplete keratinization observed in the keratin pearls of squamous cell carcinoma. Careful evaluation of the clinical data, including the number and distribution of the lesions and the pattern of inheritance, is necessary in some cases to establish an unequivocal diagnosis.

Trichofolliculoma

This benign tumor is often confused with a sebaceous (pilar) cyst. Clinically, *trichofolliculoma* appears as a slightly elevated, small nodule with a central area of umbilication that is the opening of a keratin-filled, dilated follicle. The presence of small white hairs growing from the central pore is strong clinical evidence that the small nodule is a trichofolliculoma (fig. 5-81A). The lesions grow slowly and range in size from 4 to 5 mm (80).

Microscopically, the tumor is composed of a centrally dilated, cystic structure lined by keratinizing, stratified squamous epithelium that is continuous with the epidermis. The cystic structure is a dilated hair follicle filled with keratinous material (fig. 5-81B,C). As a rule, several small birefringent hair shafts are present in the lumen of the follicle. The large cystic follicle typically is surrounded by branching strands of basaloid epithelial cells showing variable degrees

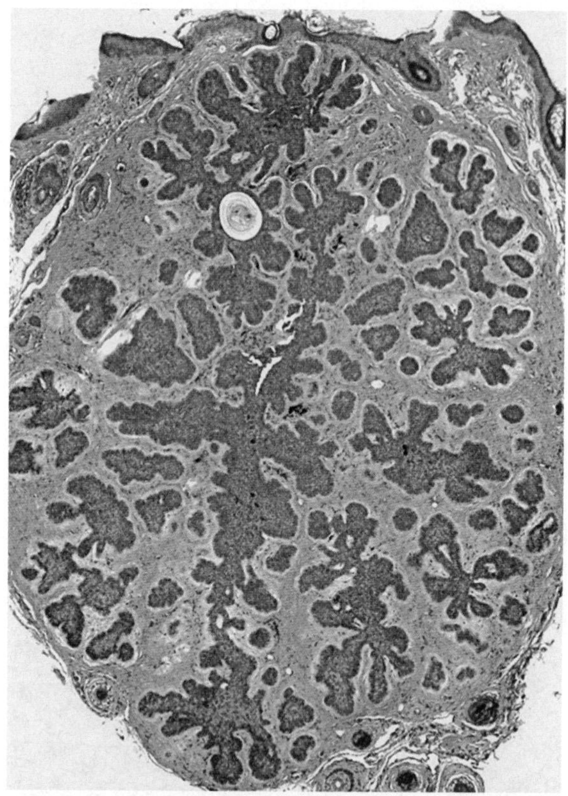

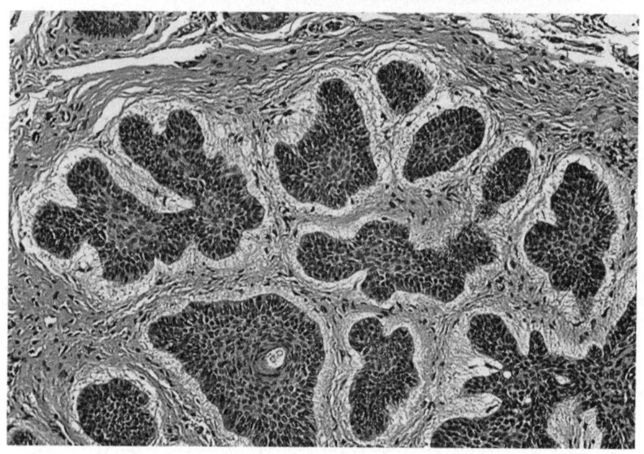

Figure 5-80

TRICHOEPITHELIOMA OF EYELID

Top: Solitary trichoepithelioma of eyelid.

Bottom: Well-demarcated dermal nodule with pilar differentiation. No mitoses were present.

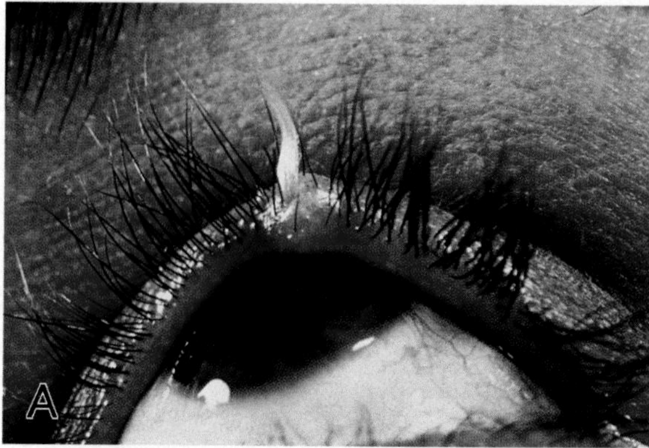

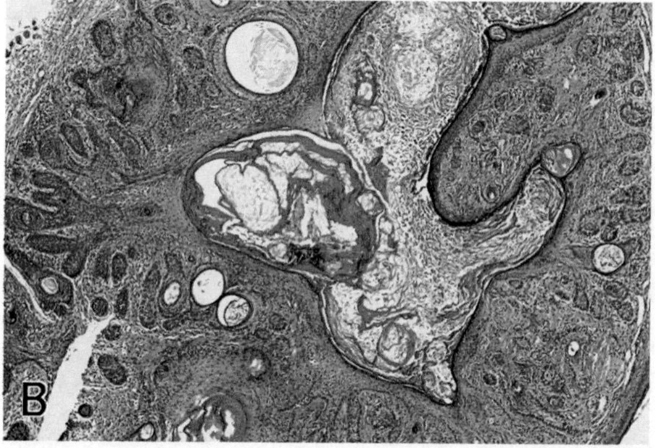

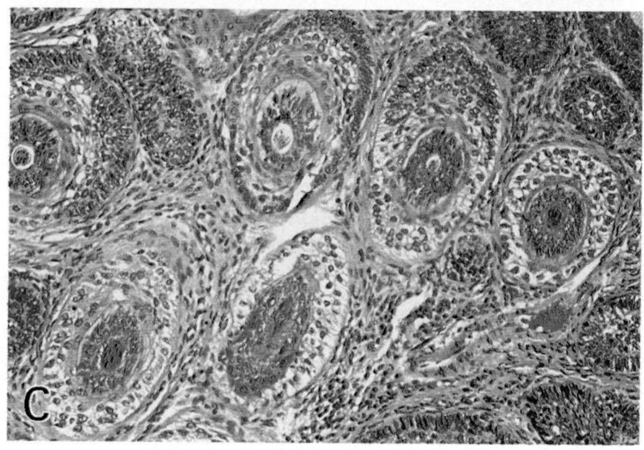

Figure 5-81

TRICHOFOLLICULOMA OF EYELID

A: Trichofolliculoma of upper lid contains white hair.

B: Keratin-filled cystic cavity is surrounded by immature hair follicles.

C: High-power view of the hair follicles.

of abortive pilar formation (secondary "immature" hair structures). The lesion has abundant connective tissue stroma that is sharply demarcated from the adjacent dermis. Histochemically, abundant glycogen is present in the walls of the branching abortive, hair follicles (80).

Trichilemmoma

Trichilemmoma is a benign tumor of the hair follicle that arises from the outer hair sheath (trichilemma); it is mostly composed of glycogen-rich clear cells. Hidayat and Font (81)

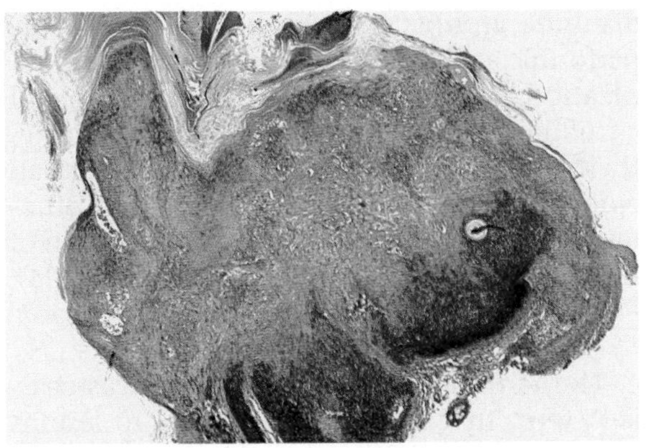

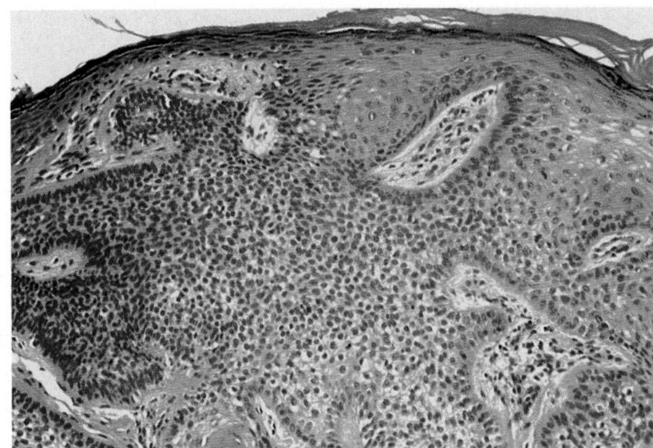

Figure 5-82

TRICHILEMMOMA OF EYELID

Left: Numerous glycogen-rich cells are at the base of the lesion (periodic acid–Schiff [PAS] stain).
Right: High-power view shows a plate-like attachment to the epidermis.

reviewed 107 cases: 31 involved the ophthalmic region; 28, the eyelid; and 3, the eyebrow. All lesions were solitary, small, and asymptomatic. Unlike basal cell carcinoma of the eyelid, trichilemmoma rarely involves the lid margin or the inner canthus. The median age of the patients in this series was 56 years.

Histologically, there is a lobular acanthosis composed mainly of glycogen-rich cells (fig. 5-82). The periphery of the tumor lobules often shows palisading of columnar cells, with a distinct basal membrane. Usually, several hair follicles are observed within the lesion. Frequently, the center of the lesion has areas of hyalinization that contain epithelial islands with squamoid differentiation. The tumor is frequently misinterpreted histologically as a basal cell carcinoma. It may also be confused with a squamous cell carcinoma, adnexal carcinoma, sebaceous neoplasm, or seborrheic keratosis.

Pilomatrixoma

Pilomatrixoma, also known as *calcifying epithelioma of Malherbe*, is a solid or cystic, freely movable, subcutaneous nodule covered by normal skin. The lesion is usually solitary and has a peculiar pink to purple discoloration (fig. 5-83A). The face and upper extremities are the most common sites of involvement. The lesion tends to occur in children: 40 percent of the lesions are first noted in patients 10 years of age or younger, and an additional 20 percent appear in patients between ages 11 and 20 years. The upper eyelid and the eyebrow are sites of predilection for this tumor (82).

The tumor is a well-demarcated nodule that involves the lower dermis and extends into the subcutaneous tissue (fig. 5-83B). It is composed of irregular epithelial islands containing basophilic cells and shadow cells. The basophilic cells are characteristically located at the periphery of the epithelial islands, and the shadow cells appear toward the center (fig. 5-83C). With aging, the number of basophilic cells decreases owing to their transformation into shadow cells. Most of the tumors contain varying amounts of calcium; this is especially noticeable in tumors composed predominantly of shadow cells. The calcium initially appears as basophilic granules within the cytoplasm of shadow cells. The masses of calcified shadow cells often act as a foreign body, eliciting a giant cell granulomatous reaction. Areas of ossification are observed in approximately 15 to 20 percent of the tumors. Occasionally, the basophilic cells display moderate nuclear pleomorphism and increased mitotic activity. Rare examples of malignant transformation have been reported. The malignant tumors have pleomorphic basaloid cells with prominent nucleoli. Abnormal mitoses are frequent, as is infiltration by the tumor cells into the adjacent tissues (83).

Histochemical studies provide evidence that pilomatrixoma develops from hair matrix cells. A strongly positive reaction for sulfhydryl or

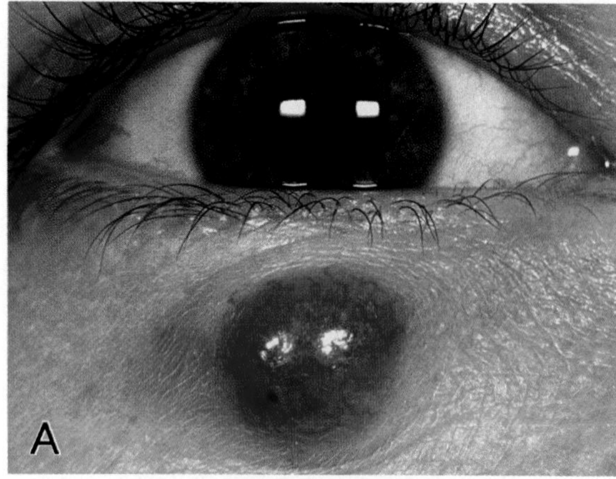

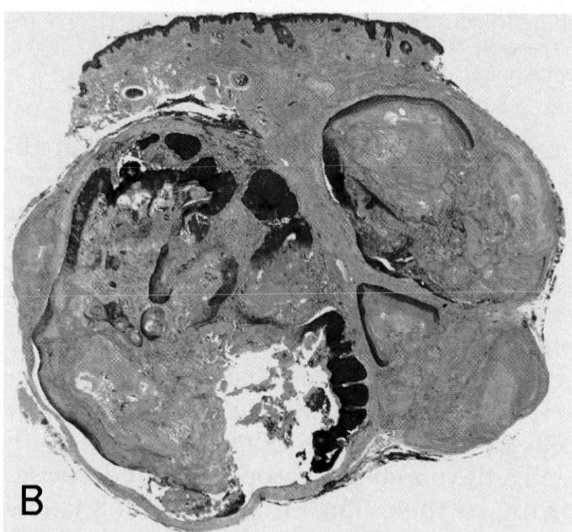

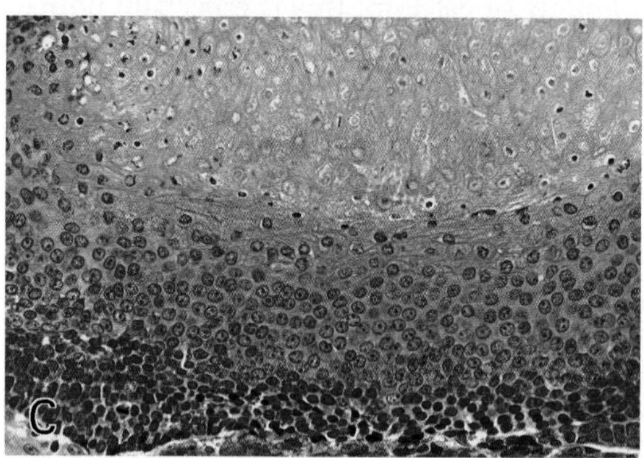

Figure 5-83

PILOMATRIXOMA OF EYELID

A: Clinical appearance of pilomatrixoma.

B: Low-power microscopic view of a dermal nodule.

C: High-power view shows both basophilic and shadow cells.

disulfide groups has been observed with the performic acid-Schiff stain, indicative of keratinization. Additionally, the demonstration of citrulline in the cells of pilomatrixoma indicates their capacity to form hair keratin rather than epidermal keratin. Electron microscopic studies have also provided evidence of the origin of the tumor from primitive hair matrix cells (84).

ADNEXAL CARCINOMA

The term *adnexal carcinoma* is a "wastebasket" term that should be restricted to lesions that histologically bear a striking resemblance to basal cell carcinoma and exhibit a similar biologic behavior but in which the exact site of origin (from the epidermis or adnexal structures) cannot be determined with certainty.

VASCULAR TUMORS

Primary angiomatous lesions of the eyelid include hamartomas that may be present at birth or become clinically apparent 1 to 2 weeks after birth (congenital lesions); hamartomas that appear later in childhood or in early adulthood (developmental lesions); and a group of secondary angiomatous lesions that arise at any age (acquired lesions). The capillary hemangioma of infancy and the nevus flammeus (port wine stain) are the most important congenital lesions. Cavernous hemangiomas are not usually present in the neonatal period and are considered here as developmental lesions. Vascular and other soft tissue tumors arising in the eyelids are summarized in Table 5-8.

Capillary Hemangioma and Nevus Flammeus

Capillary hemangioma, also referred to as *juvenile hemangioma, strawberry nevus, nevus vasculosus*, and *benign hemangioendothelioma of childhood*, is the most common form of hemangioma. It has been estimated to occur in 1/200 infants (85). The lesion usually appears at birth or becomes manifest in the first or second week of life. Typically, it is reddish purple, elevated, and of soft consistency with small surface invaginations. Most hemangiomas are superficial lesions that have a predilection for the head and neck.

Involvement of the eyelid margin is common. Deeply located lesions involving the skin of the eyelid or elsewhere may impart a slight violaceous discoloration or no change in color to the overlying skin, and therefore may be misdiagnosed clinically. Involvement of the eyelid may be associated with concomitant involvement of the conjunctiva, orbit, or both. Juvenile hemangioma is believed to be an immature form of capillary hemangioma.

Capillary hemangioma of childhood must be differentiated from *nevus flammeus (port wine stain)*. The latter is often associated with Sturge-Weber syndrome. Nevus flammeus is always present at birth, and it may become darker and more prominent with the passage of time. The skin lesion is flat and has a deeper, more purple hue than the cherry-red appearance observed in capillary hemangioma. Additionally, unlike capillary hemangioma, nevus flammeus does not blanch on pressure, or enlarge and become hypertrophic. Histopathologic examination shows the presence of large, dilated cavernous spaces in the dermis and not the small blood vessels observed in capillary hemangioma.

The natural history and evolution of capillary hemangioma are quite characteristic. Although the lesions are described as congenital, they usually appear within the first 2 weeks after birth and rapidly enlarge in the first 6 months of life. Regression occurs over a period of several years and usually is accompanied by fading of the color of the lesion from red to a dull grayish red, with concomitant wrinkling of the overlying skin ("crepe paper" change). About 30 percent of lesions completely regress by age 3 years and by age 7 years, 75 to 90 percent totally regress (86). This characteristic involutional tendency, coupled with the histopathologic features, makes capillary hemangioma a distinct separate entity.

Histologically, the lesion is composed of lobules of capillaries interspersed with sparse fibrous septa. The capillaries may infiltrate the underlying skeletal muscle and subcutaneous tissues. Frequently, a moderate number of mitotic figures are observed. Early, immature lesions have plump endothelial cells that tend to obliterate the vascular lumens. Reticulin stains establish that the proliferation of endothelial cells lies inside the capillary basement membrane. As the lesion matures, blood flow is established and the capillary endothelium becomes progressively attenuated and resembles that seen in the adult type of capillary hemangioma. Regression of the capillary hemangioma is accompanied by progressive interstitial fibrosis, with thickening of the fibrous septa and peripheral replacement of the tumor lobules by adipose tissue. Areas of perivascular fibrosis may lead to complete obliteration of the capillary channels. The terms *angiofibroma* and *angiolipoma* have been used for these stages of regression of capillary hemangiomas.

Table 5-8

TUMORS OF SOFT TISSUE ORIGIN OF THE EYELID[a]

Type of Tumor	Number of Cases
Benign	
Capillary hemangioma	11
Neurofibroma	10
Cavernous hemangioma	10
Fibrous histiocytoma	3
Glomus tumor	2
Intravascular papillary endothelial hyperplasia	2
Nevus flammeus	1
Malignant	
Kaposi's sarcoma	8
Rhabdomyosarcoma	3
Hemangiopericytoma	2
Pleomorphic liposarcoma	1
Malignant fibrous histiocytoma	1

[a]Frequency distribution of 54 tumors from the Doheny Eye Institute files collected between 1970 and 2000.

Despite the increased number of mitoses and the infiltrative growth pattern of the lesion, it should not be classified as malignant. Capillary hemangioma is a benign vascular tumor that does not spontaneously evolve into an angiosarcoma. The management of these lesions varies with the rate of growth as well as the location of the mass. The general approach is to observe and do nothing for smaller lesions that do not produce functional compromise. Rapidly enlarging lesions that cause functional impairment or pose a serious cosmetic problem should be treated. Different modalities of therapy include cryotherapy, injection of sclerosing agents, and irradiation; however, most of these therapeutic approaches are inadequate or cause unacceptable results. Systemic steroids have been advocated by some in an effort to obviate surgery and to induce regression of the lesion (87). Intralesional corticosteroid injections also appear to decrease tumor size (88).

Cavernous Hemangioma

Cavernous hemangioma occurs less frequently than does capillary hemangioma. Typically, these lesions do not appear in the neonatal period but usually arise in the second to fourth decades; occasionally, they become clinically manifest late in the first decade of life. They differ from capillary hemangiomas in several important respects. The lesions of cavernous hemangioma slowly but progressively enlarge, are less circumscribed (with the exception of the well-encapsulated orbital masses), and have no tendency for spontaneous regression. The color of a cavernous hemangioma usually depends on its depth. Superficially located lesions are dark blue, caused by dilatation and engorgement of blood vessels. Deeply located lesions may display little or no change in the color of the overlying skin. Superficial eyelid cavernous hemangiomas are usually well circumscribed but not encapsulated, in contrast to orbital lesions. Cavernous hemangiomas in other parts of the body may be more deeply situated and have more diffuse infiltrative features.

Secondary changes observed in cavernous hemangioma include foci of calcification, fibrosis, hemosiderin deposits, and scattered lymphoplasmacytic infiltrates. Dystrophic calcification with phlebolith formation is a frequent and highly specific finding. The phlebolith is a round mass of dystrophic calcification within an organizing thrombus.

Cavernous hemangiomas are composed of large, dilated, blood-filled vascular spaces that are lined by a flat layer of endothelium. The tumor may have an ill-defined lobular arrangement or a more diffuse, haphazard pattern. The intervascular stroma may show areas of fibrosis and scattered chronic inflammatory cells. By electron microscopy, the walls of the cavernous spaces often demonstrate smooth muscle cells, a feature not shared by capillary hemangiomas. In contrast to capillary hemangiomas, most cavernous hemangiomas require surgery. Following local excision of the lesion, recurrences are rare. Malignant transformation does not occur.

The association of an extensive cavernous hemangioma with thrombocytopenic purpura is known as the *Kasabach-Merritt syndrome* (89). Typically, this syndrome occurs in infants, and the onset of purpuric manifestations is heralded by rapid enlargement of the tumor. The pathogenesis of this syndrome is poorly understood, but it is believed that a consumption coagulopathy as well as sequestration of platelets within the tumor may be pathogenetically important.

Two other syndromes are associated with cavernous hemangiomas. The *blue rubber bleb nevus syndrome* is characterized by cutaneous cavernous hemangiomas that typically are soft, compressible, bluish, and associated with similar gastrointestinal hemangiomas that lead to severe bleeding and chronic anemia, complicating the course of the disease. The hemangiomas compress easily with pressure, leaving a flaccid, wrinkled appearance to the overlying skin (90). *Maffucci's syndrome* is a rare mesodermal dysplasia characterized by multiple cavernous hemangiomas as well as numerous enchondromas and exostoses, mainly involving the bones of the hands (91).

Lymphangioma

Lymphangiomas, like hemangiomas, are hamartomatous growths that can involve the eyelid and ocular adnexa. Lymphangiomas tend to involve the bulbar conjunctiva as well as the eyelid and orbit. Eyelid lesions are typically more diffuse but easier to manage than are orbital lesions. Lymphangiomas of the eyelid may be associated with concomitant conjunctival and facial lesions. Unlike capillary hemangiomas, lymphangiomas of the lid are slowly progressive lesions with no tendency for spontaneous regression.

Histopathologically, three types of lymphangiomas are encountered: *dermal* (*lymphangioma circumscriptum*), *cavernous*, and *cystic*. The latter often involves the neck (*cystic hygroma*). Cavernous lymphangioma is the most frequent type encountered in the ocular adnexa and the orbit. Microscopically, this tumor is composed of irregular, anastomosing lymphatic channels lined by a flat layer of endothelial cells. The stroma is usually hypocellular and loose. Older lesions may show areas of fibrosis intermixed with hemosiderin deposits and focal lymphoplasmacytic infiltrates. A highly characteristic feature of lymphangioma is the presence of well-developed lymphoid follicles displaying prominent germinal centers. Electron microscopy details vessel walls lined by a single layer of endothelial cells, without associated pericytes. Additionally, the endothelial cells are invested with an interrupted basement membrane (92). In some lesions, the larger lymphatic spaces may also possess fascicles of poorly developed smooth muscle cells. Lymphangiomas do not communicate with the systemic circulation but may contain smaller blood vessels scattered throughout the periphery of the mass. In a few instances, however, lymphangiomas evolve into hemangioma (*hemangiolymphangioma*). In general, cellular atypia is minimal or absent. Spontaneous malignant transformation of a lymphangioma is extremely rare.

Glomus Tumor

Glomus tumor, also known as *glomangioma*, is a benign, vascular, hamartomatous lesion that appears clinically as a solitary, reddish purple nodule that is usually tender and measures only a few millimeters in diameter. Glomus tumors may be solitary or multiple.

Multiple glomus tumors microscopically resemble cavernous hemangiomas and contain irregularly dilated vascular channels that are surrounded by a narrow rim of one to three layers of glomus cells. Because of the prominent vascular component, they are often referred to as glomangiomas. In contrast, solitary glomus tumors are more circumscribed and more cellular, with a large collection of glomus cells forming a prominent perivascular mantle.

Immunohistochemical stains reveal that the endothelial cell markers (factor VIII and *Ulex europaeus*) are consistently nonreactive. The glomus cells stain for antibodies against muscle-specific actin and vimentin, substantiating that glomus cells are probably of mesenchymal origin and may represent specialized vascular smooth muscle. Ultrastructurally, the polygonal cells are invested with a continuous basal lamina containing intracytoplasmic, 8-nm filaments with dense bodies and subplasmalemmal micropinocytotic vesicles (caveolae) (93).

Cutaneous Angiosarcoma

Cutaneous angiosarcoma is uncommon and tends to involve the head, especially the face and scalp, of elderly individuals. The lesions may be solitary, but in about half the cases they are multicentric and appear as raised, reddish purple or violaceous plaques and nodules that resemble blood blisters; they may ulcerate and bleed spontaneously. In some instances, a solitary, reddish blue, elevated nodule is localized to the eyelid.

Moderately to well-differentiated tumors are composed of irregular, anastomosing, vascular channels lined by atypical, plump endothelial cells with hyperchromatic nuclei that often pile up and display intraluminal papillary tufts. The histologic appearance varies with the degree of differentiation of the tumor. Poorly differentiated tumors are composed of pleomorphic anaplastic cells that may be difficult to distinguish from carcinoma or fibrosarcoma. Reticulin stains help outline the vascular structures and establish that the tumor cells lie on the luminal side of the vessels.

Malignant transformation in a preexisting benign vascular tumor is unusual. In a series of 28 cases of cutaneous angiosarcomas, 4 occurred in preexisting benign lesions; 3 arose in children, all of whom had nevus flammeus; and 1 arose in an irradiated lymphangioma (94).

The fatality rate is approximately 40 percent as the result of multiple recurrences and distant metastases, especially to the lung and liver (95). Approximately 15 to 20 percent of patients develop regional lymph node metastasis. Control of the tumor is difficult because it responds poorly to radiotherapy; since it is frequently multicentric, it cannot be readily excised (especially when it occurs on the face). Wide excision has been recommended for solitary lesions.

Other unusual vascular tumors, including hemangiopericytomas and Kaposi's sarcoma, are discussed in chapters 8 and 2. Benign and malignant neurogenic tumors are discussed in detail in chapter 8.

XANTHOMATOUS LESIONS

Localized xanthomatous lesions that involve the eyelids include xanthelasma and fibrous histiocytoma (fibrous xanthoma). The most common generalized xanthomatous lesions with eyelid involvement are tuberous xanthoma, juvenile xanthogranuloma, histiocytosis X, and lipoid proteinosis. Xanthomas and other tumors occurring in the eyelids are summarized in Tables 5-9 and 5-10.

Table 5-9

MISCELLANEOUS TUMORS OF THE EYELID[a]

Type of Tumor	Number of Cases
Benign	
Xanthoma	5
Phakomatous choristoma	4
Necrobiotic xanthogranuloma	4
Langerhans cell histiocytosis	3
Juvenile xanthogranuloma	2
Granular cell tumor	2
Nodular fasciitis	1
Angiofibroma	1
Malignant	
Merkel cell tumor	4
Metastasis	
Metastatic adenocarcinoma	7
Site	
Unknown	4
Prostate	1
Breast	1
Lung	1
Others	
Rhabdomyomatous mesenchymal hamartoma	1
Kimura's disease	1

[a]Frequency distribution of 35 tumors from the Doheny Eye Institute files collected between 1970 and 2000.

Table 5-10

TUMORS OF THE LYMPHOCYTIC OR HEMATOPOIETIC ORIGIN OF THE EYELID[a]

Type of Tumor	Number of Cases
Benign	
Reactive lymphoid hyperplasia	3
Atypical lymphoid hyperplasia	2
Malignant	
Lymphoma	17
Lymphoplasmacytic	9
Anaplastic large cell	3
Immunoblastic	2
AIDS-large cell	1
Mycosis fungoides	2
Miscellaneous	
Lymphomatoid granulomatosis	1

[a]Frequency distribution of 23 tumors from the Doheny Eye Institute files collected between 1970 and 2000.

Xanthelasma

Xanthelasma is a localized, reactive lesion composed of foamy histiocytes; it is the most common form of cutaneous xanthoma. About two thirds of patients with xanthelasma are normolipemic, but these lesions occur in patients with hyperlipidemia as well. Xanthelasmas tend to occur in middle-aged or elderly patients. They are usually bilateral and appear as flat or slightly elevated, yellowish tan, soft plaques, located on the inner canthi. Most lesions are locally excised for cosmetic reasons.

Microscopically, the plaques are composed of focal collections of lipid-laden histiocytes (xanthoma cells) that are distributed mainly around the blood vessels and adnexal structures of the papillary and reticular dermis. Fibrosis and inflammatory cell infiltration are minimal. The lesions are superficially located and almost never extend into the subcutis.

Fibrous Histiocytoma

The eyelid is an unusual location for *fibrous histiocytoma*, also referred to as *fibrous xanthoma*, *dermatofibroma*, and *sclerosing hemangioma* (96). This lesion has a predilection, however, to occur in the orbit. Other ocular sites of involvement include the tarsus, the corneoscleral limbus, the conjunctiva, and the lacrimal sac. The eyelid lesion usually appears as a 10- to 15-mm, freely movable, deeply located, solid (occasionally cystic) mass covered by intact skin. The cutaneous type of fibrous histiocytoma differs slightly in its microscopic appearance from the deep type.

Microscopic examination of cutaneous fibrous histiocytoma shows a nodular, cellular proliferation involving the dermis and subcutis. The margins are poorly defined, and the lesion consists of interlacing fascicles of fibroblastic cells that exhibit a vague storiform pattern. Scattered, large histiocytic cells are intermixed with the spindle cell proliferation. Multinucleated giant cells of the foreign body or Touton type are common.

Tuberous Xanthoma

Tuberous xanthoma is a subcutaneous, plaque-like lesion with a predilection for the buttocks, elbows, knees, and fingers. These lesions are observed in patients with types II and III hyperlipidemia. They differ significantly from xanthelasmata in that the lesions are more deeply located and display foamy histiocytes intermixed with multinucleated Touton-type giant cells, as well as extracellular cholesterol deposits, moderate fibrosis, and inflammation. The association of tuberous xanthoma with hyperlipidemia suggests that this is a reactive, non-neoplastic lesion. There is evidence that the lipid within the xanthomatous lesion is derived from the blood.

Juvenile Xanthogranuloma

Juvenile xanthogranuloma is a non-neoplastic, self-limited, histiocytic proliferation of unknown etiology that usually occurs in infants 2 years of age or younger. It has been called *nevoxanthoendothelioma*; however, the term *juvenile xanthogranuloma* seems more appropriate. The eyelid lesion typically appears as an elevated, orange or reddish brown nodule, which may be solitary or part of a generalized cutaneous eruption. The most common sites of involvement are the head and neck, and 24 percent of the cases involve the eyelid. Zimmerman (97) emphasized a striking difference in the age distribution of 32 cases with uveal involvement, compared with the 12 cases with solitary eyelid lesions: 85 percent of patients with uveal involvement were infants less than 1 year of age, and 64 percent were 17 months of age or younger; in contrast, only 2 patients with eyelid lesions were infants less than 1 year old, 7 were between 17 months and 5 years of age, and the remaining 3 patients were 11, 19, and 30 years old.

The early cutaneous lesions show a monomorphous infiltrate of histiocytes intermixed with lymphocytes, mononuclear cells, and scattered eosinophils. Some of the histiocytes display pale, vacuolated cytoplasm indicative of early lipidization. In mature lesions a mixed population of histiocytes, lymphocytes, eosinophils, and multinucleated foreign body–type giant cells, some of the Touton type, are observed. The Touton giant cells have a wreath of nuclei encircling a portion of nonlipid-containing cytoplasm. Older lesions have a more pronounced fibroblastic proliferation, with areas of scarring. The histologic picture of the cutaneous and eyelid lesions is notably different from that seen in the uvea. The eyelid lesions typically are less vascularized and contain greater numbers of spindle-shaped cells, histiocytes, and Touton giant cells than do the uveal lesions.

The prognosis of patients with juvenile xanthogranuloma is excellent except for the intraocular complications of iris lesions (98). Although juvenile xanthogranuloma has been reported to be associated with neurofibromatosis (99), it is not related to the histiocytosis X group of lesions and the latter rarely involves the eyelids (97).

Other Xanthogranulomatous Lesions

There are other xanthogranulomatous lesions that involve the eyelids: *necrobiotic xanthogranuloma* (figs. 5-84, 5-85) and *Erdheim-Chester disease*. The former displays foci of necrobiosis surrounded by histiocytes and Touton giant cells (fig. 5-85). The necrobiotic foci may contain cholesterol. Erdheim-Chester disease is a systemic disorder with xanthogranulomatous infiltration (fig. 5-86).

LIPOID PROTEINOSIS

Lipoid proteinosis, also known as *hyalinosis cutis et mucosae* and *Urbach-Wiethe syndrome*, is a rare condition, inherited in an autosomal recessive fashion. Involvement of the eyelids (fig. 5-87A) is characterized by the formation of small nodules that tend to occupy the entire margin of all four lids. The nodules occasionally become confluent and have a waxy or yellowish appearance (100). Occasionally, they present as a row of nodules with a beaded appearance.

Microscopic examination of early lesions shows thickening of the capillary walls with deposition of hyaline material mainly around the basement membrane (fig. 5-87B,C). In fully developed lesions, a homogeneous, eosinophilic, hyaline mantle surrounds the dermal vessels and extends into the papillary and reticular dermis. Similar deposits surround the sweat glands and hair follicles as well as the smooth muscle of the arrectores pilorum.

The hyaline material of lipoid proteinosis is strongly PAS positive and diastase-resistant. Stains for mucopolysaccharide (alcian blue at ph 2.5) are slightly positive. This material is sensitive to hyaluronidase digestion, suggesting that the acid mucopolysaccharide is mainly hyaluronic acid. Stains for amyloid (Congo red and crystal violet) give slightly positive results. The results of lipid stains are variable. Sudan III and IV stains display small lipid droplets throughout the hyaline material, particularly around the blood vessels, indicating the presence of neutral fat. On frozen sections the lipid is not birefringent. The Schultz reaction for cholesterol is

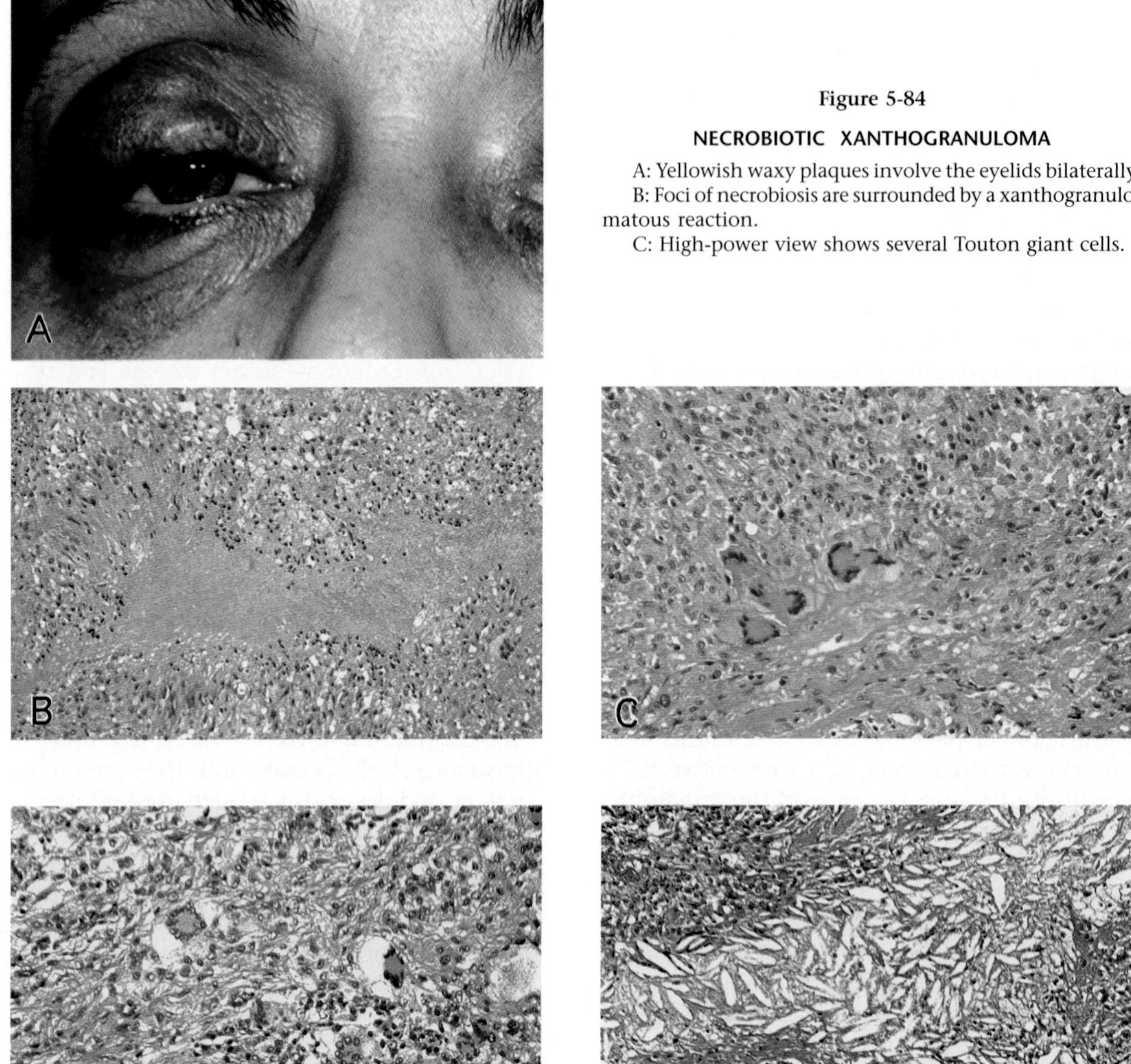

Figure 5-84

NECROBIOTIC XANTHOGRANULOMA

A: Yellowish waxy plaques involve the eyelids bilaterally.

B: Foci of necrobiosis are surrounded by a xanthogranulomatous reaction.

C: High-power view shows several Touton giant cells.

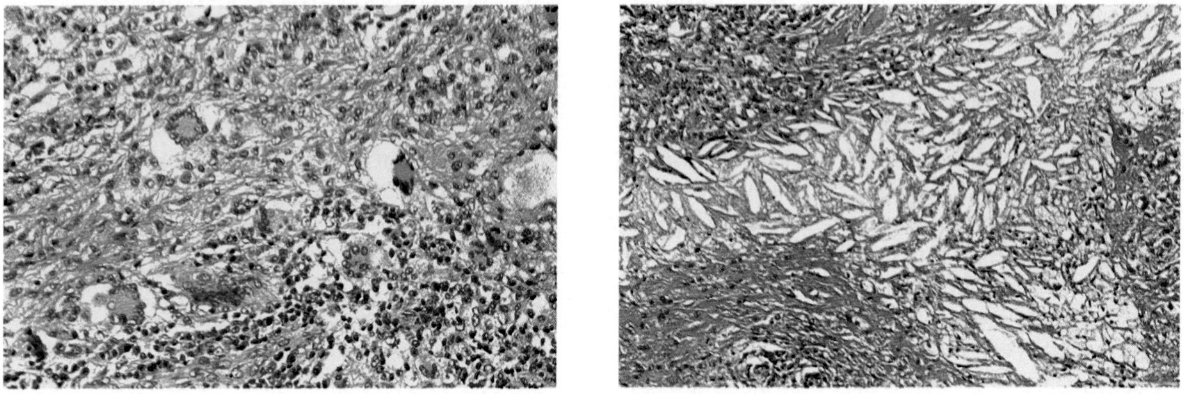

Figure 5-85

NECROBIOTIC XANTHOGRANULOMA

Left: Touton giant cells are seen.

Right: A focus of necrobiosis of collagen contains masses of cholesterol crystals.

often positive. Histochemical stains for phospholipids demonstrate that they are absent or present only in small amounts.

Electron microscopy shows that the hyaline material is composed of 5- to 10-nm filaments that appear to be generated by the fibroblasts. These cells have dilated cisternae of rough-surfaced endoplasmic reticulum containing amorphous and filamentous material. The filaments are curved and branching and anastomose with each other (in contrast to the filaments of amyloid, which are straight and nonbranching). A highly characteristic feature of the hyaline material is the close relationship of the filaments to the basement membrane of the capillaries. Typically, a network of haphazardly arranged filaments is concentrically arranged around the capillaries and embedded between the layers of reduplicated basement membrane. Similar filamentous material and amorphous deposits are found interspersed diffusely among normal collagen fibers throughout the dermis. Thicker filaments, measuring up to 30 nm in diameter, may be intermixed with thin, immature collagen fibrils. It has been postulated that the abnormal hyaline material is produced either by the splitting of collagen fibrils into smaller filaments and protofilaments or by the defective polymerization of protofilaments into larger collagenous fibrils (101).

MISCELLANEOUS LESIONS

Mycosis Fungoides

Mycosis fungoides is a form of cutaneous malignant lymphoma that arises from thymus-dependent lymphocytes (T cells). Clinically, the disease is divided into three stages: erythematous, plaque, and tumor (fig. 5-88, left). In the tumor stage, visceral manifestations consisting of hepatosplenomegaly and lymphadenopathy are frequently seen. Stenson and Ramsay (102) studied 30 patients with biopsy-proved mycosis fungoides and summarized the ocular abnormalities. Eleven of the 30 patients, most of whom were in the tumor stage of the disease,

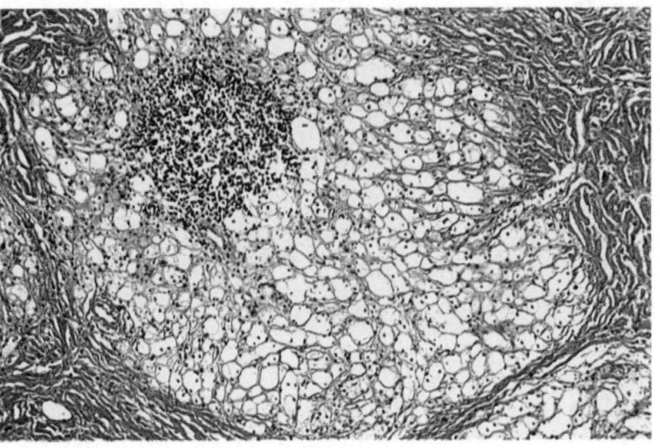

Figure 5-86

ERDHEIM-CHESTER DISEASE

Section of a retroperitoneal mass showing a diffuse xanthogranulomatous process.

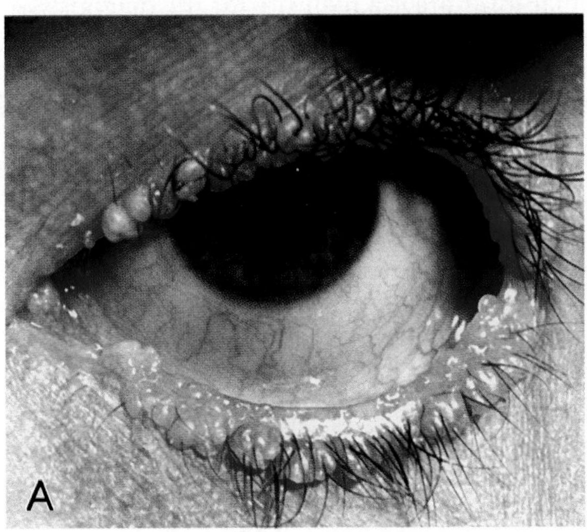

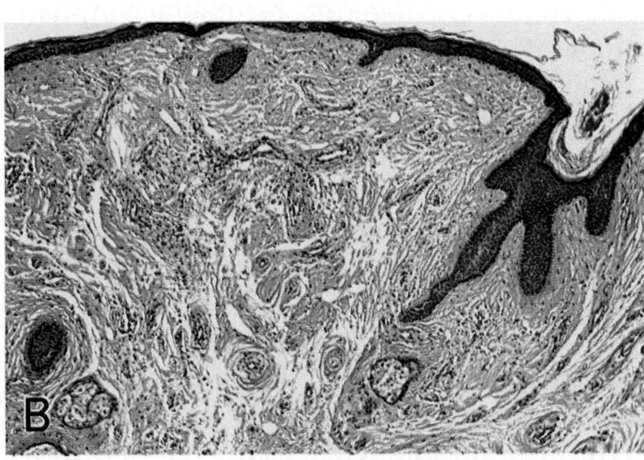

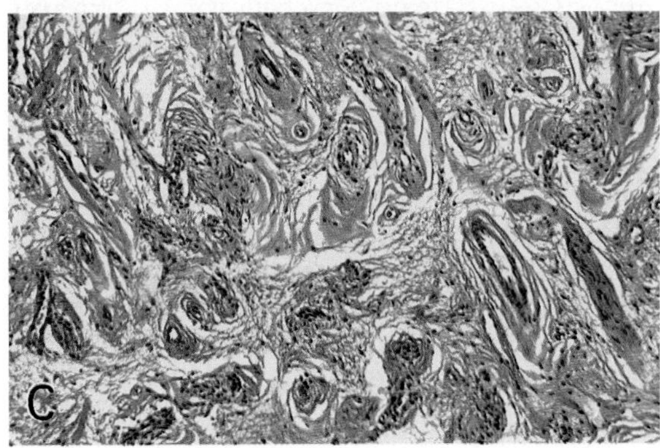

Figure 5-87

LIPOID PROTEINOSIS

A: Clinical features.

B,C: A hyaline mantle surrounds dermal blood vessels, which are radiating toward the upper dermis.

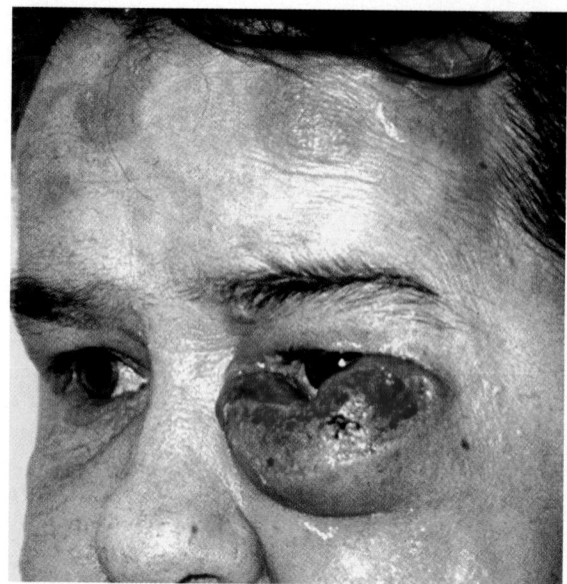

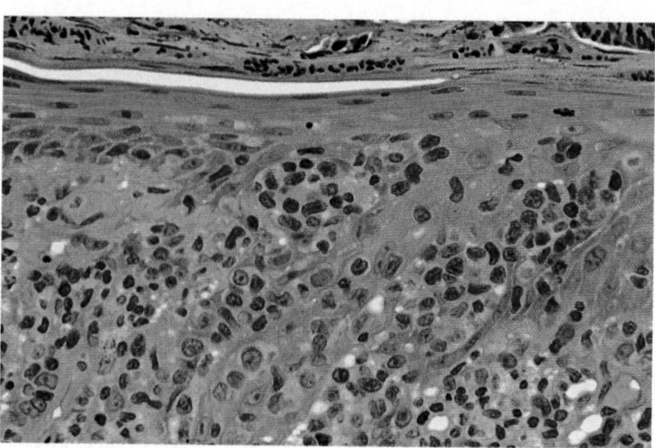

Figure 5-88

MYCOSIS FUNGOIDES

Left: The eyelid is involved. A biopsy site is seen in the left lower eyelid.

Above: Epidermal involvement by T-cell lymphoma forming Pautrier abscesses.

had ophthalmologic changes believed to be directly related to the disease. The eyelid was the most common site of involvement; eight patients had solitary or multiple eyelid tumors that ranged in size from a few millimeters to 10 cm in diameter. A rare variant of mycosis fungoides is *Sézary's syndrome*, characterized by generalized erythroderma, peripheral lymphadenopathy, hepatosplenomegaly, and abnormal circulating T cells ("Sézary cells").

Microscopic examination of the erythematous stage of mycosis fungoides may disclose nonspecific changes similar to those observed in other inflammatory dermatoses. In the plaque stage, the histologic features are usually diagnostic. The dermis contains a polymorphic cellular infiltrate composed of histiocytes, lymphoid cells, eosinophils, plasma cells, and a variable number of highly characteristic, atypical lymphoreticular cells, referred to as mycosis cells. The mycosis cells vary in size and cytologic appearance. The small variant measures from 10 to 15 µm and displays a hyperchromatic nucleus without nucleoli and scanty cytoplasm. The nucleus often has a crenated appearance due to the multiple irregular clefts in the nuclear membrane. The small mycosis cell (Lutzner cell) has a multilobulated, cerebriform nucleus with deep lobulations of the nuclear membrane. This cell is highly characteristic, but not pathognomonic, of mycosis fungoides (103,104). The large variant of the mycosis cell, which measures 20 to 30 µm in diameter, has abundant, vacuolated, amphophilic cytoplasm with an irregularly clefted nucleus and multiple nucleoli. Binucleated or multinucleated forms of the large mycosis cell are occasionally observed.

Epidermal involvement by the atypical cellular infiltrate is a requisite for the diagnosis of mycosis fungoides. The epidermis and the hair follicles may be extensively infiltrated with mycosis cells, which are distributed either singly or in small clusters (Pautrier abscesses) (fig. 5-88, right). Thus, the diagnosis of mycosis fungoides depends upon the presence of an atypical, pleomorphic, mononuclear cell infiltrate containing large and small cell variants of the mycosis cell, intermixed with a polymorphic inflammatory infiltrate, and involvement of both the dermis and the epidermis. In the tumor stage, the infiltrate is composed of large atypical anaplastic cells that have a monomorphic appearance. In some instances, the histologic picture resembles that observed in other malignant lymphomas of the skin.

Lymphomatoid Granulomatosis

Lymphomatoid granulomatosis was first described by Liebow and colleagues in 1972 (105) as "angiocentric and angiodestructive lymphoreticular proliferative and granulomatous disease involving predominantly the lungs." The ophthalmic manifestations of lymphomatoid granulomatosis are unusual and include bilateral uveitis, atypical lymphoma of the eyelid (106), scleritis and episcleritis, atypical lymphoplasmacytic choroidal infiltrates, central retinal artery occlusion, and bilateral peripheral retinal vasculitis with posterior uveitis. There is central nervous system involvement in 19 percent of patients, which includes mental confusion, ataxia, hemiparesis and seizures, diplopia, transient blindness, proptosis, deafness, and vertigo. Signs of cranial neuropathies occur in approximately 11 percent of patients (107).

The dermis is usually replaced by a polymorphic, atypical lymphoreticular infiltrate with plasmacytoid cells, often associated with necrotizing vasculitis. The vasculitis tends to affect the deep vessels in the dermis and subcutaneous tissues, usually under the areas of ulceration. The affected vessels are lined by swollen endothelial cells with fibrinoid deposits in the vessel walls and occasional organized thrombi. Lymphomatoid granulomatosis can be differentiated from Wegener's granulomatosis by the presence of a polymorphic lymphoreticular infiltrate and the absence of multinucleated giant cells.

Lymphomatoid granulomatosis is fatal in approximately two thirds of patients (median survival time is only 14 months). Progression to malignant lymphoma invariably occurs, especially if appropriate treatment with cyclophosphamide and prednisone is not instituted. Originally, the disease was regarded as a form of vasculitis that could evolve into malignant lymphoma. Currently, it is regarded as a form of T-cell lymphoma with predominant involvement of the lungs, typically causing angiocentric and angiodestructive lesions.

Lymphomatoid granulomatosis may be confused with mycosis fungoides because the polymorphic infiltrate is associated with large atypical lymphoreticular cells. Mycosis fungoides, however, is characterized by a tendency for the neoplastic T cells to invade the overlying epidermis (Pautrier abscesses) and by the absence of vasculitis.

Nodular Fasciitis

Nodular fascitis, also known as *pseudosarcomatous fasciitis*, *proliferative fasciitis*, *infiltrative fasciitis*, and *pseudosarcomatous fibromatosis*, is a benign, reactive proliferation of fibroblasts and vascular elements that involve the facial and subcutaneous tissues. Clinically, it appears as a rapidly growing nodule (fig. 5-89A) that has been present for only a few weeks and often is associated with tenderness or slight pain. It most commonly affects young adults between 20 and 35 years of age. Both sexes are equally affected. The lesions grow rapidly; in 45 percent of patients, the preoperative duration of the lesion was less than 1 month, and in 30 percent, it was less than 2 weeks (108).

Histologically, the lesions are composed of plump, stellate or spindle-shaped fibroblasts, arranged either in parallel fascicles or haphazardly, which resemble growing fibroblasts in tissue culture. The fibroblasts show little variation in size and shape, and have oval nuclei and slender cytoplasmic processes. Most lesions display large cystoid spaces containing a variable amount of intercellular myxoid ground substance (some of which is hyaluronic acid), serous exudate, or both (fig. 5-89B,C). The irregular bundles and fascicles of fibroblasts are often accompanied by a dense reticulin network and small amounts of mature birefringent collagen. Typically, there is a proliferation of slit-like vascular spaces or well-formed capillaries, sometimes with extravasation of erythrocytes, resembling the histologic features of Kaposi's sarcoma. Frequently, scattered lymphocytes and mononuclear cells are seen at the periphery of the nodule. Other lesions have small collections of lipid-laden macrophages and multinucleated giant cells as well as small areas of hemorrhage. The histologic appearance of nodular fasciitis correlates well with the preoperative duration of the lesion; late lesions of nodular fasciitis may exhibit areas of hyaline fibrosis.

Electron microscopic studies have shown that the elongated bipolar cells contain abundant cisternae of rough-surfaced endoplasmic reticulum, some of which are filled with granular, electron-dense deposits. Many of the cells have intracytoplasmic bundles of microfilaments with focal fusiform densities, as well as occasional desmosomes. The plasma membrane displays numerous micropinocytotic vesicles and focal basement membrane formation. Occasional subplasmalemmal collections of actin-like filaments are observed. All of these ultrastructural features are typical of myofibroblasts (109).

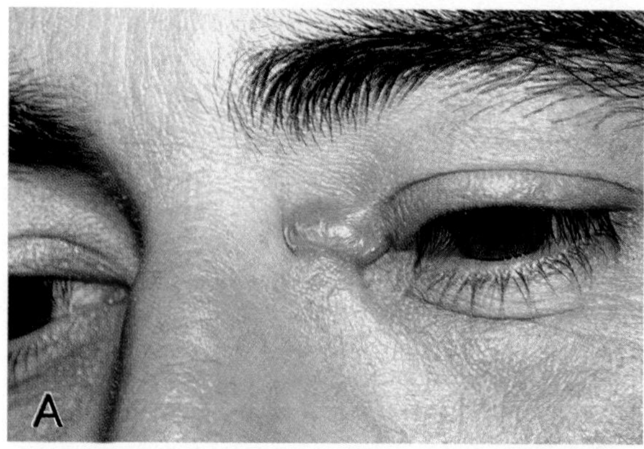

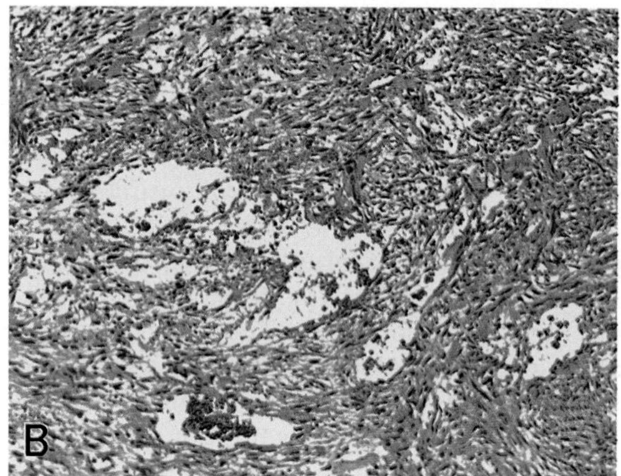

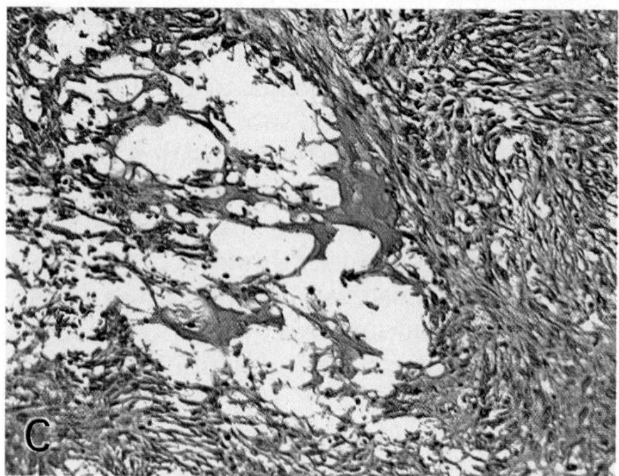

Figure 5-89

NODULAR FASCIITIS

A: Nodule at the left inner canthus.
B,C: Cystoid changes and florid myofibroblastic proliferations are seen.

Nodular fasciitis must be differentiated histopathologically from several benign and malignant fibrous lesions. These include fibroma, fibrosarcoma, fibromatosis, fibrous histiocytoma, myxoma, neurofibroma, and neurilemmoma. Local excision is the treatment of choice; recurrences are rare, occurring in about 1 to 2 percent of cases, usually as a result of incomplete excision of the lesion.

Juvenile Fibromatosis

The fibromatoses comprise a broad group of benign fibrous tissue proliferations that share similar histologic features and exhibit a biologic behavior intermediate between benign fibrous lesions and fibrosarcoma. The lesions are usually nonencapsulated fibrous tumors that have a tendency for local recurrence but do not metastasize. Rarely, they regress spontaneously. They are most common in children and young adults.

Hidayat and Font (110) reported a series of six cases of *juvenile fibromatosis* of the periorbital region and eyelid. The median age of the patients at the time of diagnosis was 8 years. The tumors had a median size of 15 mm. A definite propensity for the tumor to involve the infraorbital region and lower eyelid was observed. Two of the six tumors in their series recurred after excision. Histopathologically, the tumors were composed of interlacing fascicles of fibroblasts with oval, plump, vesicular nuclei and ill-defined cytoplasm. Three tumors had a distinct lobular pattern with dilated, thin-walled blood vessels located in the interlobular fibrous septa. Mitotic activity was minimal. Three tumors exhibited a peculiar leiomyomatous appearance, resembling that observed in cases of congenital generalized fibromatosis. Ultrastructurally, juvenile fibromatosis shows cells with the features of fibroblasts intermixed with a few cells displaying features of myofibroblasts.

Local excision of the mass is recommended as the initial therapy. Wide local re-excision is indicated for recurrent tumors.

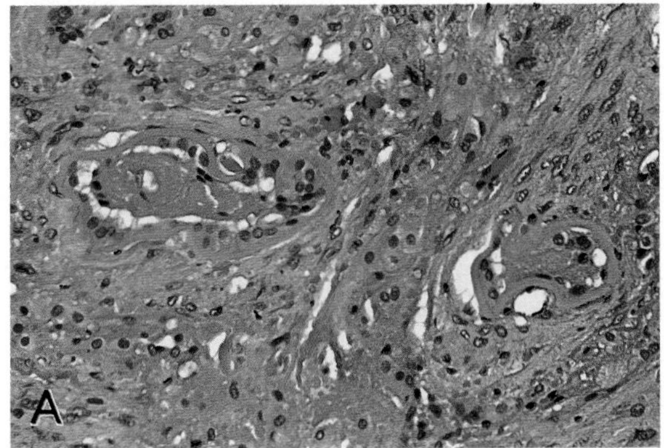

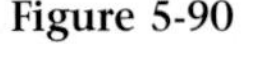

Figure 5-90

PHAKOMATOUS CHORISTOMA

A: Tubular structures are lined by cuboidal epithelial cells.

B: PAS-positive basement membrane surrounds proliferated lens epithelial cells.

C: Swollen degenerated cells resemble the "bladder" cells of cataractous lens.

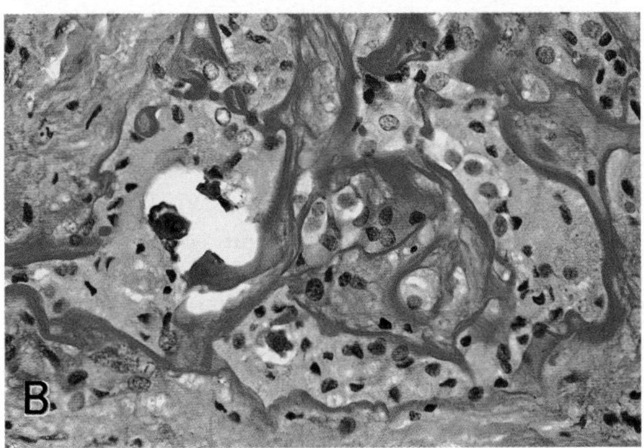

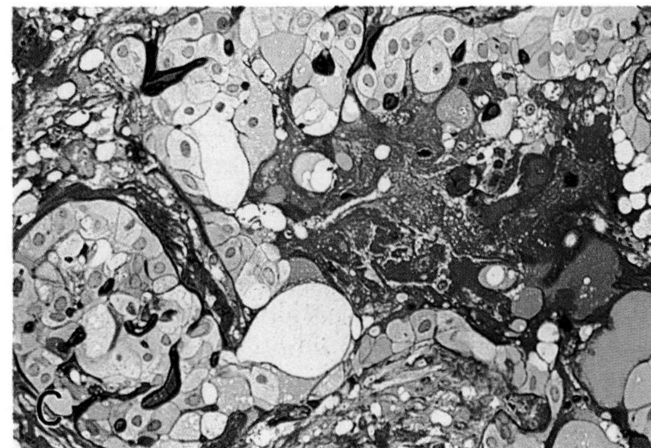

Phakomatous Choristoma

Zimmerman (111) first described three infants who had a peculiar choristomatous lesion that involved the lower eyelid. Following Zimmerman's original description, several additional cases of this unusual tumor of the eyelid have been reported (112). This mass occurs in infants either at birth or in the first 6 months of life; in each case the localized, enlarging mass involves the lower eyelid nasally. The lid masses ranged from 10 to 17 mm in diameter.

The lesions are composed of dense, collagenous tissue that contains small nests and islands of cuboidal cells; these cells are surrounded by a thick, irregular, PAS-positive basement membrane (fig. 5-90A,B). Swollen cells resembling the "bladder" cells of human cataractous lenses are observed within the epithelial islands (fig. 5-90C). Small foci of dystrophic calcification, in some cases containing numerous psammoma bodies, have also been noted. The epithelial cells are positive for alpha, beta, and gamma crystalline of the lens protein (112).

The combination of light and electron microscopic findings is highly reminiscent of the pathologic changes observed in human congenital cataracts. It has been suggested, therefore, that the lesion is a choristoma of lenticular anlage that probably results from displacement and migration of the inferior lens placode cells into the mesodermal tissues of the lower eyelid. An alternative explanation is that the lesion may originate from an additional locus of lens vesicle from the primitive surface ectoderm forming the lower eyelid. The specific localization of the lesion in the lower eyelid nasally probably is determined by the ventronasal location of the patent embryonic choroidal fissure, the closure of which is not complete until the 18-mm stage of embryonic development.

Granular Cell Tumor

Granular cell tumors are commonly referred to as *granular cell myoblastomas*. They are slow-growing, nonencapsulated, painless growths that occur in virtually every organ of the body but most frequently involve the tongue and skin. Granular cell tumors arise in the eyelid and brow (113–115), the conjunctiva, the caruncle, the lacrimal sac, and the orbit.

When the eyelid is involved, the lesion usually appears as a small, well-circumscribed, slightly elevated nodule located at the lid margin. The tumor cells are embedded in dense collagenous tissue and display abundant, granular, acidophilic cytoplasm and small, paracentral or eccentric nuclei.

Merkel Cell Tumor

In 1875, Friedrich Merkel described clear, nondendritic, oval cells oriented parallel to the skin surface and located in the deeper layers of the epidermis, adjacent to hair follicles, where they formed complexes with nerve endings. In the eyelids, these cells are common, and form clusters (Merkel touch spots) along the lid margin between the cilia (116). They are best identified with the electron microscope.

Although *Merkel cell tumor* of the skin is uncommon, in recent years, it has been recognized with increasing frequency. It is a highly aggressive neoplasm with a potential for local recurrence and metastasis. The age distribution of the reported cases ranges from 54 to 95 years, with a mean age of 75 years, and 62.5 percent occur in females. The upper eyelid is involved more often than the lower.

Clinically, the eyelid tumors present as painless, cutaneous nodules with violaceous or reddish blue overlying skin, resembling an angiomatous lesion (fig. 5-91A). Telangiectatic vessels are frequently observed on the surface of the mass.

The tumor cells have round to oval, uniform nuclei with finely dispersed chromatin and one to three small, inconspicuous nucleoli (fig. 5-91B,C) (117). The cells possess scanty cytoplasm. Mitotic figures are usually numerous. The tumor cells infiltrate the dermis and are arranged in diffuse sheets or a trabecular pattern. They may also form pseudorosettes or pseudoglandular structures. The epidermis is usually spared, but involvement of the hair follicles may be observed. Merkel cell tumor is a poorly differentiated, cutaneous neoplasm and thus the differential diagnosis includes malignant lymphoma, metastatic oat cell carcinoma, amelanotic melanoma, and sebaceous gland carcinoma.

Ultrastructural examination reveals 80- to 200-nm, membrane-bound, dense core granules (fig. 5-91D); perinuclear microfilaments (7 to 9 nm in diameter); desmosomes; hemidesmosomes; and focal basal lamina formation (117). Another ultrastructural feature observed in normal Merkel cells, as well as in some Merkel cell tumors, is the presence of intranuclear rodlets. Warner et al. (118) described straight cytoplasmic processes ("spikes") containing actin-like filaments that abut the plasmalemmae of adjacent cells. Other ultrastructural features include numerous polyribosomes and prominent Golgi lamellae. Mitochondria and rough-surfaced endoplasmic reticulum are relatively scarce.

Immunohistochemical studies are helpful in establishing the diagnosis of Merkel cell tumor. Immunoreactivity to antibodies for cytokeratins, neuron-specific enolase, and synaptophysin (fig. 5-92), and a negative reaction for leukocyte common antigen are highly suggestive of Merkel cell carcinoma. The positive results of immunohistochemical staining are similar to those observed in other neuroendocrine tumors from other anatomic locations, including those with metastasis to the skin.

The treatment of choice is wide surgical excision of the mass with frozen section control of the margins. Because of the relatively small numbers of cases with eyelid involvement and incomplete follow-up data, general guidelines regarding the response to radiotherapy and chemotherapy are not available. It is generally agreed, however, that aggressive management of local recurrences and regional adenopathy is appropriate and likely to improve the prognosis and survival rate of the patient.

Intravascular Papillary Endothelial Hyperplasia

Intravascular papillary endothelial hyperplasia is an exuberant proliferation of endothelial cells that was first described by Masson as "vegetant intravascular hemangioendothelioma" (119). Most cases develop within vascular channels of the deep dermis or subcutis. Intravascular papillary endothelial hyperplasia also arises in hemangiomas, hematomas, arteriovenous malformations, and rarely, lymphangiomas.

In the eyelid and brow, the lesions appear as reddish purple nodules or masses, some of which are movable and occur in the subcutaneous

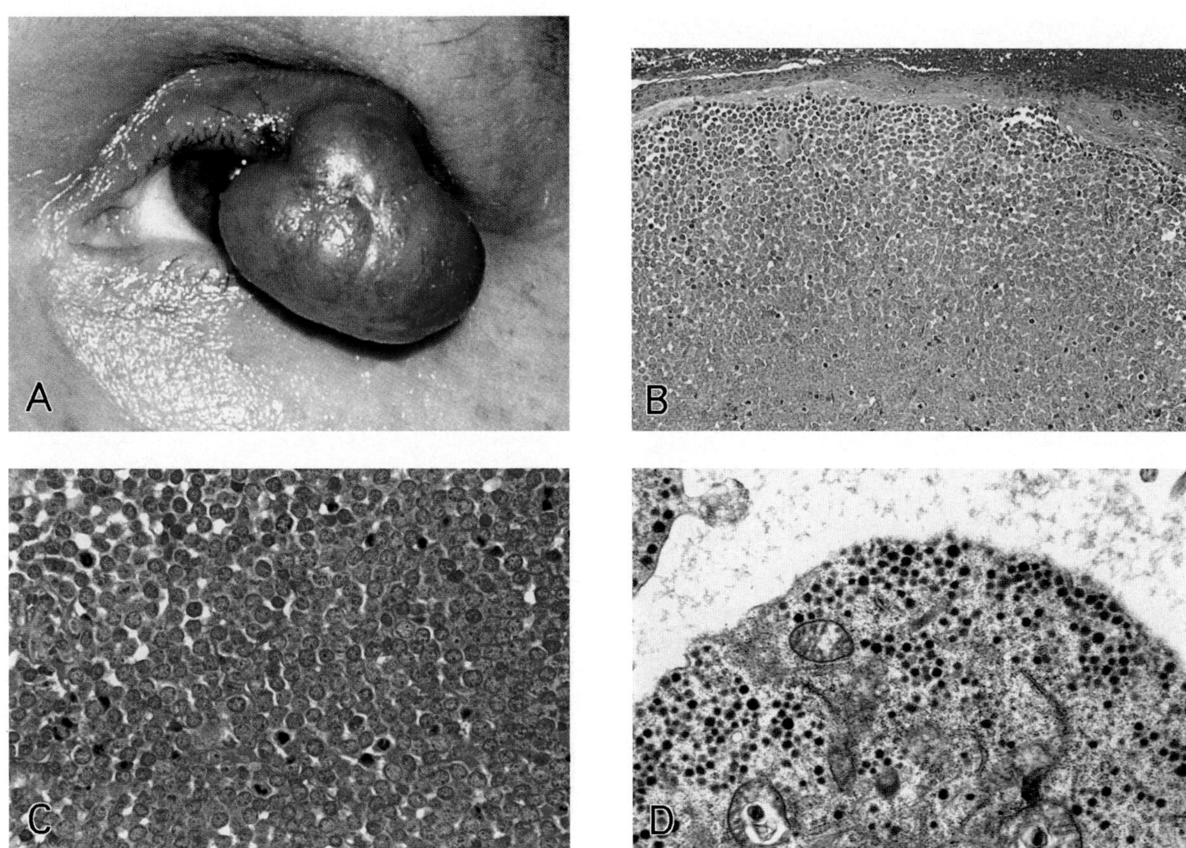

Figure 5-91

MERKEL CELL CARCINOMA

A: Typical large angiomatous-like nodule.

B,C: Low- and high-power magnification depicts the typical histologic appearance of Merkel cell carcinoma: round to oval nuclei with fine uniform euchromatin.

D: Electron micrograph shows dense core membrane-bound granules.

tissues. Most lesions are located within a distended vein, but arteries are also involved. The intraluminal mass, which is intimately attached to the vessel wall, has a collagenous core that forms papillary tufts lined by a single layer of flat endothelial cells. In some lesions, several concentric layers of endothelial cells are centered on cores of fibrin and collagen (120). The intraluminal mass is composed of spindle-shaped cells that have features of endothelial cells: a polarized basement membrane with numerous micropinocytotic vesicles under the plasmalemma. Occasional cells have features of pericytes. The lesion appears to represent an unusual, exuberant proliferation of vascular endothelium as a cellular response to the organization of a thrombus. Intravascular papillary endothelial hyperplasia is occasionally confused with angiosarcoma.

Erdheim-Chester Disease

The ophthalmologic manifestations of *Erdheim-Chester disease* include bilateral xanthelasma, thinning of the skin of the eyelids, exophthalmos, ophthalmoplegia, bilateral enhancing masses on CT scan of the orbit, swelling of the optic disc, optic atrophy, and retinal striae. Elevated blood lipid levels have been observed in some patients.

Visceral lesions have been reported; these include involvement of the lungs (pulmonary infiltrates by foamy histiocytes containing cholesterol, pleural effusion, and pulmonary

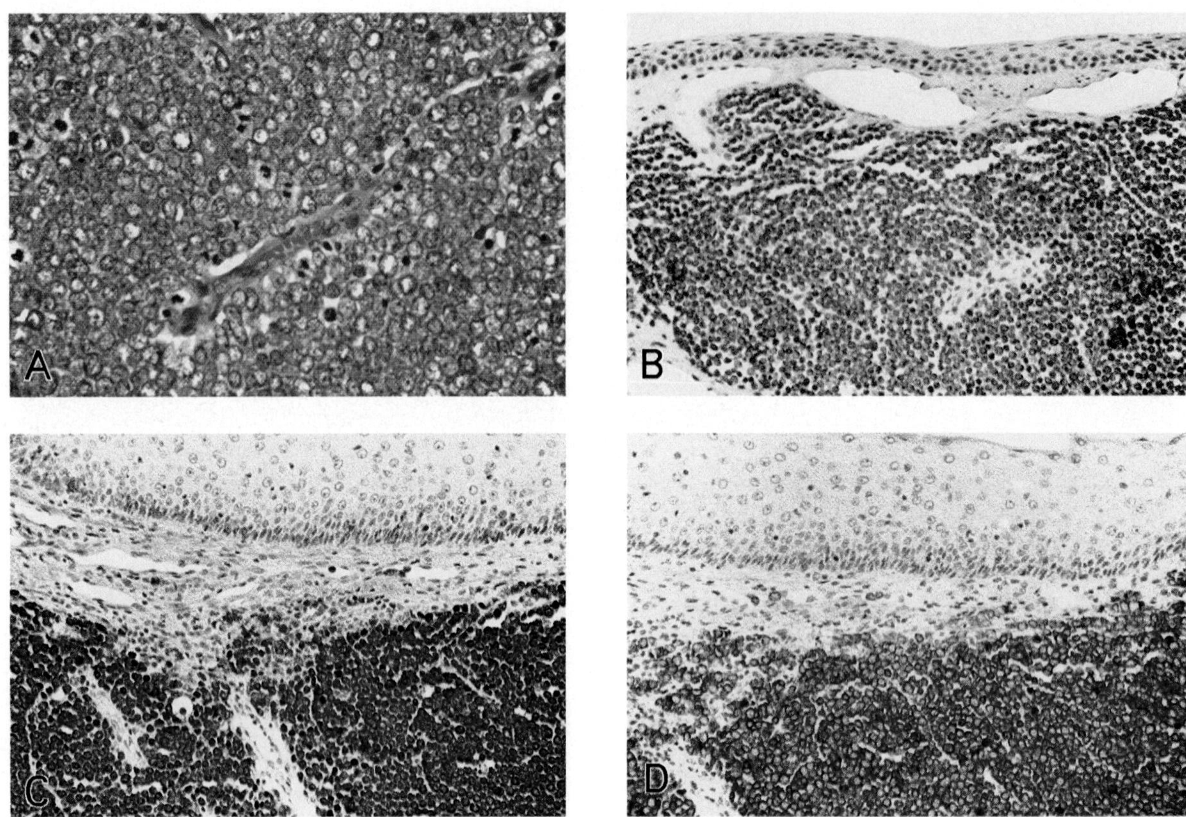

Figure 5-92

MERKEL CELL CARCINOMA

Immunoreactivity of the tumor cells for cytokeratin 20 (A), neuron-specific enolase (B), synaptophysin (C), and H&E (D).

fibrosis), the heart (cardiac decompensation and pericardial effusion), and kidneys (congenital megacalices, hydronephrosis, hydroureter, and chronic lipogranulomatous pyelonephritis). In some cases, a retroperitoneal xanthogranuloma has been reported (121).

Histopathologically, Erdheim-Chester disease is a fibrosing xanthogranulomatous process with an admixture of xanthomatous histiocytes; numerous multinucleated giant cells, mostly of the Touton type; and areas of fibrosis with collagenization (see fig. 5-86). Erdheim-Chester disease is unrelated to the histiocytosis X group of diseases. S-100 protein is positive in the histiocytes of the histiocytosis X group (121,123), in contrast to the histiocytes of other xanthogranulomatous lesions, including Erdheim-Chester disease, which fail to stain with this immunocytochemical marker.

Necrobiotic Xanthogranuloma with Paraproteinemia

Roberts and Winkelmann (124) described the ophthalmic features of *necrobiotic xanthogranuloma* in 16 patients: eyelid lesions, orbital masses, conjunctival involvement, keratitis, scleritis, episcleritis, and anterior uveitis. Although the eyelid lesions resemble xanthelasma, they are deep, firm, and indurated on palpation, and they may extend into the orbit.

There is extensive granulomatous replacement of the dermis, subcutaneous tissue, or both, with a polymorphic infiltrate composed of foamy histiocytes, multinucleated giant cells, and lymphocytes. Areas of necrobiosis of collagen are present, either as palisading granulomas surrounding necrobiotic foci or as broad bands dividing the process into lobules. A highly characteristic finding is the presence of

Table 5-11

SYSTEMIC FINDINGS OF 63 PATIENTS WITH CARNEY'S COMPLEX[a]

Systemic Finding	Number of Patients	Percent
Spotty skin pigmentation	44	70
Myxomas		
Cardiac	44	70
Skin	29	46
Breast	13	21
Cushing's syndrome	22	35
Testicular tumors	12	44
Pituitary adenoma	6	10

[a]Data from reference 130.

cholesterol clefts within the foci of necrobiotic collagen. Multinucleated Touton-type giant cells are numerous in the granulomatous areas, as well as close to the areas of necrobiotic collagen (see figs. 5-84, 5-85); foreign body–type giant cells of irregular size, shape, and nuclear grouping that have a bizarre, atypical appearance are often observed. Involvement of the subcutaneous tissues with a granulomatous panniculitis is common.

Significant but inconsistent findings are the presence of lymphoid follicles, some with prominent germinal centers; foci of plasma cells; and cholesterol clefts (125). The cytoplasm of the giant cells and histiocytes contains a PAS-positive, diastase-resistant mucopolysaccharide, often in a ring-like pattern (125). Oil red-O and Sudan IV stains demonstrate lipid droplets within the giant cells and histiocytes as well as in the areas of necrobiosis.

The histiocytic cells of the infiltrate stain with OKM1 (a marker for monocytes and null cells), MAC387 (a macrophage marker), but not for S-100 protein which differentiates these macrophages from the S-100-protein–positive cells of Langerhans cell histiocytosis and sinus histiocytosis of Rosai and Dorfman. Significant numbers of helper/inducer T cells and small numbers of suppressor/cytotoxic T cells are present; collections of B cells and an increased number of plasma cells are also described (125).

Paraproteinemia occurs in approximately 80 percent of patients. Other patients have demonstrable cryoglobulinemia, and some have evidence of complement consumption. Examination of the bone marrow occasionally reveals a lymphoproliferative disorder such as multiple myeloma or B-cell malignant lymphoma, or an increased number of atypical plasma cells.

The clinical course of necrobiotic xanthogranuloma is often chronic and gradually progressive. Treatment is difficult to assess in view of the small number of reported cases, but some reports indicate that the cutaneous and orbital lesions may respond to chemotherapy and/or steroids for the associated lymphoproliferative disorder. Radiation therapy has been reported to be effective in a patient with eyelid and orbital involvement (126).

Carney's Complex

This interesting and unusual disease complex was first recognized by Carney and his associates in 1985 (127). Children and young adults have various combinations of cutaneous and cardiac myxomas, multiple pigmented skin lesions, endocrine overactivity including Cushing's syndrome due to primary pigmented nodular adrenocortical hyperplasia, male sexual precocity associated with Sertoli or Leydig cell tumors of the testis, and acromegaly or gigantism due to growth hormone–secreting pituitary adenomas (127–129).

Kennedy and associates (130) assessed the systemic and ophthalmic findings in 63 patients (27 males and 36 females) with Carney's complex. Of these, 44 (70 percent) had facial and eyelid lentigines, 17 (27 percent) had pigmented lesions on the caruncle or conjunctival semilunar fold, and 10 (16 percent) had eyelid myxomas (Table 5-11). The pigmented lesions from this study and Carney's initial series (127) consisted histologically of a range of benign melanocytic lesions, including lentigo (hyperpigmentation of the basal layer of the epidermis, hyperplasia of melanocytes with or without elongation of rete ridges), junctional or compound nevi, ephelis, blue nevus, and combinations of the above occurring in individual patients.

Eyelid myxomas, found in up to 70 percent of patient's with Carney's complex, are single, multiple, or bilateral (131). The myxomas are nonencapsulated and consist of dermal pools of slightly basophilic ground substance (most of which is hyaluronic acid), containing widely separated stellate- and spindle-shaped cells. The differential diagnosis includes other benign and malignant neoplasms, such as peripheral nerve sheath tumors, fibrous histiocytomas, hemangiopericytomas, rhabdomyosarcomas, pleomorphic adenomas, and adnexal skin tumors. Sporadic eyelid myxomas occur as a rare tumor in patients without Carney's complex.

Other cutaneous lesions described rarely in Carney's complex include trichofolliculoma with myxoid stroma (three patients); acanthosis nigricans, milia-like keratinous cysts, and scleroderma circumscripta (morphea) (two patients each); and keratinous trichilemmal cyst (one patient) (127).

The diagnosis of Carney's complex is established by the presence of two or more of the following lesions: cardiac myxoma, cutaneous myxoma, mammary myxoid fibroadenoma, spotty mucocutaneous pigmentation, primary pigmented nodular adrenocortical hyperplasia, testicular tumors, and growth hormone–secreting pituitary adenoma. If patients present with facial/eyelid signs (pigmented lesions or myxomas), this clinical appearance should precipitate a thorough search for other findings of the complex, including cardiac myxoma, testicular tumors in males, adrenal hyperplasia, and pituitary and soft tissue tumors. Furthermore, first-degree relatives (parents, siblings, and children) should be investigated to exclude the possibility of cardiac myxomas (128–132).

METASTATIC TUMORS

Metastases to the eyelid are uncommon. The primary sites are the breast, cutaneous melanoma, lung, stomach, colon, thyroid, parotid, and trachea. Mammary carcinomas metastatic to the eyelids have a "histiocytoid" histologic appearance or more typical morphologic features of metastatic breast carcinoma. On microscopic examination, the histiocytoid tumor cells exhibit a uniform appearance, with bland, round to oval nuclei having a distinct nuclear membrane, uniform chromatin, and inconspicuous nucleoli. The cytoplasm is abundant and amphophilic, with a ground-glass appearance, and contains small and large vacuoles. The tumor cells are embedded in a ground substance containing coarse collagen fibrils. The cells are arranged singly or in small groups. Occasionally, they are arranged in rows of single cells. Mitotic figures are generally absent or sparse. These histiocytoid features may lead to misinterpretations, resulting in initial diagnoses of xanthelasma, xanthoma, histiocytoma, granular cell myoblastoma, and blastomycosis. The cytoplasmic vacuoles contain variable amounts of hyaluronidase-resistant Alcian blue–positive material that also stains vividly with the PAS and mucicarmine techniques.

Malignant tumors from various sites can metastasize to the eyelids. Breast cancer appears to be the most common primary tumor, and can involve four eyelids (133). Eyelid metastases originate in cutaneous melanoma, gastrointestinal system, esophagus, testis, choroidal melanoma, lumbosacral chordoma, osteogenic sarcoma, and renal cell carcinoma (134–146). In a series of 31 patients with metastatic disease to the eyelids, metastasis was present predominantly in women whose mean age was 69 years, and the most common sites were breast (35 percent), skin (16 percent), and gastrointestinal and urogenital tracts (10 percent each) (142). Breast carcinoma can present as lesions simulating inflammatory processes (145).

REFERENCES

Benign Epithelial Tumors

1. Boniuk M, Zimmerman LE. Eyelid tumors with reference to lesions confused with squamous cell carcinoma. II. Inverted follicular keratosis. Arch Ophthalmol 1963;69:698–707.
2. Goette DK. Benign lichenoid keratosis. Arch Dermatol 1980;116:780–2.
3. Tegner E. Solitary lichen planus simulating malignant lesions. Acta Derm Venereol 1979;59:263–6.
4. Berman A, Herszenson S, Winkelmann RK. The involuting lichenoid plaque. Arch Dermatol 1982;118:93–6.
5. Weinstock MA, Olbricht SM, Arndt KA, Kwan TH. Well-demarcated papules and plaques in sun-exposed areas. Multiple large-cell acanthomas. Arch Dermatol 1987;123:1075–6.
6. Boniuk M, Zimmerman LE. Eyelid tumors with reference to lesions confused with squamous cell carcinoma. 3. Keratoacanthoma. Arch Ophthalmol 1967;77:29–40.
7. Stewart WB, Nicholson DH, Hamilton G, Tenzel RR, Spencer WH. Eyelid tumors and renal transplantation. Arch Ophthalmol 1980;98:1771–2.

Precancerous Epithelial Lesions

8. Graham JH, Helwig EB, Johnson WC. Premalignant cutaneous and mucocutaneous diseases. In: Graham JH, Johnson WC, Helwig EB, eds. Dermal pathology. Hagerstown, MD: Harper & Row; 1972:561–624.
9. Lund HZ. How often does squamous cell carcinoma of the skin metastasize? Arch Dermatol 1965;92:635–7.
10. Graham JH, Helwig EB. Bowen's disease and its relationship to systemic cancer. AMA Arch Dermatol 1959;80:133–59.
11. Lynch HT, Anderson DE, Smith JL Jr, Howell JB, Krush AL. Xeroderma pigmentosum, malignant melanoma and congenital ichthyosis. A family study. Arch Dermatol 1967;96:625–35.
12. Guerrier CJ, Lutzner MA, Devico V, Prunieras M. An electron microscopical study of the skin in 18 cases of xeroderma pigmentosum. Dermatologia 1973;146:211–21.

Malignant Epithelial Tumors

13. Aurora AL, Blodi FC. Lesions of the eyelids. A clinicopathological study. Surv Ophthalmol 1970;15:94–104.
14. Doxanas MT, Green WR, Iliff CE. Factors in the successful surgical management of basal cell carcinoma of the eyelids. Am J Ophthalmol 1981;91:726–36.
15. Wiggs EO. Morphea-form basal cell carcinomas of the canthi. Trans Sect Ophthalmol Am Acad Ophthalmol Otolaryngol 1975;79:649–53.
16. Doxanas MT, Green WR. Adult lid lesions: basal cell carcinoma. Paper presented at the 38th meeting of the Wilmer Residents' Association, Baltimore, April 1979.
17. Farmer ER, Helwig EB. Metastatic basal cell carcinoma: a clinicopathologic study of seventeen cases. Cancer 1980;46:748–57.
18. Michel M. [Syndrome of multiple nevoid basocellular cancer.] Pediatrie 1968;23:601–3. (French.)
19. Kahn LB, Gordon W. The naevoid basal cell naevus syndrome—report of a case. S Afr Med J 1967;41:832–5.
20. Geeraets WJ. Ocular syndromes, 3rd ed. Philadelphia: Lea & Febiger; 1976:199.
21. Southwick GJ, Schwartz RA. The basal cell nevus syndrome: disasters occurring among a series of 36 patients. Cancer 1979;44:2294–305.
22. Zackheim HS, Loud AV, Howell AB. Nevoid basal cell carcinoma syndrome. Some histologic observations on the cutaneous lesions. Arch Dermatol 1966;93:317–23.
23. Mason JK, Helwig EB, Graham JH. Pathology of the nevoid basal cell carcinoma syndrome. Arch Pathol 1965;79:401–8.
24. Lederman M. Discussion of carcinomas of conjunctiva and eyelild. In: Boniuk M, ed. Ocular and adnexal tumors. St. Louis: CV Mosby; 1964:101–22.
25. Kwitko ML, Boniuk M, Zimmerman LE. Eyelid tumors with reference to lesions confused with squamous cell carcinoma. I. Incidence and errors in diagnosis. Arch Ophthalmol 1963;69:693–7.
26. Johnson WC, Helwig EB. Adenoid squamous cell carcinoma (adenoacanthoma). A clinicopathologic study of 155 patients. Cancer 1966;19:1639–50.

Melanocytic Tumors

27. Mishima Y. Macromolecular changes in pigmentary disorders. Arch Dermatol 1965;91:519–57.
28. Hashimoto K, Bale GF. An electron microscopic study of balloon cell nevus. Cancer 1972;30:530–40.

29. Schreiner E, Wolff K. [Ultrastructure of benign juvenile melanoma.] Arch Klin Exp Dermatol 1970;237:749–68. (German.)
30. Reed WB, Becker WS Sr, Becker WS Jr, Nickel WR. Giant pigmented nevi, melanoma, and leptomeningeal melanocytosis: a clinical and histopathological study. Arch Dermatol 1965;91:100–19.
31. Rodriguez HA, Ackerman LV. Cellular blue nevus. Clinicopathologic study of forty-five cases. Cancer 1968;21:393–405.
32. Blodi FC, Widner RR. The melanotic freckle (Hutchinson) of the lids. Surv Ophthalmol 1968;13:23–30.
33. Clark WH Jr, Mastrangelo MJ, Ainsworth AM, Berd D, Bellet RE, Bernardino EA. Current concepts of the biology of human cutaneous malignant melanoma. Adv Cancer Res 1977;24: 267–338.
34. Breslow A. Thickness, cross-sectional areas and depths of invasion in the prognosis of cutaneous melanoma. Ann Surg 1970;172:902–8.
35. Clark WH Jr, Mihm MC Jr. Lentigo maligna and lentigo-maligna melanoma. Am J Pathol 1969;55:39–67.
36. Grossniklaus HE, McLean IW. Cutaneous melanoma of the eyelid. Clinicopathologic features. Ophthalmology 1991;98:1867–73.
37. Tahery DP, Golberg R, Moy RL. Malignant melanoma of the eyelid. A report of eight cases and a review of the literature. J Am Acad Dermatol 1992;27:17–21.
38. Clark WH Jr, Reimer RR, Greene M, Ainsworth AM, Mastrangelo MJ. Origin of familial malignant melanoma from heritable melanocytic lesions. The B-K mole syndrome. Arch Dermatol 1978;114:732–8.

Benign Sebaceous Gland Tumors

39. Lloyd KM, Dennis M. Cowden's disease. A possible new symptom complex with multiple system involvement. Ann Intern Med 1963;58: 136–42.
40. Brownstein MH, Mehregan AH, Bikowski JB, Lupulescu A, Patterson JC. The dermatopathology of Cowden's syndrome. Br J Dermatol 1979;100:667–73.
41. Thyresson HN, Doyle JA. Cowden's disease (multiple hamartoma syndrome). Mayo Clin Proc 1981;56:179–84.
42. Finan MC, Connolly SM. Sebaceous gland tumors and systemic disease: a clinicopathologic analysis. Medicine 1984;63:232–42.
43. Cohen PR, Kohn SR, Kurzrock R. Association of sebaceous gland tumors and internal malignancy: the Muir-Torre syndrome. Am J Med 1991;90:606–13.
44. Gardner EJ. Follow-up study of family group exhibiting dominant inheritance for syndrome including intestinal polyps, osteomas, fibromas and epidermal cysts. Am J Hum Genet 1962;14:376–90.
45. Oldfield MC. The association of familial polyposis of the colon with multiple sebaceous cysts. Br J Surg 1954;41:534–41.

Sebaceous Gland Carcinoma

46. Welch RB, Duke JR. Lesions of the lids; a statistical note. Am J Ophthalmol 1958;45:415–26.
47. Ginsberg J. Present status of meibomian gland carcinoma. Arch Ophthalmol 1965;73:271–7.
48. Boniuk M, Zimmerman LE. Sebaceous carcinoma of the eyelid, eyebrow, caruncle and orbit. Trans Am Acad Ophthalmol Otolaryngol 1968;72:619–42.
49. Ni C, Kuo P. Meibomian gland carcinoma. A clinicopathological study of 156 cases with long-period follow-up of 100 cases. Jpn J Ophthalmol 1979;23:388–401.
50. Ni C, Guo BK. Pathological classification of meibomian gland carcinomas of the eyelids: clinical and pathologic study of 156 cases. Chin Med J 1979;92:671–6.
51. Ni C, Searl SS, Kuo PK, et al. Sebaceous gland carcinomas of the ocular adnexa. Int Ophthalmol Clin 1982;22:23–61.
52. Rulon DB, Helwig EB. Cutaneous sebaceous neoplasms. Cancer 1974;33:82–102.
53. Rumelt S, Hogan NR, Rubin PA, Jakobiec FA. Four-eyelid sebaceous cell carcinoma following irradiation. Arch Ophthalmol 1998;116:1670–2.
54. Rao NA, McLean IW, Zimmerman LE. Sebaceous carcinoma of the eyelids and caruncle: correlation of clinicopathologic features with prognosis. In: Jakobiec FA, ed. Ocular and adnexal tumors. Birmingham, AL: Aesculapius Publishers; 1978:461.
55. Rao NA, Hidayat AA, McLean IW, Zimmerman LE. Sebaceous carcinoma of the occular adnexa. A clinicopathologic study of 104 cases, with five-year follow-up data. Hum Pathol 1982;13:113–22.
56. Niizuma K. Lipid droplet of sebaceous carcinoma. Electron microscopic study utilizing glycol methacrylate-glutaraldehyde-urea procedure. Arch Dermatol Res 1977;260:111–9.
57. Sinard JH. Immunohistochemical distinction of ocular sebaceous carcinoma from basal cell and squamous cell carcinoma. Arch Ophthalmol 1999;117:776–83.
58. Sugiki H, Ansai S, Imaizumi T, Hozumi Y, Kondo S. Ocular sebaceous carcinoma. Two unusual cases, and their histochemical and immunohistochemical findings. Dermatology 1996;192:364–7.

59. Niu Y, Zhou Z, Liu F, Wang H. Expression of P16 protein and Bcl-2 protein in malignant eyelid tumors. Chin Med J 2002;115:21–5.
60. Gonzalez-Fernandez F, Kaltreider SA, Patnaik BD, et al. Sebaceous carcinoma. Tumor progression through mutational inactivation of p53. Ophthalmology 1998;105:497–506.
61. Cho KJ, Khang SK, Koh JS, Chung JH, Lee SS. Sebaceous carcinoma of the eyelids: frequent expression of c-erB-2 oncoprotein. J Korean Med Sci 2000;15:545–50.
62. Yen MT, Tse DT, Wu X, Wolfson AH. Radiation therapy for local control of eyelid sebaceous cell carcinoma: report of two cases and review of the literature. Ophthal Plast Reconstr Surg 2000;16:211–5.

Tumors of Eccrine and Apocrine Glands

63. Hashimoto K, Gross BG, Lever WF. Syringoma. Histochemical and electron microscopic studies. J Invest Dermatol 1966;46:150–66.
64. Hashimoto K, DiBella RJ, Borsuk GM, Lever WF. Eruptive hidradenoma and syringoma. Histological, histochemical, and electron microscopic studies. Arch Dermatol 1967;96:500–19.
65. Daicker B, Gafner E. Apocrine mixed tumour of the lid. Ophthalmologica 1975;170:548–53.
66. Boniuk M, Halpert B. Clear cell hidradenoma or myoepithelioma of the eyelid. Arch Ophthalmol 1964;72:59–63.
67. Ferry AP, Haddad HM. Eccrine acrospiroma (porosyringoma) of the eyelid. Arch Ophthalmol 1970;83:591–3.
68. Hashimoto K, DiBella RJ, Lever WF. Clear cell hidradenoma. Histologic, histochemical and electron microscopic studies. Arch Dermatol 1967;96:18–38.
69. Wright JD, Font RL. Mucinous sweat gland adenocarcinoma of eyelid: a clinicopathologic study of 21 cases with histochemical and electron microscopic observations. Cancer 1979;44:1757–68.
70. Wick MR, Swanson PE. Primary adenoid cystic carcinoma of the skin. A clinical, histological, and immunocytochemical comparison with adenoid cystic carcinoma of salivary glands and adenoid basal cell carcinoma. Am J Dermatopathol 1986;8:2–13.
71. Rosen Y, Kim B, Yermakov VA. Eccrine sweat gland tumor of clear cell origin involving the eyelids. Cancer 1975;36:1034–41.
72. Grizzard WS, Torezynski E, Edwards WC. Adenocarcinoma of eccrine sweat glands. Arch Ophthalmol 1976;94:2119–23.
73. Jakobiec FA, Austin P, Iwamoto T, Trokel SL, Marguardt MD, Harrison W. Primary infiltrating signet ring carcinoma of the eyelids. Ophthalmology 1983;90:291–9.
74. Steinbrecher JS, Silverberg SG. Signet-ring cell carcinoma of the breast. The mucinous variant of infiltrating lobular carcinoma? Cancer 1976;37:828–40.
75. Aurora AL, Luxenberg MN. Case report of adenocarcinoma of glands of Moll. Am J Ophthalmol 1970;70:984–90.
76. Ni C, Wagoner M, Kieval S, Albert DM. Tumours of the Moll's glands. Br J Ophthalmol 1984;68:502–6.
77. Futrell JW, Krueger GR, Chretien PB, Ketcham S. Multiple primary sweat gland carcinomas. Cancer 1971;28:688–91.
78. Shintaku M, Tsuta K, Yoshida H, Tsubura A, Nakashima Y, Noda K. Apocrine adenocarcinoma of the eyelid with aggressive biological behavior: report of a case. Pathol Int 2002;52:169–73.

Tumors of the Pilar Structures

79. Wolken SH, Spivey BE, Blodi FC. Hereditary adenoid cystic epithelioma (Brooke's tumor). Am J Ophthalmol 1968;68:26–34.
80. Gray HR, Helwig EB. Trichofolliculoma. Arch Dermatol 1962;86:619–25.
81. Hidayat AA, Font RL. Trichilemmoma of eyelid and eyebrow. A clinicopathologic study of 31 cases. Arch Ophthalmol 1980;98:844–7.
82. Boniuk M, Zimmerman LE. Pilomatrixoma (benign calcifying epithelioma) of the eyelids and eyebrow. Arch Ophthalmol 1963;70:399–406.
83. Hardisson D, Linares MD, Cuevas-Santos J, Contreras F. Pilomatrix carcinoma: a clinicopathologic study of six cases and review of the literature. Am J Dermatopathol 2001;23:394–401.
84. McGavran MH. Ultrastructure of pilomatrixoma (calcifying epithelioma). Cancer 1965;18:1445–56.

Vascular Tumors

85. Tompkins VN, Walsh TS Jr. Some observations on the strawberry nevus of infants. Cancer 1956;9:869–904.
86. Margileth AM, Museles M. Current concepts in diagnosis and management of congenital cutaneous hemangiomas. Pediatrics 1965;36:410–6.
87. Hiles DA, Pilchard WA. Corticosteroid control of neonatal hemangiomas of the orbit and ocular adnexa. Am J Ophthalmol 1971;71:1003–8.
88. Kushner BJ. Intralesional corticosteroid injection for infantile adnexal hemangioma. Am J Ophthalmol 1982;93:496–506.

89. Kasabach HH, Merritt KK. Capillary hemangioma with extensive purpura. Report of a case. Am J Dis Child 1940;59:1063–70.
90. Bean WB. Vascular spiders and related lesions of the skin. Springfield, Ill: Charles C Thomas; 1958.
91. Bean WB. Dyschondroplasia and hemangiomata (Maffucci's syndrome). II. AMA Arch Intern Med 1958;102:544–50.
92. Jones IS, Jakobiec FA. Vascular tumors, malformations and degenerations. In: Jones IS, Jakobiec FA, eds. Diseases of the orbit. Hagerstown, MD, Harper & Row; 1979:269–308.
93. Saxe SJ, Grossniklaus HE, Wojno TH, Hertzler GL, Boniuk M, Font RL. Glomus cell tumor of the eyelild. Ophthalmology 1993;100:139–43.
94. Girard C, Johnson WC, Graham JH. Cutaneous angiosarcomas. Cancer 1970;26:868–83.
95. Rosai J, Sumner HW, Kostianovsky M, Perez-Mesa C. Angiosarcoma of the skin. A clinicopathologic and fine ultrastructural study. Hum Pathol 1976;7:83–109.

Xanthomatous Lesions

96. John T, Yanoff M, Scheie HG. Eyelid fibrous histiocytoma. Ophthalmology 1981;88:1193–5.
97. Zimmerman LE. Ocular lesions of juvenile xanthogranuloma. Nevoxanthoendothelioma. Am J Ophthalmol 1965;60:1011–35.
98. Zamir E, Wang RC, Krishnakumar S, Aiello Leverant A, Dugel PU, Rao NA. Juvenile xanthogranuloma masquerading as pediatric chronic uveitis: a clinicopathologic study. Surv Ophthalmol 2001;46:164–71.
99. Newell GB, Stone OJ, Mullins JF. Juvenile xanthogranuloma and neurofibromatosis. Arch Dermatol 1973;107:262.
100. Charlin C, Fernandez FL. Le syndrome d'Urbach-Wiethe. Arch Ophtalmol (Paris) 1975;35:521–6.
101. Hashimoto K, Klingmuller G, Rodermund OE. Hyalinosis cutis et mucosae. An electron microscopic study. Acta Dermatol 1972;52:179–95.

Miscellaneous Lesions

102. Stenson S, Ramsay DL. Ocular findings in mycosis fungoides. Arch Ophthalmol 1981;99:272–7.
103. Flaxman BA, Zelazny G, van Scott EJ. Nonspecificity of characteristic cells in mycosis fungoides. Arch Dermatol 1971;104:141–7.
104. Lutzner MA, Hobbs JW, Horvath P. Ultrastructure of abnormal cells in Sezary syndrome, mycosis fungoides and parapsoriasis en plaque. Arch Dermatol 1971;103:375–86.
105. Liebow AA, Carrington CR, Friedman PJ. Lymphomatoid granulomatosis. Hum Pathol 1972;3:457–8.
106. Katzenstein AL, Carrington CB, Liebow AA. Lymphomatoid granulomatosis: a clinicopathologic study of 152 cases. Cancer 1979;43:360–73.
107. Font RL, Rosenbaum PS, Smith JL Jr. Lymphomatoid granulomatous of eyelid and brow with progression to lymphoma. J Am Acad Dermatol 1990;23(Pt 2):334–7.
108. Enzinger FM, Weiss SW. Benign tumors and tumor-like lesions of blood vessels. In Enzinger FM, Weiss SW, eds. Soft tissue tumors. St. Louis: CV Mosby Co; 1983:379–421.
109. Wirman JA. Nodular fasciitis, a lesion of myofibroblasts: an ultrastructural study. Cancer 1976;38:2378–89.
110. Hidayat AA, Font RL. Juvenile fibromatosis of the periorbital region and eyelid. A clinicopathologic study of six cases. Arch Ophthalmol 1980;98:280–5.
111. Zimmerman LE. Phakomatous choristoma of the eyelid. A tumor of lenticular anlage. Am J Ophthalmol 1971;1(Pt 1):169–77.
112. Ellis FJ, Eagle RC Jr, Shields JA, Shields CL, Fessler JN, Takemoto LJ. Phakomatous choristoma (Zimmerman's tumor). Immunohistochemical confirmation of lens-specific proteins. Ophthalmology 1993;100:955–60.
113. Blodi FC. Unusual myogenic tumors around the eye. AMA Arch Ophthalmol 1956;56:698–701.
114. Friedman Z, Eden E, Neumann E. Granular cell myoblastoma of the eyelid margin. Br J Ophthalmol 1973;57:757–60.
115. Rubenzik R, Tenzel RR. Granular cell myoblastoma of the lid: case report. Ann Ophthalmol 1976;8:421–2.
116. Singh AD, Eagle RC Jr, Shields CL, Shields JA. Merkel cell carcinoma of the eyelids. Int Ophthalmol Clin 1993;33:11–7.
117. Beyer CK, Goodman M, Dickersin GR, Dougherty M. Merkel cell tumor of the eyelid. A clinicopathologic case report. Arch Ophthalmol 1983;101:1098–101.
118. Warner TF, Uno H, Hafez GR, et al. Merkel cells and Merkel cell tumors. Ultrastructure, immunocytochemistry and review of the literature. Cancer 1983;52:238–45.
119. Masson P. Hemangioendothelioma vegetant intravasculaire. Bull Soc Anat Paris 1923;93:517–23.
120. Font RL, Wheeler TM, Boniuk M. Intravascular papillary endothelial hyperplasia of the orbit and ocular adnexa. A report of five cases. Arch Ophthalmol 1983;101:1731–6.
121. Simpson FG, Robinson PJ, Hardy GJ, Losowsky MS. Erdheim-Chester disease associated with retroperitoneal xanthogranuloma. Br J Radiol 1979;52:232–5.

122. Weiss SW, Langloss JM, Enzinger FM. Value of S-100 protein in the diagnosis of soft tissue tumors with particular reference to benign and malignant Schwann cell tumors. Lab Invest 1983;49:299–308.
123. Kahn HJ, Marks A, Thom H, Baumal R. Role of antibody to S100 protein in diagnostic pathology. Am J Clin Pathol 1983;79:341–7.
124. Robertson DM, Winkelmann RK. Ophthalmic features of necrobiotic xanthogranuloma with paraproteinemia. Am J Ophthalmol 1984;97:173–83.
125. Finan MC, Winkelman RK. Histopathology of necrobiotic xanthogranuloma with paraproteinemia. J Cutan Pathol 1987;14:92–9.
126. Char DH, LeBoit PE, Ljung BM, Wara W. Radiation therapy for ocular necrobiotic xanthogranuloma. Arch Ophthalmol 1987;105:174–5.
127. Carney JA, Gordon H, Carpenter PC, Shenov BV, Go VL. The complex of myxomas, spotty pigmentation, and endocrine overactivity. Medicine (Baltimore) 1985;64:270–83.
128. Carney JA, Hruska LA, Beaushamp GD, Gordon H. Dominant inheritance of the complex of myxomas, spotty pigmentation, and endocrine overactivity. Mayo Clin Proc 1986;61:165–72.
129. Carney JA, Headington JT, Su WP. Cutaneous myxomas. A major component of the complex of myxomas, spotty pigmentation, and endocrine overactivity. Arch Dermatol 1986;122:790–8.
130. Kennedy RH, Waller RR, Carney JA. Ocular pigmented spots and eyelid myxomas. Am J Opthalmol 1987;104:533–8.
131. Kennedy RH, Flanagan JC, Eagle RC Jr, Carney JA. The Carney complex with ocular signs suggestive of cardiac myxoma. Am J Ophthalmol 1991;111:699–702.
132. Wallace TM, Levin HS, Ratliff NB, Hobbs RE. Evaluation and management of Carney's complex: an illustrative case. Clin J Med 1991;58:248–50, 255–6.

Metastatic Tumors

133. Douglas RS, Goldstein SM, Einhorn E, Ibarra MS, Gausas RE. Metastatic breast cancer to 4 eyelids: a clinicopathologic report. Cutis 2002;70:291–3.
134. Hartstein ME, Biesman B, Kincaid MC. Cutaneous malignant melanoma metastatic to the eyelid. Ophthalmic Surg Lasers 1998;29:993–5.
135. Bachymeyer C, Alovor G, Chatelain D, et al. Cystic metastasis of the pancreas indicating relapse of Merkel cell carcinoma. Pancreas 2002;24:103–5.
136. Kuchle M, Holbach L, Schlotzer-Schrehardt U. Gastric adenocarcinoma presenting as an eyelid and conjunctival mass. Eur J Ophthalmol 1992;2:3–9.
137. Esmaeli B, Cleary KL, Ho L, Safar S, Prieto VG. Leiomyosarcoma of the esophagus metastatic to the eyelid: a clinicopathologic report. Ophthal Plast Reconstr Surg 2002;18:159–61.
138. Ham JA, Carr NJ. Testicular cancer presenting as a red swollen lid. Br J Ophthalmol 1988;72:868–70.
139. Shields JA, Shields CL, Shakin EP, Kobetz LE. Metastasis of choroidal melanoma to the contralateral choroid, orbit, and eyelid. Br J Ophthalmol 1988;72:456–60.
140. Malone TJ, Folberg R, Nerad JA. Lumbosacral chordoma metastatic to the eyelid. Ophthalmology 1987;94:966–70.
141. Newman NM, DiLoreto DA. Metastasis of primary osteogenic sarcoma to the eyelid. Am J Ophthalmol 1987;104:659–60.
142. Mansour AM, Hidayat AA. Metastatic eyelid disease. Ophthalmology 1987;94:667–70.
143. Arnold AC, Bullock JD, Foos RY. Metastatic eyelid carcinoma. Ophthalmology 1985;92:114–9.
144. Castro PA, Albert DM, Wang WJ, Ni C. Tumors metastatic to the eye and adnexa. Int Ophthalmol Clin 1982;22:189–223.
145. Mottow-Lippa L, Jakobiec FA, Iwamoto T. Pseudoinflammatory metastatic breast carcinoma of the orbit and lids. Ophthalmology 1981;88:575–80.
146. Kindermann WR, Shields JA, Eiferman RA, Stephens RF, Hirsch SE. Metastatic renal cell carcinoma to the eye and adnexae: a report of three cases and review of the literature. Ophthalmology 1981;88:1347–50.

6 TUMORS OF THE LACRIMAL GLAND

ANATOMY AND HISTOLOGY

The lacrimal gland is a nonencapsulated, multilobulated, secretory structure located in the lacrimal gland fossa behind the supertemporal orbital rim. The lateral edge of the levator palpebrae aponeurosis divides the lacrimal gland into a superficial, palpebral, subconjunctival lobe and a deeper orbital lobe. The gland develops superolaterally from solid epithelial evaginated cords of conjunctiva. The lacrimal gland tissue consists of ectodermal glandular units surrounded by mesenchymal myoepithelial and fibrous tissue. Differentiation of the lacrimal gland is completed 3 or 4 years postnatally. The normal weight of the lacrimal gland in the adult is 6 to 10 g, and it measures 2.0 x 1.2 x 0.5 cm.

Histologically, the lacrimal gland is divided into acini and ducts (fig. 6-1). The secretory acini consist of cuboidal zymogen-bearing cells, surrounded externally by myoepithelial cells. Individual acini and lobules of acini are separated from each other by intralobular and interlobular connective tissue. Mucus-secreting cells are not present. The interlobular ducts converge into main ducts that open into the supertemporal fornix. Plasma cells and lymphocytes are lightly dispersed among the secretory acini of the lacrimal gland. Occasionally, small lymphoid aggregates without well-defined germinal centers are observed. The plasma cells of the lacrimal gland secrete immunoglobulin (Ig)A, which binds to a secretory piece during the passage across the ducts of the gland. Approximately 40 percent of the lymphocytes present in the normal lacrimal gland are T cells. A thin layer of connective tissue, or pseudocapsule, facilitates the distinction of the lacrimal gland from the surrounding orbital tissues.

The lacrimal artery, a branch of the ophthalmic artery, provides the blood supply to the lacrimal gland. Several anastomoses exist between this system from the internal carotid artery and the external carotid system. The venous system drains into the superior ophthalmic vein. The lymphatic channels drain into the regional preauricular and cervical lymph nodes.

In addition to the main lacrimal gland, accessory lacrimal glands are present as the glands of Krause, found along the conjunctival fornices, and the glands of Wolfring, found along the superior tarsal border of the upper eyelid. Lobules of secretory units may be found within the caruncle (Popoff glands).

CLASSIFICATION AND FREQUENCY

Lesions and tumors of the lacrimal gland comprise 5 to 18 percent of all orbital masses studied histologically (1,2). Lacrimal gland lesions are basically grouped into epithelial and nonepithelial lesions, the relative frequencies of which have varied through the years. Currently, nonepithelial lesions represent approximately two thirds of biopsied lacrimal gland masses (1,3). These nonepithelial lesions include inflammatory diseases and infections.

Although lacrimal and salivary glands differ in embryologic origin, and because lacrimal gland tumors are relatively much less common,

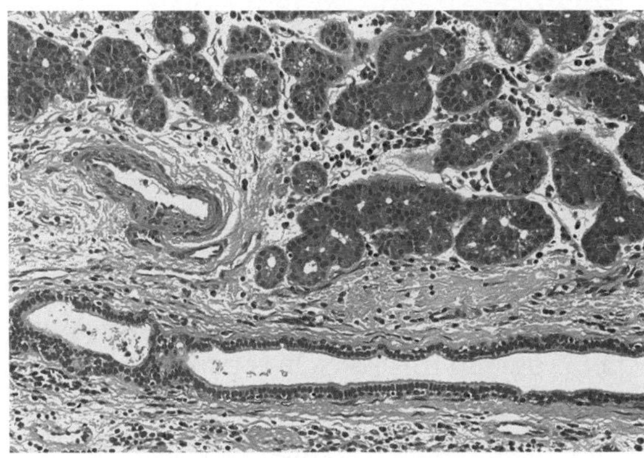

Figure 6-1

NORMAL LACRIMAL GLAND

Acini with periodic acid–Schiff (PAS)-positive granules (zymogen) and ducts.

Table 6-1

CLASSIFICATION OF LACRIMAL GLAND TUMORS

Benign Epithelial Tumors
- Pleomorphic adenoma (mixed tumor)
- Oncocytoma (oxyphilic adenoma)
- Warthin's tumor (papillary cystadenoma lymphomatosum)
- Myoepithelioma

Malignant Epithelial Tumors
- Adenoid cystic carcinoma
- Malignant mixed tumor (carcinoma in pleomorphic adenoma)
- Adenocarcinoma (not otherwise specified)
- Basal cell adenocarcinoma
- Acinic cell carcinoma
- Ductal adenocarcinoma
- Cystadenocarcinoma
- Polymorphous low-grade carcinoma
- Mucinous adenocarcinoma
- Mucoepidermoid carcinoma
- Squamous cell carcinoma
- Spindle cell carcinoma
- Carcinosarcoma
- Sebaceous carcinoma
- Epithelial-myoepithelial carcinoma
- Lymphoepithelioma-like carcinoma
- Oncocytic carcinoma

Lymphoid Tumors
- Reactive lymphoid hyperplasia
- Malignant lymphoma

Mesenchymal Tumors
- Hemangioma
- Hemangiopericytoma
- Neurofibroma and schwannoma
- Solitary fibrous tumor
- Lipoma

Secondary and Metastatic Tumors

Tumor-Like Conditions
- Chronic dacryoadenitis
- Benign lymphoepithelial lesion
- Inflammatory pseudotumor
- Lacrimal duct cyst (dacryops)
- Ectopic lacrimal gland

the classification of epithelial tumors is based on salivary gland tumors (4,5). The classification scheme used in this Fascicle is mainly based on the histologic features seen by light microscopy following the World Health Organization (WHO) classification of salivary gland tumors (6). Table 6-1 is a comprehensive list of published tumors of the lacrimal gland. The cellular classification shown in Table 6-2 also parallels that of salivary gland tumors.

Table 6-2

CELLULAR CLASSIFICATION OF MALIGNANT LACRIMAL GLAND TUMORS

Low-Grade Malignancies
- Acinic cell carcinoma
- Mucoepidermoid carcinoma (grades I or II)
- Basal cell adenocarcinoma
- Polymorphous low-grade carcinoma
- Cystadenocarcinoma
- Mucinous adenocarcinoma
- Epithelial-myoepithelial carcinoma

High-Grade Malignancies
- Adenoid cystic carcinoma
- Carcinoma in pleomorphic adenoma
- Adenocarcinoma
- Ductal adenocarcinoma
- Mucoepidermoid carcinoma (grade III)
- Squamous cell carcinoma
- Carcinosarcoma

Regarding the frequency of primary epithelial tumors, most reported series were collected at referral centers; thus, a bias towards more unusual or difficult cases is implied (Table 6-3). In recent series, the reported incidence of true primary epithelial tumors ranged from 21 to 39 percent (1,7,8), of which 29 to 55 percent were malignant epithelial tumors (7,9). Malignant neoplasms of the lacrimal gland appear to be more common in some Asian populations (10). The most frequent primary epithelial tumors are benign pleomorphic adenoma and malignant adenoid cystic carcinoma. Epithelial tumors of the lacrimal glands are extremely rare in children under the age of 10 years; during the second decade, pleomorphic adenoma and adenoid cystic carcinoma may be observed (11).

Early detection and proper diagnosis of malignant lacrimal gland tumors influence the management, prognosis, and survival of the patient. An adequate initial approach to benign and malignant epithelial tumors of the lacrimal gland influences life expectancy. Duration of more than 10 months, absence of pain, and the demonstration by computerized tomography (CT) of a smoothly contoured, expanding, round globular mass without calcification favor a benign epithelial tumor, and an excisional biopsy of the entire, intact lacrimal gland should be performed (12). Painful tumors of shorter duration that are associated with calcification and invasion of bone are suggestive of a carcinoma and favor

Table 6-3

FREQUENCY OF LACRIMAL GLAND TUMORS

	Font & Gamel 1978 (9) No. (%)	Shields et al. 1989 (1) No. (%)	Ni et al. 1992 (10) No. (%)	Wright et al. 1992 (7) No. (%)	Henderson 1994 (13) No. (%)	Font et al. 1998 (8) No. (%)
Epithelial						
Benign pleomorphic adenoma	136 (51)[a]	17 (53)	140 (52)	78 (61)	25 (38)	17 (38)
Myoepithelioma	–	–	2 (1)	–	–	–
Malignant						
Malignant mixed tumor	34 (13)	3 (9)	25 (9)	6 (5)	10 (15)	7 (16)
Adenoid cystic carcinoma	70 (26)	2 (6)	68 (25)	38 (30)	22 (33)	12 (27)
Adenocarcinoma (de novo)[b]	25 (9)	2 (6)	–	4 (3)	5 (7)	2 (4)
Others	–	–	37 (13)[c]	2[d] (2)	4[e] (6)	3[f] (7)
Cysts (Dacryops)	NS[g]	8 (25)	NS	NS	NS	4 (9)
Total epithelial (%)[h]	265	32 (23)	272 (70)	128	66	45 (37)
Nonepithelial						
Inflammatory	NS	90	NS	NS	NS	58
Lymphoid	NS	19	NS	NS	NS	17
Nonspecified	NS	1	NS	NS	NS	NS
Total nonepithelial (%)[h]	–	110 (77)	118 (30)	–	–	75 (63)
Total	265	142	390	128	66	120

[a]Percent of epithelial tumors.
[b]Not otherwise specified.
[c]Polymorphous low-grade carcinoma (3), carcinosarcoma (1).
[d]Squamous cell carcinoma (1), mucoepidermoid carcinoma (1).
[e]Squamous cell carcinoma (2), mucoepidermoid carcinoma (2).
[f]Metastatic.
[g]NS = not stated.
[h]Percent of all lacrimal gland lesions.

an incisional biopsy followed by complete resection of affected tissues and radiotherapy (7).

The simultaneous (synchronous) or "temporally displaced" (metachronous) presentation of epithelial tumors of the lacrimal and salivary glands is a rare event (14a). The tumors may represent pleomorphic adenomas or carcinomas. Patients with tumors of the lacrimal gland that metastasize to the parotid gland appear to have a better prognosis than those with a primary tumor of the parotid gland and dissemination to the lacrimal gland.

BENIGN EPITHELIAL TUMORS

Pleomorphic Adenoma (Benign Mixed Tumor)

Definition. *Pleomorphic adenoma* is a well-circumscribed benign tumor characterized by a pleomorphic or mixed appearance of proliferated epithelial ducts and myxoid, mucoid, or cartilaginous areas containing myoepithelial cells. The tumor appears to arise from a progenitor ductal cell capable of both epithelial and myoepithelial differentiation (15).

General Features. Pleomorphic adenoma is the most common epithelial tumor of the lacrimal gland and constitutes more than 50 percent of primary tumors. It usually arises from the orbital lobe (90 percent) (12), occasionally from the palpebral lobe of the main lacrimal gland (10 percent) (16,17), and rarely from accessory lacrimal glands (18). The tumor may develop at any age, but the average age of patients at presentation is at about 40 years, with a range of 6 to 79 years (12,19,20). There is neither sex nor side predilection.

Clinical Features. Most patients present with a slowly progressive, painless mass at the supertemporal orbit (fig. 6-2). The eye is usually displaced downward and inward. The mean

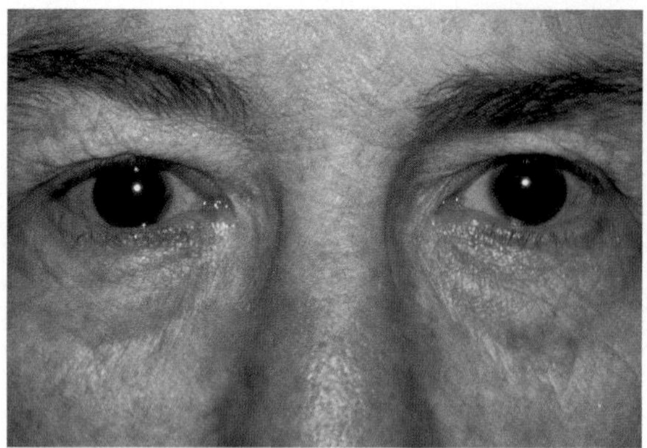

Figure 6-2

PLEOMORPHIC ADENOMA

Tumor of the right lacrimal gland.

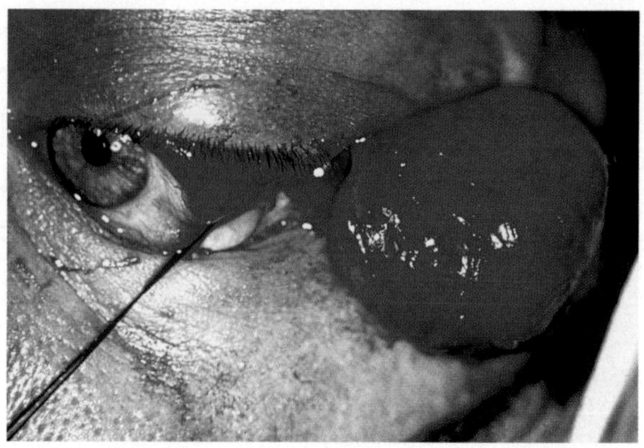

Figure 6-4

PLEOMORPHIC ADENOMA

An encapsulated nodular mass is seen at surgery.

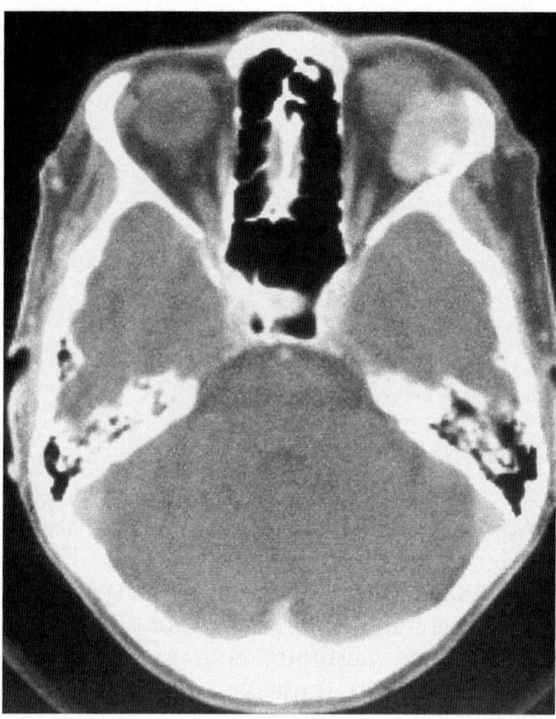

Figure 6-3

PLEOMORPHIC ADENOMA

Axial computerized tomography (CT) scan shows a well-encapsulated oval mass without bone involvement.

duration of symptoms before consultation is approximately 2 years. Patients with orbital lobe tumors have a shorter duration of symptoms. CT scans and magnetic resonance imaging (MRI) show a well-delimited, round to oval mass that may indent and erode the adjacent bone but not produce irregular destruction (fig. 6-3) (21–23). Radiologic evidence of calcification is rare (12).

Gross Findings. Pleomorphic adenomas are pseudoencapsulated, smooth surfaced, "knobby" tumors (fig. 6-4). The cut surface shows alternating mucinous and fibrous areas with occasional cystic structures. A layer of compressed connective tissue surrounds the tumor and focal small tumor projections referred as "bosselations" (fig. 6-5). These projections should be differentiated from small ruptures during the surgical procedure (fig. 6-6).

Microscopic Findings. The characteristic features are the presence of epithelium-lined duct-like structures and an outer layer of darker myoepithelial cells (fig. 6-7). The size of the duct lumen is variable and may contain inspissated, eosinophilic, periodic acid–Schiff (PAS)-positive material. Mucoid, basophilic material accumulates among the myoepithelial cells, between the epithelial duct-like structures. In some instances, foci of chondroid-like material and even calcification are observed. Variations of this general pattern may occur. The epithelial cells may form solid cords and even show foci of squamous transformation and cysts. In some cases, most of the tumor is represented by spindle-shaped myoepithelial cells, which are clearly differentiated from the cuboidal, eosinophilic, epithelial duct-lining cells. Extracellular fibrillar deposits resembling amyloid and crystalline structures of oxalate or tyrosine may be found in the tumor

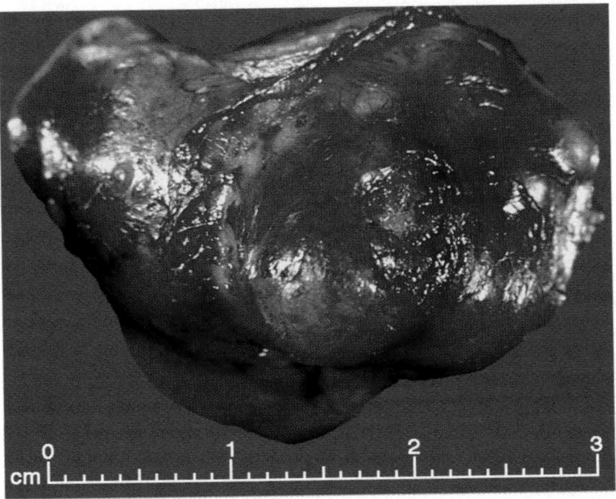

Figure 6-5

PLEOMORPHIC ADENOMA

Focal tumor expansion (bosselation) under the thick connective tissue capsule.

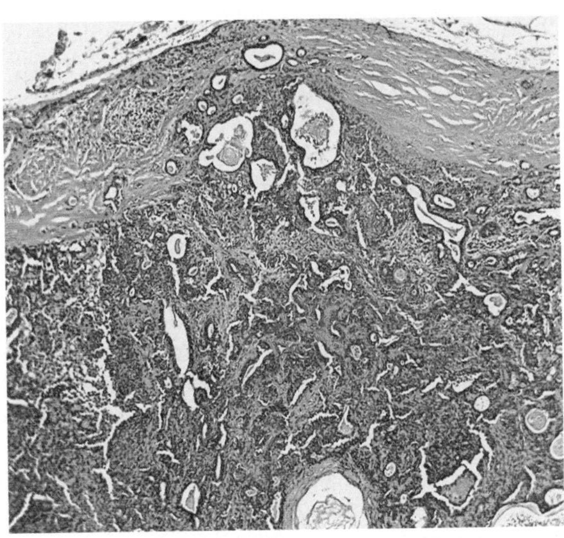

Figure 6-6

PLEOMORPHIC ADENOMA

Multinodular mass with a small rupture of the capsule on the right.

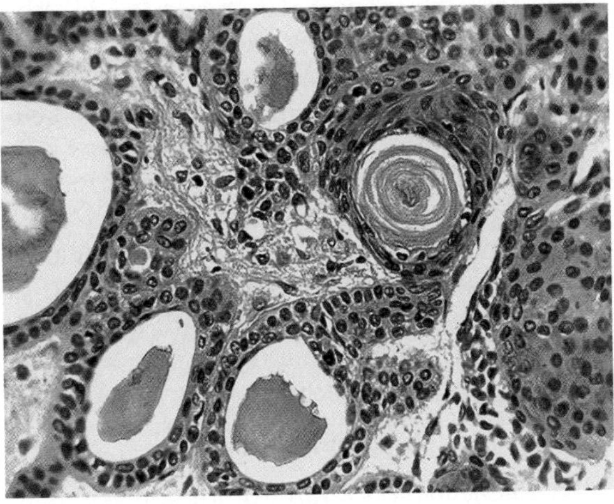

Figure 6-7

PLEOMORPHIC ADENOMA

Ducts are lined by cuboidal epithelial cells and myxoid stroma.

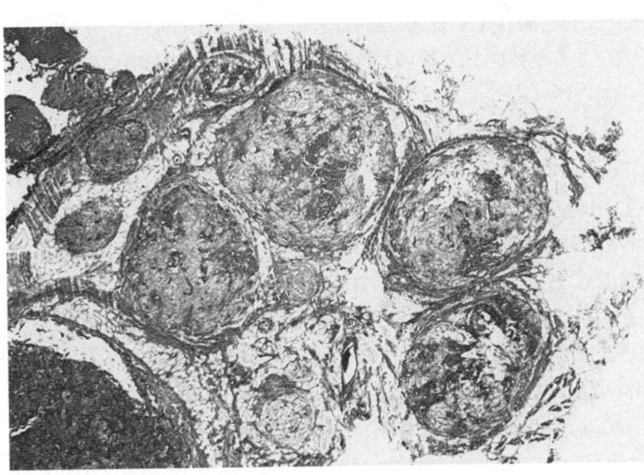

Figure 6-8

RECURRENT PLEOMORPHIC ADENOMA

Multiple, pale-stained nodules within the orbital fat.

matrix. The recurrent tumor has the same growth pattern as the original (fig. 6-8).

Immunohistochemical Findings. Cytokeratin is expressed in epithelial cells and occasionally in myoepithelial cells (24). Muscle-specific antigen may stain stromal myoepithelial cells. A few myoepithelial cells express glial fibrillary acidic protein (GFAP).

Ultrastructural Findings. The epithelial cell lining of the ducts resembles that of the normal intralobular ducts, but with fewer secretory granules (15). The outer, darker myoepithelial cells retain epithelial features, with focal myofilament bundles at the cell periphery, attachment plaques, and intercellular junctions.

Cytologic Findings. Fine-needle aspiration biopsy is rarely indicated for the diagnosis of pleomorphic adenoma of the lacrimal gland (25,26). Examination of imprints or squash preparations reveals a cellular tumor with a chondromyxoid background and epithelial cells intermingled with mesenchymal cells in a fibrillary matrix. The epithelial cells have round nuclei surrounded by pale cytoplasm. The nuclei of stromal cells are oval or elongated.

Differential Diagnosis. The microscopic diagnosis of pleomorphic adenoma is simple. The few myoepithelial adenomas and oncocytic adenomas of the lacrimal gland are easily differentiated from pleomorphic adenoma. Solid duct-like or squamous epithelial areas may suggest malignant change; however, these focal features in an otherwise typical pleomorphic adenoma do not have prognostic significance. Similarly, the focal small projections at the periphery of the tumor (bosselations) should not be interpreted as malignant invasion.

Special Studies. Pleomorphic adenomas are DNA diploid tumors with low expression of the *p53* gene (27). *P21ras* expression is apparently related to progression of pleomorphic adenoma (28). One study showed recurrent chromosomal abnormalities involving chromosomes 3, 8, 9, and 12, similar to those found in salivary gland tumors (29,30).

Treatment and Prognosis. The sensitivity of preoperative clinical and radiologic diagnosis of pleomorphic adenoma of the lacrimal gland is approximately 90 percent (12). Pleomorphic adenomas of the orbital lobe of the lacrimal gland should be removed intact, including an adequate margin of normal tissue, via a lateral orbitotomy, without previous incisional biopsy. Tumors of the palpebral lobe are excised through a transseptal approach. The overall 15-year recurrence rate is less than 3 percent if the tumor is totally removed at the initial surgery, in contrast to 32 percent if the tumor is biopsied prior to removal (9,12). Despite the observation of recurrences, the survival rate at 15 years is almost 100 percent (12). Longstanding, recurrent, and incompletely excised tumors may undergo malignant transformation. The actuarial estimate of malignant transformation is 10 percent by 20 years after initial treatment and 20 percent by 30 years (9).

Oncocytoma (Oncocytic Adenoma, Oxyphilic Adenoma)

Oncocytomas are epithelial tumors composed of cells of large size with finely granular acidophilic cytoplasm that, by electron microscopy and immunohistochemical studies, are extremely rich in mitochondria. Based on the histologic features, these lesions are designated *oncocytic hyperplasia, oncocytic adenoma,* and *oncocytic carcinoma*. Oxyphilic cells may be present as part of other epithelial tumors. Oncocytic adenoma and carcinoma of the main and accessory lacrimal glands are exceedingly rare (31–33): less than 10 cases have been reported, and only 1 was considered malignant (34).

Warthin's Tumor (Adenolymphoma)

Warthin's tumor is a benign neoplasm composed of cystic, papillary, epithelial structures associated with a variable amount of lymphoid cells. Although Warthin's tumor accounts for approximately 10 percent of epithelial neoplasms of the salivary glands, only two cases, one in the lacrimal grand and another from the eyelid, have been reported in the eye (35,36). The lacrimal gland tumor was observed in a 62-year-old woman with a 2-year history of painless exophthalmos (35). CT scan disclosed a well-circumscribed, round, cyst-like mass. Microscopically, the epithelial component consisted of solid and cystic spaces that contained papillae lined by columnar cells with abundant eosinophilic cytoplasm. The lymphoid elements consisted of lymphocytes and plasma cells with a focal follicular arrangement. Treatment was complete excision, and no recurrences were observed.

Myoepithelioma

Myoepithelioma is a rare tumor composed almost exclusively of myoepithelial cells and characterized by several growth patterns. Some authors suggest that pleomorphic adenoma, pure epithelial adenoma, and myoepithelioma originate from a common cell precursor (36a,36b). By definition, predominantly myoepithelial tumors with prominent epithelial duct proliferation (more than 10 percent) are considered myoepithelial adenomas, a subset of pleomorphic adenomas (37). A few proven cases of myoepithelioma of the lacrimal gland have been published (38–41). A review of the reported cases reveals that the age at presentation ranges from 23 to 77 years. The lesions are well-circumscribed, apparently encapsulated, nodular masses with a white-yellow cut surface (fig. 6-9).

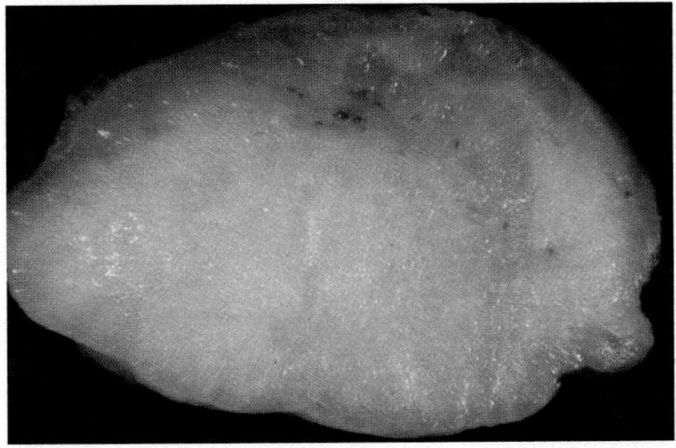

Figure 6-9

MYOEPITHELIOMA

Elongated, well-circumscribed lacrimal gland tumor has a solid yellow-white cut surface.

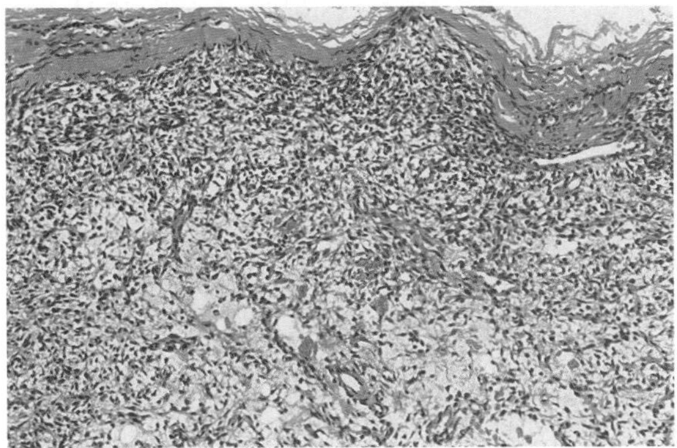

Figure 6-10

MYOEPITHELIOMA

The tumor has a connective tissue capsule and is composed of loosely arranged spindle-shaped cells.

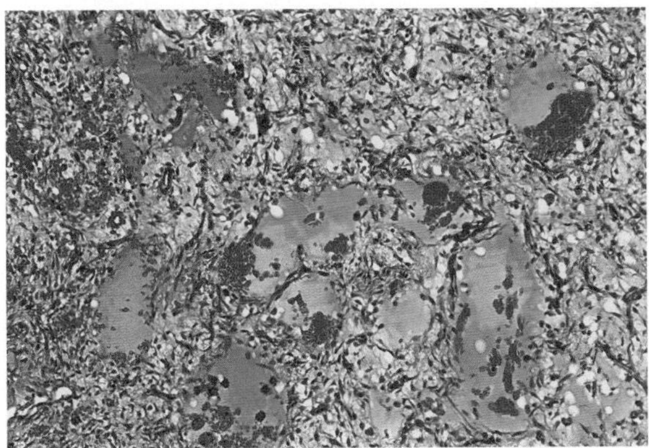

Figure 6-11

MYOEPITHELIOMA

The spindle cells have a mesenchymal appearance.

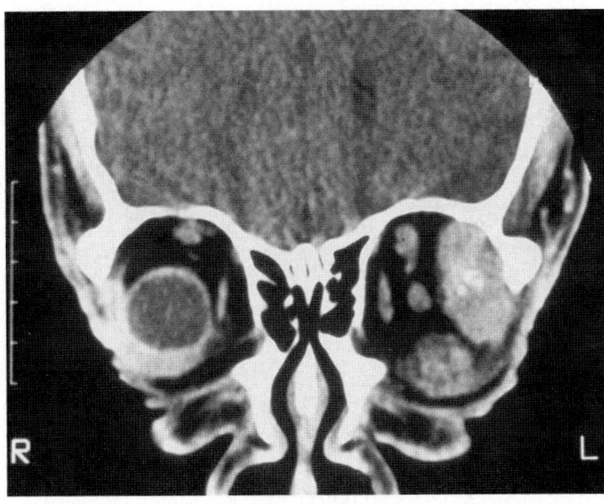

Figure 6-12

EPITHELIAL-MYOEPITHELIAL CARCINOMA

Coronal CT scan shows a large well-circumscribed mass with heterogeneous internal density in the left lacrimal gland fossa.

Histologically, the tumors are mainly composed of spindle cells with scanty eosinophilic cytoplasm (figs. 6-10, 6-11). Other myoepithelioma cell types include epithelial or epithelioid, plasmacytoid or polygonal, and clear cell myoepithelioma. The diagnosis is based on light microscopic features and immunohistochemical findings. Myoepithelial cells are immunoreactive for alpha-actin, muscle-specific actin, cytokeratin, GFAP, vimentin, and S-100 protein.

Most myoepitheliomas of the lacrimal gland are benign and the prognosis is not different from that of pleomorphic adenoma. Ostrowski et al. (42) described a *clear cell epithelial-myoepithelial carcinoma* arising from a pleomorphic adenoma (figs. 6-12–6-16). The tumor consisted of lobules of clear cells with an eccentric nucleus and well-defined cytoplasm. The cells contained glycogen and reacted with cytokeratin and alpha-actin antibodies. The patient was free of local and systemic disease 2½ years after exenteration.

MALIGNANT EPITHELIAL TUMORS

Adenoid Cystic Carcinoma

Definition. *Adenoid cystic carcinoma* is an infiltrative, highly malignant epithelial tumor composed of small neoplastic cells. It has been

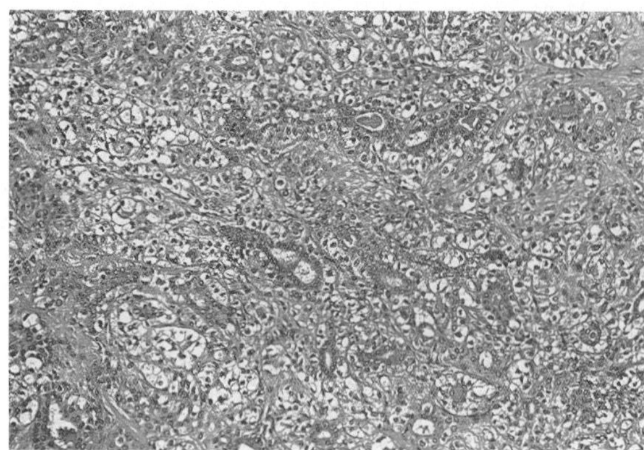

Figure 6-13

EPITHELIAL-MYOEPITHELIAL CARCINOMA

The two-cell population consists of duct-like epithelial cells and clear cells.

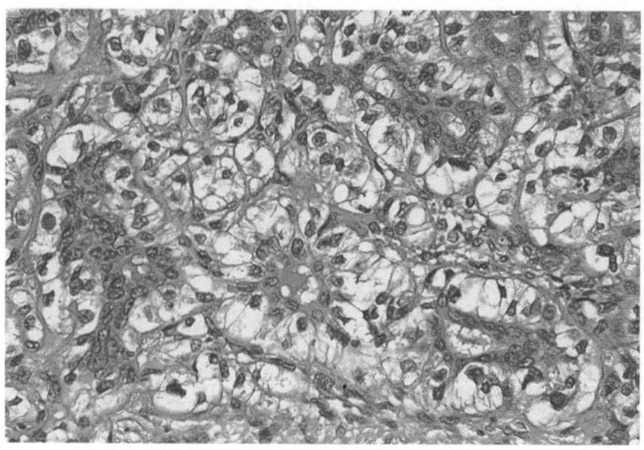

Figure 6-14

EPITHELIAL-MYOEPITHELIAL CARCINOMA

The eosinophilic cuboidal epithelial cells are surrounded by larger polygonal cells with pale or clear cytoplasm.

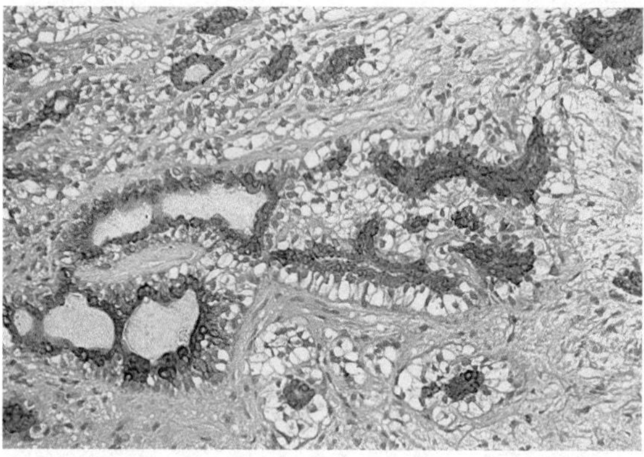

Figure 6-15

CYTOKERATIN IN EPITHELIAL-MYOEPITHELIAL CARCINOMA

The epithelial component is clearly differentiated from the clear myoepithelial cells.

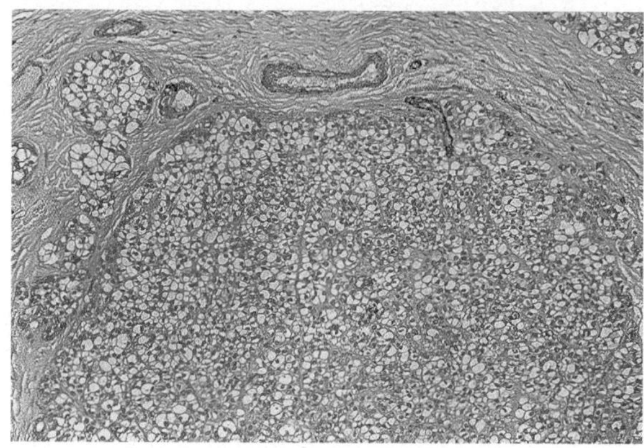

Figure 6-16

EPITHELIAL-MYOEPITHELIAL CARCINOMA

The clear cells show focal immunoreactivity for alpha-actin. The walls of the vessel above serve as a positive control.

suggested that this tumor originates from intralobular duct cells at the transition zone between the acini and the ducts (42a). Adenoid cystic carcinoma occurs with greater frequency in the lacrimal gland than in salivary glands.

General Features. In a series of lacrimal gland tumors, adenoid cystic carcinoma comprised approximately 25 percent of primary epithelial tumors (43). It is the second most common epithelial tumor and the most frequent malignant epithelial tumor. Tumor-related deaths occur as a result of direct invasion into the middle cranial fossa and hematogenous metastasis to the lungs (44). Dissemination to the regional lymph nodes is uncommon. The mean age of the patients is approximately 40 years (43–44b). Adenoid cystic carcinoma may develop in children and adolescents (mean age, 14 years; range, 6 to 18 years) (45). In this younger group, tumor affects predominately females (82 percent).

Clinical Features. Characteristically, patients present with a short history (less than 1 year) of pain, numbness, ptosis, motility disturbances, and diplopia (fig. 6-17) (44a). CT scans disclose a round mass with an irregular contour (fig. 6-18). Calcification of the mass is evident in about one third of cases (44a). Either erosion or sclerotic

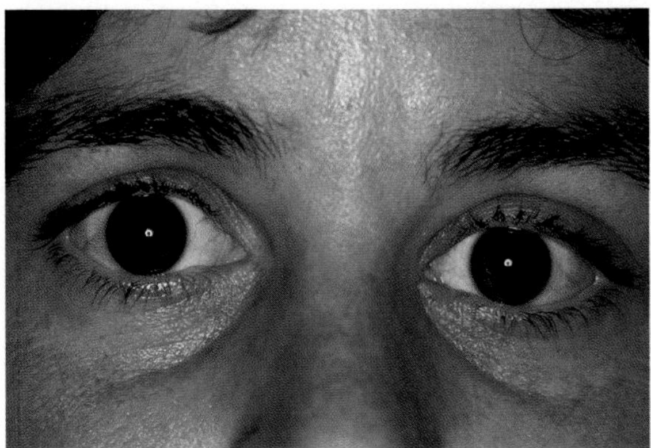

Figure 6-17

ADENOID CYSTIC CARCINOMA

This young woman noted an enlargement of the supertemporal region of the upper eyelid and eyebrow on the left side.

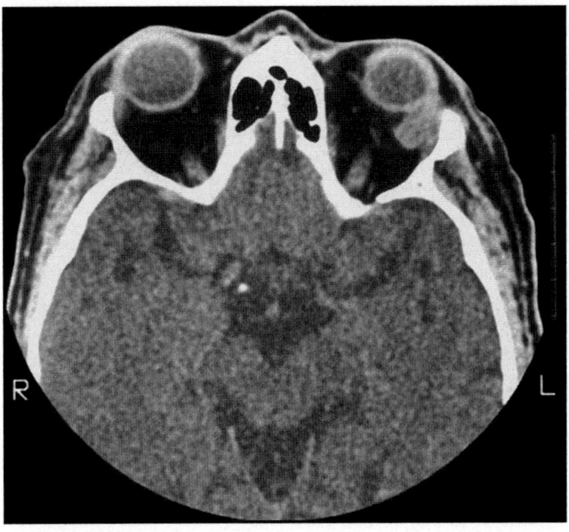

Figure 6-18

ADENOID CYSTIC CARCINOMA

Axial CT scan shows a circumscribed mass with some irregular borders in the lacrimal gland fossa.

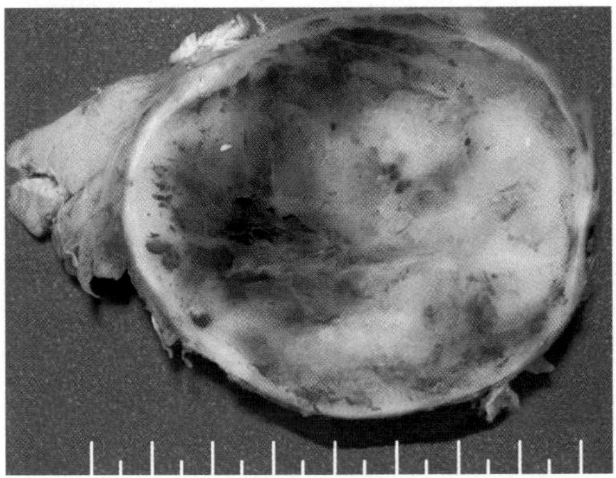

Figure 6-19

ADENOID CYSTIC CARCINOMA

The tumor appears deceptively well circumscribed but the cut surface shows irregularity and foci of hemorrhage.

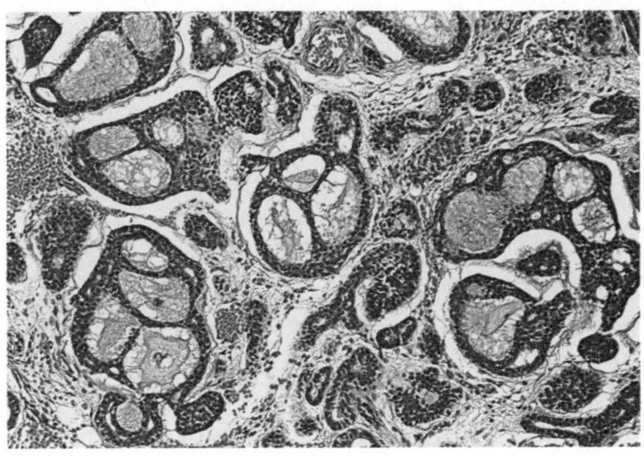

Figure 6-20

ADENOID CYSTIC CARCINOMA

An island of small neoplastic cells has multiple pseudocystic structures.

bone changes are observed in more than 80 percent of the cases, and bone invasion or extraorbital spread is demonstrated in 36 percent. MRI may aid in the evaluation of perineural invasion and intracranial extension.

Gross and Microscopic Findings. Grossly, the tumors have a deceptively circumscribed, globular, round appearance (fig. 6-19). A grayish white surface is seen on cross section. Histologically, adenoid cystic carcinoma is characterized by aggregates or a cord-like arrangement of small neoplastic epithelial cells with cystic spaces that contain mucinous material (figs. 6-20, 6-21). Elongated cords of cells separated by hyalinized stroma may be present. Adenoid cystic carcinoma displays a variety of architectural patterns (43): cribriform or "Swiss cheese" (fig. 6-22), sclerosing "cylindromatous carcinoma" (fig. 6-23), basaloid or solid (fig. 6-24), comedo-carcinoma (fig. 6-25), and tubular or ductal (fig. 6-26). Most commonly, there is an admixture of two or more patterns.

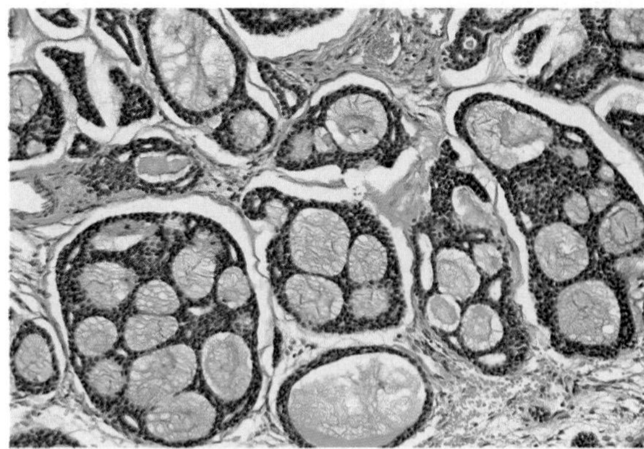

Figure 6-21

ADENOID CYSTIC CARCINOMA

The content of the pseudocystic structures stains for mucin (Morat pentachrome stain).

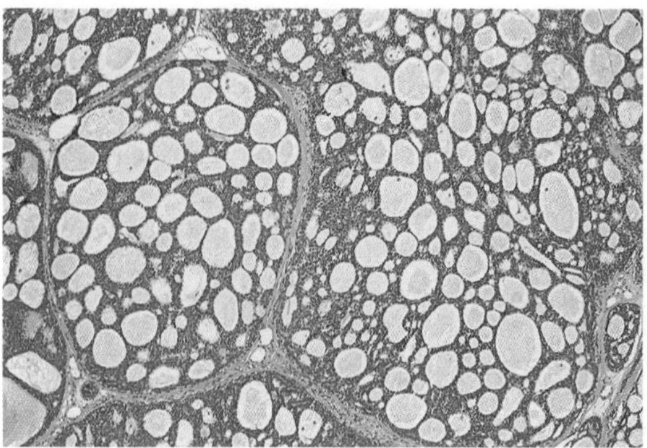

Figure 6-22

ADENOID CYSTIC CARCINOMA

Cribriform "Swiss-cheese" pattern, with lobules of neoplastic epithelial cells and multiple round spaces containing glycosaminoglycans.

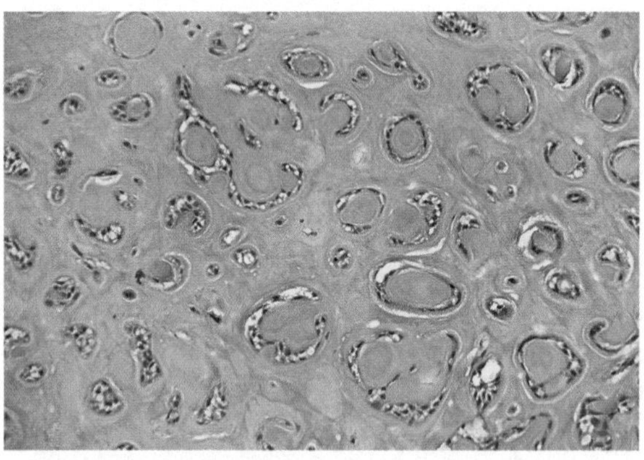

Figure 6-23

ADENOID CYSTIC CARCINOMA

The sclerosing pattern consists of abundant hyalinized stroma between the epithelial proliferations.

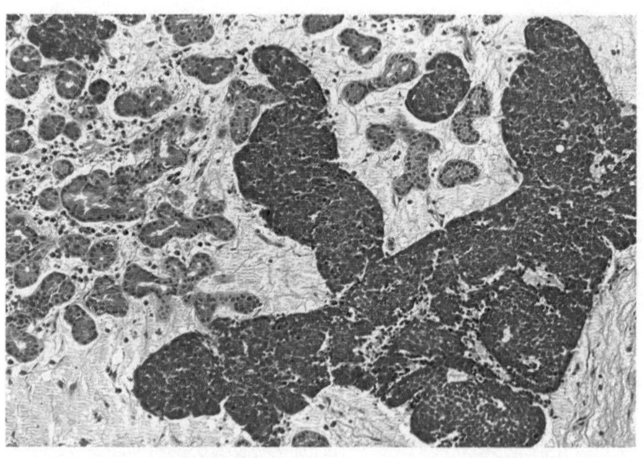

Figure 6-24

ADENOID CYSTIC CARCINOMA

The solid pattern shows lobular islands of cells with hyperchromatic nuclei infiltrating the remaining normal lacrimal gland tissue (left).

The presence of solid basaloid sheets should be noted in the diagnosis and labeled basaloid or nonbasaloid, accordingly (46). The small neoplastic cells are highly invasive and extension along nerves and vessels is usually evident (fig. 6-27). Bone tissue samples should be studied to rule out tumor invasion.

Immunohistochemical Findings. In one case of adenoid cystic carcinoma arising from a pleomorphic adenoma, the tumor demonstrated cytokeratin-positive epithelial cells and muscle-specific actin–positive myoepithelial cells (42a). GFAP was negative.

Ultrastructural Findings. Adenoid cystic carcinoma of the lacrimal gland consists of three different cell types: type 1, small cuboidal cells containing either small duct-like granules (1A), or large acinus-like granules (1B); type 2, cells showing bundles of tonofilaments; and type 3, cells that display features of myoepithelium (46a). Adenoid spaces are surrounded by multilaminar basement membrane.

Cytologic Findings. Fine-needle aspiration biopsy specimens and touch-imprints from incisional biopsy specimens disclose clusters of

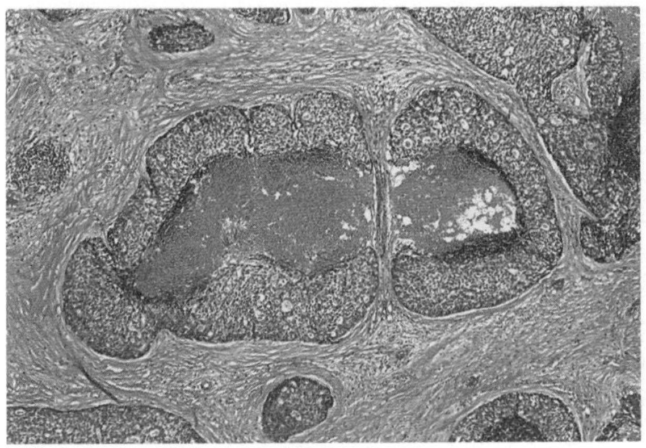

Figure 6-25

ADENOID CYSTIC CARCINOMA

The solid lobules have central areas of necrosis resembling comedo-type carcinoma.

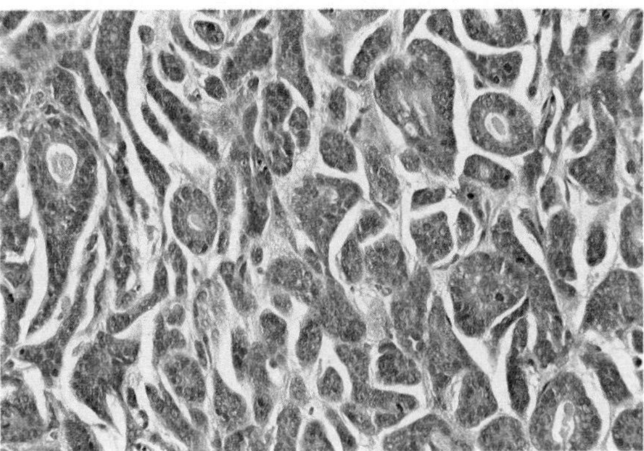

Figure 6-26

ADENOID CYSTIC CARCINOMA

Tubular or duct-like pattern.

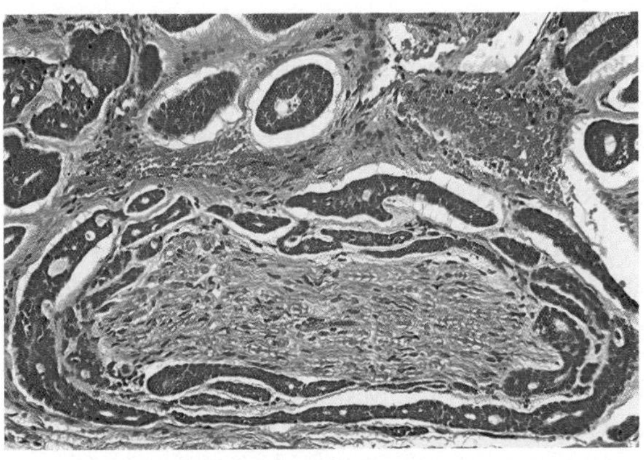

Figure 6-27

ADENOID CYSTIC CARCINOMA

A characteristic feature is perineural and intraneural invasion.

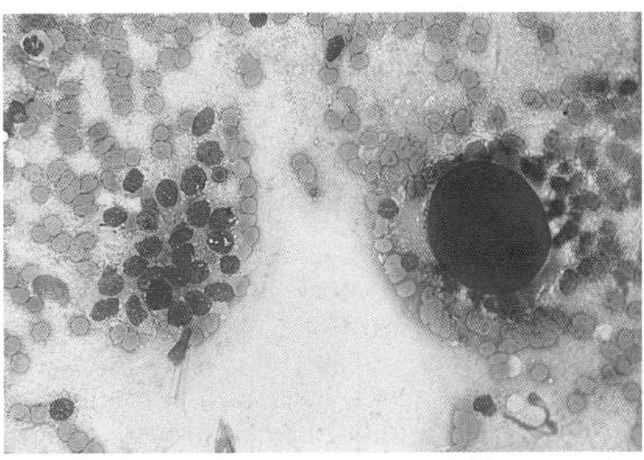

Figure 6-28

ADENOID CYSTIC CARCINOMA

Cytologic smear shows a cluster of cells with granular cytoplasm and a hyaline core surrounded by one layer of tumor cells.

epithelial cells and acellular hyaline material (fig. 6-28) (46b). The small cuboidal cells vary little in size.

Differential Diagnosis. The diagnosis of adenoid cystic carcinoma presents little difficulty. In some cases, the mucoid material and the cuffing of myoepithelial cells mimics a pleomorphic adenoma (fig. 6-29). Rarely, tumors with a predominant basaloid pattern are confused with basal cell adenocarcinoma or infiltrative basal cell carcinoma of the eyelid. The appropriate diagnosis is important because basaloid adenoid cystic carcinoma is a high-grade tumor, and basal cell adenocarcinoma is a low-grade malignancy. The unusual pleomorphic low-grade adenocarcinoma may have a similar histologic pattern. The expression of C-kit, a transmembrane receptor tyrosine kinase, in adenoid cystic carcinoma helps distinguish it from other low-grade tumors (47).

Special Studies. DNA analysis of salivary gland adenoid cystic carcinoma shows that tumor to be aneuploid (48). The expression of p53 may correlate with prognosis (49).

Treatment and Prognosis. Adenoid cystic carcinoma may be graded according to the proportion of the basaloid pattern (grade I, 0 percent; grade II, 25 percent or less; grade III, 25

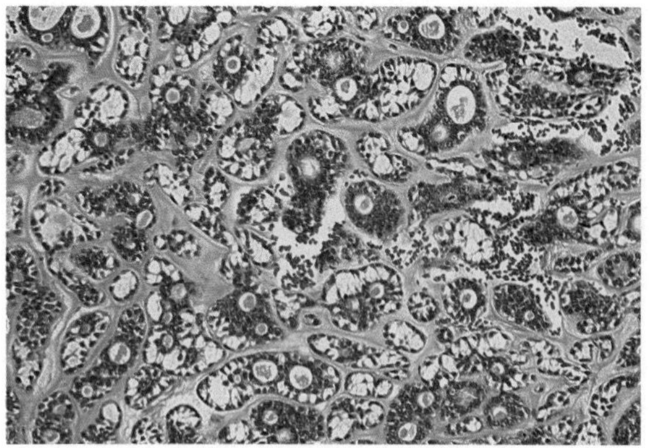

Figure 6-29

ADENOID CYSTIC CARCINOMA

The prominent, clear cell myoepithelial proliferation may be confused with other tumors.

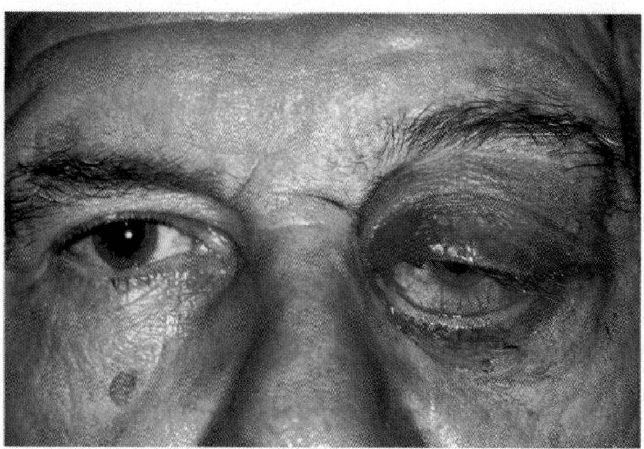

Figure 6-30

MALIGNANT MIXED TUMOR

A sudden increase of proptosis of the left eye in a patient with a history of painless, progressive proptosis of 5 years' duration.

to 50 percent; and grade IV, 50 percent or more). A higher grade, increased mitotic count, necrosis, hemorrhage, and perineural and vascular invasion are poor survival indicators. The reported recurrence rates are as high as 75 percent, with an interval range of 0.2 to 9.3 years (44a). Most of the recurrences involve the orbital bones, intraorbital structures, and direct intracranial extension. In the past, there was a higher incidence of metastasis for adenoid cystic carcinoma of the lacrimal gland, with a 10-year survival rate of 20 percent and a median survival period of 5 years (43,46). Recent series show a 15-year survival rate of 46 percent using combined therapies (50). In children and adolescents, the median survival time is greater than 10 years (45). Less aggressive histologic features may account for the better prognosis in this younger age group. Patients with adenoid cystic carcinoma arising from pleomorphic adenoma have a better prognosis and longer survival period.

The best treatment for adenoid cystic carcinoma of the lacrimal gland is still debated. The traditional recommended treatment has been complete en block excision of the tumor and adjacent compromised tissues. Recent clinical studies, however, suggest that complete excision without extensive bone removal, followed by high doses of radiotherapy, may be effective in local control to prevent intracranial invasion and death (44a). Combined therapy of intracarotid cisplatin and intravenous doxorubicin hydrochloride as an adjunct to surgery and radiotherapy may result in better tumor control (51). Patients who undergo exenteration do not have an increased survival rate (43).

Malignant Mixed Tumor

Definition. *Malignant mixed tumor*, also called *carcinoma in pleomorphic adenoma* or *pleomorphic carcinoma*, is a pleomorphic adenoma that shows cytologic features of carcinoma and invasive growth (52). Malignant mixed tumors are the third most frequent epithelial lacrimal gland tumor, after pleomorphic adenoma and adenoid cystic carcinoma.

General and Clinical Features. The incidence in different series of lacrimal gland tumors has ranged from 4 to 24 percent. The patients are approximately 5 to 12 years older than those with pleomorphic adenoma (52,53). Patients with malignant mixed tumor of the lacrimal gland present in three clinical settings: patients who have a long history of a slowly growing mass of the lacrimal gland fossa that suddenly becomes symptomatic (fig. 6-30); patients not known to have a previous tumor of the lacrimal gland who develop a rapidly growing mass associated with pain; and patients who, after one or more recurrences of pleomorphic adenoma over a period of several years, undergo a malignant transformation in one of the recurrences. CT may show a circumscribed mass corresponding to the original benign mixed tumor and dense areas of invasive carcinoma (fig. 6-31) (54). In all cases

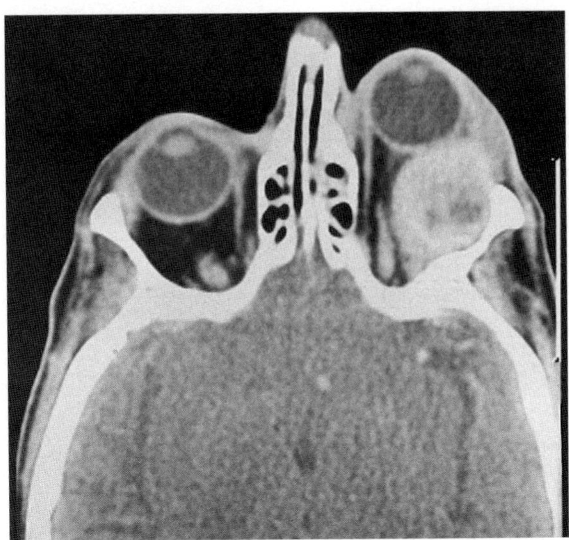

Figure 6-31

MALIGNANT MIXED TUMOR

Axial CT scan of the orbit discloses a large, round to oval, well-circumscribed mass that compresses and thins the lateral orbital bones.

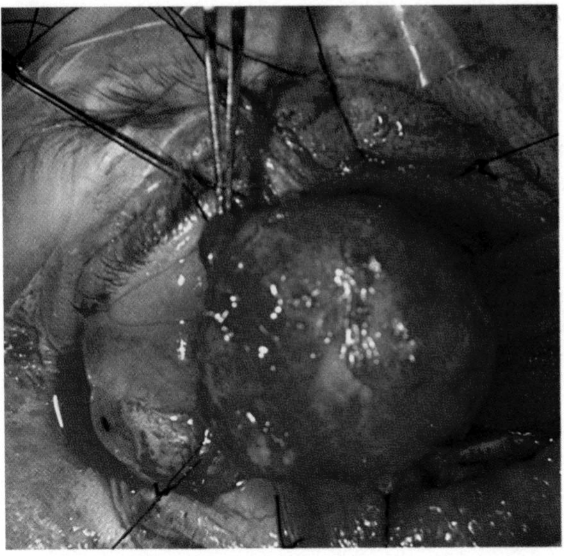

Figure 6-32

MALIGNANT MIXED TUMOR

Intraoperative appearance of the tumor shows a round mass with an irregular surface.

of suspected malignant mixed tumor, regional lymph nodes should be carefully evaluated for any evidence of metastasis.

Gross and Microscopic Findings. Grossly, the tumor may appear partially well circumscribed and nodular (fig. 6-32). The cut surface may show areas indistinguishable from pleomorphic adenoma as well as infiltration of the surrounding tissues (fig. 6-33). The histologic types of carcinoma include adenocarcinoma, adenoid cystic carcinoma, squamous cell carcinoma, and undifferentiated carcinoma (figs. 6-34–6-36). Rarely, the only histologic evidence of pleomorphic adenoma is the presence of large areas of hyalinized stroma containing myoepithelial cells and a few duct structures. Sarcomatous areas and foci of sebaceous carcinoma may be seen and may be the only finding of malignancy. Tumors composed of carcinomatous and sarcomatous elements are classified as carcinosarcoma.

Differential Diagnosis. The main difficulty in diagnosing a malignant mixed tumor is identifying remnants of pleomorphic adenoma in carcinoma, or recognizing malignant transformation in pleomorphic adenoma. A precedent pleomorphic adenoma is suspected by clinical history. The presence of a hyaline and acellular area together with cartilage-like tissue is suggestive of a carcinoma arising from a pleomorphic adenoma. The main criteria for malignancy in a pleomorphic adenoma are frank carcinomatous infiltrative areas and foci of necrosis.

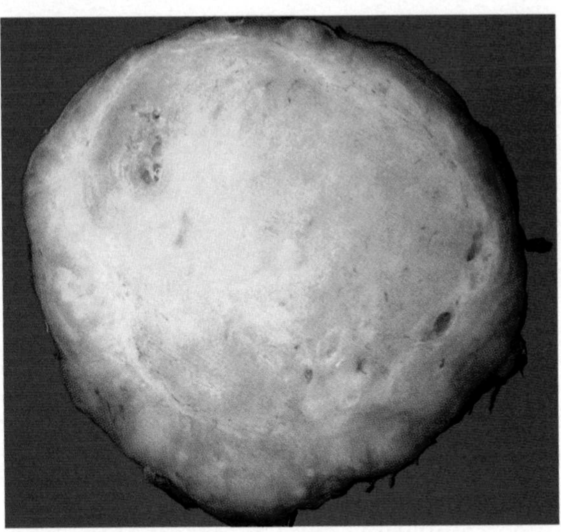

Figure 6-33

MALIGNANT MIXED TUMOR

The tumor is yellowish, has a large central nodule, and has cystic areas, which correspond to a benign mixed tumor. The periphery of the mass shows multiple white nodules that are carcinomatous foci.

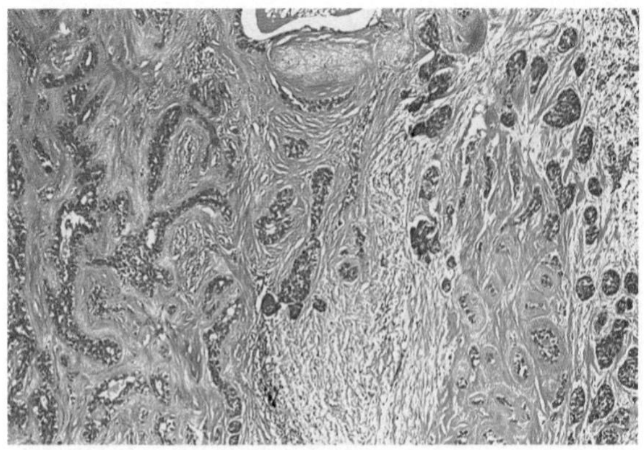

Figure 6-34

MALIGNANT MIXED TUMOR

Low-power view discloses three distinct zones from left to right: pleomorphic adenoma, borderline zone, and frank carcinoma.

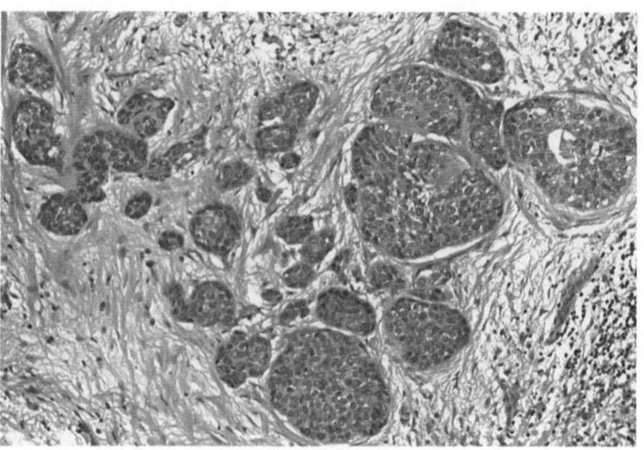

Figure 6-36

MALIGNANT MIXED TUMOR

The predominant malignant component of the tumor depicted in figure 6-34 is an adenoid cystic carcinoma with a prominent sclerosing pattern.

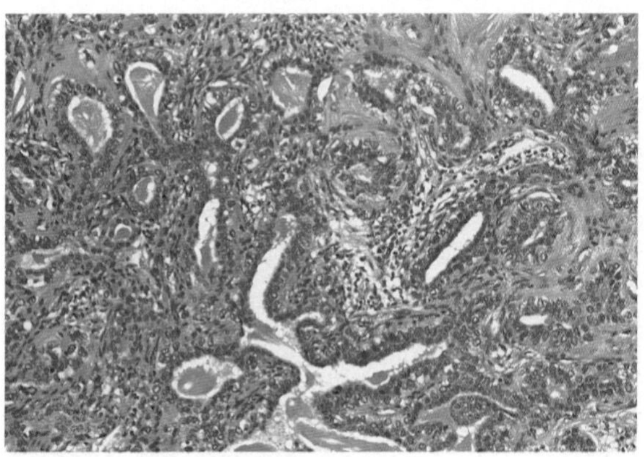

Figure 6-35

MALIGNANT MIXED TUMOR

Classic benign epithelial proliferation of the pleomorphic adenoma component.

Hypercellularity, some pleomorphism, and occasional mitotic figures, as well as focal expansion into the adjacent tissues (bosselations) should not be interpreted as indicative of malignant pleomorphic carcinoma. Carcinosarcomas may resemble a chondrosarcoma.

Treatment and Prognosis. The prognosis of patients with malignant mixed tumor is poor, with a mean survival period of 3 years after diagnosis (54a,54b). The treatment is complete excision and should include free surgical margins and regional lymph node dissection.

Primary Adenocarcinoma

Primary adenocarcinoma (otherwise unclassified) of the lacrimal gland arising unassociated with a preexisting pleomorphic adenoma accounts for 5 to 10 percent of the epithelial tumors of the lacrimal gland (55–57a) Heaps et al. (57) reviewed 13 cases from multiple institutions. Most patients were white males with an average age of 50 years (range, 31 to 78 years). The most common symptoms were palpable mass, pain, and proptosis of 3 weeks' to 20 years' duration before diagnosis.

Grossly, the tumors have irregular borders. The cut surface is white or yellow-white with hemorrhagic and necrotic zones (fig. 6-37). Other tumors are friable and rupture during surgery (fig. 6-38). These tumors often display different growth patterns. The features in common are the presence of glandular or duct-like structures and the presence of infiltrative growth (fig. 6-39). Fine-needle aspiration cytology may be useful to provide a diagnosis (figs. 6-40, 6-41).

Treatment includes complete excision including exenteration, followed by radiotherapy and chemotherapy in a few cases. Font and Gamel (9) reported 19 cases among 256 epithelial tumors of the lacrimal gland; 93 percent of the patients had recurrence of their lacrimal gland tumors and the 5-year survival rate was 34 percent.

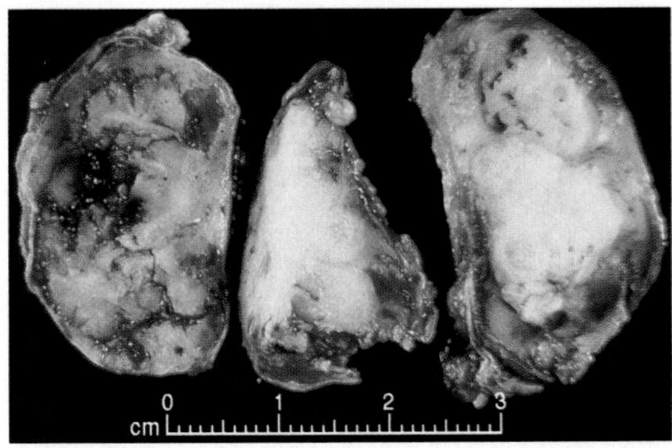

Figure 6-37

ADENOCARCINOMA

The cut surface of this tumor shows irregular, white, multinodular areas with necrosis and hemorrhage.

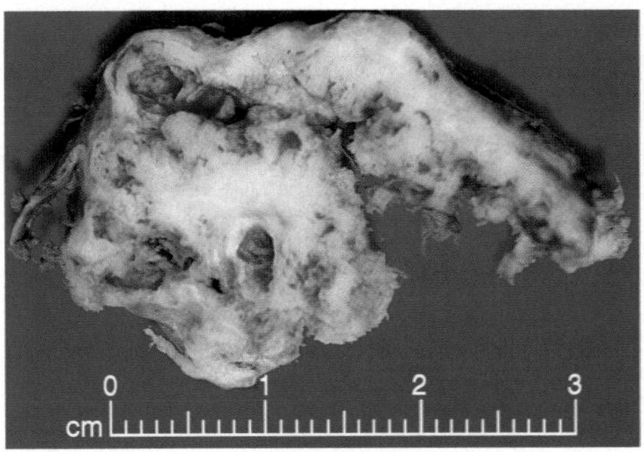

Figure 6-38

ADENOCARCINOMA

Friable, white tumor with necrosis. A fibrous capsule is seen in some areas.

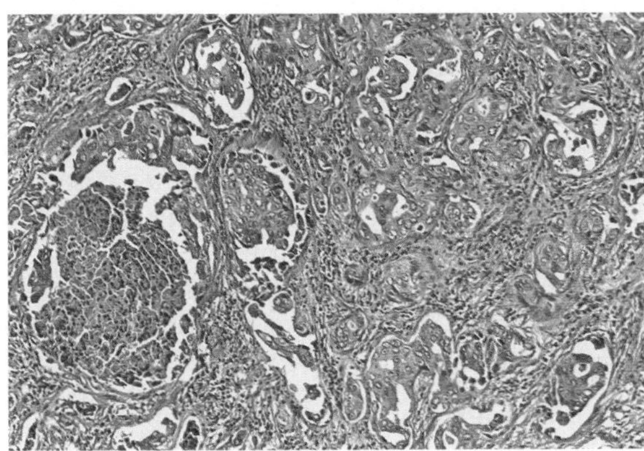

Figure 6-39

ADENOCARCINOMA

Infiltrating epithelial tumor with duct-like structures, central necrosis in some foci, and scattered mitotic figures.

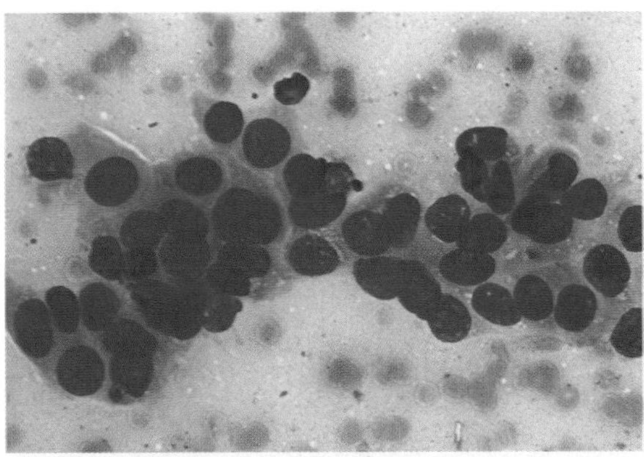

Figure 6-40

ADENOCARCINOMA

Fine-needle aspiration biopsy of an adenocarcinoma of the lacrimal gland discloses clusters of large cells with atypical, variably sized nuclei.

Mucoepidermoid Carcinoma

Mucoepidermoid carcinoma of the lacrimal gland comprises 1 to 2 percent of all lacrimal gland tumors. The average age of the patients is 49.3 years, range 12 to 79 years (58–60). Females are more frequently affected than males in a ratio of 3 to 2. The duration of symptoms does not correlate with histologic grade or prognosis (fig. 6-42).

Microscopically, these tumors are composed of islands of neoplastic squamous elements, including keratinization, with evidence of mucus secretion (fig. 6-43). Mucoepidermoid carcinomas are classified as low-grade (grades 1 and 2) or high-grade (grade 3) malignancies according to the nuclear to cytoplasmic ratio, mitotic activity, mucin production, and epidermoid predominance. Grade 3 tumors, with numerous mitotic figures and fewer mucin-secreting cells, are associated with local or regional invasion and dissemination.

Treatment of high-grade tumors is wide local excision with histologic examination of regional lymph nodes and radiotherapy. Metastatic work-up should include the search for metastasis to the lung and mediastinum. Two cases of an oxyphilic (oncocytic) variant of mucoepidermoid carcinoma of the lacrimal gland have been

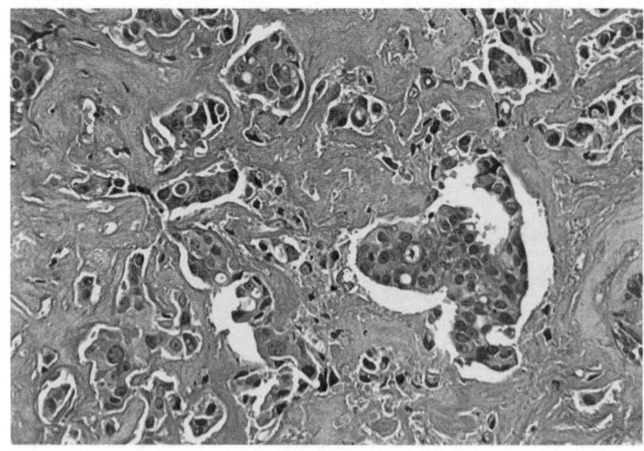

Figure 6-41

ADENOCARCINOMA

Adenocarcinomatous foci in the sclerosing hyalinized extracellular matrix.

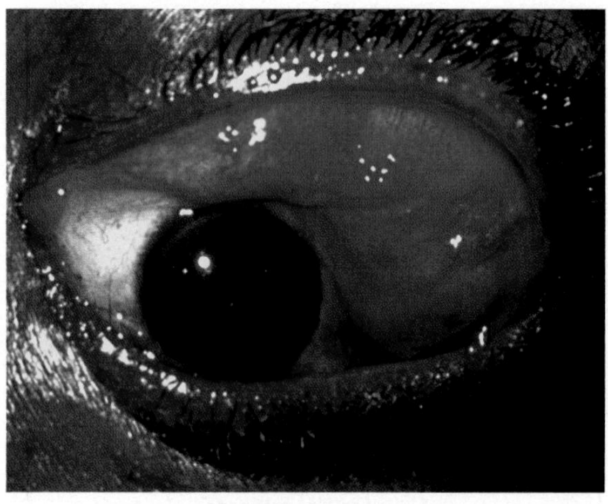

Figure 6-42

MUCOEPIDERMOID CARCINOMA

Mucoepidermoid carcinoma arises from the palpebral lobe of the lacrimal gland.

described in the literature (61). These two tumors manifested aggressive metastatic behavior that resulted in the death of the patients.

MISCELLANEOUS MALIGNANT EPITHELIAL TUMORS

Although the types of lacrimal gland tumors are more limited than those of the salivary glands, recently, there have reports identifying specific subtypes of adenocarcinomas and carcinomas. Those not discussed here are mentioned in reviews of series of cases from one

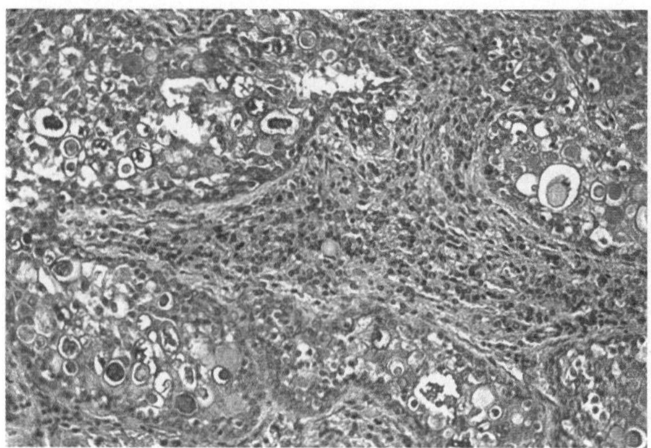

Figure 6-43

MUCOEPIDERMOID CARCINOMA

Alcian blue stain highlights the mucous cells within islands of cuboidal intermediate epithelial cells.

institution or are limited to single case reports. They include basal cell adenocarcinoma (62), squamous cell carcinoma (62a,62b), polymorphous low-grade carcinoma (63), cystadenocarcinoma, mucinous adenocarcinoma, spindle cell carcinoma (63a), carcinosarcoma, and lymphoepithelioma-like carcinoma (64,65). Since most of these tumors are extremely rare in the lacrimal gland, the behavior and prognosis are based on similar tumors of the salivary glands.

Primary Ductal Adenocarcinoma

Primary ductal adenocarcinoma originates from the excretory portion of the salivary duct. The three reported patients with primary ductal adenocarcinoma arising from the lacrimal gland were aged 52, 67, and 68 years; two were male and one female (55,66,67). Although the tumors may appear circumscribed grossly, they are highly infiltrative and usually solid with occasional cystic areas. The cells are cuboidal or polygonal, with eosinophilic cytoplasm and apocrine features. The duct-like structures are embedded in a collagenous matrix. Comedonecrosis and a high rate of mitosis are characteristically found. Alcian blue and mucicarmine stains are negative for mucin cell secretion. The differential diagnosis includes papillary cystadenocarcinoma, polymorphous low-grade adenocarcinoma, mucinous adenocarcinoma, and mucoepidermoid carcinoma.

This high-grade tumor is best managed with complete en block excision and radiotherapy;

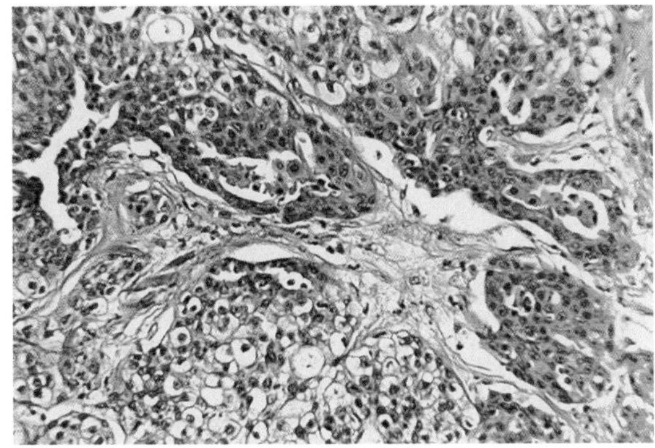

Figure 6-44

ADENOCARCINOMA WITH SEBACEOUS DIFFERENTIATION

There are foci of cells with clear multivacuolated cytoplasm.

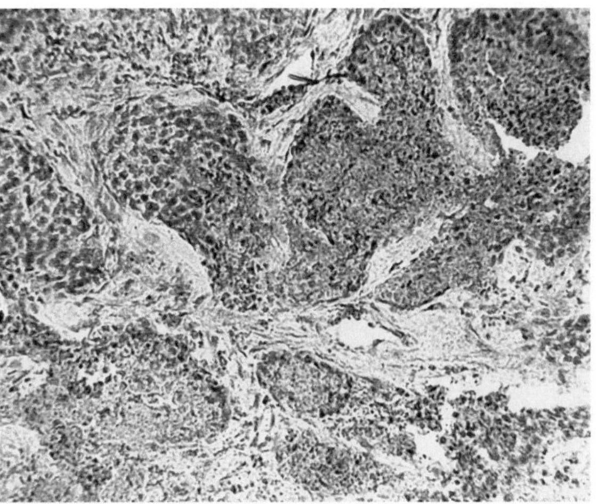

Figure 6-45

ADENOCARCINOMA WITH SEBACEOUS DIFFERENTIATION

Oil red-O stain reveals the presence of lipid within the clear cells.

in addition, lymph node dissection or regional radiotherapy may be considered. One reported patient had nodal metastasis, and another developed a recurrence with subdural invasion (66,67).

Acinic Cell Carcinoma

A few cases of *acinic cell carcinoma* of the lacrimal gland have been reported (68-70). The patients range in age from 18 to 59 years. The tumors are multinodular or infiltrative. Acinic cell carcinoma is composed mainly of small, basophilic, acinus-like cells. There are four growth patterns: solid, microcystic, papillary-cystic, and follicular. The supporting stroma frequently contains a lymphocytic infiltrate. These tumors may secrete mucus. Acinic cell carcinomas of the salivary gland frequently recur, and recurrences have been associated with increased metastatic potential. Recurrent tumors may invade the cranial cavity. Encapsulation, low mitotic counts, and absence of neural and vascular invasion indicate a more favorable prognosis. Treatment is complete surgical excision.

Sebaceous Adenocarcinoma

Although foci of sebaceous differentiation are found on rare occasion in adenocarcinomas of the lacrimal gland (figs. 6-44, 6-45), a primary sebaceous carcinoma occurs very rarely (71–75). This tumor should be differentiated from secondary involvement from an eyelid sebaceous carcinoma. There is a tendency to early recurrence and dissemination to regional lymph nodes.

LYMPHOID TUMORS

The normally present lymphoid cells within the stroma of the lacrimal gland are considered part of the mucosa-associated lymphoid tissue (MALT). Thus, *reactive lymphoid hyperplasia* and *lymphoma* may develop within the lacrimal gland (76–76b). Lacrimal gland involvement may be unilateral or bilateral. The duration of symptoms varies from 1 to 12 months. Patients with lymphoma are generally older (sixth to seventh decades; range, 25 to 78 years) (76a). Clinically they present with a nontender lesion. Prominent contrast-enhanced CT shows a well-demarcated oblong mass, suggesting the diagnosis of an inflammatory lesion or a lymphoid tumor. The diagnosis of malignant lymphoma is established from an incisional biopsy that should provide tissue sample adequate enough to apply all currently available techniques. Fine-needle aspiration biopsy can identify malignant lymphoid lesions of the lacrimal gland and serves as a valuable adjunct in the assessment of this lesion (77). The histopathologic features do not differ from lymphoid proliferations of the orbit; the most frequent type is extranodal marginal B-cell non-Hodgkin's lymphoma. One third to half of patients with lymphoma of the

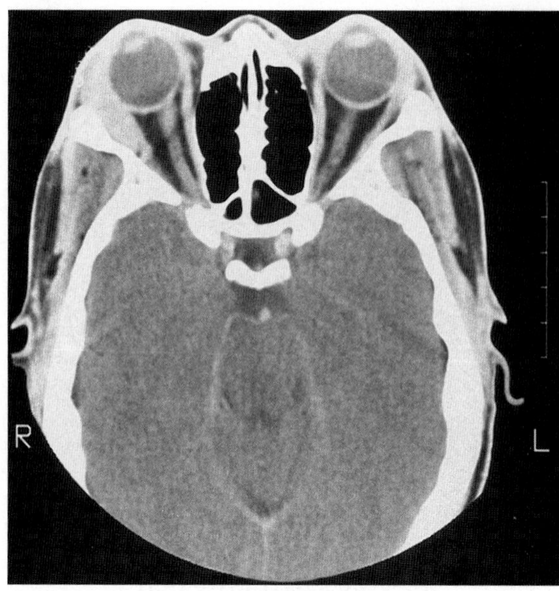

Figure 6-46

CHRONIC DACRYOADENITIS

Axial CT scan shows an elongated mass between the right globe and the lateral orbital wall.

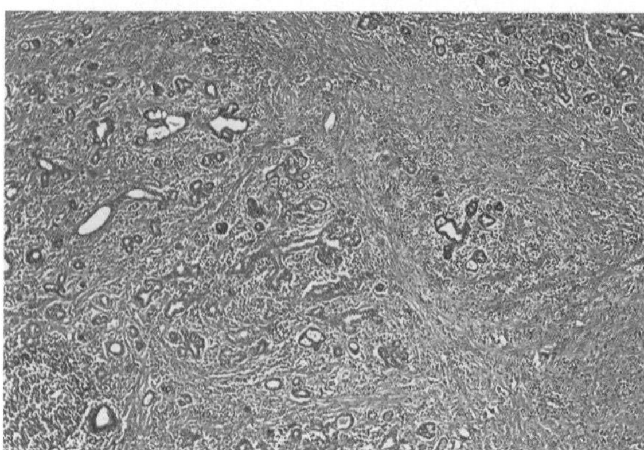

Figure 6-47

CHRONIC DACRYOADENITIS

The acini are atrophic. The remaining ducts show fibrosis of the interlobular septa and a chronic inflammatory infiltrate.

lacrimal gland have or will develop systemic disease. Therefore, evaluation for systemic involvement is mandatory. The treatment for local orbital disease is radiotherapy; chemotherapeutic regimens are required for systemic disease. Rarely, Hodgkin's disease, plasmacytoma, and other types of plasma cell dyscrasias may involve the lacrimal gland (78–81).

MESENCHYMAL TUMORS

Soft tissue tumors rarely arise within the lacrimal gland; most frequently, they arise around the lacrimal gland area. The reported cases include *hemangioma* (82,83), *hemangiopericytoma* (84), *peripheral nerve tumors* (85), and *solitary fibrous tumor*, among others (86).

SECONDARY AND METASTATIC TUMORS

Direct invasion into the lacrimal gland may result from tumors arising from the eyelid and conjunctiva, or tumors that originate in bone adjacent to the lacrimal gland fossa. In addition, the lacrimal gland may be the site of hematogenous metastases (87,88). Secondary and metastatic tumors should be differentiated from primary tumors affecting the lacrimal gland.

TUMOR-LIKE LESIONS

Chronic Dacryoadenitis

Chronic inflammation of the lacrimal gland is broadly termed *chronic dacyroadenitis* (88a). The diagnosis of idiopathic nonspecific chronic inflammation (*lacrimal gland pseudotumor*) is made after excluding systemic and local causes. Patients present with pain, swelling and redness of the eyelid, ptosis, motility disturbances, and proptosis (88a,88b). Typically, the gland has an oblong and contoured shape that can be demonstrated by CT scan and MRI (fig. 6-46). The acini are atrophic and the stroma shows periductal and interlobular fibrosis; an inflammatory infiltrate composed of lymphocytes and plasma cells with lymphoid follicles and perivasculitis is also present (fig. 6-47). Treatment is corticosteroids with the addition of radiotherapy for recurrent disease. Surgical excision or debulking could be considered for locally enlarged lacrimal glands (89).

Noninfectious dacryoadenitis may be associated with other systemic diseases such as sarcoidosis, Wegener's granulomatosis, systemic lupus erythematosus, or autoimmune diseases (3). Sarcoidosis may affect the palpebral and orbital lobes of the lacrimal gland. Involvement of the lacrimal gland is demonstrated by gallium scanning in 80 percent of patients with systemic sarcoidosis.

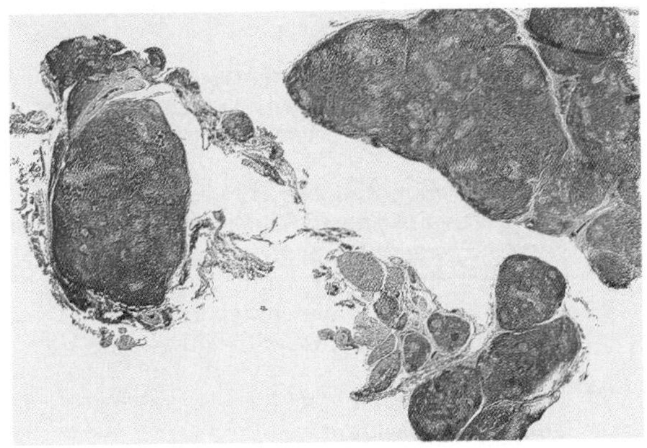

Figure 6-48

BENIGN LYMPHOEPITHELIAL LESION

Lobules of lacrimal gland are replaced by a dense lymphocytic infiltrate with clear areas.

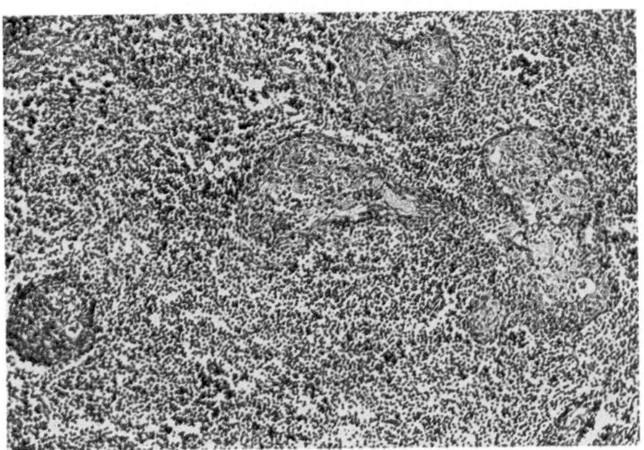

Figure 6-49

BENIGN LYMPHOEPITHELIAL LESION

The clear areas surrounded by lymphocytes represent an epithelial duct cell proliferation.

Benign Lymphoepithelial Lesion

Benign lymphoepithelial lesion refers to a peculiar chronic inflammatory infiltrate of the lacrimal gland seen in patients with Sjögren's syndrome (90). Sheets of lymphocytes and plasma cells, which may have follicular centers, replace the lacrimal gland lobules; acini are atrophic (figs. 6-48, 6-49). The epithelial lining of the remaining ducts may proliferate into solid cellular nests. The lymphocytes are B cells and T-helper cells. Epstein-Barr antigens have been detected in the lacrimal gland of patients with Sjögren's syndrome. The development of malignant lymphoma is rare (92).

Lacrimal Gland Cysts

Simple cysts of the orbital lobe are rare (93–95). The term *dacryops* refers to a closed cyst of the palpebral lobe of the lacrimal gland (fig. 6-50) (95). In addition, cysts may develop from the accessory lacrimal glands of Krause and Wolfring, and from ectopic (choristomatous) lacrimal gland tissue (95a). Lacrimal ducts may become ectatic secondary to inflammation or scarring due to idiopathic inflammatory disease, trauma, or surgery. Rarely, tumors may cause dacryops by infiltrating and compressing the lacrimal gland ducts. The cysts are noted after everting the upper eyelid; they are whitish blue and transilluminate. Echography and CT scans demonstrate the cystic nature of the mass.

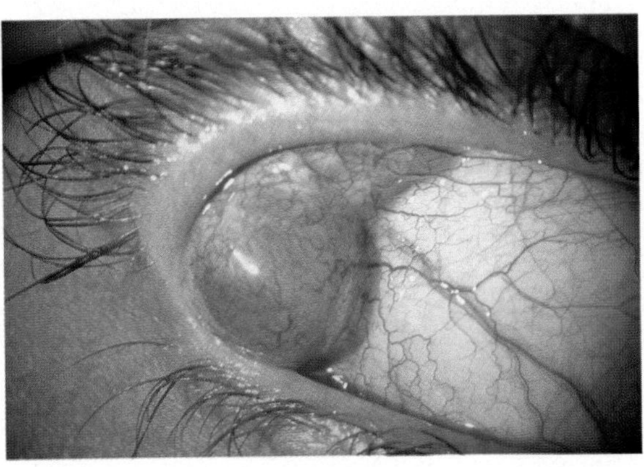

Figure 6-50

DACRYOPS

A large cyst at the outer canthal area arises from the palpebral lobe of the lacrimal gland.

The cysts are lined by a double layer of cuboidal cells (fig. 6-51). Mucin-producing goblet cells may be observed, representing the normal terminal duct of the lacrimal gland. The lumen may show inspissated laminated concretions that contain epithelial cells, and which stain for mucin and immunoglobulin (IgA). Bilateral cases have been associated with trachoma. The differential diagnosis includes conjunctival cysts, epidermoid cysts, dermoid cysts, and adnexal cutaneous cysts.

Treatment of symptomatic or cosmetically unacceptable lacrimal gland cysts is complete surgical excision. Aspiration or partial excisions usually result in recurrence of the cysts.

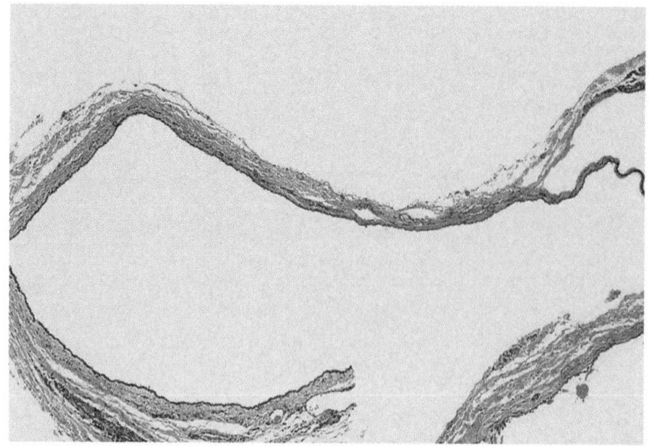

Figure 6-51

DACRYOPS

A large cystic cavity is lined by regular cuboidal epithelial cells.

STAGING AND GRADING OF LACRIMAL GLAND TUMORS

The system presented in Table 6-4 was recommended by the Task Force for Staging of Cancer of the Eye of the American Joint Committee on Cancer (96).

Table 6-4

STAGING AND GRADING OF LACRIMAL GLAND TUMORS

Primary Tumor (T)	
TX	Primary tumor cannot be assessed
T0	No evidence of primary tumor
T1	Tumor 2.5 cm or less in greatest dimension limited to the lacrimal gland
T2	Tumor 2.5 cm or less in greatest dimension invading the periosteum of the fossa of the lacrimal gland
T3	Tumor more than 2.5 cm but not more than 5 cm in greatest dimension
T3a	Tumor limited to the lacrimal gland
T3b	Tumor invades the periosteum of the fossa of the lacrimal gland
T4	Tumor more than 5 cm in greatest dimension
T4a	Tumor invades the orbital soft tissues, optic nerve, or globe without bone invasion
T4b	Tumor invades the orbital soft tissues, optic nerve, or globe with bone invasion
Regional Lymph Nodes (N)	
NX	Regional lymph nodes cannot be assessed
N0	No regional lymph node metastasis
N1	Regional lymph node metastasis
Distant Metastasis (M)	
MX	Distant metastasis cannot be assessed
M0	No distant metastasis
M1	Distant metastasis
	Note: no stage grouping is presently recommended.
Microscopic Grade (G)	
GX	Grade cannot be assessed
G1	Well differentiated
G2	Moderately differentiated (includes adenoid cystic carcinoma without prominent basaloid pattern)
G3	Poorly differentiated (includes adenoid cystic carcinoma with prominent basaloid pattern)
G4	Undifferentiated

REFERENCES

Classification and Frequency

1. Shields CL, Shields JA, Eagle RC, Rathmell JP. Clinicopathologic review of 142 cases of lacrimal gland lesions. Ophthalmology 1989;96:431–5.
2. Ni C, Ma X. [Histopathologic classification of 1921 orbital tumors.] Yan Ke Xue Bao 1995;11: 101–4. (Chinese.)
3. Jakobiec FA, Bilyk JR, Font RL. Orbit. In Spencer WH, ed. Ophthalmic pathology. An atlas and textbook, 4th ed. Philadelphia: WB Sauders Co; 1996:2485–525.
4. Forrest AW. Epithelial lacrimal gland tumors: pathology as a guide to prognosis. Trans Am Acad Ophthalmol 1954;58:848–66.
5. Zimmerman LE, Sanders TE, Ackerman LV. Epithelial tumors of the lacrimal gland: prognostic and therapeutic significance and histologic types. Int Ophthalmol Clin 1962;2:337–67.
6. Seifert G, Sobin LH. The World Health Organization's Histological Classification of Salivary Gland Tumors. A commentary on the second edition. Cancer 1992;70:379–85.
7. Wright JE, Rose GE, Garner A. Primary malignant neoplasms of the lacrimal gland. Br J Ophthalmol 1992;76:401–7.
8. Font RL, Smith SL, Bryan RG. Malignant epithelial tumors of the lacrimal gland: a clinicopathologic study of 21 cases. Arch Ophthalmol 1998;116:613–6.
9. Font RL, Gamel JW. Epithelial tumors of the lacrimal gland: an analysis of 265 cases. In: Jakobiec FA, ed. Ocular and adnexal tumors. Birmingham, AL: Aesculapius Publishing Co; 1978:787–805.
10. Ni C. [Primary epithelial lacrimal gland tumors: the pathologic classification of 272 cases.] Yan Ke Xue Bao 1994;10:201–5. (Chinese.)
11. Nicholson DH, Green WR. Pediatric ocular tumors. New York: Masson Publishing USA, Inc; 1981:293–5.
12. Rose GE, Wright JE. Pleomorphic adenoma of the lacrimal gland. Br J Ophthalmol 1992;76:395–400.
13. Henderson JW. Orbital tumors, 3rd ed. New York: Raven Press; 1994.
14. Klijanienko J, El-Naggar AK, Servois V, et al. Histologically similar, synchronous or metachronous, lacrimal salivary-type and parotid gland tumors: a series of 11 cases. Head Neck 1999;21:512–6.

14a. Iwamoto T, Jakobiec FA. A comparative ultrastructural study of the normal lacrimal gland and its epithelial tumors. Hum Pathol 1982;13:236–62.

Pleomorphic Adenoma

15. Iwamoto T, Jakobiec FA. A comparative ultrastructural study of the normal lacrimal gland and its epithelial tumors. Hum Pathol 1982;13:236–62.
16. Parks SL, Glover AT. Benign mixed tumors arising in the palpebral lobe of the lacrimal gland. Ophthalmology 1990;97:526–30.
17. Vangveeravong S, Katz SE, Rootman J, White V. Tumors arising in the palpebral lobe of the lacrimal gland. Ophthalmology 1996;103:1606–12.
18. Tong JT, Flanagan JC, Eagle RC Jr, Mazzoli RA. Benign mixed tumor arising from an accessory lacrimal gland of Wolfring. Ophthal Plast Reconstr Surg 1995;11:136–8.
19. Faktorovich EG, Crawford JB, Char DH, Kong C. Benign mixed tumor (pleomorphic adenoma) of the lacrimal gland in a 6-year-old boy. Am J Ophthalmol 1996;122:446–7.
20. Mercado GJ, Gunduz K, Shields CL, Shields JA, Eagle RC. Pleomorphic adenoma of the lacrimal gland in a teenager. Arch Ophthalmol 1998;116:962–3.
21. Jakobiec FA, Yeo JH, Trokel SL, et al. Combined clinical and computed tomographic diagnosis of primary lacrimal fossa lesions. Am J Ophthalmol 1982;94:785–807.
22. Lemke AJ, Hosten N, Grote A, Felix R. [Differentiation of lacrimal gland tumors with high resolution computerized tomography in comparison with magnetic resonance tomography.] Ophthalmologe 1996;93:284–91. (German.)
23. Mafee MF, Edward DP, Koeller KK, Dorodi S. Lacrimal gland tumors and simulating lesions. Clinicopathologic and MR imaging features. Radiol Clin North Am 1999;37:219–39.
24. Grossniklaus HE, Abbuhl MF, McLean IW. Immunohistologic properties of benign and malignant mixed tumor of the lacrimal gland. Am J Ophthalmol 1990;110:540–9.
25. Sturgis CD, Silverman JF, Kennerdell JS, Raab SS. Fine-needle aspiration for the diagnosis of primary epithelial tumors of the lacrimal gland and ocular adnexa. Diagn Cytopathol 2001;24:86–9.
26. Lakhey M, Thakur SK, Mishra A, Rani S. Pleomorphic adenoma of lacrimal gland: diagnosis based on fine needle aspiration cytology. Indian J Pathol Microbiol 2001;44:333–5.

27. Zhao P, Sun X. [Quantitative analyses of DNA content and P53 gene product expression from epithelial lacrimal gland tumors.] Zhonghua Yan Ke Za Zhi 1996;32:424–8. (Chinese.)
28. Zheng L, He S, Fan Z, Han C. [Relationship between expression of P21ras and cellular DNA in pleomorphic adenoma of lacrimal gland.] Yan Ke Xue Bao 1996;12:54–7. (Chinese.)
29. Jin Y, Mertens F, Limon J, et al. Characteristic karyotypic features in lacrimal and salivary gland carcinomas. Br J Cancer 1994;70:42–7.
30. Hrynchak M, White V, Berean K, Horsman D. Cytogenetic findings in seven lacrimal gland neoplasms. Cancer Genet Cytogenet 1994;75: 133–8.

Oncocytoma

31. Biggs SL, Font RL. Oncocytic lesions of the caruncle and other ocular adnexa. Arch Ophthalmol 1977;95:474–8.
32. Riedel K, Stefani FH, Kampik A. [Oncocytoma of the ocular adnexa.] Klin Monatsbl Augenheilkd 1983;182:544–8. (German.)
33. Pecorella I, Garner A. Ostensible oncocytoma of accessory lacrimal glands. Histopathology 1997;30:264–70.
34. Dorello U. Carcinoma oncocitario della ghlandola lacrimale. Riv ONO 1961;36:452–61.

Warthin's Tumor

35. Bonavolonta G, Tranfa F, Staibano S, Di Matteo G, Orabona P, De Rosa G. Warthin tumor of the lacrimal gland. Am J Ophthalmol 1997;124: 857–8.
36. Mathur A, Mehrotra ML, Dhaliwal U. Warthin's tumor of the eye lid. Indian J Ophthalmol 1989;37:193.
36a. Iwamoto T, Jakobiec FA. A comparative ultrastructural study of the normal lacrimal gland and its epithelial tumors. Hum Pathol 1982;13: 236–62.
36b. Grossniklaus HE, Abbuhl MF, McLean IW. Immunohistologic properties of benign and malignant mixed tumor of the lacrimal gland. Am J Ophthalmol 1990;110:540–9.

Myoepithelioma

37. Dardick I, Thomas MJ, van Nostrand AW. Myoepithelioma—new concepts of histology and classification: a light and electron microscopic study. Ultrastruct Pathol 1989;13:187–224.
38. Heathcote JG, Hurwitz JJ, Dardick I. A spindle-cell myoepithelioma of the lacrimal gland. Arch Ophthalmol 1990;108:1135–9.
39. Font RL, Garner A. Myoepithelioma of the lacrimal gland: report of a case with spindle cell morphology. Br J Ophthalmol 1992;76:634–6.
40. Grossniklaus HE, Wojno TH, Wilson MW, Someren AO. Myoepithelioma of the lacrimal gland. Arch Ophthalmol 1997;115:1588–90.
41. Okudela K, Ito T, Iida MI, Kameda Y, Furuno K, Kitamura H. Myoepithelioma of the lacrimal gland: report of a case with potentially malignant transformation. Pathol Int 2000;50:238–43.
42. Ostrowski ML, Font RL, Halpern J, Nicolitz E, Barnes R. Clear cell epithelial-myoepithelial carcinoma arising in pleomorphic adenoma of the lacrimal gland. Ophthalmology 1994;101: 925–30.

Adenoid Cystic Carcinoma

42a. Grossniklaus HE, Abbuhl MF, McLean IW. Immunohistologic properties of benign and malignant mixed tumor of the lacrimal gland. Am J Ophthalmol 1990;110:540–9.
43. Font RL, Gamel JW. Adenoid cystic carcinoma of the lacrimal gland: a clinicopathologic study of 79 cases. In: Nicholson D, ed. Ocular pathology update. New York: Masson Publishing USA; 1980:277–83.
44. Lee DA, Campbell RJ, Waller RR, Ilstrup DM. A clinicopathologic study of primary adenoid cystic carcinoma of the lacrimal gland. Ophthalmology 1985;92:128–34.
44a. Wright JE, Rose GE, Garner A. Primary malignant neoplasms of the lacrimal gland. Br J Ophthalmol 1992;76:401–7.
44b. Font RL, Smith SL, Bryan RG. Malignant epithelial tumors of the lacrimal gland: a clinicopathologic study of 21 cases. Arch Ophthalmol 1998;116:613–6.
45. Tellado MV, McLean IW, Specht CS, Varga J. Adenoid cystic carcinomas of the lacrimal gland in childhood and adolescence. Ophthalmology 1997;104:1622–5.
46. Gamel JW, Font RL. Adenoid cystic carcinoma of the lacrimal gland: the clinical significance of a basaloid histologic pattern. Hum Pathol 1982;13:219–25.
46a. Iwamoto T, Jakobiec FA. A comparative ultrastructural study of the normal lacrimal gland and its epithelial tumors. Hum Pathol 1982;13: 236–62.
46b. Sturgis CD, Silverman JF, Kennerdell JS, Raab SS. Fine-needle aspiration for the diagnosis of primary epithelial tumors of the lacrimal gland and ocular adnexa. Diagn Cytopathol 2001;24: 86–9.
47. Penner CR, Folpe AL, Budnick SD. C-kit expression distinguishes salivary gland adenoid cystic carcinoma from polymorphous low-grade adenocarcinoma. Mod Pathol 2002;15:687–91.
48. Franzen G, Nordgard S, Boysen M, Larsen PL, Halvorsen TB, Clausen OP. DNA content in adenoid cystic carcinomas. Head Neck 1995;17: 49–55.
49. Yamamoto Y, Wistuba II, Kishimoto Y, et al. DNA analysis at p53 locus in adenoid cystic carcinoma: comparison of molecular study and p53 immunostaining. Pathol Int 1998;48:273–80.

50. Umeno H, Miyajima Y, Mori K, Nakashima T. [Clinicopathological study of 54 cases of adenoid cystic carcinoma in the head and neck.] Nippon Jibiinkoka Gakkai Kaiho 1997;100: 1442–9. (Japanese.)
51. Meldrum ML, Tse DT, Benedetto P. Neoadjuvant intracarotid chemotherapy for treatment of advanced adenocystic carcinoma of the lacrimal gland. Arch Ophthalmol 1998;116:315–21.

Malignant Mixed Tumor

52. Perzin KH, Jakobiec FA, Livolsi VA, Desjardins L. Lacrimal gland malignant mixed tumors (carcinomas arising in benign mixed tumors): a clinico-pathologic study. Cancer 1980;45: 2593–606.
53. Henderson JW, Farrow GM. Primary malignant mixed tumors of the lacrimal gland. Report of 10 cases. Ophthalmology 1980;87:466–75.
54. Font RL, Patipa M, Rosenbaum PS, Smith S, Berg L. Correlation of computed tomographic and histopathologic features in malignant transformation of benign mixed tumor of lacrimal gland. Surv Ophthalmol 1990;34:449–52.
54a. Wright JE, Rose GE, Garner A. Primary malignant neoplasms of the lacrimal gland. Br J Ophthalmol 1992;76:401–7.
54b. Font RL, Smith SL, Bryan RG. Malignant epithelial tumors of the lacrimal gland: a clinicopathologic study of 21 cases. Arch Ophthalmol 1998;116:613–6.

Primary Adenocarcinoma

55. Paulino AF, Huvos AG. Epithelial tumors of the lacrimal glands: a clinicopathologic study. Ann Diagn Pathol 1999;3:199–204.
56. Henderson JW. Orbital tumors, 3rd ed. New York: Raven Press; 1994.
57. Heaps RS, Miller NR, Albert DM, Green WR, Vitale S. Primary adenocarcinoma of the lacrimal gland. A retrospective study. Ophthalmology 1993;100:1856–60.
57a. Font RL, Gamel JW. Epithelial tumors of the lacrimal gland: an analysis of 265 cases. In: Jakobiec FA, ed. Ocular and adnexal tumors. Birmingham, AL: Aesculapius Publishing Co; 1978:787–805.

Mucoepidermoid Carcinoma

58. Wagoner MD, Chuo N, Gonder JR, Grove AS Jr, Albert DM. Mucoepidermoid carcinoma of the lacrimal gland. Ann Ophthalmol 1982;14:383–4, 386.
59. Sofinski SJ, Brown BZ, Rao N, Wan WL. Mucoepidermoid carcinoma of the lacrimal gland. Case report and review of the literature. Ophthal Plast Reconstr Surg 1986;2:147–51.
60. Eviatar JA, Hornblass A. Mucoepidermoid carcinoma of the lacrimal gland: 25 cases and a review and update of the literature. Ophthal Plast Reconstr Surg 1993;9:170–81.
61. Pulitzer DR, Eckert ER. Mucoepidermoid carcinoma of the lacrimal gland. An oxyphilic variant. Arch Ophthalmol 1987;105:1406–9.

Miscellaneous Carcinomas

62. Khalil M, Arthurs B. Basal cell adenocarcinoma of the lacrimal gland. Ophthalmology 2000;107: 164–8.
62a. Wright JE, Rose GE, Garner A. Primary malignant neoplasms of the lacrimal gland. Br J Ophthalmol 1992;76:401–7.
62b. Henderson JW. Orbital tumors, 3rd ed. New York: Raven Press; 1994.
63. Ni C, Kuo PK, Dryja TP. Histopathological classification of 272 primary epithelial tumors of the lacrimal gland. Chin Med J (Engl) 1992;105: 481–5.
63a. Paulino AF, Huvos AG. Epithelial tumors of the lacrimal glands: a clinicopathologic study. Ann Diagn Pathol 1999;3:199–204.
64. Bloching M, Hinze R, Berghaus A. Lymphoepithelioma-like carcinoma of the lacrimal gland. Eur Arch Otorhinolaryngol 2000;257:399–401.
65. Rao NA, Kaiser E, Quiros PA, Sadun AA, See RF. Lymphoepithelial carcinoma of the lacrimal gland. Arch Ophthalmol 2002;120:1745–8.
66. Katz SE, Rootman J, Dolman PJ, White VA, Berean KW. Primary ductal adenocarcinoma of the lacrimal gland. Ophthalmology 1996;103: 157–62.
67. Nasu M, Haisa T, Kondo T, Matsubara O. Primary ductal adenocarcinoma of the lacrimal gland. Pathol Int 1998;48:981–4.
68. De Rosa G, Zeppa P, Tranfa F, Bonavolonta G. Acinic cell carcinoma arising in a lacrimal gland. First case report. Cancer 1986;57:1988–91.
69. Rosenbaum PS, Mahadevia PS, Goodman LA, Kress Y. Acinic cell carcinoma of the lacrimal gland. Arch Ophthalmol 1995;113:781–5.
70. Jang J, Kie JH, Lee SY, et al. Acinic cell carcinoma of the lacrimal gland with intracranial extension: a case report. Ophthal Plast Reconstr Surg 2001;17:454–7.
71. Shields JA, Font RL. Meibomian gland carcinoma presenting as a lacrimal gland tumor. Arch Ophthalmol 1974;92:304–6.
72. Rodgers IR, Jakobiec FA, Gingold MP, Hornblass A, Krebs W. Anaplastic carcinoma of the lacrimal gland presenting with recurrent subconjunctival hemorrhages and displaying incipient sebaceous differentiation. Ophthal Plast Reconstr Surg 1991;7:229–37.

73. Konrad EA, Thiel HJ. Adenocarcinoma of the lacrimal gland with sebaceous differentiation. A clinical study using light and electron-microscopy. Graefes Arch Chin Exp Ophthalmol 1983;221:81–5.
74. Harvey PA, Parsons MA, Rennie IG. Primary sebaceous carcinoma of lacrimal gland: a previously unreported primary neoplasm. Eye 1994; 8:592–5.
75. Briscoe D, Mahmood S, Bonshek R, Jackson A, Leatherbarrow R. Primary sebaceous carcinoma of the lacrimal gland. Br J Ophthalmol 2001;85:625–6.

Lymphoid Lesions

76. Polito E, Leccisotti A. Prognosis of orbital lymphoid hyperplasia. Graefes Arch Clin Exp Ophthalmol 1996;234:150–4.
76a. Jakobiec FA, Bilyk JR, Font RL. Orbit. In Spencer WH, ed. Ophthalmic pathology. An atlas and textbook, 4th ed. Philadelphia: WB Sauders Co; 1996:2485–525.
76b. Shields CL, Shields JA, Eagle RC, Rathmell JP. Clinicopathologic review of 142 cases of lacrimal gland lesions. Ophthalmology 1989;96:431–5.
77. Jeffrey PB, Cartwright D, Atwater SK, Char DH, Miller TR. Lacrimal gland lymphoma: a cytomorphologic and immunophenotypic study. Diagn Cytopathol 1995;12:215–22.
78. Patel S, Rootman J. Nodular sclerosing Hodgkin's disease of the orbit. Ophthalmology 1983;90:1433–6.
79. Chim CS, Ng I, Trendell-Smith NJ, Liang R. Primary extramedullary plasmacytoma of the lacrimal gland. Leuk Lymphoma 2001;42:831–4.
80. Little JM. Waldenstrom's macroglobulinemia in the lacrimal gland. Trans Am Acad Ophthalmol Otorhinolaryngol 1967;71:875–9.
81. Krishnan K, Adams PT. Bilateral orbital tumors and lacrimal gland involvement in Waldenstrom's macroglobulinemia. Eur J Haematol 1995;55:205–6.

Mesenchymal Tumors

82. Basar D, Ozman M. Hemangioma of the lacrimal gland. Report of a case. Am J Ophthalmol 1966;62:343–4.
83. Kargi S, Ozdal P, Kargi E, Koybasioglu F. Hemangioma of the lacrimal gland. Plast Reconstr Surg 2001;108:1829–30.
84. Burnstine MA, Morton AD, Font RL, et al. Lacrimal gland hemangiopericytoma. Orbit 1998;17:179–88.
85. McDonald P, Jakobiec FA, Hornblass A, Iwamoto T. Benign peripheral nerve sheath tumors (neurofibromas) of the lacrimal gland. Ophthalmology 1983;90:1403–13.
86. Scott IU, Tanenbaum M, Rubin D, Lores E. Solitary fibrous tumor of the lacrimal gland fossa. Ophthalmology 1996;103:1613–8.

Secondary and Metastatic Tumors

87. Harris DC, Clark CV, Bartholomew RS. Carcinoid tumour in the lacrimal gland. Doc Ophthalmol 1989;73:43–51.
88. Shields JA, Shields CL, Eagle RC Jr, Singh AD, Armstrong T. Metastatic renal cell carcinoma to the palpebral lobe of the lacrimal gland. Ophthal Plast Reconstr Surg 2001;17:191–4.
88a. Jakobiec FA, Bilyk JR, Font RL. Orbit. In Spencer WH, ed. Ophthalmic pathology. An atlas and textbook, 4th ed. Philadelphia: WB Sauders Co; 1996:2485–525.
88b. Shields CL, Shields JA, Eagle RC, Rathmell JP. Clinicopathologic review of 142 cases of lacrimal gland lesions. Ophthalmology 1989;96:431–5.

Tumor-Like Lesions

89. Mombaerts I, Schlingemann RO, Goldschmeding R, Noorduyn LA, Koornneef L. The surgical management of lacrimal gland pseudotumors. Ophthalmology 1996;103:1619–27.
90. Font RL, Yanoff M, Zimmerman LE. Benign lymphoepithelial lesion of the lacrimal gland and its relationship to Sjogren's syndrome. Am J Clin Pathol 1967;48:365–76.
91. Pepose JS, Akata RF, Pflugfelder SC, Voigt W. Mononuclear cell phenotypes and immunoglobulin gene rearrangements in lacrimal gland biopsies from patients with Sjogren's syndrome. Ophthalmology 1990;97:1599–605.
92. Font RL, Laucirica R, Rosenbaum PS, Patrinely JR, Boniuk M. Malignant lymphoma of the ocular adnexa associated with the benign lymphoepithelial lesion of the parotid glands. Report of two cases. Ophthalmology 1992;99: 1582–7.
93. Smith S, Rootman J. Lacrimal duct cysts. Presentation and management. Surv Ophthalmol 1986;30:245–50.
94. Bullock JD, Fleishman JA, Rosset JS. Lacrimal ductal cysts. Ophthalmology 1986;93:1355–60.
95. Duke-Elder S, MacFaul PA. The ocular adnexa, Vol XIII. In: Duke-Elder S, ed. System of ophthalmology. London: Henry Kimptom; 1974: 638–43.
95a. Jakobiec FA, Bilyk JR, Font RL. Orbit. In Spencer WH, ed. Ophthalmic pathology. An atlas and textbook, 4th ed. Philadelphia: WB Sauders Co; 1996:2485–525.

Staging and Grading

96. American Joint Committee on Cancer. AJCC cancer staging manual, 5th ed. Philadelphia: Lippincott-Raven; 1997.

7 TUMORS OF THE LACRIMAL DRAINAGE SYSTEM

ANATOMY AND HISTOLOGY

The lacrimal drainage system is composed of an upper and a lower punctum, two lacrimal canaliculi, a lacrimal sac, and a nasolacrimal duct. The tears are drained from the ocular surface into the canaliculi through the puncta. The upper punctum is located at the medial end of the upper eyelid margin, 6 mm lateral to the medial canthus (fig. 7-1). The lower punctum is located at the lower eyelid margin, 6.5 mm lateral to the canthus. Each punctum is a round or transversely oval aperture, measuring about 0.33 mm, and surrounded by connective tissue and skeletal muscle fibers. Extending from each punctum is the canaliculus, a small tubular structure measuring about 0.5 mm in diameter. The canaliculus has two portions: a vertical portion, approximately 2 mm in length, and a horizontal portion, about 8 mm in length. The vertical portion bends medially at a right angle to continue with the horizontal portion. Both upper and lower canaliculi narrow abruptly and turn medially to join before entering the lacrimal sac through its lateral wall. The opening in the lateral wall is called the internal lacrimal punctum. In some cases, the two canaliculi may not join, and each may enter the sac individually.

The lacrimal sac measures about 13 to 15 mm in length. It is located in the lacrimal fossa of the medial orbital wall and is surrounded by loose connective tissue that contains a rich venous plexus and lacrimal fascia. The sac is composed of a fundus, which is located above the medial canthus, and a body, located below the canthus. The downward extension of the sac forms the nasolacrimal duct (fig. 7-1). The duct is about 17 mm long, with the upper 12 mm enclosed in a bony canal. The duct terminates inferiorly as the lacrimal ostium, which opens on the lateral wall of the inferior nasal meatus.

Histologically, the tubular canaliculus is lined by nonkeratinizing, stratified squamous epithelium (fig. 7-2). The wall of the canaliculus contains collagenous and elastic tissue. In contrast, the lacrimal sac is lined by a stratified columnar epithelium that contains scattered goblet cells; in some areas, this epithelium may be ciliated (figs. 7-3, 7-4). The epithelial lining rests on a basement membrane. The subepithelial tissue contains scattered lymphocytes. The nasolacrimal duct has histologic features similar to those noted in the sac.

CLASSIFICATION AND FREQUENCY

Primary lacrimal sac tumors include those arising from the epithelium or the mesenchymal components of the sac. Secondary tumors involving the sac originate in the adjacent maxillary and ethmoid sinuses, in the nose, or in the orbit. Tumors that arise from these sites may

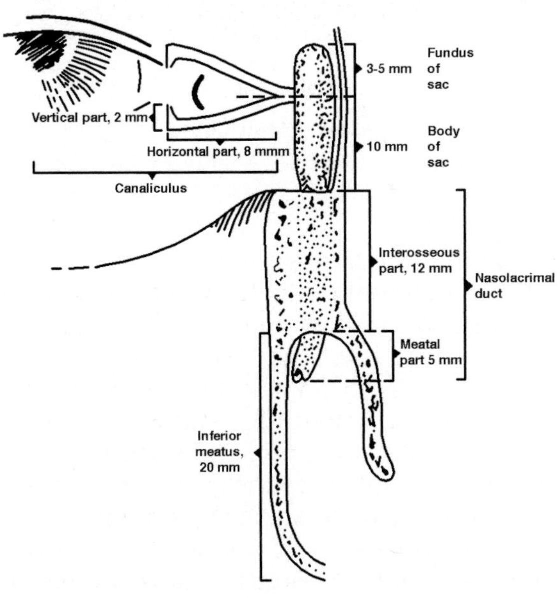

Figure 7-1

LACRIMAL DRAINAGE SYSTEM

The measurements of the adult lacrimal drainage system. (Fig. 60 from Jones LT. The lacrimal apparatus. In: Jones LT, Reeh MJ, Wirtschapter JD, eds. Ophthalmic anatomy: a manual with some clinical application. Rochester, MN: American Academy of Ophthalmology and Otolaryngology; 1970:225.)

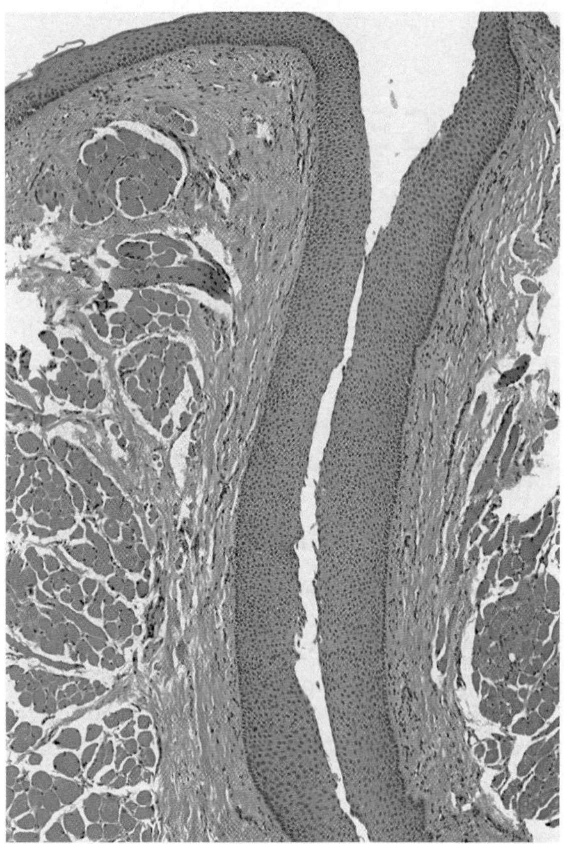

Figure 7-2

NORMAL CANALICULUS

The canaliculus is lined by stratified nonkeratinized epithelium.

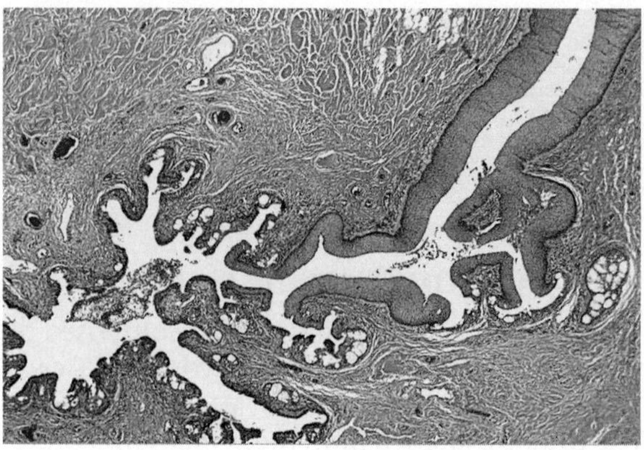

Figure 7-3

LACRIMAL SAC AND CANALICULUS

The canaliculus on the right has nonkeratinized squamous epithelium and the sac on the left, stratified columnar epithelium containing goblet cells.

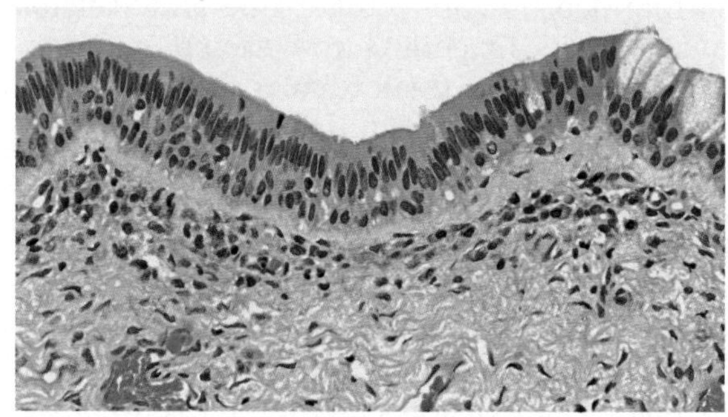

Figure 7-4

LACRIMAL SAC

Higher magnification of the sac seen in figure 7-3 shows stratified columnar epithelium containing goblet cells.

extend into the lacrimal sac and may present with clinical features similar to those observed in primary lacrimal sac tumors, including signs associated with nasolacrimal system obstruction.

The majority of primary tumors arise from the epithelium. Among these epithelial tumors, malignant tumors are more common than benign tumors. Primary epithelial tumors account for 73 percent of all lacrimal sac tumors, followed by mesenchymal tumors (14 percent), lymphoid lesions (8 percent), malignant melanoma (4 percent), and others (1 percent) (1–17). The distribution of lacrimal sac tumors on file at the American Registry of Ophthalmic Pathology and those seen at the Doheny Eye Institute are summarized in Tables 7-1 and 7-2.

Although several investigators have classified lacrimal sac tumors into primary epithelial and mesenchymal neoplasms, Ryan and Font (2) proposed an in-depth classification of the epithelial tumors based on histopathologic features combined with growth pattern. These investigators based their classification system on their study of 27 primary epithelial tumors of the lacrimal sac. They divided these neoplasms into three major groups: papillomas, papillomas with foci of carcinoma changes, and carcinomas. Based on their histologic features the papillomas were subdivided into three types: 1) squamous cell papillomas, 2) transitional cell papillomas, and 3) mixed cell papillomas that exhibited features of both squamous and transitional cell papillomas. Moreover, based on their growth patterns, these benign tumors were grouped as

Table 7-1

FREQUENCY DISTRIBUTION OF 35 LACRIMAL SAC TUMORS COLLECTED BETWEEN 1984 AND 1989 AT THE AMERICAN REGISTRY OF OPHTHALMIC PATHOLOGY, ARMED FORCES INSTITUTE OF PATHOLOGY

Type of Tumor	Number of Cases
Epithelial	
Papilloma	9
Oncocytoma	3
Carcinoma	17
Lymphoid	
Reactive lymphoid hyperplasia	2
Lymphoma	4

Table 7-2

FREQUENCY DISTRIBUTION OF 28 LACRIMAL SAC TUMORS COLLECTED BETWEEN 1970 AND 2000 AT THE DOHENY EYE INSTITUTE

Type of Tumor	Number of Cases
Benign Epithelial Tumors	
Transitional cell papilloma	3
Oncocytoma	1
Malignant Epithelial Tumors	
Transition cell carcinoma	5
Adenoid cystic carcinoma	4
Mucoepidermoid cancer	2
Adenocarcinoma	3
Squamous cell carcinoma	3
Nonepithelial Tumors	
Lymphoid lesions	5[a]
Granular cell tumor	1
Primary melanoma	1

[a]Two of these cases were lymphomas, and one was chronic lymphocytic leukemia. The remaining two revealed atypical lymphoid hyperplasia.

exophytic, inverted, or mixed growth pattern. Papillomas with foci of carcinoma change were similarly divided into various subtypes, based on their histologic features and growth patterns, as summarized in Table 7-3.

Carcinomas that arise de novo are divided into papillary and nonpapillary types. Based on their histologic features, these carcinomas are further subdivided into squamous carcinomas, transitional carcinomas, or adenocarcinomas (Table 7-2). Stefanyzyn et al. (3) identified additional histologic types of both benign and malignant epithelial tumors, based on their review of 82 epithelial tumors filed in the American Registry of Ophthalmic Pathology at the Armed Forces Institute of Pathology (AFIP). From the same institute, Pe'er and his co-workers (17) reported 33 nonepithelial tumors, including mesenchymal and lymphoid lesions. These epithelial and nonepithelial tumors are summarized in Tables 7-4 and 7-5.

The above three large reported series from the American Registry of Ophthalmic Pathology of the AFIP reveal that epithelial tumors are more common than nonepithelial tumors of the lacrimal sac (2,3,17). Based on such reported case series, the original classification proposed by Ryan and Font can be expanded to include additional histologic types of both benign and malignant epithelial neoplasms of the lacrimal sac. Moreover, the nonepithelial tumors include diverse histologic types. Thus the classification of lacrimal sac tumors may require the inclusion of varieties of both epithelial and nonepithelial tumors, as summarized in Table 7-6.

Table 7-3

CLASSIFICATION OF LACRIMAL SAC EPITHELIAL TUMORS[a]

Tumors	Number of Cases
Papilloma	11
Growth pattern	
Exophytic	6
Inverted	3
Mixed	2
Histologic features	
Squamous	3
Transitional	7
Mixed	1
Papilloma with Foci of Carcinoma	7
Growth pattern	
Exophytic	0
Inverted	3
Mixed	4
Histologic features	
Squamous	3
Transitional	3
Mixed	1
Carcinoma	9
Growth pattern	
Papillary	2
Nonpapillary	7
Histologic features	
Squamous	6
Transitional	2
Oncocytic	1

[a]Modified from Table 3 from reference 2.

Table 7-4

HISTOPATHOLOGIC CLASSIFICATION OF LACRIMAL SAC EPITHELIAL TUMORS[a]

Benign (38 cases)		Malignant (44 cases)	
Squamous papilloma	19	Papilloma with foci of carcinoma	6
Transitional papilloma	13	Squamous carcinoma	22
		Transitional carcinoma	5
Oncocytoma	4	Mucoepidermoid carcinoma	3
Benign mixed carcinoma	2	Adenoid cystic carcinoma	3
		Adenocarcinoma	2
		Oncocytic carcinoma	2
		Poorly differentiated carcinoma	1

[a]Data from reference 3.

Table 7-5

HISTOPATHOLOGIC CLASSIFICATION OF LACRIMAL SAC NONEPITHELIAL TUMORS[a]

Fibrous histiocytoma	13
Lymphoid lesion[b]	10
Melanoma	6
Hemangiopericytoma	1
Lipoma	1
Granulocytic sarcoma	1
Neurofibroma	1

[a]Based on data from reference 17.
[b]Of the 10 lymphoid lesions, 8 were lymphomas and 2 were atypical lymphoid hyperplasia.

Table 7-6

HISTOLOGIC CLASSIFICATION OF LACRIMAL SAC TUMORS BASED ON PREVIOUSLY REPORTED SERIES OF CASES FROM THE AMERICAN REGISTRY OF OPHTHALMIC PATHOLOGY, ARMED FORCES INSTITUTE OF PATHOLOGY

Epithelial Tumors
- Papillomas
  - Growth pattern
    - Exophytic
    - Inverted
    - Mixed
  - Histologic features
    - Squamous
    - Transitional
    - Squamous mixed with transitional features
    - Oncocytic
    - Benign mixed tumor
- Papillomas with foci of carcinoma
  - Growth pattern
    - Exophytic
    - Inverted
    - Exophytic mixed with inverted pattern
  - Histologic features
    - Squamous
    - Transitional
    - Squamous mixed with transitional features
- Carcinomas
  - Growth pattern
    - Papillary
    - Nonpapillary
  - Histologic features
    - Squamous
    - Transitional
    - Mucoepidermoid
    - Adenoid cystic
    - Adenocarcinoma
    - Oncocytic
    - Poorly differentiated

Nonepithelial Tumors
- Mesenchymal tumor
- Lymphoid and hematopoietic tumor
- Melanoma
- Others

Lacrimal sac tumors may be slightly more common in men than in women: of the 38 benign epithelial tumors on file with the AFIP, 23 occurred in men and 15 in women. There were 44 malignant epithelial tumors: 24 in men and 20 in women. Similarly, of the 33 nonepithelial tumors, 17 occurred in men and 15 in women (2,3,17).

EPITHELIAL TUMORS (PAPILLOMAS AND CARCINOMAS OF THE LACRIMAL SAC)

Epithelial tumors of the lacrimal sac are divided, based on their histologic features, into papillomas of squamous cell, transitional cell, mixed squamous and transitional cell, and oncocytic type. In addition to these benign tumors, pleomorphic adenomas also develop in the lacrimal sac. Malignant epithelial tumors include papillomas with foci of carcinoma change and carcinomas that arise de novo (Table 7-6).

Benign Epithelial Tumors

Definition. Benign epithelial tumors of the lacrimal sac are mostly *papillomas*, exhibiting either stratified squamous epithelium or transitional epithelium, or a mixture of both. Rarely,

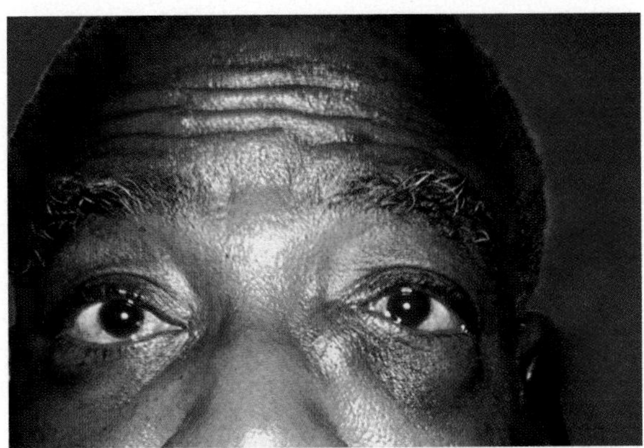

Figure 7-5

ONCOCYTOMA

Clinical appearance of oncocytoma of the left lacrimal sac.

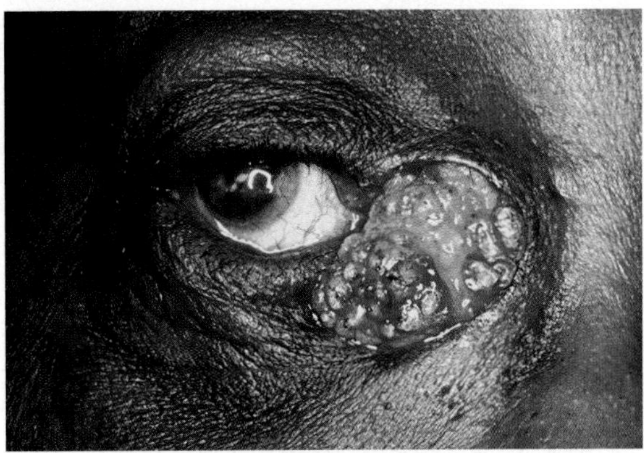

Figure 7-6

RECURRENT PAPILLOMA

Recurrent papilloma of the lacrimal sac ulcerates the overlying skin.

other histologic features are seen in these benign tumors, such as oncocytic cells or features of benign mixed tumor. Cytologic examination reveals small nuclei without hyperchromasia and infiltrative features; some papillomas, however, show invasive acanthosis.

General Features. In a large series of lacrimal sac tumors reported by Stefanyszyn et al. (3), the mean age of patients with benign epithelial tumors was 52 years: 44 years for patients with benign papillomas, 47 years for patients with squamous cell papillomas, and 40 years for those with transitional cell papillomas. The age range of these patients was 9 to 88 years. In contrast, most patients with oncocytoma and benign mixed tumor were older, with mean ages of 72 and 67 years, respectively, and an age range of 55 to 80 years.

The pathogenesis of these lacrimal sac tumors is not clear; however, immunohistochemical and polymerase chain reaction analyses reveal evidence of the presence of human papilloma virus (HPV) infection, particularly in papillomas composed of squamous epithelium (18).

Clinical Features. Signs and symptoms are virtually similar in patients with the various histologic types of lacrimal sac tumors; these include epiphora, recurrent episodes of dacryocystitis, and the presence of a mass in the region of the lacrimal sac (fig. 7-5). Patients present with the insidious onset of dacryostenosis and/or dacryocystitis. In the AFIP series, more than half of the patients complained of chronic epiphora or tearing, more than a third of the patients had a history of chronic dacryocystitis, and one third of the patients presented with a lacrimal sac mass or mucocele (2,3). Bleeding from the puncta or nose occurs in some cases, particularly in patients with malignant neoplasms (2,3). The usual sequence of clinical events is the presence of epiphora, followed by recurrent bouts of dacryocystitis, development of a lacrimal sac mass, and in some cases, epistaxis (3). The slow growth of the tumor, coupled with the obstructive symptoms, often masquerades as chronic dacryocystitis. Frequently, the dacryocystitis does not respond to antibiotics and anti-inflammatory agents (16). Recurrent tumors may cause ulceration of overlying skin (fig. 7-6). The presence of epistaxis and pain could be an ominous sign, suggestive of a malignant tumor.

Investigations are usually directed at determining the patency of the lacrimal drainage system by dacryocystogram, Jones testing, lacrimal syringing, telescopic nasal endoscopy, and computerized tomography (CT). The radiologic investigations that are most useful in the diagnosis of the tumors are the dacryocystogram and CT scan (3). The dacryocystogram may reveal a filling defect in conjunction with delayed drainage of the contrast material. The lacrimal sac may be distended and have a mottled density. The CT scan is better at delineating tumor extent and is helpful in follow-up examinations after surgery or radiation.

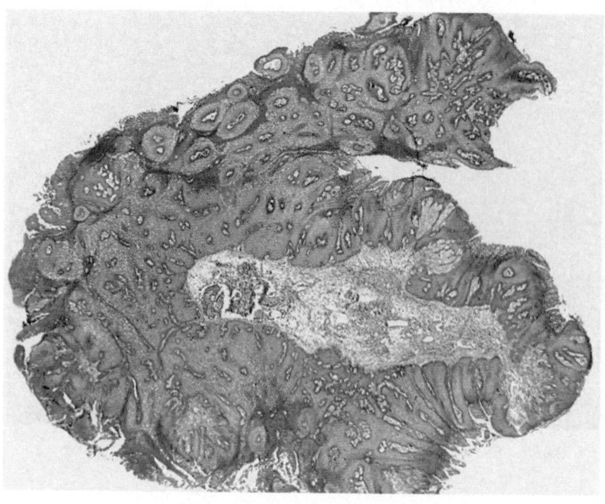

Figure 7-7

SQUAMOUS CELL PAPILLOMA

Squamous cell papilloma with exophytic pattern.

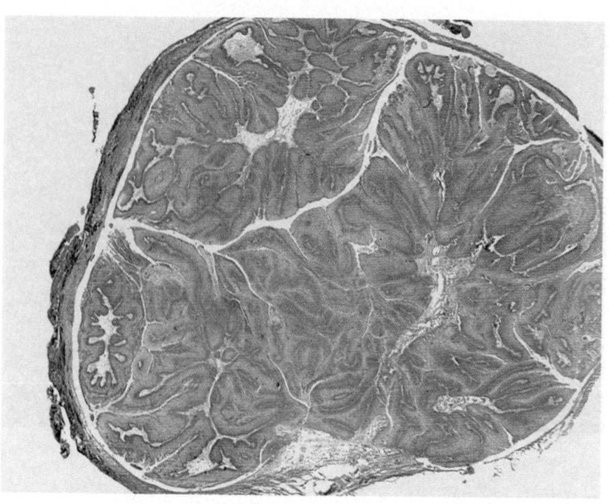

Figure 7-8

SQUAMOUS CELL PAPILLOMA

Squamous cell papilloma with inverted pattern fills the lacrimal sac.

Microscopic Findings. Papillomas arising from the epithelium of the lacrimal sac exhibit three distinct growth patterns: exophytic (fig. 7-7), inverted (fig. 7-8), and mixed. Exophytic papillomas are fungiform masses with projecting, finger-like proliferations of acanthotic epithelium. In inverted papillomas, areas of acanthotic of surface epithelium invade the underlying stroma. Papillomas with mixed growth pattern have a combination of exophytic and inverted patterns. The epithelial lining of these papillomas can be squamous (fig. 7-7), transitional (figs. 7-9–7-11), or a mixture of these two epithelia. Squamous papillomas are composed of acanthotic, stratified, squamous epithelium with occasional foci of dyskeratosis. Transitional cell papillomas have epithelial cells resembling those normally present in the mucosa of the lacrimal sac: that is, stratified columnar epithelium containing goblet cells (fig. 7-12) and, in some instances, fine cilia. Numerous neutrophils are scattered within the epithelium. Papillomas with mixed histologic patterns are made up of acanthotic, stratified, squamous epithelium and of stratified columnar epithelium containing few or several goblet cells.

Although papillomas are classified based on both their histologic features and their growth patterns, the latter may have biologic significance, particularly with the occurrence of focal carcinomatous changes (fig. 7-13). Unlike exophytic tumors, papillomas with an inverted or mixed growth pattern may contain foci of malignancy, or they may develop into carcinoma (2). In the study reported by Ryan and Font (2), none of the six exophytic papillomas developed into carcinoma; however, 7 of the 12 papillomas that exhibited an inverted or mixed growth pattern either revealed foci of carcinoma or developed into carcinoma. In contrast, Stefanyszyn et al. (3) found that carcinoma developed in both exophytic and inverted papillomas and carcinoma was seen in both squamous and transitional cell papillomas.

Benign oncocytomas consist of large epithelial cells that contain abundant granular eosinophilic cytoplasm and a round to oval paracentral nucleus (19–21). The oncocytes form cords, nests, and tubules, surrounded by mucin-filled cystic spaces (figs. 7-14, 7-15). These oncocytes contain numerous abnormal-appearing mitochondria. Occasional tumors may contain lymphoid follicles similar to a Warthin's tumor of the salivary gland.

Benign mixed tumor of the lacrimal sac is rare; in their series of 82 epithelial tumors of the sac, Stefanyszyn et al. (3) found only 2 cases exhibiting features of benign mixed tumor. These tumors were made up of proliferating cuboidal cells that formed ducts in a hyalinized stroma. Histologic examination revealed features similar to pleomorphic adenoma of the lacrimal gland.

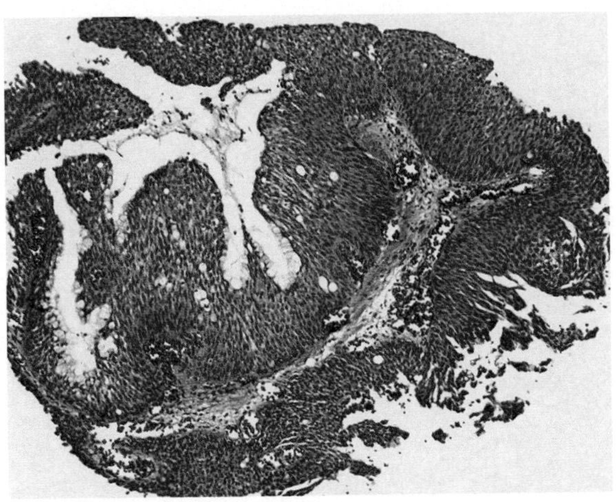

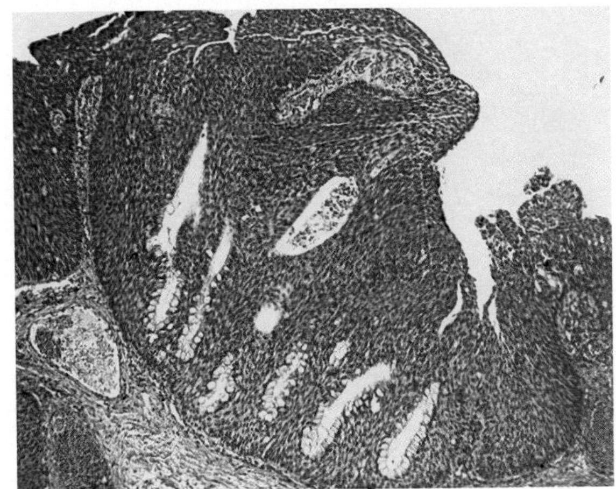

Figure 7-9

TRANSITIONAL CELL PAPILLOMA

Left: Transitional cell papilloma of the lacrimal sac with focal goblet cell hyperplasia.
Right: In another example, the cystic spaces show goblet cell hyperplasia.

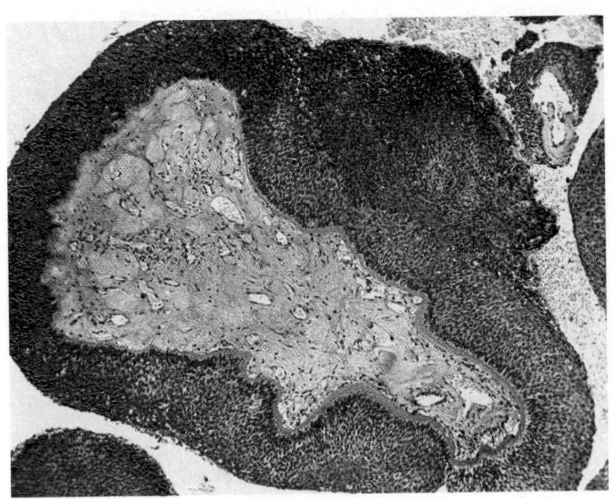

Figure 7-10

TRANSITIONAL CELL PAPILLOMA

Transitional cell papilloma with exophytic pattern. The periodic acid–Schiff (PAS)-positive material in the epithelium is glycogen.

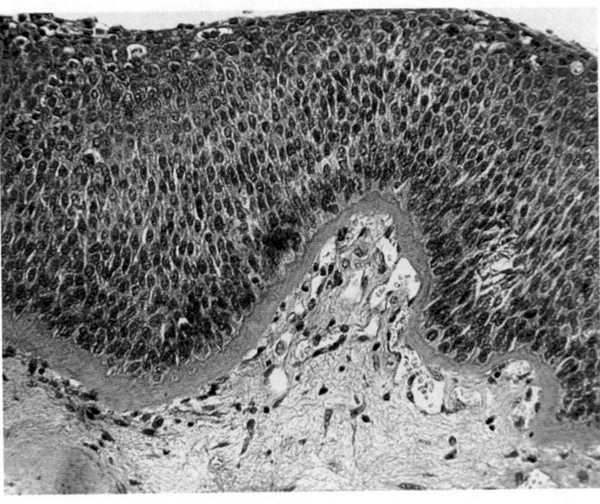

Figure 7-11

TRANSITIONAL CELL PAPILLOMA

The basement membrane is thickened (PAS positive).

Treatment and Prognosis. Benign lacrimal sac tumors are usually managed by dacryocystorhinostomy with simple excision of the mass. Between 10 and 40 percent of patients who undergo such surgical excision have a recurrence of the tumor. Most recurrences are of the inverted type of papilloma, even after wide excision (1,2). Recurrent tumors may also reveal foci of carcinomatous change (2).

Malignant Epithelial Tumors

Definition. Carcinomas of the lacrimal sac include papillomas with foci of carcinoma, recurrent papillomas with focal carcinomatous change, and carcinomas arising de novo into papillary and nonpapillary growth patterns (2).

General Features. Patients with malignant epithelial tumors of the lacrimal sac are generally older than those with benign tumors. The mean age of patients with carcinoma is 58

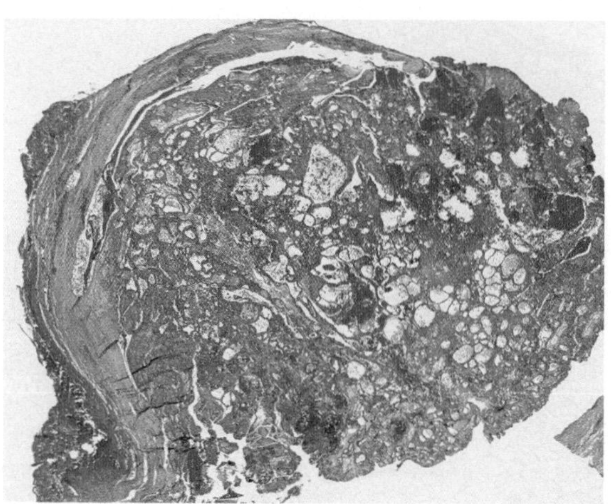
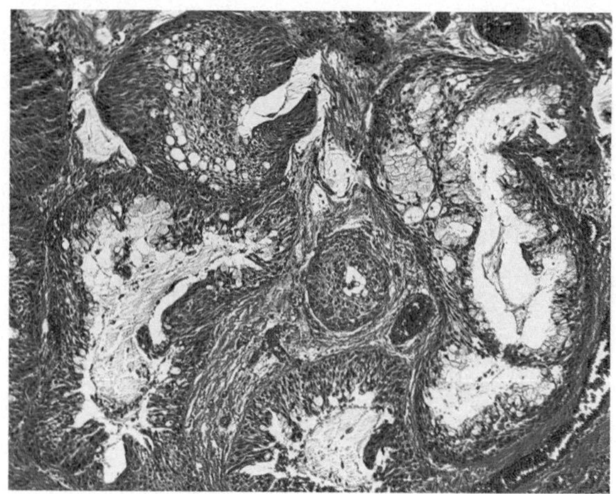

Figure 7-12

TRANSITIONAL CELL PAPILLOMA

Left: The papilloma has an inverted pattern and goblet cell hyperplasia with mucus-filled cystic spaces.
Right: Inverted pattern and areas of goblet cell hyperplasia.

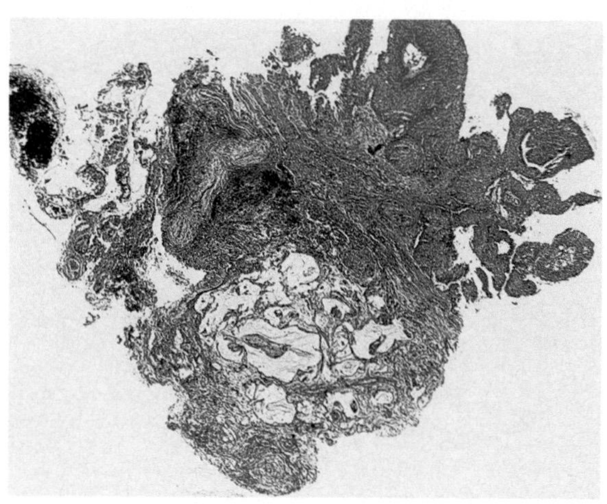
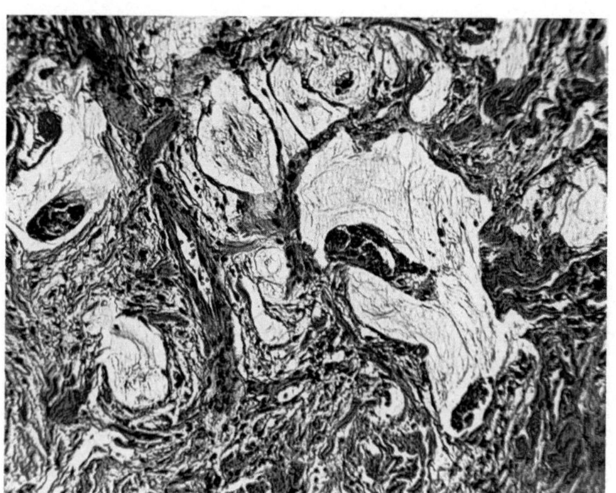

Figure 7-13

EXOPHYTIC PAPILLOMA

Left: An infiltrating mucus-secreting adenocarcinoma is at the base of an exophytic papilloma.
Right: High-power view shows mucin-filled pools containing epithelial islands.

years; however, the age range is from 16 to 89 years (3). With a mean age of 63 years, patients with squamous cell carcinoma are older than those with transitional cell carcinoma (mean, 47 years). The mean age of patients with oncocytic adenocarcinoma is 79 years. In contrast, patients with adenoid cystic carcinoma are relatively young, with a mean age of 51 years and an age range of 38 to 64 years (3).

Clinical Features. Patients with malignant epithelial tumors of the lacrimal sac present with signs and symptoms similar to those seen with benign tumors, except that epistaxis is often noted with malignancy (16). These tumors may also present as an ulcerated mass at the medial canthus (figs. 7-16, 7-17). Since the normal lacrimal sac is a small structure, it may not be visualized by either CT scan or magnetic resonance imaging (MRI), whereas such scans of sac malignancies may show a mass (fig. 7-18). An MRI of epithelial carcinoma may reveal a preseptal mass in the medial orbit that, on T1-

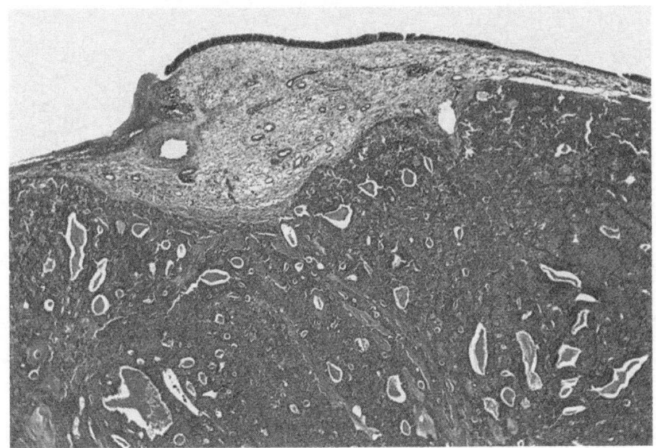

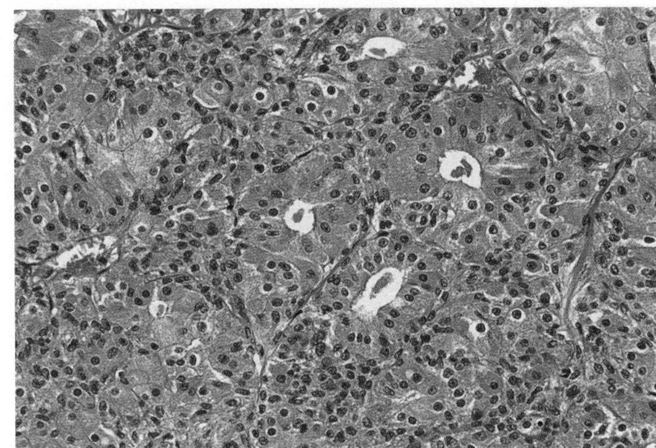

Figure 7-14

ONCOCYTOMA

Left: The oncocytes in the glandular pattern display marked acidophilia of the cytoplasm.
Right: High-power view of the tubular structures lined with oncocytes.

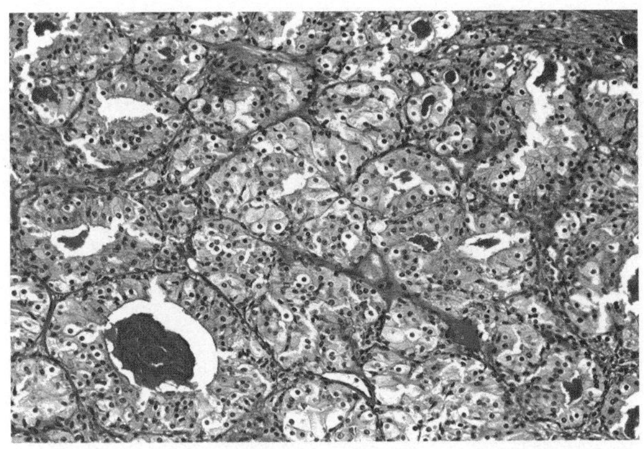

Figure 7-15

ONCOCYTOMA

PAS-positive material is present in the lumens of the tubules.

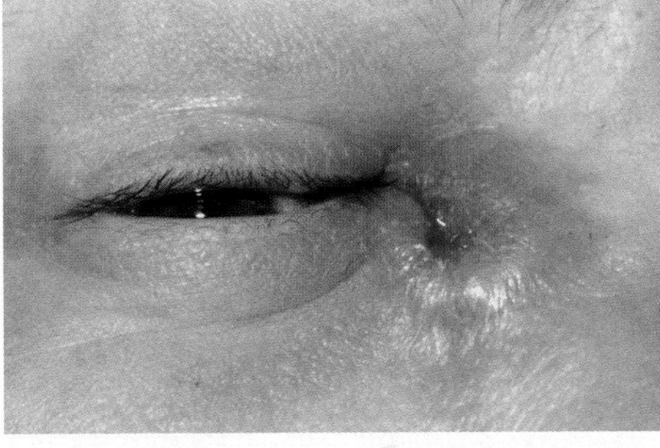

Figure 7-16

MUCOEPIDERMOID CARCINOMA

The ulcerated mass extends from the medial canthus to the bridge of the nose.

weighted imaging, shows isointense to normal brain and enhances moderately after contrast administration. On proton density-weighted imaging, squamous cell carcinomas of the lacrimal sac are isointense to normal muscle, but on T2-weighted sequences, these carcinomas are of low signal intensity (22).

Microscopic Findings. Based on their histologic features, carcinomas are classified as squamous, transitional, or adenocarcinoma. Other rare histologic types of carcinoma are sometimes noted; these include mucoepidermoid carcinoma (figs. 7-19–7-22), adenoid cystic carcinoma, oncocytic carcinoma, and poorly differentiated carcinoma (figs. 7-3, 7-23–7-28). Of all these histologic types of epithelial malignancy, the most frequent is squamous cell carcinoma (figs. 7-23–7-30), followed by papillomas with focal carcinomatous change and transitional cell carcinomas (2). These malignant tumors may show vascular invasion (2).

Squamous cell carcinomas have a wide range of differentiation, including the formation of keratin pearls, atypical squamous cells with abundant eosinophilic cytoplasm, pleomorphic nuclei, and prominent nucleoli. Mitotic figures are frequently seen, and the neoplastic cells invade the lacrimal sac wall. Necrosis and infiltration of

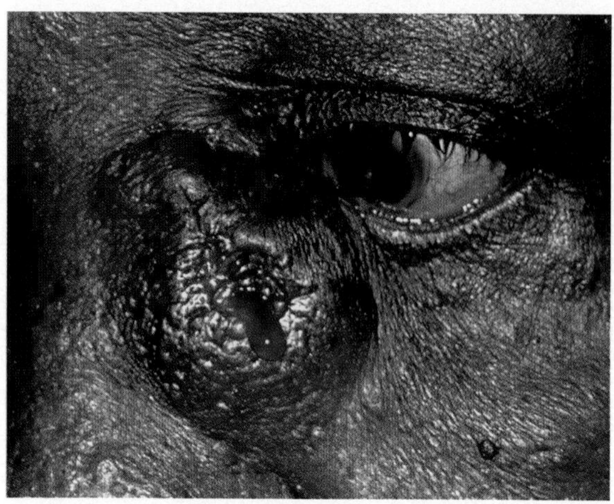

Figure 7-17

MUCOEPIDERMOID CARCINOMA

The mass involves the left inner canthus.

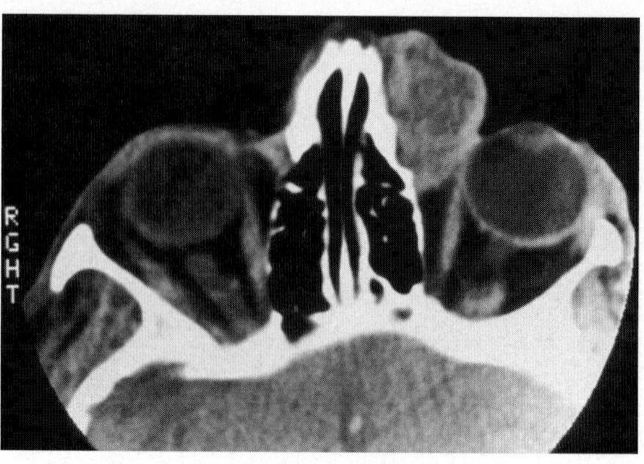

Figure 7-18

MUCOEPIDERMOID CARCINOMA

Computerized tomography (CT) shows a large mass involving the left inner canthus.

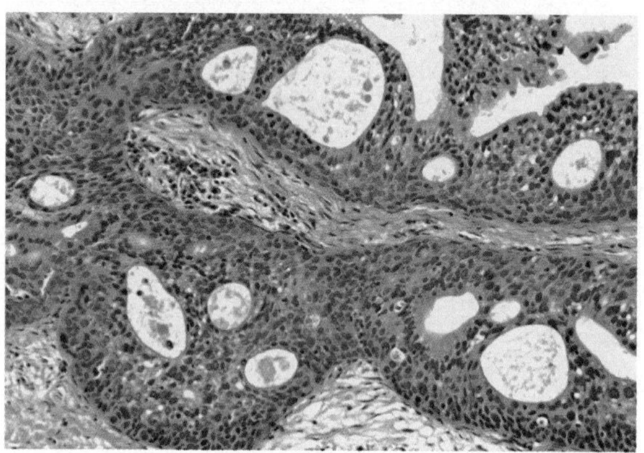

Figure 7-19

MUCOEPIDERMOID CARCINOMA

The glandular tumor has microcystic spaces.

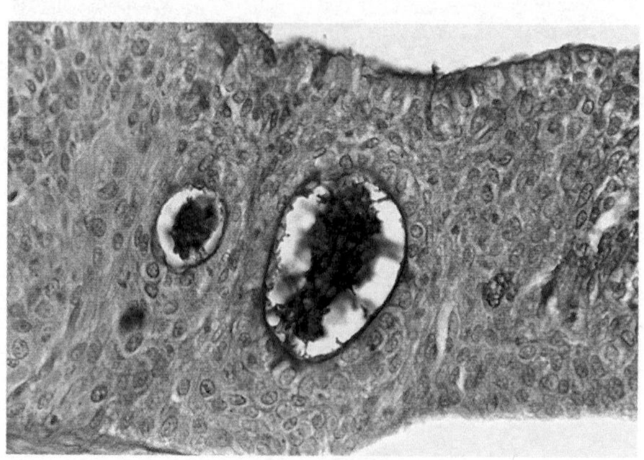

Figure 7-20

MUCOEPIDERMOID CARCINOMA

The microcystic spaces contain mucopolysaccharides, revealed with the Alcian blue stain.

inflammatory cells may be present. Some have a papillary growth pattern; others have a nonpapillary, infiltrative growth pattern (2).

Transitional cell carcinomas have a papillary growth pattern (figs. 7-31–7-33); histologically, they resemble transitional cell carcinomas of the urinary bladder. The lining epithelium shows pleomorphism, hyperchromatic nuclei, and prominent nucleoli. Mitotic figures are present.

Mucoepidermoid carcinomas have both epidermoid and mucous-secreting cells. Cystic spaces filled with mucinous material are usually noted. The mucinous material stains with the Alcian blue and mucicarmine stains. Mucoepidermoid carcinomas have a lower rate of metastasis than adenocarcinomas or adenoid cystic carcinomas (25).

Adenoid cystic carcinomas have two different histologic patterns: cribriform and basaloid (16,28). These tumors resemble adenoid cystic carcinomas of the lacrimal gland. The basaloid or solid pattern may confer a bad prognosis.

Oncocytic adenocarcinomas are composed of cells with granular eosinophilic cytoplasm, an infiltrative pattern, and nuclear atypia, and cells that form a pseudoglandular pattern (3, 29). The tumor cells infiltrate the lacrimal sac

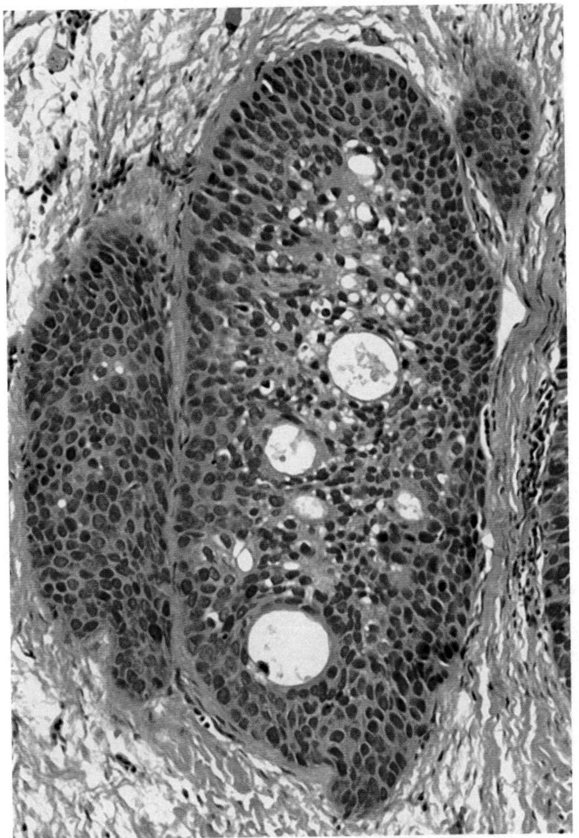

Figure 7-21

MUCOEPIDERMOID CARCINOMA

The infiltrating tumor lobules have microcystic spaces in the center.

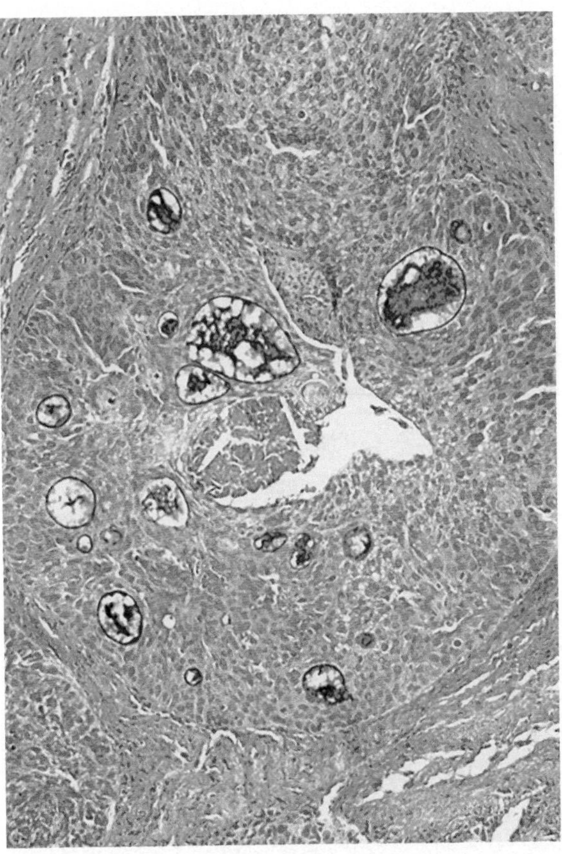

Figure 7-22

MUCOEPIDERMOID CARCINOMA

The microcystic spaces in the tumor lobule show Alcian blue–positive mucopolysaccharides.

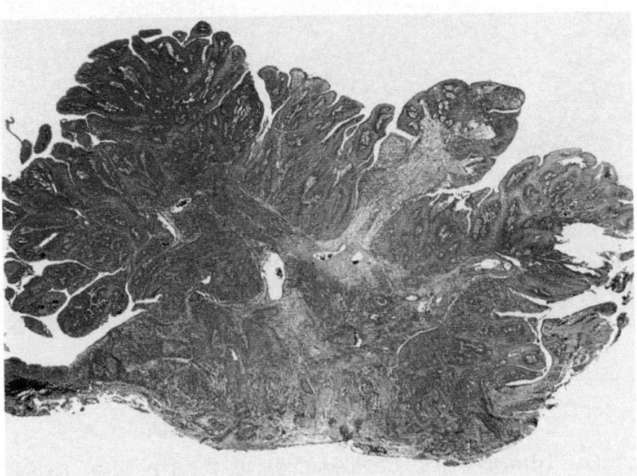

Figure 7-23

PAPILLARY SQUAMOUS CELL CARCINOMA

Invasion at the base of a papillary carcinoma.

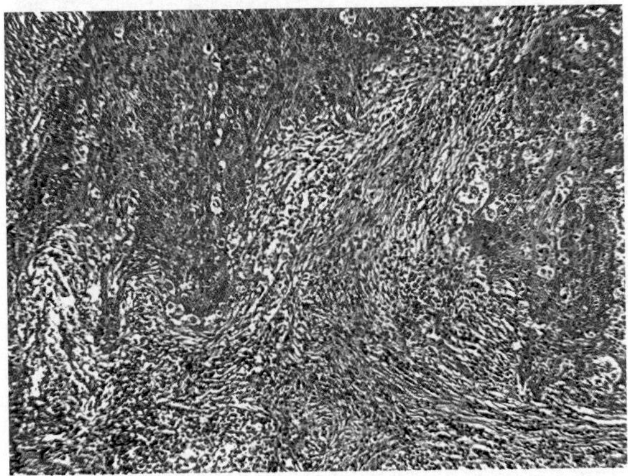

Figure 7-24

PAPILLARY SQUAMOUS CELL CARCINOMA

Higher magnification of figure 7-23 reveals glands of infiltrating squamous cell carcinoma. The stroma shows scarring and chronic inflammatory cell infiltration.

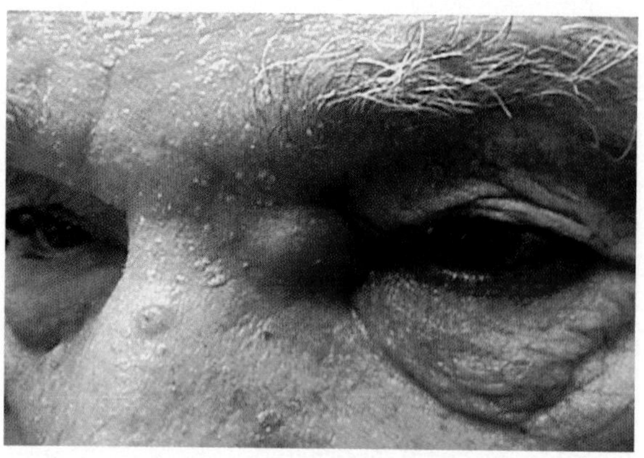

Figure 7-25

SQUAMOUS CELL CARCINOMA

The tumor is located in the left medial canthus.

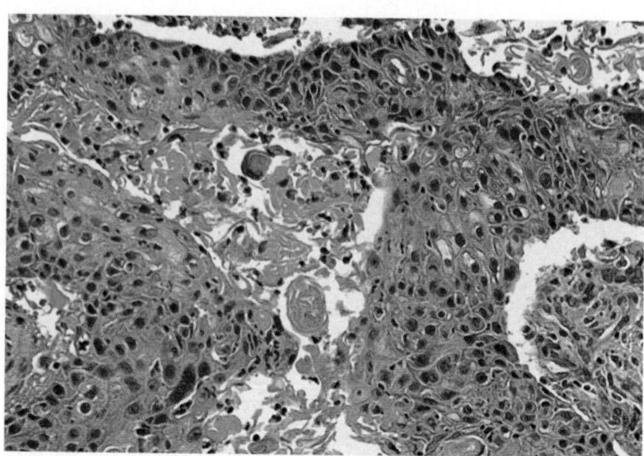

Figure 7-26

SQUAMOUS CELL CARCINOMA

Infiltrating carcinoma with hyperchromatic nuclei and keratin formation.

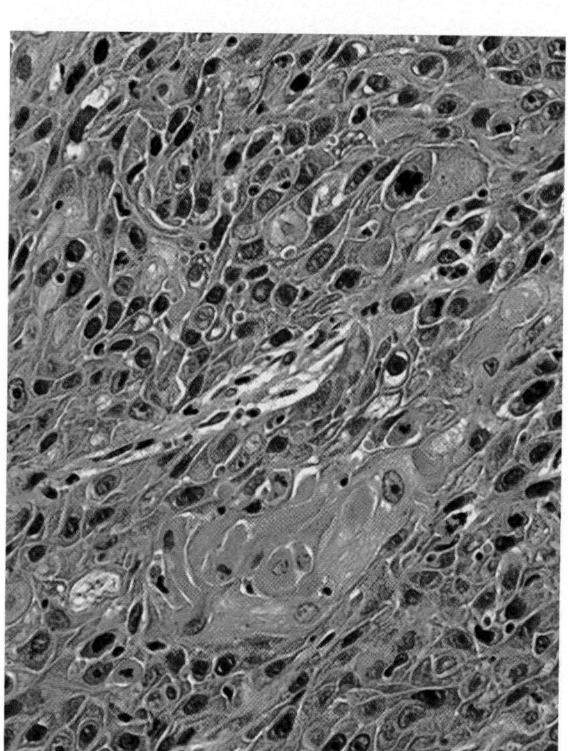

Figure 7-27

SQUAMOUS CELL CARCINOMA

Higher magnification of the tumor shown in figure 7-26 shows squamous differentiation.

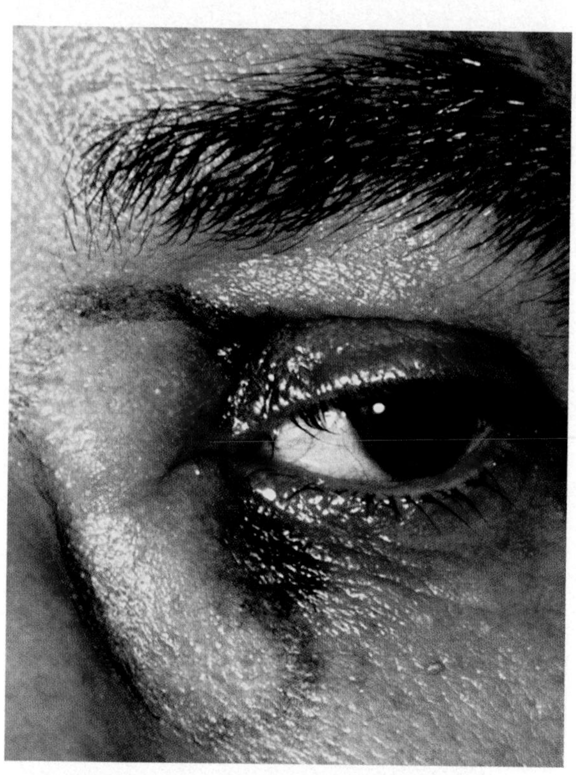

Figure 7-28

SQUAMOUS CELL CARCINOMA

The tumor is localized mainly above the left medial canthal ligament.

wall. There are a large number of abnormal mitochondria. The mitochondrial cristae are usually fragmented and irregularly oriented. In contrast, adenocarcinomas of the lacrimal sac have a glandular or trabecular pattern and pleomorphic cells.

Treatment and Prognosis. Malignant tumors require more extensive surgical excision that

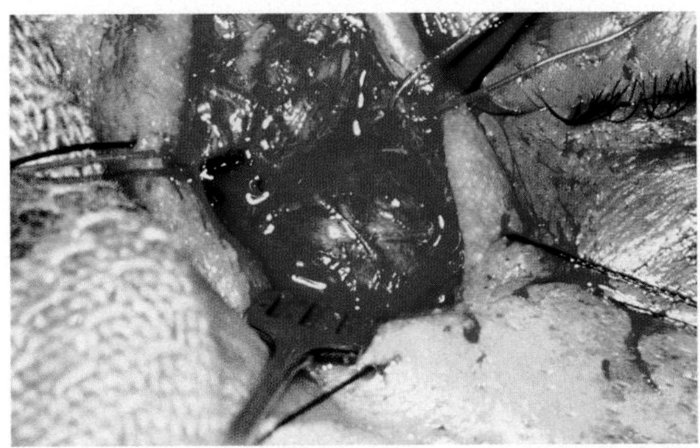

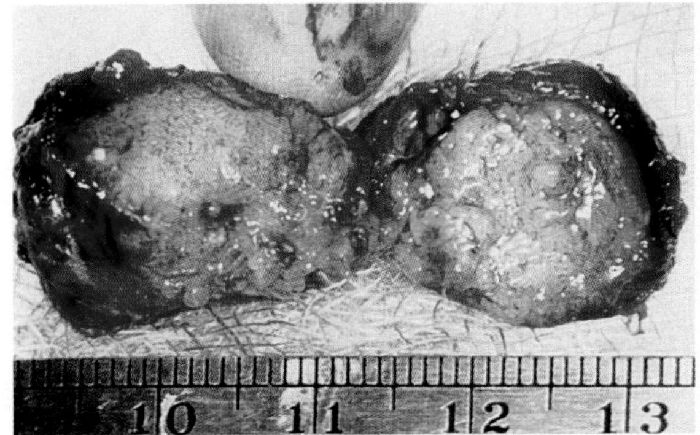

Figure 7-29

SQUAMOUS CELL CARCINOMA

Left: Surgically exposed mass at the medial canthus.
Right: Gross appearance of the sectioned mass.

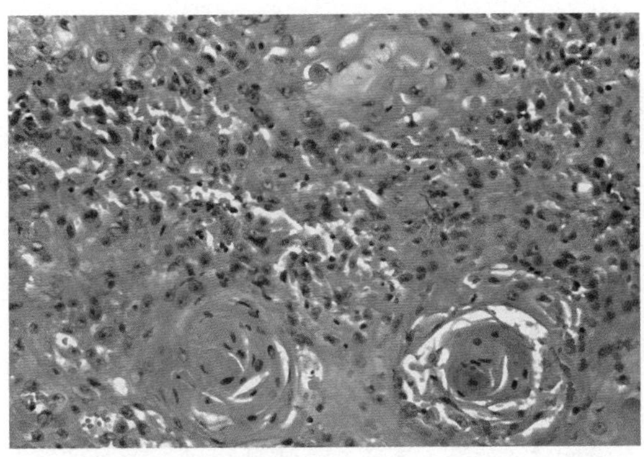

Figure 7-30

SQUAMOUS CELL CARCINOMA

The mass shows squamous differentiation with formations of squamous pearls.

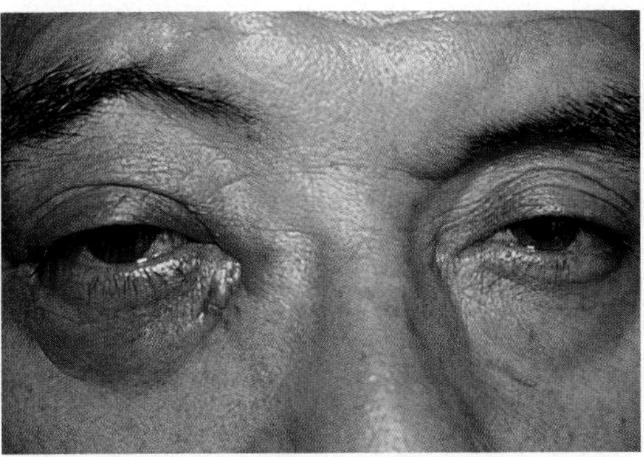

Figure 7-31

TRANSITIONAL CELL CARCINOMA

The mass is located at the right medial canthus.

includes the canaliculi, the sac, and the nasolacrimal duct. Because these tumors tend to extend down the nasolacrimal duct, lateral rhinotomy is recommended. In a large series reported by Ni (4), malignant neoplasms managed with wide excision and lateral rhinotomy had a recurrence rate of 12.5 percent, compared to a rate of 43.7 percent in patients whose neoplasms were managed with localized lacrimal sac excision. Preoperative and/or postoperative radiation, in the range of 3,000 to 5,000 rad, is recommended for the treatment of malignant epithelial tumors. Larger, more extensive malignant lacrimal sac tumors require radical surgery, including exenteration, lymph node dissection, and paranasal sinus resection.

Epithelial malignant tumors often recur (50 percent recurrence rate) (2,3). These tumors may invade blood vessels, and tumor emboli may be present in the lymphatic vessels (figs. 7-34, 7-35). In a series of 71 lacrimal sac carcinomas, Ni (4) found a mortality rate of 13.6 percent in patients with papillary squamous cell carcinoma, 50 percent in patients with invasive squamous cell carcinoma, and 100 percent in patients with transitional cell carcinoma. The overall mortality rate, however, in patients managed with wide surgical excision and radiation was 37.5 percent.

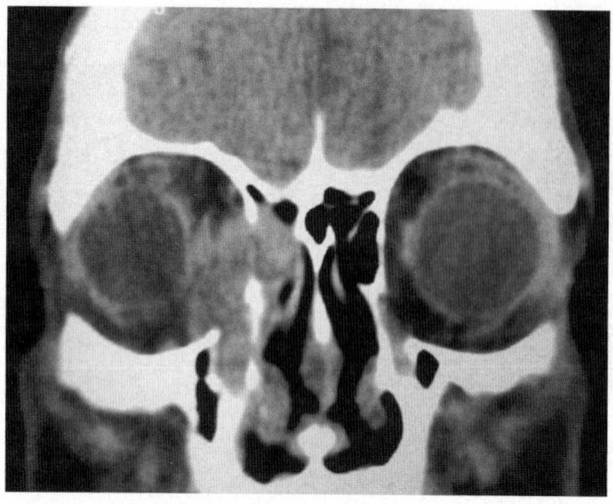

Figure 7-32

TRANSITIONAL CELL CARCINOMA

CT shows a right medial canthal mass with destruction of the medial orbital bony wall.

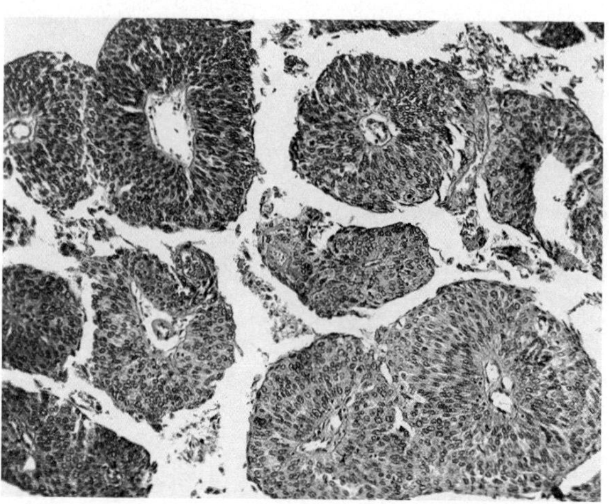

Figure 7-33

TRANSITIONAL CELL CARCINOMA

Papillary type of transitional cell carcinoma.

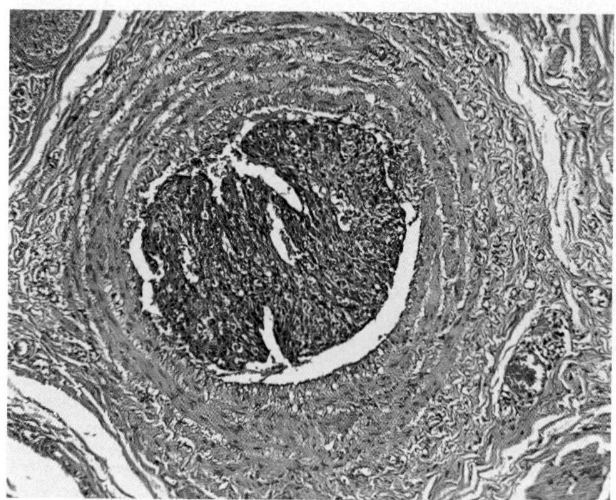

Figure 7-34

CARCINOMA OF THE LACRIMAL SAC

The lumen of a vein is invaded by carcinoma.

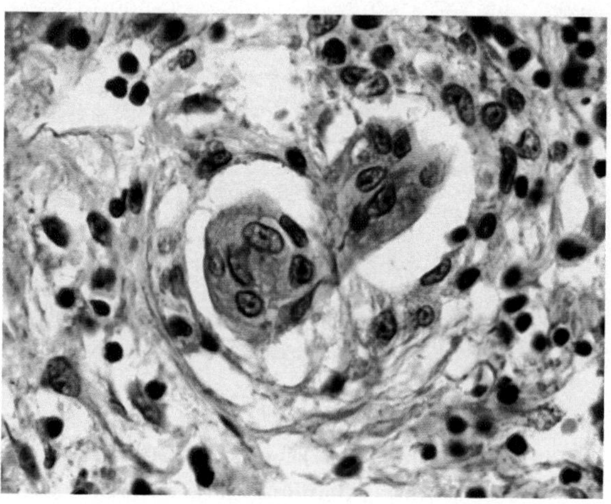

Figure 7-35

CARCINOMA OF THE LACRIMAL SAC

Emboli of tumor cells in lymphatic vessels.

Lymphatic spread occurred in 27 percent and hematogenous metastases to the lungs or esophagus in 9.1 percent of patients.

NONEPITHELIAL TUMORS

Definition. There are several types of primary nonepithelial benign and malignant tumors of the lacrimal sac, including *fibrous histiocytoma, hemangiopericytoma, angiosarcoma, neurilemmoma, lymphoma,* and *melanoma* (30–48). Fibrous histiocytoma is the most common of these tumors, followed by lymphoid lesions and melanoma. Histologically, these tumors arise primarily from the walls of the lacrimal sac.

General Features. The mean age of patients with lacrimal sac fibrous histiocytoma is 34 years, with an age range of 9 to 60 years. For the two other common tumors, lymphoma and melanoma, the median patient age is 54 and 64 years, respectively, with a range of 39 to 79 years (3,17).

Clinical Features. Similar to epithelial tumors of the lacrimal sac, nonepithelial tumors present as a mass with signs of obstruction, leading to epiphora. In contrast, the most common initial manifestations in patients with malignant nonepithelial lacrimal sac tumors are mass, epiphora, and bloody discharge. As with epithelial malignant neoplasms of the sac, melanomas of the sac may cause a bloody nasal discharge and bleeding from the punctum (17).

Microscopic Findings, Treatment and Prognosis. Fibrous histiocytoma of the sac is composed of two intermixed cell types: large histiocytic cells, showing abundant eosinophilic cytoplasm and round to oval plump nuclei, and fibroblastic cells arranged in fascicles and bundles (fig. 7-36). No mitoses are seen, but there are occasional histiocytes with vacuolated cytoplasm. A characteristic storiform pattern is common. Ultrastructurally, there are two types of neoplastic cells: the histiocytic cells with numerous electron-lucent cytoplasmic inclusions, and the fibroblasts with indented nuclei and prominent profiles of rough-surfaced endoplastic reticulum.

Pe'er and co-workers (17) reported 35 cases of nonepithelial tumors of the lacrimal sac of which 10 were lymphoid lesions; 2, atypical lymphoid hyperplasia; and 8, malignant lymphomas. Five of the lymphomas were of the diffuse large cell type, one was a diffuse small cleaved cell type, one was a small noncleaved cell type, and one was a malignant small lymphocytic lymphoma. Primary natural killer cell lymphomas originating in the lacrimal sac have also been reported (44), as well as angiotropic lymphoma, sinus histiocytosis, and leukemia (16,45).

Presumably, malignant melanoma of the sac arises from melanocytic cells located either within the epithelium of the lacrimal sac or in the underlying stroma (figs. 7-37, 7-38) (16,47, 48). Patients range from 38 to 79 years (4). Histologic examination reveals features resembling poorly differentiated carcinoma or malignant lymphoma. The degree of pigmentation varies, and a few cases have amelanotic tumor cells. Such tumors are immunoreactive for HMB45 and S-100 protein. Patients with melanomas have a poor prognosis, despite the use of wide surgical excision, radiotherapy, and chemotherapy. The tumors are highly invasive, extending into the nasolacrimal duct and in some patients, into the orbit (4,16).

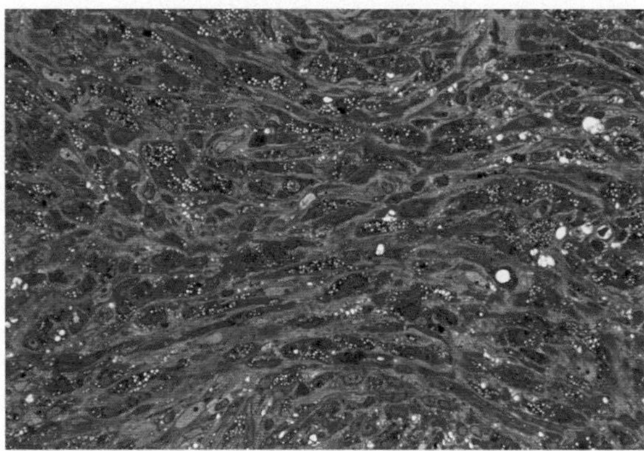

Figure 7-36

FIBROUS HISTIOCYTOMA

The histiocytic cells show evidence of lipidization of the cytoplasm (toluidine blue stain [1-µm section]).

Hemangiopericytomas of the lacrimal sac have a prominent vascular pattern of sinusoidal spaces separated by solid areas composed of spindle-shaped cells. Histologically, some hemangiopericytomas simulate a fibrous histiocytoma or solitary fibrous tumor (4,16,17). Ultrastructurally, the neoplastic cells have an ovoid nucleus, a prominent nucleolus, and elongated cytoplasmic processes. The tumor cells show an interrupted basement membrane, rough-surfaced endoplasmic reticulum, and an irregular nuclear border. The stroma contains collagen fibers. Hemangiopericytomas have the potential to recur and undergo malignant change. Late recurrence, up to 15 years after first surgery, has been noted. The tumor histologically classified as benign can recur. Other vascular tumors listed in the literature include capillary angioma, angiofibroma, hemangioendothelioma, glomus tumor, Kaposi's sarcoma, and angiosarcoma (16).

Solitary fibrous tumor of the lacrimal sac is rare, and in two reported cases the patients were 23 and 34 years of age (30). This tumor is a slow-growing, painless mass in the medial canthus. Histologically, the tumor has a hemangiopericytoma-like appearance and a diffuse sclerosing pattern. The cells express CD34. Solitary fibrous tumor of the sac may recur after incomplete excision; complete excision is required for management.

Granular cell tumor also occurs in the lacrimal sac, however, this is rare (37). This benign

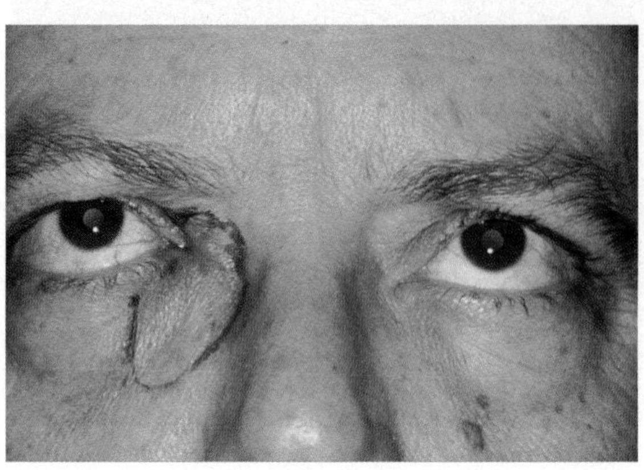

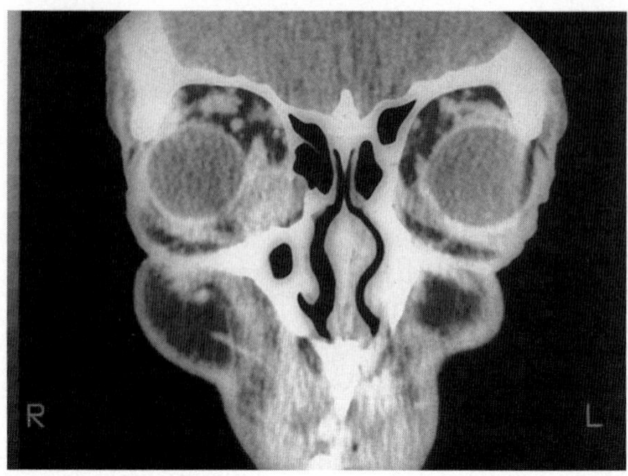

Figure 7-37

PRIMARY MELANOMA

Left: The edges of the tumor are outlined.
Right: CT shows the mass involving the right lacrimal sac.

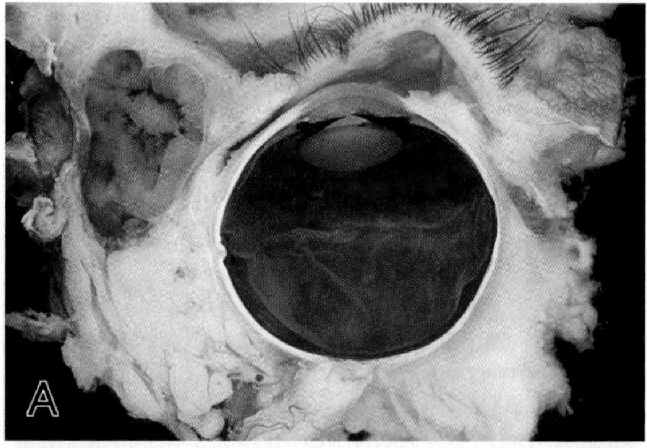

Figure 7-38

PRIMARY MELANOMA

A: Exenteration specimen (horizontal section) shows the dark brown mass involving the lacrimal sac region.

B: Epithelioid melanoma cells with increased mitotic activity.

C: The tumor cells contain a moderate amount of melanin pigment in the cytoplasm.

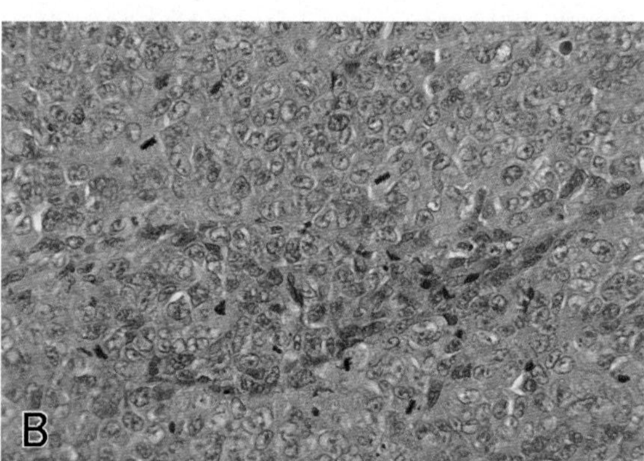

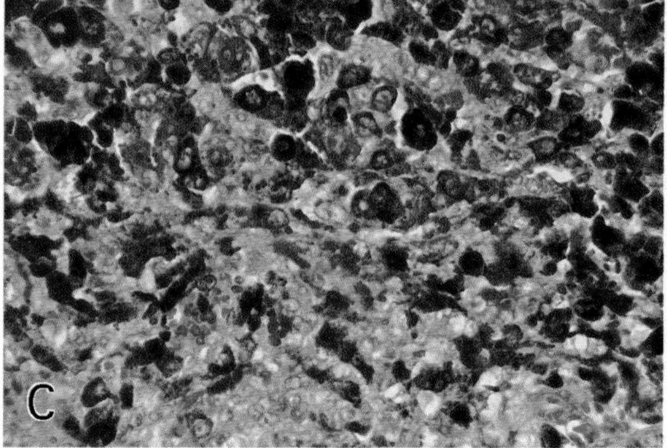

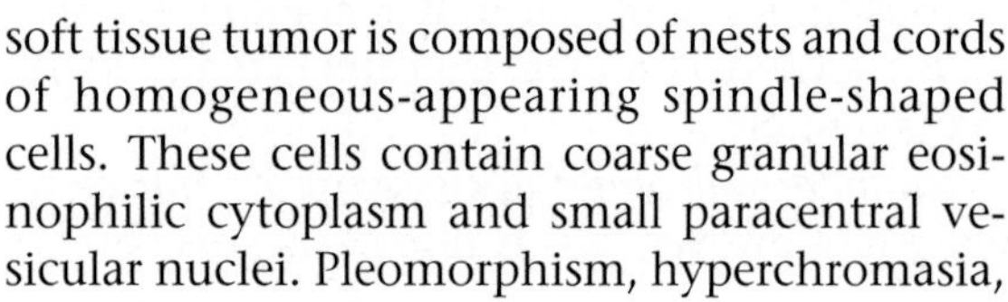

soft tissue tumor is composed of nests and cords of homogeneous-appearing spindle-shaped cells. These cells contain coarse granular eosinophilic cytoplasm and small paracentral vesicular nuclei. Pleomorphism, hyperchromasia, necrosis, and mitotic figures are not seen. The neoplastic cells stain with periodic acid–Schiff (PAS) and for S-100 protein. Electron microscopy discloses tumor cells packed with numerous degenerating lysosomes.

REFERENCES

1. Duke-Elder S. Tumors of the lacrimal passages. In: Text-book of ophthalmology, vol 5. St. Louis: CV Mosby; 1952:5279–368.
2. Ryan SJ, Font RL. Primary epithelial neoplasms of the lacrimal sac. Am J Ophthalmol 1973;76: 73–88.
3. Stefanyszyn MA, Hidayat AA, Pe'er JJ, Flanagan JC. Lacrimal sac tumors. Ophthal Plast Reconstr Surg 1994;10:169–84.
4. Ni C, D'Amico DJ, Fan CQ, Kuo PK. Tumors of the lacrimal sac: a clinicopathological analysis of 82 cases. Int Ophthalmol Clin 1982;22:121–40.
5. Cole SH, Ferry AP. Fibrous histiocytoma (fibrous xanthoma) of the lacrimal sac. Arch Ophthalmol 1978;96:1647–9.
6. Marback RL, Kincaid MC, Green WR, Iliff WJ. Fibrous histiocytoma of the lacrimal sac. Am J Ophthalmol 1982;93:511–7.
7. Howcroft MJ, Hurwitz JJ. Lacrimal sac fibroma. Can J Ophthalmol 1980;15:196–7.
8. Sen DK, Mohan H. Fibroma of the lacrimal sac. J Pediatr Ophthalmol Strabismus 1980;17:410–1.
9. Gurney N, Chalkley T, O'Grady R. Lacrimal sac hemangiopericytoma. Am J Ophthalmol 1971;71:757–9.
10. Harry J, Ashton N. The pathology of tumours of the lacrimal sac. Trans Ophthalmol Soc UK 1969;88:19–35.
11. Jones IS. Tumors of the lacrimal sac. Am J Ophthalmol 1956;42:561–6.
12. Duguid IM. Malignant melanoma of the lacrimal sac. Br J Ophthalmol 1964;48:394–8.
13. Farkas TG, Lamberson RE. Malignant melanoma of the lacrimal sac. Am J Ophthalmol 1968; 66:45–8.
14. Thomas A, Sujatha S, Ramakrishan PM, Sudarsanam D. Malignant melanoma of the lacrimal sac. Eur Arch Ophthalmol 1975;3:84–6.
15. Yamade S, Kitagawa A. Malignant melanoma of the lacrimal sac. Ophthalmologica 1978;177: 30–3.
16. Font R. Eyelids and lacrimal drainage system. In: Spencer WH, ed. Ophthalmic pathology: an atlas and textbook. Philadelphia: WB Saunders; 1996:2218–437.
17. Pe'er JJ, Stefanyszn M, Hidayat AA. Nonepithelial tumors of the lacrimal sac. Am J Ophthalmol 1994;118:650–8.
18. Nakamura Y, Mashima Y, Kameyama K, Mukai M, Oguchi Y. Detection of human papillomavirus infection in squamous tumors of the conjunctiva and lacrimal sac by immunohistochemistry, in situ hybridisation, and polymerase chain reaction. Br J Ophthalmol 1997;81:308–13.
19. Chen LJ, Liao SL, Kao SC, Wu CT, Hou PK, Chen MS. Oncocytic adenomatous hyperplasia of the lacrimal sac: a case report and review of the literature. Ophthal Plast Reconstr Surg 1998;14: 436–40.
20. Domanski H, Ljungberg O, Andersson LO, Schele B. Oxyphil cell adenoma (oncocytoma) of the lacrimal sac. Review of the literature. Acta Ophthalmol (Copenh) 1994;72:393–6.
21. Lamping KA, Albert DM, Ni C, Fournier G. Oxyphil cell adenomas. Three case reports. Arch Ophthalmol 1984;102;263–5.
22. Rahangdale SR, Castillo M, Shockley W. MR in squamous cell carcinoma of the lacrimal sac. AJNR Am J Neuroradiol 1995;16:1262–4.
23. Ni C, Wagoner MD, Wang WJ, Albert DM, Fan CO, Robinson N. Mucoepidermoid carcinomas of the lacrimal sac. Arch Ophthalmol 1983;101: 1572–4.
24. Blake J, Mullaney J, Gillan J. Lacrimal sac mucoepidermoid carcinoma. Br J Ophthalmol 1986;70:681–5.
25. Bambirra EA, Miranda D, Rayes A. Mucoepidermoid tumor of the lacrimal sac. Arch Ophthalmol 1981;99:2149–50.
26. Kohn R, Nofsinger K, Freedman SI. Rapid recurrence of papillary squamous cell carcinoma of the canaliculus. Am J Ophthalmol 1981;92:363–7.
27. Bonder D, Fischer MJ, Levine MR. Squamous cell carcinoma of the lacrimal sac. Ophthalmology 1983;90:1133–5.
28. Kincaid MC, Meis JM, Lee MW. Adenoid cystic carcinoma of the lacrimal sac. Ophthalmology 96:1655–8.
29. Peretz WL, Ettinghausen SE, Gray GF. Oncocytic adenocarcinoma of the lacrimal sac. Arch Ophthalmol 1978;96:303–4.
30. Woo KI, Suh YL, Kim YD. Solitary fibrous tumor of the lacrimal sac. Ophthal Plast Reconstr Surg 1999;15:450–3.
31. Schenck NL, Ogura JH, Pratt LL. Cancer of the lacrimal sac. Presentation of five cases and review of the literature. Ann Otol Rhinol Laryngol 1973;82:153–61.
32. Charles NC, Palu RN, Jagirdar JS. Hemangiopericytoma of the lacrimal sac. Arch Ophthalmol 1998;116:1677–80.
33. Geiger K, Witschel H. Haemangiopericytoma of the lacrimal sac. Orbit 1994;13:91–6.

34. Carnevali L, Trimarchi F, Rosso R, Stringa M. Haemangiopericytoma of the lacrimal sac: a case report. Br J Ophthalmol 1988;72:782–5.
35. Ferry AP, Kaltreider SA. Cavernous hemangioma of the lacrimal sac. Am J Ophthalmol 1990;110: 316–8.
36. Roth SI, August CZ, Lissner GS, O'Grady RB. Hemangiopericytoma of the lacrimal sac. Ophthalmology 1991;98:925–7.
37. Sabet SJ, Tarbet KJ, Lemke BN, Smith ME, Albert DM. Granular cell tumor of the lacrimal sac and nasolacrimal duct: no invasive behavior with incomplete resection. Ophthalmology 2000;107:1992–4.
38. Choi G, Lee U, Won NH. Fibrous histiocytoma of the lacrimal sac. Head Neck 1997;19:72–5.
39. Cole SH, Ferry AP. Fibrous histiocytoma (fibrous xanthoma) of the lacrimal sac. Arch Ophthalmol 1978;96:1647–9.
40. Marback RL, Kincaid MC, Green WR, Iliff WJ. Fibrous histiocytoma of the lacrimal sac. Am J Ophthalmol 1982;93:511–7.
41. Nakamura K, Uehara S, Omagari J, et al. Primary non-Hodgkin's lymphoma of the lacrimal sac: a case report and a review of the literature. Cancer 1997;80:2151–5.
42. Benger RS, Frueh BR. Lacrimal drainage obstruction from lacrimal sac infiltration by lymphocytic neoplasia. Am J Ophthalmol 1986;101: 242–5.
43. Karesh JW, Perman KI, Rodrigues MM. Dacryocystitis associated with malignant lymphoma of the lacrimal sac. Ophthalmology 1993;100: 669–73.
44. Mori T, Tokuhira M, Mori S, et al. Primary natural killer cell lymphoma of the lacrimal sac. Ann Hematol 2001;80:607–10.
45. O'Connor SR, Tan JH, Walewska R, Brown LJ, Lauder I. Angiotropic lymphoma occurring in a lacrimal sac oncocytoma. J Clin Pathol 2002; 55:787–8.
46. Dolman PJ, Harris GJ, Weiland LH. Sinus histiocytosis involving the lacrimal sac and duct. A clincopathologic case report. Arch Ophthalmol 1991;109:1582–4.
47. Lee HM, Kang HJ, Choi G, et al. Two cases of primary malignant melanoma of the lacrimal sac. Head Neck 2001;23:809–13.
48. McNab AA, McKelvie P. Malignant melanoma of the lacrimal sac complicating primary acquired melanosis of the conjunctiva. Ophthalmic Surg Lasers 1997;28:501–4.

8 TUMORS OF THE ORBIT

ANATOMY AND HISTOLOGY

The orbits are pyramid-like structures limited by bony walls that protect and contain the eyeball and its adnexa. The distance from the apex posteriorly to the orbital rim anteriorly varies from 40 to 50 mm, and the volume is 30 cm^3. Seven bones comprise the orbital walls: frontal, greater and lesser wings of the sphenoid, ethmoid, palatine, maxilla, zygomatic, and lacrimal. Bones that form the roof, medial wall, and floor of the orbit separate the intraorbital tissues from the paranasal sinuses. The bony wall is thinnest at the medial aspect of the orbit, overlying the ethmoidal sinus. The only fibrocartilaginous structure of the orbit is the trochlea of the tendon of the superior oblique muscle, which is located in the upper nasal quadrant. Supertemporally, behind the orbital rim, a depression of the sphenoidal bone is the fossa that contains the orbital lobe of the lacrimal gland.

Several apertures in the orbital bones allow the passage of blood vessels and nerves. At the apex of the orbit, the optic foramen or canal transmits the optic nerve, the ophthalmic artery, and accompanying sympathetic nerve fibers. The superior orbital fissure transmits divisions of the fifth cranial nerve, sympathetic nerve fibers, and the superior ophthalmic vein before it enters the cavernous sinus and communicates with the middle cranial fossa. The inferior orbital fissure carries the maxillary division of the trigeminal nerve and venous connections between the orbit and the pterygoid fossa.

The contents of the orbit include the globe, optic nerve and meningeal sheaths, extraocular striated muscles, levator palpebrae superioris muscle and tendons, connective tissue fascia, and fat (fig. 8-1). Connective tissue septa divide and connect orbital fat lobules and compartments. The striated muscles of the orbit include the four rectus muscles, and the inferior and superior oblique muscles. The four rectus muscles arise at the orbital apex, surround the optic canal to form the annulus of Zinn, and run anteriorly to their scleral insertion in front of the equator of the globe. The resultant funnel-shaped muscle cone divides the orbit into an intraconal and extraconal space. The former is limited anteriorly by the posterior eyewall and includes the optic nerve, blood vessels, and nerves that supply the eye. The levator palpebrae superioris arises at the orbital apex and runs anteriorly to attach to the superior rectus muscle by dense fascia.

Several central and peripheral nerves traverse the orbit, generally in a posterior-anterior direction. The frontal nerve runs under the roof of the orbit and exits from the superior orbital rim to supply sensation to the skin of the eyelid and periorbital regions. Most peripheral nerves

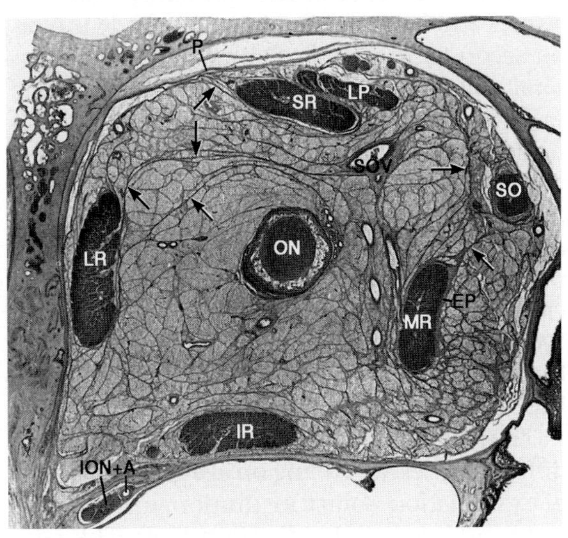

Figure 8-1

CONTENT OF THE ORBIT

Coronal section of the posterior orbit discloses the orbital bony wall, periosteum (P), adipose tissue and fasciae (arrows), extraocular muscles (SR, superior rectus muscle; LP, levator palpebrae superioris muscle; LR, lateral rectus muscle; MR, medial rectus muscle; SO, superior oblique muscle; IR, inferior rectus muscle), peripheral nerves and blood vessels (ION+A, inferior orbital nerve and artery; SOV, superior orbital vein), and the optic nerve (ON).

consist of sensory fibers from the ophthalmic and maxillary divisions of the trigeminal nerve. The ciliary ganglion, which transmits parasympathetic and sympathetic nerve fibers, is an 11-mm, flat, oval structure that lies between the optic nerve and the lateral rectus muscle.

The blood supply of the orbit comes from branches of the external and internal carotid arteries. The lateral orbit and forehead are supplied by the superficial temporal artery, a branch of the external carotid artery. The supraorbital and lacrimal arteries arise from the internal carotid arteries. The venous system of the orbit drains to the superior ophthalmic vein, which is joined by other veins coming from the eye, and by the inferior ophthalmic vein at the orbital apex. The veins drain posteriorly into the cavernous sinus and inferiorly into the pterygoid plexus. There are no identifiable lymphatic vessels or lymph nodes in the orbit. The tissues from the most anterior part of the orbit drain into the lymphatics of the conjunctiva and eyelid.

CLASSIFICATION AND FREQUENCY

Tumors of the orbit arise primarily from soft tissues and bones. Other tumors invade the orbit secondarily from ocular adnexa and periorbital structures. In addition, metastases to the orbit originate from various organs. The classification of primary tumors of the orbit is based mainly on the line of differentiation of the tumor (1). Each type is further divided into a benign and a malignant group. In some categories, an intermediate group is incorporated. The classification used here is a modification of the World Health Organization "Histological Typing of Tumors of the Eye and Its Adnexa" published in 1998 (2).

The frequency of orbital tumors varies among different series depending on age group, method of examination, source institution, medical specialty, and geographic location (3,4). The relative frequencies of different orbital tumors in children and adults are listed in Table 8-1 (5–7). About half of tumors occurring in children are cystic. Every physician involved in the clinical evaluation and diagnosis of ocular and adnexal tumors should entertain the diagnosis of rhabdomyosarcoma. Despite its aggressive behavior, early diagnosis and institution of treatment of rhabdomyosarcoma result in almost 95 percent survival. Other pediatric tumors include capillary hemangioma, mesenchymal lesions, histiocytic lesions, and leukemia.

Table 8-1

COMPARATIVE FREQUENCY OF ORBITAL TUMORS OBTAINED FROM SEVERAL SERIES IN CHILDREN AND ADULTS[a]

	General	Children	Adults
Cystic lesions	12%	26%	3%
Mesenchymal and adipose lesions	3%	3%	<1%
Rhabdomyosarcoma	1%	9%	NA[b]
Vasculogenic lesions	9%	15%	14%
Peripheral nerve tumors	3%	5%	NA
Optic nerve and meninges	5%	13%	5%
Osseous and cartilaginous lesions	4%	4%	<1%
Primary melanocytic lesions	<1%	<1%	1%
Lacrimal gland lesions	6%	2%	3%
Lymphoid tumors and leukemia	8%	4%	28%
Histiocytic and related lesions	<1%	2%	NA
Secondary and metastatic tumors	14%	5%	26%
Inflammatory lesions	12%	8%	11%
Thyroid ophthalmopathy	17%	NA	NA
Other	8%	5%	NA

[a]Total % is more than 100% because of rounding.
[b]NA = not available.

Inflammatory pseudotumors, lymphoid proliferations, and cavernous hemangioma are the most frequent causes of an intraorbital mass in adults. The incidence of malignant tumors increases with age, from approximately 22 percent in children to 63 percent in older adults (8). The average annual incidence for all malignant orbital tumors is 2 cases/million population (9).

Based on clinicopathologic correlations, orbital tumors may be divided into cystic and solid groups; the latter are circumscribed and diffuse or infiltrative. The most common cystic lesions of the orbit are dermoid cysts, conjunctival cysts, and mucoceles. Circumscribed intraconal lesions include optic nerve tumors, vascular lesions such as cavernous hemangioma and hemangiopericytoma, and benign peripheral nerve tumors. Diffuse or infiltrative tumors include lymphoid

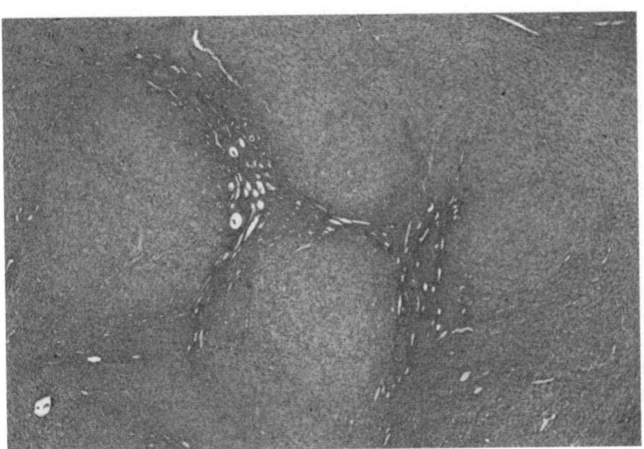

Figure 8-2

JUVENILE FIBROMATOSIS

Low-power microscopic view reveals a multinodular proliferation of spindle-shaped cells.

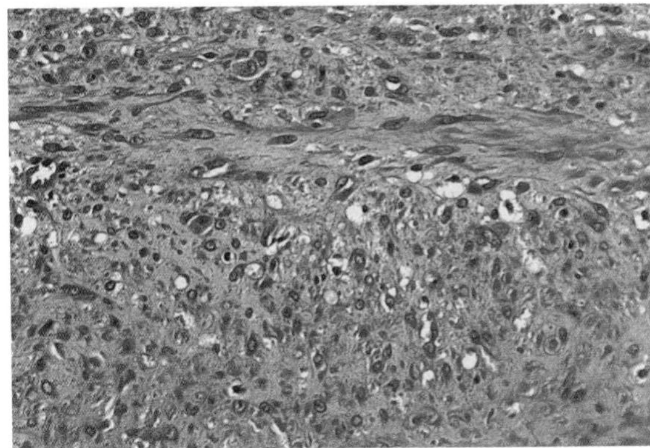

Figure 8-3

JUVENILE FIBROMATOSIS

Masson trichrome stain shows the fuchsinophilic cytoplasm of the myofibroblasts.

lesions, metastases, capillary hemangiomas, and lymphangiomas, and usually involve the extraconal space. Bone tumors, although rare, include a wide variety of osseous, fibro-osseous, and cartilaginous tumors.

It is important to emphasize the correlation between tissue-type location within the orbit and histologic tumor type. Extraocular muscles are mainly affected by some metastatic tumors, lymphoid proliferations, inflammatory pseudotumors, and vascular malformations. Secondary tumors invading the orbital structures originate from the eyelid and conjunctiva, globe, paranasal sinuses, and intracranial cavity. Basal cell carcinoma of the eyelid is the most frequent secondary orbital tumor in adults. In underdeveloped countries, neglected, longstanding retinoblastoma frequently invades the orbit.

The following discussion emphasizes aspects of soft tissues and bone lesions especially relevant to the orbit. For a more comprehensive discussion and illustrations of many of the pathologic entities mentioned in this Fascicle, the reader is referred to the Fascicles *Tumors of the Soft Tissues*, *Tumors of the Bone and Joints*, and *Tumors of the Lymph Nodes and Spleen* (9a,b,c).

FIBROUS TUMORS

Fibromatosis

Fibromatoses are a group of well-differentiated, nonencapsulated, fibrous tissue proliferations that have a tendency to invade locally and recur (10). Several terms have been used to refer to special entities and subgroups of fibromatoses. Rarely, the orbit is infiltrated by deep fibromatosis (11,12). The patients are usually children; occasionally, young adults have retroperitoneal fibromatosis (13). Histopathologically, the lesions are characterized by infiltrative growth consisting of highly differentiated fibrous tissue.

Infantile myofibromatosis, a rare benign disorder of childhood, has been reported in the orbit (14). Histologic sections show a spindle cell tumor with whorled fascicles of plump myofibroblasts entrapped in a dense collagenous stroma. Hidayat and Font (15) reported six cases of *juvenile fibromatosis* of the periorbital region. Light microscopy reveals a lobulated arrangement of interlacing fascicles of fibroblasts with oval, plump, vesicular nuclei and ill-defined cytoplasm (figs. 8-2, 8-3).

The appropriate treatment of this group of lesions is excisional biopsy. Although they can recur after excision, there are no reported cases of metastases (15).

Nodular Fasciitis

Nodular fasciitis is an idiopathic, benign reactive, pseudosarcomatous proliferation that can simulate a neoplasia clinically and histologically (16). It occurs in young adults and occasionally in children. Generally, the lesion is located superficially or in the anterior orbit (17). Patients present with a rapidly enlarging, palpable, well-circumscribed nodule (fig. 8-4).

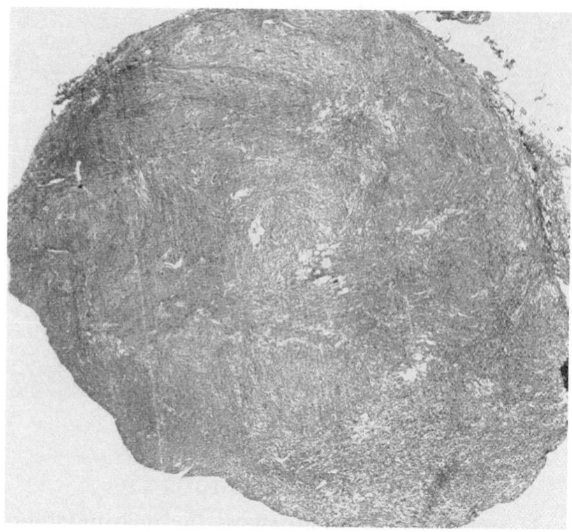

Figure 8-4

NODULAR FASCIITIS

The nodular appearance consists of dense areas and loose foci.

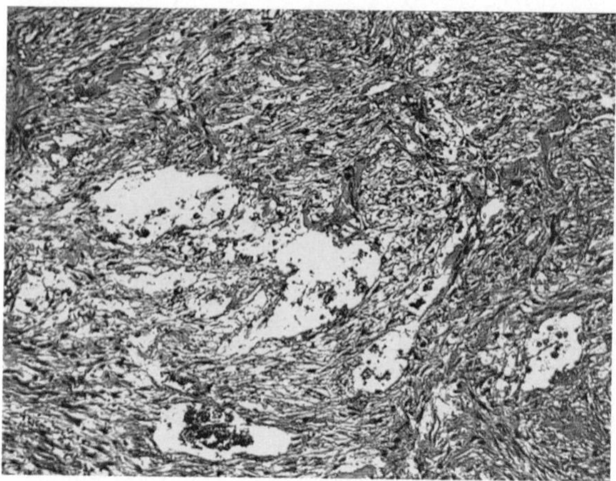

Figure 8-5

NODULAR FASCIITIS

The loose foci have plump and slender spindle-shaped cells and myxoid degeneration.

The typical microscopic appearance is a lesion composed of plump, mitotically active, stellate- or spindle-shaped fibroblasts, often arranged in parallel bundles and extending in all directions, resembling growing fibroblasts in tissue culture (fig. 8-5). Newly formed thin vessels run through the lesion. Immunohistochemistry demonstrates mixed immunophenotypes of fibroblasts and myofibroblasts that focally stain for muscle-specific antigen, smooth muscle actin, and desmin (18). The presence of actin-like filaments with fusiform densities is confirmed by electron microscopy (18).

Nodular fasciitis should be differentiated from fibrous histiocytoma, fibromatosis, and low-grade fibrosarcoma. Treatment is surgical excision; spontaneous regression may occur (19). Recurrences are rare.

Fibroma

Benign lesions composed of differentiated fibroblasts in a dense collagenous stroma are called *fibromas*. A few cases have been described in the orbit (20). Lesions with the histopathologic diagnosis of "fibroma" have been reported in patients of all ages (20,21). Some of the reported cases may be either other mesenchymal lesions or fibrohistiocytic reparative processes. The finding of inflammatory cells may suggest a burned-out pseudotumor.

Fibrous Histiocytoma

Definition and General Features. *Fibrous histiocytomas* are a diverse group of mesenchymal tumors that show fibroblastic differentiation (22). They are classified histologically as benign, locally aggressive, and malignant (23). Fibrous histiocytoma is one of the most common mesenchymal tumors of the orbit (23).

Clinical Features. In the largest series of orbital fibrous histiocytomas from the Armed Forces Institute of Pathology (AFIP), the mean age of the patients was 43 years, with a range of 4 to 85 years (23). Proptosis was the most common finding, followed by mass, decreased vision, diplopia, and pain. Patients with benign tumors had a longer duration of symptoms than those with malignant variants. The lesions occurred more often in the upper orbit.

Computerized tomography (CT) reveals a well-circumscribed lesion in benign tumors, whereas more aggressive malignant fibrous histiocytomas tend to have infiltrating margins and may involve bone (24). On magnetic resonance imaging (MRI), benign lesions tend to be homogeneous on T1-, T2-, and postgadolinium T1-weighted images, whereas malignant lesions are heterogeneous with low signals on

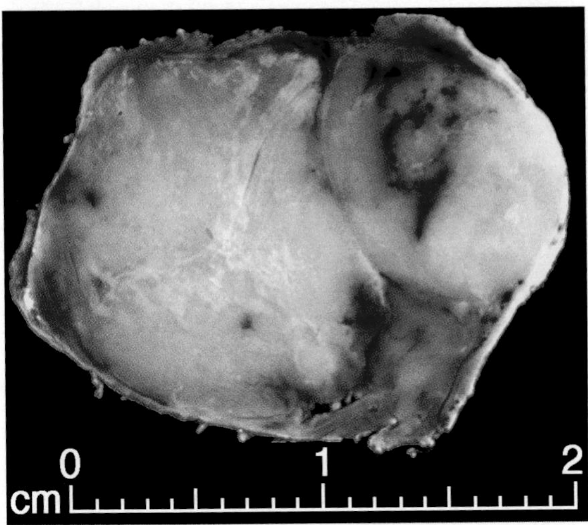

Figure 8-6

BENIGN FIBROUS HISTIOCYTOMA

Well-circumscribed solid nodules have dense white collagen bands and focal hemorrhage.

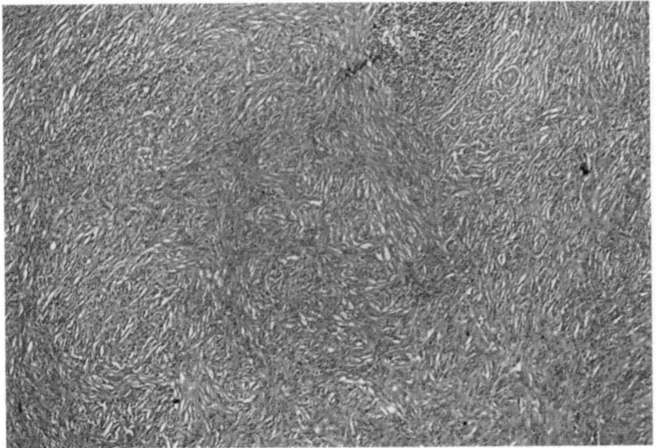

Figure 8-7

BENIGN FIBROUS HISTIOCYTOMA

Low-power microscopic view of a lesion with a storiform pattern. The tumor is permeated by occasional foci of lymphocytes.

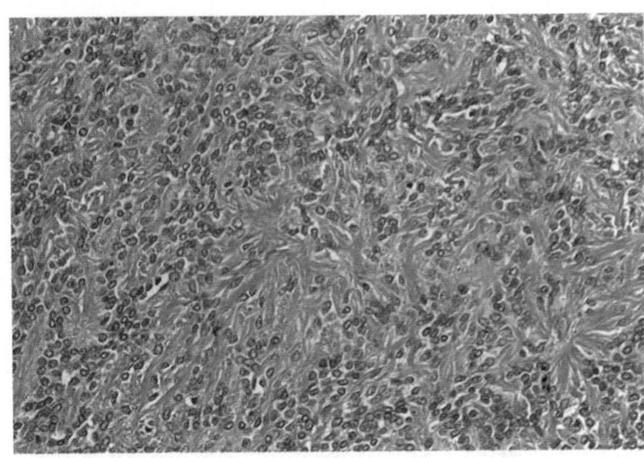

Figure 8-8

BENIGN FIBROUS HISTIOCYTOMA

Plump cells and extracellular deposits of collagen are seen.

T2-weighted images. A low T2-weighted signal comprising part or all of a fibrous lesion correlates with a dense collagen component. Areas of hyperintensity on T2-weighted images correspond with a more cellular matrix of fibroblasts and other mesenchymal cells (24).

Gross Findings. The gross appearance of fibrous histiocytoma varies considerably (23). Benign tumors are well-circumscribed, occasionally encapsulated lesions made up of grayish white or yellowish tan tissue (fig. 8-6). Cystic, hemorrhagic, or mucoid areas may be present. Malignant fibrous histiocytomas and locally aggressive tumors display infiltrating margins.

Microscopic Findings. The tumors are composed of spindle-shaped fibroblast-like cells that have storiform pattern focally and plump histiocyte-like cells (figs. 8-7, 8-8). Additional cell types include foamy xanthomatous cells, multinucleated histiocyte-like cells, chronic inflammatory cells, and macrophages containing hemosiderin. The stroma is composed of collagen fibers that often disclose hyalinized bands and loose areas rich in mucopolysaccharides.

Benign fibrous histiocytomas are well circumscribed, have cells without atypia, and rare or no mitotic figures (23). Locally aggressive tumors display infiltrating margins and hypercellular areas, but no necrosis. No significant cellular atypia or nuclear pleomorphism is noted. Mitotic figures are fewer than 1 per high-power field or less than 20 in 40 high-power fields.

Malignant fibrous histiocytomas have infiltrating edges and one or more of the following criteria of malignancy: nuclear pleomorphism, bizarre multinucleated tumor cells, areas of necrosis, and an increased number of mitoses or abnormal mitotic figures. There are three histologic patterns in malignant fibrous histiocytomas of the orbit: storiform, pleomorphic with many giant cells, and myxoid (23).

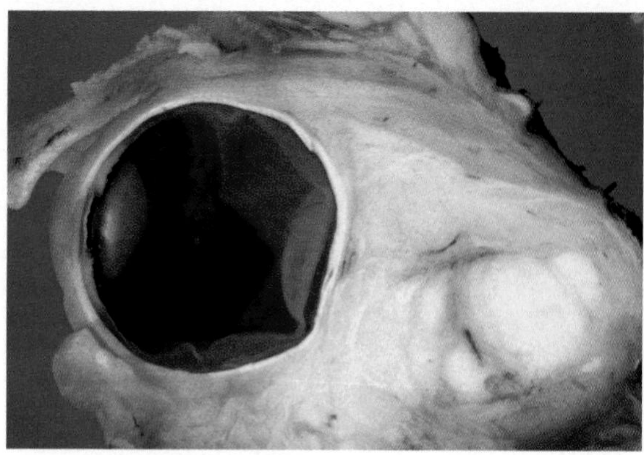

Figure 8-9

RECURRENT FIBROUS HISTIOCYTOMA

Orbital exenteration for the recurrence of the tumor shown in figure 8-8. Multiple solid white nodules are seen in the retrobulbar fat.

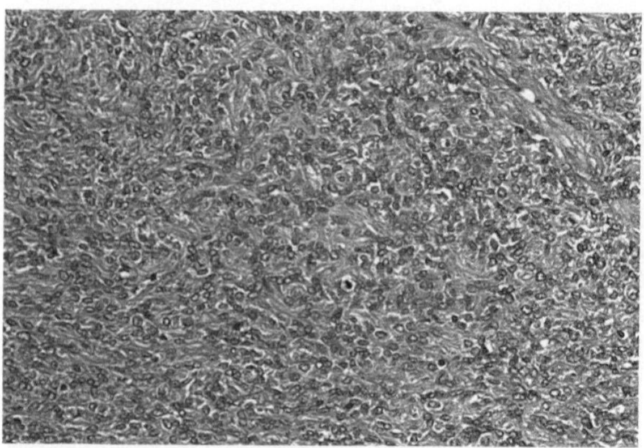

Figure 8-10

LOCALLY AGGRESSIVE FIBROUS HISTIOCYTOMA

Microscopic examination of the exenteration specimen seen in figure 8-9 disclosed a more compact cellular proliferation with occasional mitotic figures. This is consistent with a locally aggressive fibrous histiocytoma.

Immunohistochemical Findings. Fibrous histiocytomas may express factor XIIIa, CD34, focal CD68 positivity, alpha-1-antitrypsin and alpha-1-antichymotrypsin, and vimentin. High expression of Ki-67 (MIB-1) may correlate with biologic behavior and worse prognosis.

Electron Microscopic Findings. The two main cell populations are spindle-shaped cells that are indistinguishable from fibroblasts and histiocyte-like cells. The spindle cells show well-developed cisternae of rough-surfaced endoplasmic reticulum and absence of a basement membrane. Some cells have features of myofibroblasts. The histiocyte-like cells are polyhedral and contain lipid, membrane-bound structures, and dense lysosomal inclusions.

Differential Diagnosis. Orbital fibrous histiocytoma should be differentiated from fibromatosis, nodular fasciitis, fibrosarcoma, hemangiopericytoma, peripheral nerve tumors, and smooth muscle tumors. Pleomorphic variants of malignant fibrous histiocytoma must be differentiated from pleomorphic forms of other malignancies, e.g., pleomorphic leiomyosarcoma, pleomorphic liposarcoma, pleomorphic carcinoma, and atypical fibrous xanthoma. In doubtful cases, the diagnosis of fibrous histiocytoma is generally based on the absence of specific markers for other cell lineages.

Treatment and Prognosis. The biologic behavior of fibrous histiocytoma correlates with the histopathologic classification of benign, locally aggressive, or malignant (23). Complete surgical excision is the preferred management of orbital fibrous histiocytoma. Incomplete excision is associated with recurrence (fig. 8-9). Histopathologic examination of recurrent tumors disclose more cytologically aggressive variants. Orbital exenteration may be necessary in recurrent locally aggressive tumors that show a shift toward malignant cell phenotypes and malignant fibrous histiocytoma (fig. 8-10). Fatality is associated with local extension to the intracranial cavity, paranasal sinuses, and nasopharynx. Distant metastases are usually preceded by two or more local recurrences (23).

Fibrosarcoma

Fibrosarcomas of the orbit are rare. The clinical presentation varies among isolated cases of *congenital orbital fibrosarcoma, juvenile fibrosarcomas in children,* and *postradiation fibrosarcoma* (25–27). Weiner and Hidayat (27) reported five cases of juvenile fibrosarcoma of the orbit and eyelid in childhood. Histologically, these highly cellular tumors were composed of cells and fibers arranged in interlacing fascicles or a herringbone pattern. The number of mitoses was variable. Two of the five tumors recurred locally, but none metastasized.

The histologic differential diagnosis for fibrosarcoma in the pediatric age group includes rhabdomyosarcoma, infantile and juvenile fibromatosis, and nodular fasciitis. Children with fibrosarcoma of the head and neck have a much better prognosis than do adults. Initial radical excision may provide a better chance of remaining disease free. Postradiation fibrosarcomas behave more aggressively, and the prognosis is poor (26).

LIPOMATOUS TUMORS

Lipoma

Tumors arising from the adipose tissue of the orbit are rare. Although lipomas are mentioned in most series of orbital tumors, an unquestionable diagnosis is difficult to make. A *lipoma* of the orbit is a well-circumscribed, encapsulated tumor composed of lobules of mature adipocytes that are separated by thin connective tissue trabeculae.

A few cases of *spindle cell lipoma* of the orbit have been observed (28,29). They consist of bland bipolar spindle cells and hyaline bands of collagen (28,29). The spindle cells are positive for CD34 but negative for S-100 protein (28). Spindle cell lipoma of the orbit may be confused with schwannoma and diffuse neurofibroma.

Pleomorphic lipoma, resembling an anterior prolapse of the orbital fat, has recently been identified in older patients (30). Rare lipomatous tumors that may involve the orbit are the *lipomatous hamartoma* and *disseminated lipomatosis* (31).

Liposarcoma

Definition and Clinical Features. *Liposarcoma* of the orbit arises from undifferentiated or pluripotential mesenchymal cells of the connective tissue system. In two series, patients were of a median age of 51 years and presented with slowly progressive proptosis (32,33). The lesions are more commonly located in the retrobulbar space and lateral orbital wall. MRI demonstrates the characteristic bright signal on T1-weighted images and high signal intensity on T2-weighted images, suggesting abnormal fat (34). Although the lesions are not encapsulated, they may appear deceptively well circumscribed.

Microscopic Findings. Most orbital liposarcomas are well-differentiated or myxoid tumors containing spindle-shaped, stellate-shaped, and rounded lipoblasts. The lipoblasts are suspended in a myxoid matrix rich in glycosaminoglycans. There is usually a rich vascular pattern of thin, branched capillaries.

Immunohistochemical Findings. Tumor cells of myxoid and round cell liposarcoma are positive for S-100 protein in half of the cases.

Molecular Studies. Myxoid and round cell liposarcoma have a reciprocal translocation, t(12;16)(q13;p11), that results in fusion of the *CHOP* gene with the *TLS* gene. This translocation can be detected by polymerase chain reaction (PCR) for diagnostic purposes (35).

Differential Diagnosis. The distinction from other myxoid and round cell tumors of the orbit is based on the presence of lipoblastic differentiation, myxoid areas, the typical plexiform vascular pattern, and the use of immunohistochemistry to exclude other tumors such as rhabdomyosarcoma.

Treatment and Prognosis. The extent of surgical excision depends on whether the lesion is a well-differentiated, dedifferentiated, pleomorphic, or round cell liposarcoma. Recurrences are common after incomplete excision. Liposarcomas of the orbit are usually well-differentiated and small at the time of diagnosis and treatment, and the overall prognosis is generally good. Complete local surgical excision is the treatment of choice (36). Orbital exenteration may be necessary for recurrent tumors.

MYOGENIC TUMORS

Smooth Muscle Tumors

Leiomyoma. Leiomyomas of the orbit are rare, benign, smooth muscle tumors that manifest as a well-encapsulated mass. They cause slowly progressive proptosis in adults (37,38). Histopathologically, leiomyomas are solid and surrounded by a well-developed, compressed connective tissue capsule. The cells display characteristic tapered or blunt ends and cigar-shaped nuclei. They are arranged in bundles with interspersed areas of collagenization and rare foci of osseous metaplasia. The tumor cells express desmin and muscle-specific actin. These lesions may be confused with peripheral nerve sheath tumors and the spindle cell variant of fibrous histiocytoma. Orbital leiomyomas may recur after incomplete excision (39).

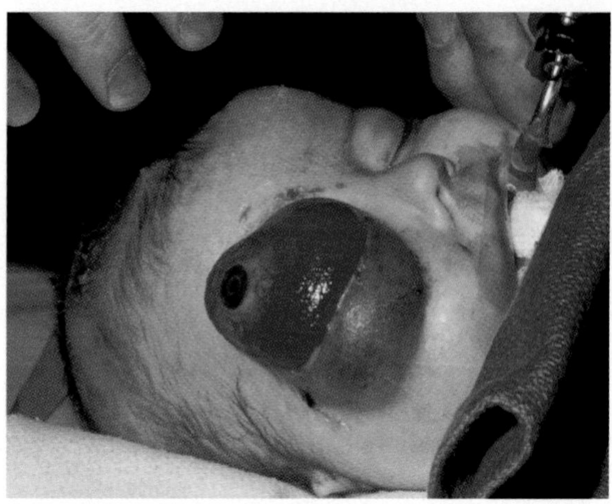

Figure 8-11

RHABDOMYOSARCOMA

This congenital rhabdomyosarcoma presented as a rapidly enlarging tumor of the right orbit in a neonate.

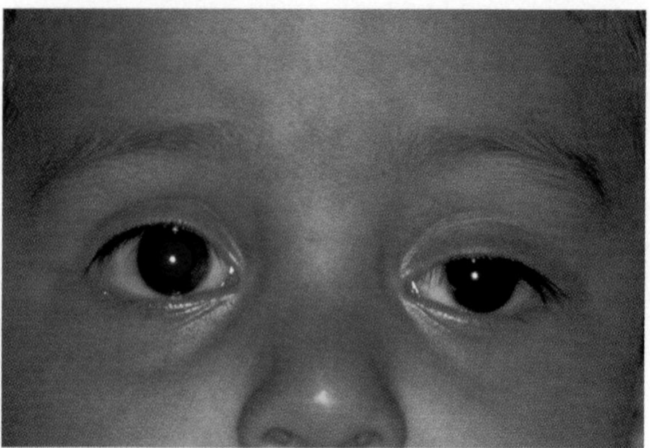

Figure 8-12

RHABDOMYOSARCOMA

A 3-year-old boy presented with a mass in the superior left orbit.

Vascular Leiomyoma. Vascular leiomyomas of the orbit are slow-growing, encapsulated masses in patients younger than 40 years of age (40). Pain and proptosis may be noted with the Valsalva maneuver. On image studies, the tumor resembles cavernous hemangioma but is usually enhanced after gadolinium injection. Histologically, interwoven bundles of spindle-shaped smooth muscle cells are interspersed with vascular spaces. The vessels vary from endothelium-lined sinusoids to dilated capillaries. The differential diagnosis includes cavernous hemangioma, hemangiopericytoma, and leiomyoma. Treatment is complete excision. Recurrences may be observed after incomplete removal.

Leiomyosarcoma. Leiomyosarcomas of the orbit typically occur in older women, and after radiation therapy for bilateral retinoblastoma (41–43). Grossly, the lesions are locally invasive. Orbital leiomyosarcomas may disclose a prominent vascular pattern. The differential diagnosis of primary orbital leiomyosarcoma includes secondary leiomyosarcomas invading the orbit from paranasal sinuses and metastatic leiomyosarcomas (44,45). Postradiation leiomyosarcoma of the orbit, when pleomorphic, may be confused with malignant fibrous histiocytoma (42). Smooth muscle actin is consistently expressed in most leiomyosarcomas. The proliferative marker Ki-67 and the expression of p53 are useful indicators of malignancy. In one study, three of four patients with postradiation leiomyosarcoma of the orbit died of metastases (42). Complete excision including exenteration, with the addition of chemotherapy and radiotherapy, is the treatment of choice.

Rhabdomyosarcoma

Definition. Rhabdomyosarcoma is a malignant tumor that arises from undifferentiated or pluripotential mesenchyme that has the capacity to differentiate into skeletal muscle. Based on histopathologic, clinical, and behavioral characteristics, the tumors are subdivided into *embryonal, alveolar,* and *pleomorphic types* (46). Undifferentiated tumors have been classified as *embryonal sarcoma.*

General Features. Orbital rhabdomyosarcoma comprises approximately 10 percent of all rhabdomyosarcoma cases (47–51). The overall prognosis of patients with rhabdomyosarcoma has greatly improved during the last decades. Rhabdomyosarcoma is the most common malignant orbital tumor in childhood (52,53).

Clinical Features. The average age of patients at presentation is 6 years, with a range of 1 month to 68 years (fig. 8-11) (54). Boys are more commonly affected. Embryonal rhabdomyosarcoma is seen most frequently in the first decade of life (median age, 6 years) while the alveolar type is observed most commonly in adolescents. Affected children often have fulminant and rapid development of proptosis and eyelid swelling.

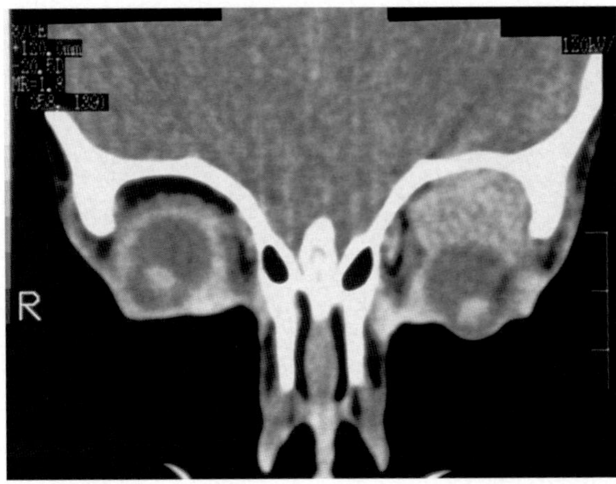

Figure 8-13

RHABDOMYOSARCOMA

Coronal CT scan revealed a large mass in the superior left orbit.

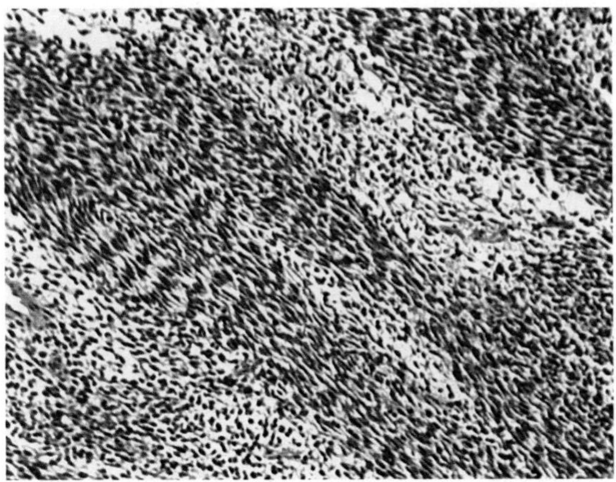

Figure 8-14

RHABDOMYOSARCOMA

Interlacing fascicles of neoplastic spindle cells in a loose stroma.

The most common locations for rhabdomyosarcoma are the supranasal quadrant and superior orbit (fig. 8-12); the alveolar type, however, affects mainly the inferior orbit and may involve the extraocular muscles. The botryoid variant of embryonal rhabdomyosarcoma appears under the conjunctival mucosa. Rhabdomyosarcomas may also arise from compartments surrounding the orbit (parameningeal sites) and secondarily extend to the orbit (55). CT scans usually show a well-circumscribed lesion, which usually enhances with contrast (fig. 8-13). MRI may distinguish rhabdomyosarcoma from well-vascularized lesions of the orbit.

Gross Findings. Grossly, rhabdomyosarcoma appears as a soft, fleshy, yellow neoplasm. The tumor may be circumscribed, and have pushing margins. The cut surface may display a myxoid appearance in tumors with abundant extracellular matrix.

Microscopic Findings. The most common variant is the embryonal form, in which fascicles of spindle cells are oriented in various directions (fig. 8-14). The stroma is frequently loose and myxoid. The cells contain hyperchromatic nuclei and are frequently bipolar, with indistinct, tapered cytoplasmic processes (fig. 8-15). Occasionally, cells with long ribbons of eosinophilic cytoplasm (tadpole cells) are noted (fig. 8-16). Cross-striations, as demonstrated with the Masson trichrome and phosphotungstic acid-hematoxylin (PTAH) stains, are seen in up to 60 percent of the neoplasms. The tumor cells may contain glycogen, confirmed by periodic acid–Schiff (PAS) stain before and after diastase digestion. The botryoid type has a subepithelial layer of densely aggregated spindle cells (Nicholson cambium layer).

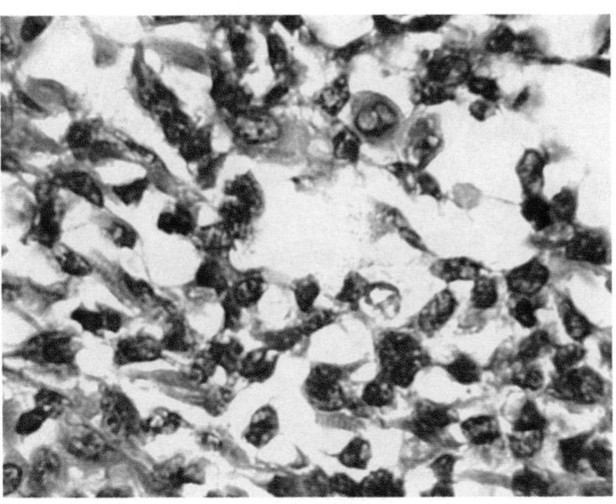

Figure 8-15

RHABDOMYOSARCOMA

Spindle-shaped and round rhabdomyoblasts with occasional striated cytoplasm (inferiorly).

The second most common histologic type is the alveolar form. The tumor is divided into round to oval spaces separated by connective tissue septa (fig. 8-17). The cells are large, round

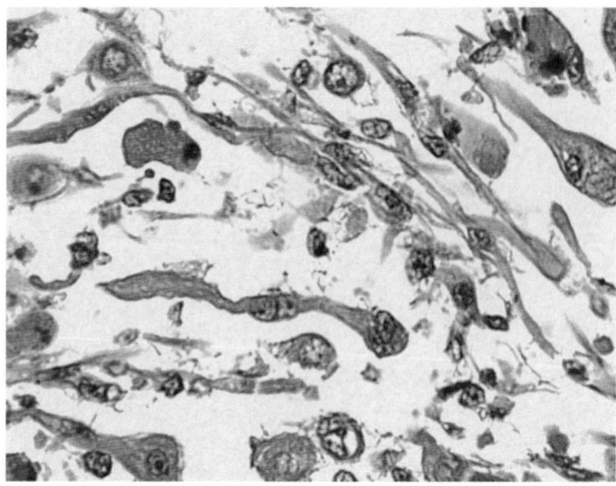

Figure 8-16

RHABDOMYOSARCOMA

Rhabdomyoblasts with asymmetric cytoplasmic expansion, the so-called tadpole cells.

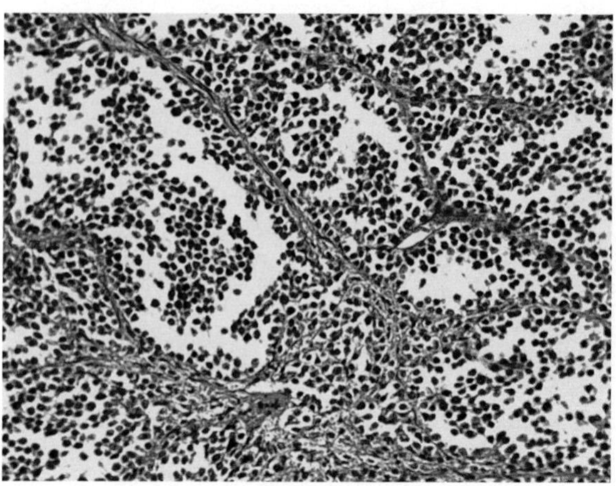

Figure 8-17

ALVEOLAR RHABDOMYOSARCOMA

Low-power microscopic view shows thin fibrous septa and loosely arranged round neoplastic cells.

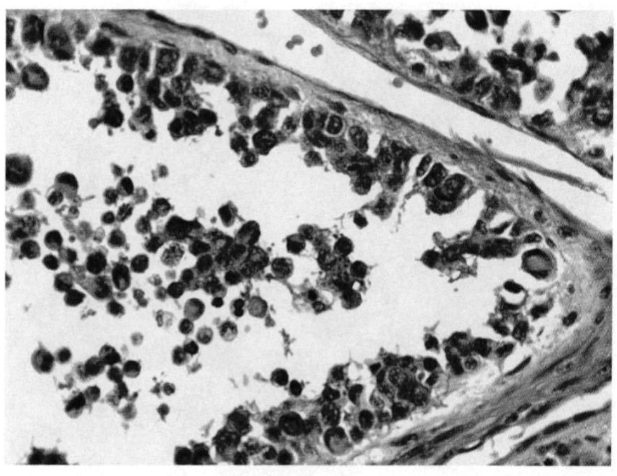

Figure 8-18

ALVEOLAR RHABDOMYOSARCOMA

Round rhabdomyoblasts with eosinophilic cytoplasm are attached to the fibrous septa.

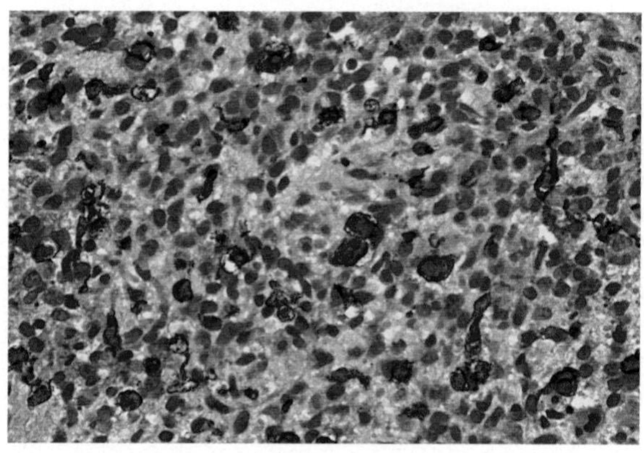

Figure 8-19

RHABDOMYOSARCOMA

The cells expressed muscle-specific antigen.

or polygonal, with abundant eosinophilic cytoplasm and one or more large vesicular nuclei (fig. 8-18).

Pleomorphic rhabdomyosarcoma is the rarest variant and shows a predilection for developing within the striated muscle of older individuals. The cells are large, elongated myoblasts or strap cells showing clear-cut cross-striations that may be highlighted with the trichrome stain.

Immunohistochemical Findings. Immunohistochemistry is used to confirm the diagnosis of rhabdomyosarcoma. Specific markers for skeletal muscle (myogenin and MyoD1) or muscle (desmin and smooth muscle actin) are positive in more than 90 percent of the cases (fig. 8-19) (56).

Electron Microscopic Findings. Electron microscopy is rarely used today for demonstrating features of myofilamentary differentiation (57). The presence of rudimentary sarcomeres is specific for rhabdomyosarcoma (figs. 8-20, 8-21).

Special Techniques. Molecular studies of embryonal rhabdomyosarcoma disclose loss of heterozygosity at chromosome 11p15.5. The alveolar type of rhabdomyosarcoma has consistent

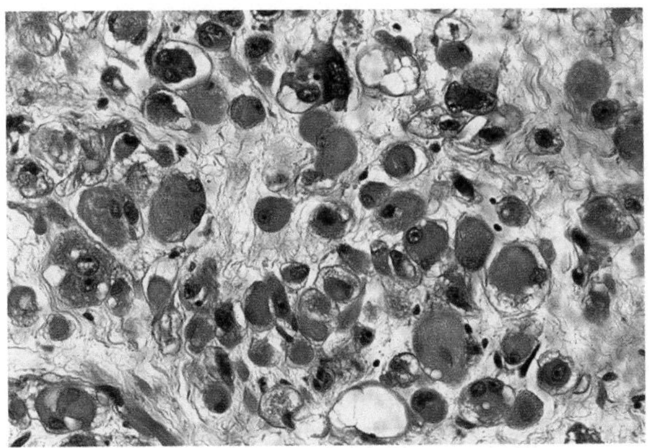

Figure 8-20

RHABDOMYOSARCOMA

Differentiated round rhabdomyoblasts have well-demarcated eosinophilic cytoplasm and an excentric nucleus.

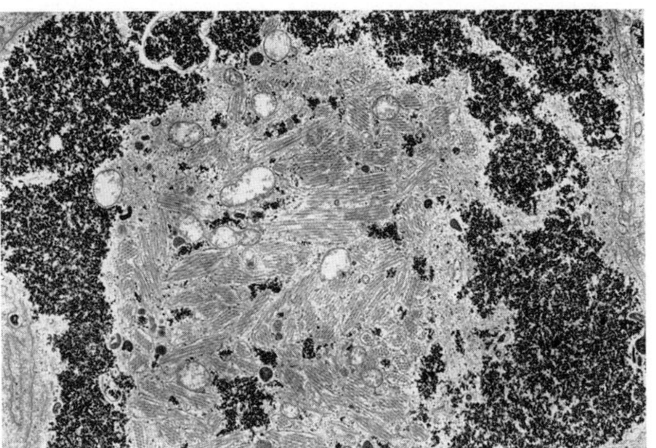

Figure 8-21

RHABDOMYOSARCOMA

Electron microscopy shows peripheral deposits of glycogen and bundles of myofilaments.

Table 8-2

IMMUNOHISTOCHEMISTRY OF MALIGNANT SMALL BLUE CELL TUMORS OF THE ORBIT IN CHILDREN

Type	Des[a]	NF	SYN	LCA	MOP	CD99	S-100	Leu-7
Rhabdomyosarcoma	+	–	–	–	–	–	–	–
Neuroblastoma	–	+	+	–	–	–	–	–
Lymphoma	–	–	+	–	–	–	–	–
Leukemia/granulocytic sarcoma	–	–	–	+	+	–	–	–
Ewing's sarcoma (FLI-1+)	–	–	–	–	–	+	–	–
PNET[b] (FLI-1+)	–	–	–	–	–	+	–	+
Round cell liposarcoma	–	–	–	–	–	–	+	–
Wilms' tumor (WT-1+)	–	–	+	–	–	–	+	–

[a]Des = desmin; NF = neurofilament; SYN = synaptophysin; LCA = leukocyte common antigen; MOP = myeloperoxidase.
[b]PNET = primitive neuroectodermal tumor.

translocations between chromosome 13 (q14) and chromosomes 2 (q35) and 1 (p36) that result in a fusion of a transcription factor (FKHR) with homeotic genes *PAX3* and *PAX7*, respectively. These translocations may be demonstrated with PCR amplification or fluorescent in situ hybridization (FISH). Embryonal rhabdomyosarcoma is usually diploid or hyperdiploid (1.4 to 1.8), and the alveolar type is tetraploid (X2).

Differential Diagnosis. Immunohistochemistry is very useful for the differentiating rhabdomyosarcoma from other malignant neoplasms observed in children, including metastatic neuroblastoma, primitive peripheral neuroectodermal tumor, extraosseous Ewing's sarcoma, lymphoma, and leukemia (Table 8-2).

Treatment and Prognosis. Any patient in whom orbital rhabdomyosarcoma is suspected based on clinical findings and imaging studies should undergo a prompt biopsy to establish the diagnosis. The biopsy should obtain a representative sample of tumor tissue for light microscopy and special studies, including fresh tissue for cytogenetic study and molecular genetics (58). Once the diagnosis is established, the treatment of choice is chemotherapy and

Table 8-3

CLINICAL AND SURGICOPATHOLOGIC GROUPING SYSTEM OF RHABDOMYOSARCOMA (INTERGROUP RHABDOMYOSARCOMA STUDIES I-III)

Group I:	Localized disease that is completely resected with no regional nodal involvement.
Group II:	
IIA:	Localized, grossly resected tumor with microscopic residual disease but no regional nodal involvement.
IIB:	Loco-regional disease with tumor-involved lymph nodes with complete resection and no residual disease.
IIC:	Loco-regional disease with involved nodes, grossly resected, but with evidence of microscopic residual and/or histologic involvement of the most distal regional node (from the primary site).
Group III:	Localized, gross residual disease including incomplete resection, or biopsy only of the primary site.
Group IV:	Distant metastatic disease present at the time of diagnosis.

Table 8-4

TNM-BASED PRETREATMENT STAGING SYSTEM OF RHABDOMYOSARCOMA

Stage I:	Localized disease involving the orbit or head and neck (excluding parameningeal sites), or nonbladder/nonprostate genitourinary region, or biliary tract.
Stage II:	Localized disease of any other primary site not included in the stage I category. Primary tumors must be less than or equal to 5 cm in diameter, and there must be no clinical regional lymph node involvement by tumor.
Stage III:	Localized disease of any other primary site not included in the stage I category. These patients differ from stage II patients by having primary tumors greater than 5 cm and/or regional node involvement.
Stage IV:	Metastatic disease at diagnosis.

radiation therapy, with orbital exenteration reserved for the small number of patients with local, persistent, or recurrent disease (59,60).

The Intergroup Rhabdomyosarcoma Studies (IRS I-III) prescribed treatment plans based on a clinical and surgicopathologic grouping system, with groups defined by the extent of disease and by pathologic review of the tumor specimens (61,62). The definitions of these clinical groups are given in Table 8-3. Most rhabdomyosarcomas of the orbit are placed in group III (48 percent). In addition to clinical grouping, the current Soft Tissue Sarcoma Committee of the Children's Oncology Group (STS-COG) protocols utilize a TNM-based pretreatment staging system (63,64). Tumor stage is determined clinically by primary tumor size and site, regional lymph node status, and the presence or absence of metastases (Table 8-4). Favorable prognostic factors are: 1) undetectable distant metastases at diagnosis; 2) primary sites in the orbit and nonparameningeal head/neck regions; 3) grossly complete surgical removal of localized tumor at the time of diagnosis; 4) embryonal/botryoid histology; 5) tumor size of 5 cm or less; and 6) patient age younger than 10 years at diagnosis.

Recurrences develop in 18 percent of patients, and metastases in 6 percent. The overall 5-year survival rate of patients with orbital rhabdomyosarcoma is greater than 95 percent. The 5-year survival rate of children with the alveolar type is 74 percent. Patients whose tumors invade the orbit from parameningeal sites have a guarded prognosis.

Miscellaneous Skeletal Muscle Tumors

Rare striated muscle neoplasms that occur in the orbit are *rhabdomyoma* and *malignant rhabdoid tumor*; the latter mimics a skeletal muscle tumor (65–67). The validity of reported cases of adult rhabdomyoma of the orbit have been questioned. Malignant rhabdoid tumor is a highly aggressive tumor of infants with distinctive histopathologic features (66). The prognosis is poor, and the treatment does not differ from that for rhabdomyosarcoma (66,67).

VASCULAR TUMORS

Capillary Hemangioma

Definition. *Capillary hemangioma of the infantile type* is an immature form of hemangioma that develops in the perinatal period. It is very common in the head and neck region. Other terms used to identify this tumor include *infantile* or *juvenile hemangioma, strawberry hemangioma,* and *benign hemangioendothelioma.*

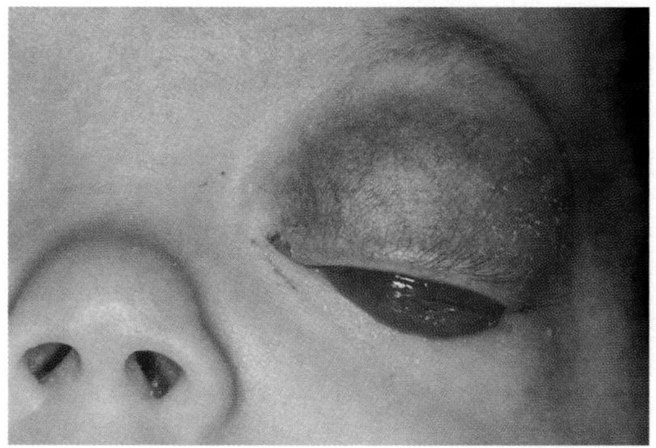

Figure 8-22

CAPILLARY HEMANGIOMA

Reddish bulky tumor of the superior left eyelid.

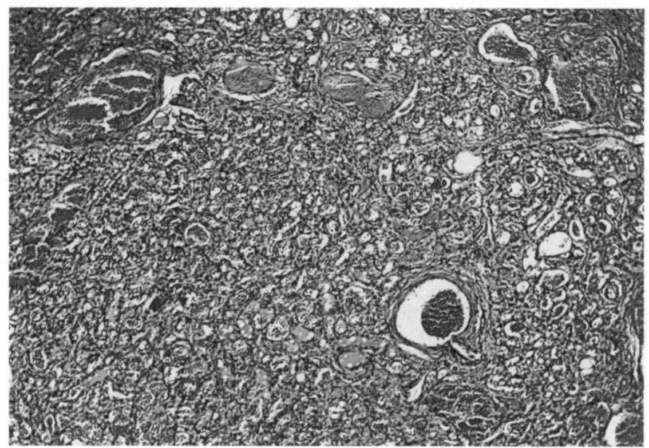

Figure 8-23

CAPILLARY HEMANGIOMA

The compact vascular tumor is composed of small blood vessels lined by endothelial cells.

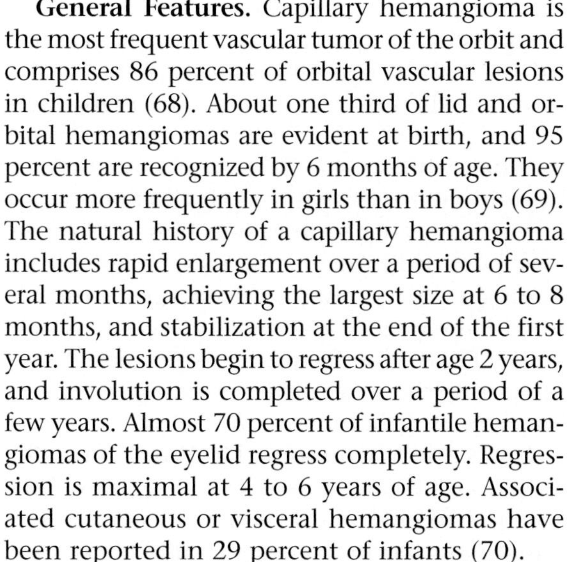

General Features. Capillary hemangioma is the most frequent vascular tumor of the orbit and comprises 86 percent of orbital vascular lesions in children (68). About one third of lid and orbital hemangiomas are evident at birth, and 95 percent are recognized by 6 months of age. They occur more frequently in girls than in boys (69). The natural history of a capillary hemangioma includes rapid enlargement over a period of several months, achieving the largest size at 6 to 8 months, and stabilization at the end of the first year. The lesions begin to regress after age 2 years, and involution is completed over a period of a few years. Almost 70 percent of infantile hemangiomas of the eyelid regress completely. Regression is maximal at 4 to 6 years of age. Associated cutaneous or visceral hemangiomas have been reported in 29 percent of infants (70).

Clinical Features. The most frequent sign is an elevated, cherry-red lesion involving the skin of the eyelid. Almost all patients with eyelid involvement have deeper lid lesions or orbital involvement (fig. 8-22). Proptosis develops over several weeks to months. Local complications during the phase of rapid growth occur in less than 5 percent of patients and include occlusion of the eye and amblyopia, bleeding, and corneal ulceration. CT discloses a diffuse expansile lesion with enhancement following injection of contrast material. MRI reveals a tumor isointense to muscle and gray matter on T1-weighted images and hyperintense on T2-weighted images. The clinical differential diagnosis includes rhabdomyosarcoma, lymphangioma, chloroma, neuroblastoma, and less common neoplasms and inflammatory conditions.

Gross and Microscopic Findings. Grossly, the lesions appear as well-vascularized, multinodular masses. Histologically, tumors in the proliferative phase are characterized by lobulated proliferations of plump endothelial cells tightly packed among inconspicuous vascular spaces (figs. 8-23, 8-24). Mitotic figures may be observed at this stage. Lesions studied in the involutional phase show dilated vascular spaces lined by flat endothelial cells. Regressed tumors have diffuse interstitial fibrosis, with disappearance of vascular lobules.

Immunohistochemical Findings. The plump and flattened lining cells are positive with endothelial markers: factor VIII-associated antigen, CD31, and *Ulex europaeus* agglutinin I.

Treatment and Prognosis. Most patients with periocular capillary hemangioma are followed clinically. Biopsy is only performed for diagnostic purposes in tumors with rapid growth (70). Excision may be indicated in well-circumscribed tumors, when the local mass is causing secondary problems (71). Nonsurgical therapies to prevent amblyopia include radiotherapy, intralesional injection of corticosteroids, injection of sclerosing solutions, administration of interferon alpha2-beta, and direct application of solid carbon dioxide (72,73).

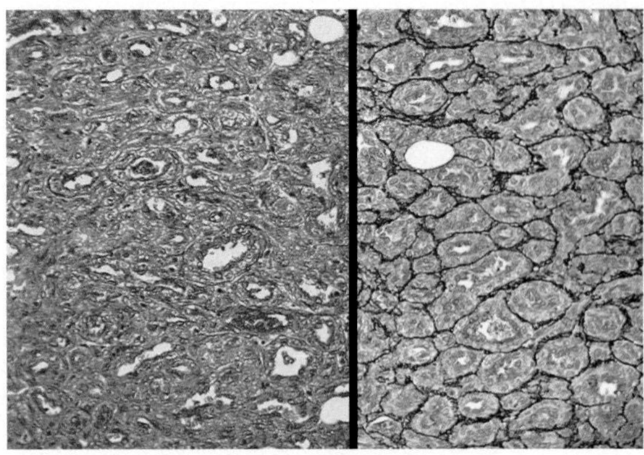

Figure 8-24

CAPILLARY HEMANGIOMA

Left: An irregular vascular pattern is seen.

Right: A reticulin stain delineates the vascular proliferation.

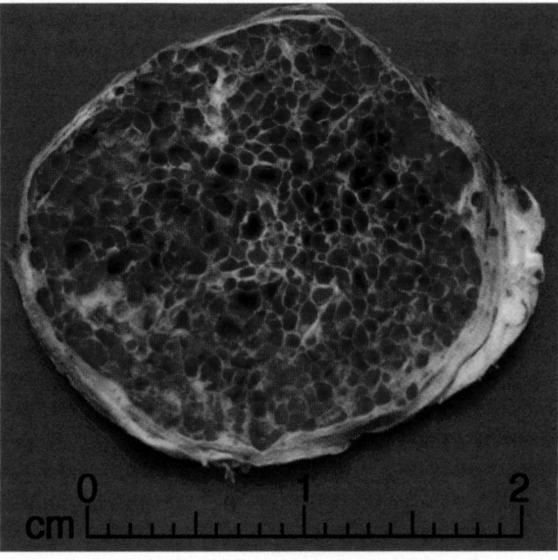

Figure 8-25

CAVERNOUS HEMANGIOMA

The well-circumscribed encapsulated mass is composed of multiple, distended vascular spaces containing blood.

Cavernous Hemangioma

Definition and General Features. *Cavernous hemangioma* is a well-circumscribed or encapsulated vascular tumor of the orbit composed of regular and large-sized vascular spaces lined by flattened endothelium (74).

Clinical Features. Two thirds of patients are women of a mean age of 42 years (range, 18 to 67 years) (74,75). Symptoms include slowly progressive, painless proptosis, and visual loss from compression of the optic nerve or pressure on the back of the eye. Ultrasonography typically reveals a circumscribed mass with high internal reflectivity and progressive attenuation of internal echoes (76). CT scan demonstrates a hyperintense mass without significant change immediately after contrast injection. MRI shows a well-defined intraconal mass. The lesions are homogeneous, isointense to muscle on the T1-weighted sequence and hyperintense to muscle on the T2-weighted sequence. After gadolinium injection, there is initial central patchy enhancement or homogeneous filling.

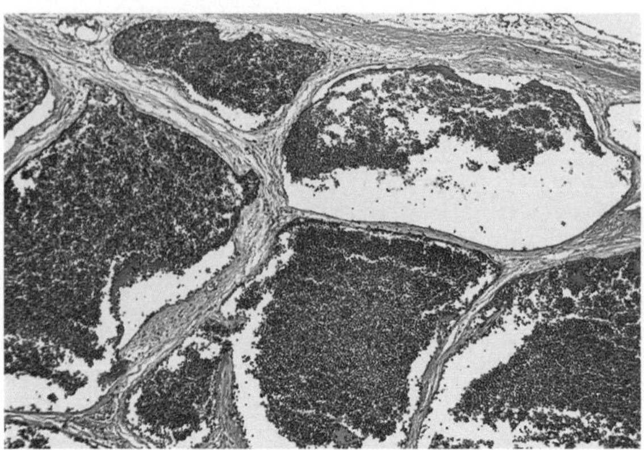

Figure 8-26

CAVERNOUS HEMANGIOMA

Large vascular spaces are lined by flat endothelial cells, separated from each other by fibrous septa.

Gross and Microscopic Findings. Typically, cavernous hemangioma is a well-circumscribed, encapsulated, red to violaceous nodular mass. The tumor has a spongy consistency, and the cut surface shows multiple, round, endothelium-lined vascular spaces containing blood (fig. 8-25).

Microscopically, the vessels are lined by endothelial cells and separated from each other by fibrous septa containing bundles of smooth muscle cells (fig. 8-26) (77). The presence of collections of lymphocytes and follicular centers should entertain the possibility of a circumscribed variant of orbital lymphangioma.

Venous angiomas are probably a variant of cavernous hemangioma in which the smooth muscle cuffs within the vascular channels are more prominent, and abundant fascicles of smooth muscle cells are found in the stroma.

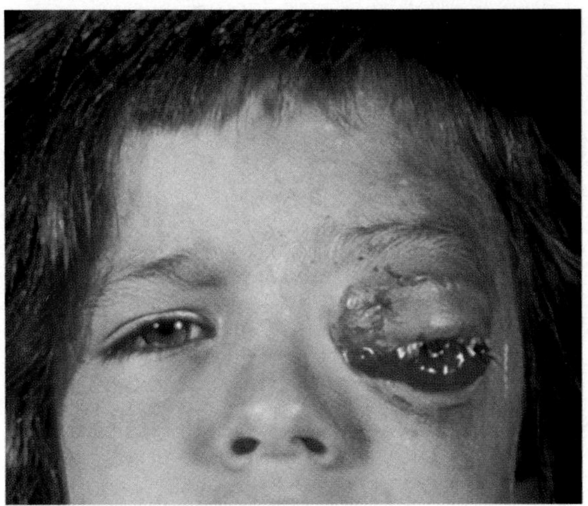

Figure 8-27

LYMPHANGIOMA

A young girl has a diffuse lymphangioma of the left orbit, conjunctiva, and eyelid.

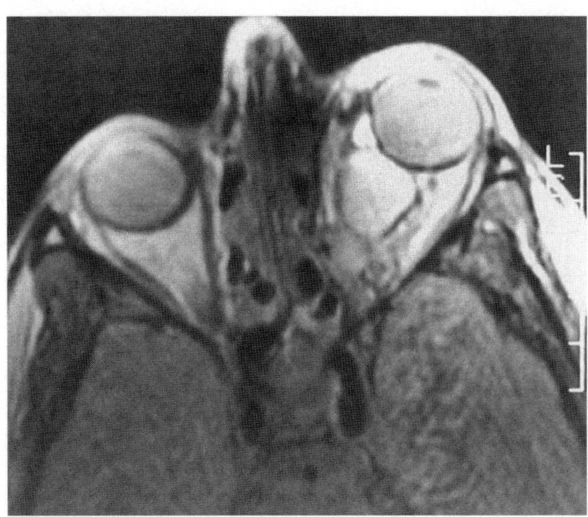

Figure 8-28

LYMPHANGIOMA

Magnetic resonance imaging (MRI) shows multiple orbital spaces.

These lesions are less well circumscribed and demonstrate contrast enhancement comparable to that observed in cavernous hemangioma.

Immunohistochemical Findings. In addition to endothelial cell markers, perivascular stromal cells express smooth muscle actin.

Treatment and Prognosis. Patients who are asymptomatic are followed without treatment. Tumors causing symptoms are easily removed without damaging other vital structures of the orbit. Following local excision no recurrences are observed (74). Venous angioma is more difficult to dissect, leading to more postoperative morbidity (78).

Lymphangioma

Definition. *Lymphangioma* is a choristomatous orbital tumor, since there are no lymphatic channels within the normal orbit (79,80). Its origin has been postulated to result from sequestration of lymphatic tissue within the orbit at some point during embryonic development. Some authors argue that orbital lymphangioma should be considered a venous-lymphatic malformation (81).

General Features. Orbital and adnexal lymphangiomas have been clinically separated into superficial, deep, and combined types (82). The superficial type affects the conjunctiva and eyelid, and is neither associated with proptosis nor loss of vision. Deeply located lesions may present with acute proptosis from hemorrhage that may cause optic nerve compression and require surgical intervention. Combined lesions are slowly progressive and may produce severe cosmetic disfigurement and decreased vision from tissue damage and/or amblyopia.

Clinical Features. Most of the cases are diagnosed between the ages of 1 and 5 years (range, birth to 44 years) and are more prevalent in females (fig. 8-27) (80). Lymphangiomas are characterized by a fluctuating clinical course, with exacerbation of proptosis due to intralesional hemorrhage and upper respiratory viral infections. A subset of diffuse lesions results in frequent anterior extension into the soft tissues of the face and forehead, other associated vascular lesions such as palatal involvement, and noncontiguous intracranial vascular abnormalities (83). MRI is more sensitive than CT in distinguishing infiltration within normal orbital tissues (fig. 8-28) (84). The lymphatic channels appear hypointensive or isointense on T1-weighted images because of the fluid content. Lesions in adults tend to be circumscribed, resembling cavernous hemangiomas (85).

Gross and Microscopic Findings. Typically, lymphangioma of the orbit is a nonencapsulated, diffuse, branching lesion that affects the orbital and periocular tissues (fig. 8-29). The

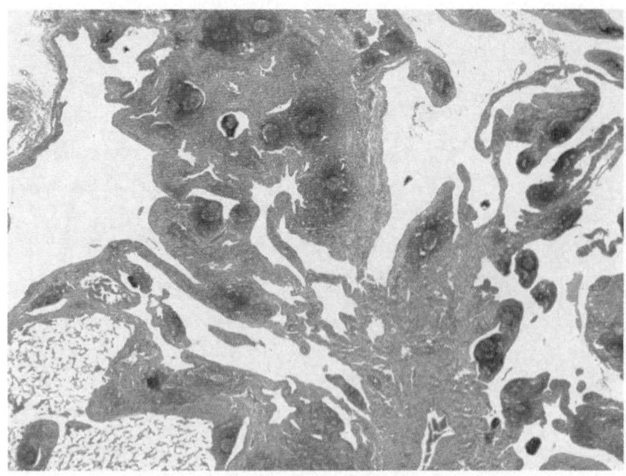

Figure 8-29

LYMPHANGIOMA

Low-power view shows large irregular spaces and lymphatic fibrous septa containing lymphocytic nodules.

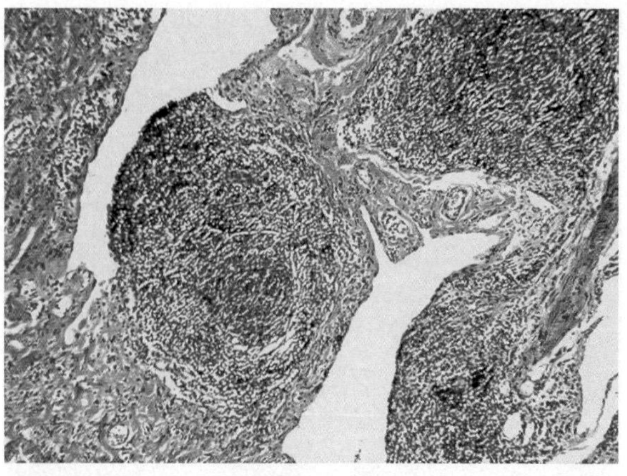

Figure 8-30

LYMPHANGIOMA

The spaces are lined by a discontinuous flat endothelial lining. Reactive lymphoid nodules are observed.

vascular spaces are lined by a monolayer of attenuated endothelium without pericytes. Well-formed lymphoid aggregates with germinal centers are usually present (fig. 8-30). Other findings are related to recent or old hemorrhage, including hemosiderin-laden macrophages, cholesterol clefts, fibrosis, and phleboliths.

Immunohistochemical Findings. Lymphatic endothelium shares the immunoprofile of other vascular tumors except for the absence of VEGF-3 expression.

Treatment and Prognosis. Diffuse orbital lymphangioma has a slowly progressive, infiltrative growth pattern with no tendency towards spontaneous involution. The lack of circumscription and free planes of cleavage make total removal difficult. Surgery is performed for functional and cosmetic reasons (86).

Hemangiopericytoma

Definition. *Hemangiopericytoma* is a tumor with a distinctive vascular pattern composed of cells resembling pericytes. Although the existence of tumors arising from pericytes has been questioned, a subset of vascular lesions exists that does not fit in any other diagnostic category (87).

Clinical Features. Hemangiopericytomas of the orbit affect mainly adults of a median age of 42 years (88). Men are affected twice as often as women. The mean duration of symptoms prior to surgery is 3 years but is less than 1 year in half of the patients. The most frequent clinical manifestations are proptosis and a palpable mass, which affects mainly the superior orbit. Hemangiopericytoma may arise from the meninges of the optic nerve (89). MRI shows rapid enhancement upon injection of contrast material (90).

Gross and Microscopic Findings. Grossly, most tumors are single and circumscribed, with an average size of 3 cm and a rubbery consistency. Microscopically, there is a rich vascular pattern of dilated branching vessels and a population of round to ovoid cells (figs. 8-31–8-33). Hemangiopericytomas of the orbit have been classified as benign, intermediate, and malignant based on the vascular pattern (evident or solid), degree of cytologic atypia, number of mitoses, and presence of necrosis (fig. 8-34) (88). Invasion of orbital tissues occurs mainly with malignant tumors.

Immunohistochemical Findings. The results of immunostaining are relatively nonspecific. Most cells express vimentin and rarely, actin. CD34 is positive but less strongly than in solitary fibrous tumor. Tumor cells are negative for factor VIII–related antigen, smooth muscle actin, and cytokeratin.

Differential Diagnosis. The vascular pattern of hemangiopericytoma may be shared by several soft tissue tumors including solitary fibrous tumor, mesenchymal chondrosarcoma, and vascular fibrous histiocytoma. Microscopically, hemangiopericytoma of the meninges of the

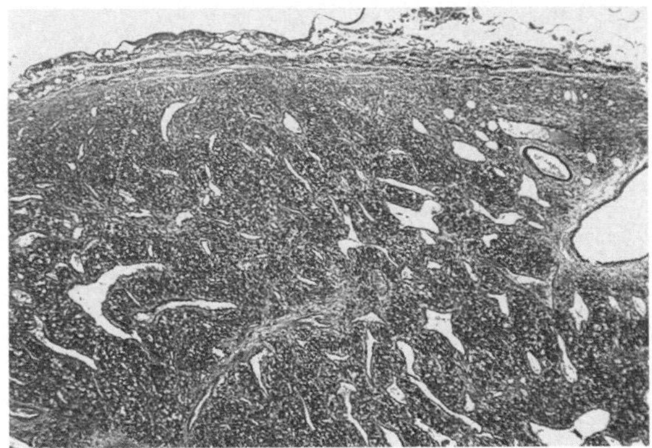

Figure 8-31

HEMANGIOPERICYTOMA

The encapsulated benign hemangiopericytoma has irregular vascular spaces, some of which resemble a staghorn configuration (Movat pentachrome stain).

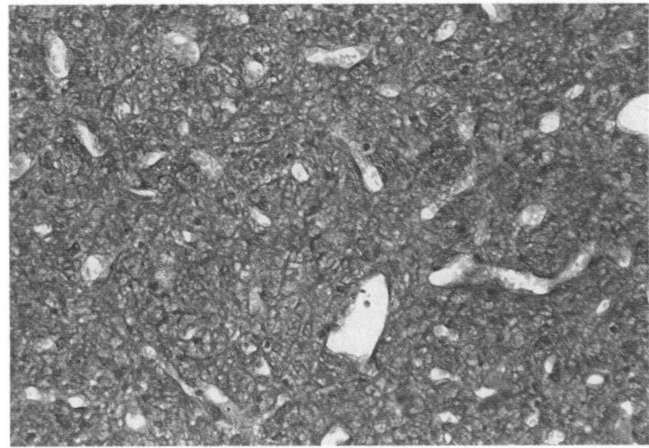

Figure 8-32

HEMANGIOPERICYTOMA

The individual cells are delineated by basement membrane material (periodic acid–Schiff [PAS] stain).

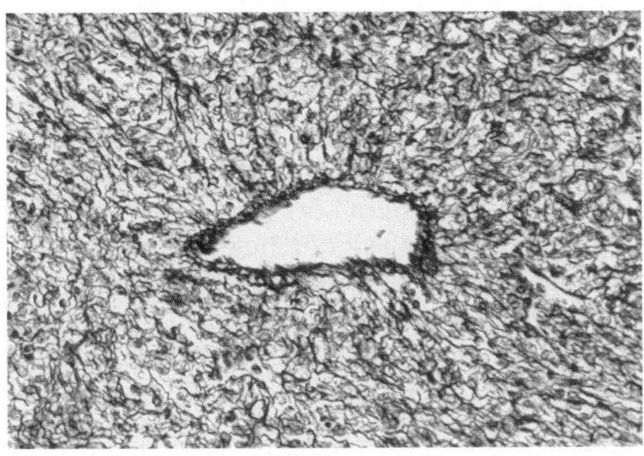

Figure 8-33

HEMANGIOPERICYTOMA

The reticulin stain demonstrates the proliferation of cells outside the vessels walls.

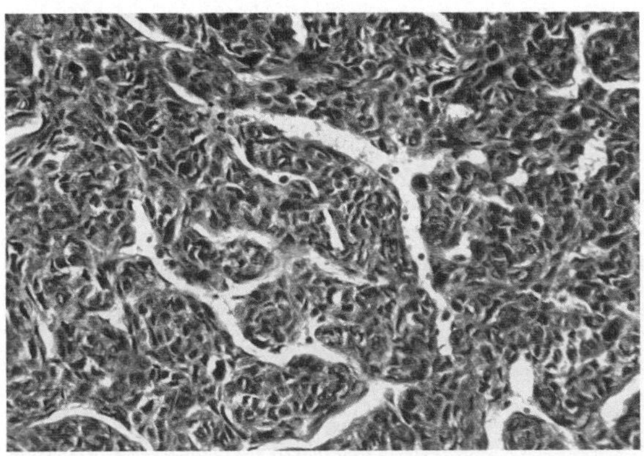

Figure 8-34

HEMANGIOPERICYTOMA

This malignant hemangiopericytoma is composed of atypical cells with hyperchromatic nuclei and mitotic figures.

optic nerve may be undistinguishable from the so-called angioblastic meningioma, which has a more aggressive behavior.

Treatment and Prognosis. The behavior of hemangiopericytoma of the orbit does not follow closely the histopathologic classification. Recurrences, found in 25 to 50 percent of the patients, are noted up to 33 years after surgery. Fifteen percent of the patients in the AFIP series died of metastatic disease 6 to 32 years after the onset of symptoms (88). Complete surgical excision and radiation therapy appear to be effective in providing tumor control (91,92).

Solitary Fibrous Tumor

Definition and General Features. *Solitary fibrous tumor* (SFT) is a rare neoplasia of mesenchymal origin that was first recognized in the pleura as a localized tumor of the pleura (93). It has been tentatively classified among perivascular tumors (94). Orbital cases have been reported with increased frequency during the last decade (95–98). These lesions may have been misdiagnosed as fibrous histiocytoma, hemangiopericytoma, or other mesenchymal orbital tumors. SFTs are generally benign, although a few cases that exhibit a malignant clinical

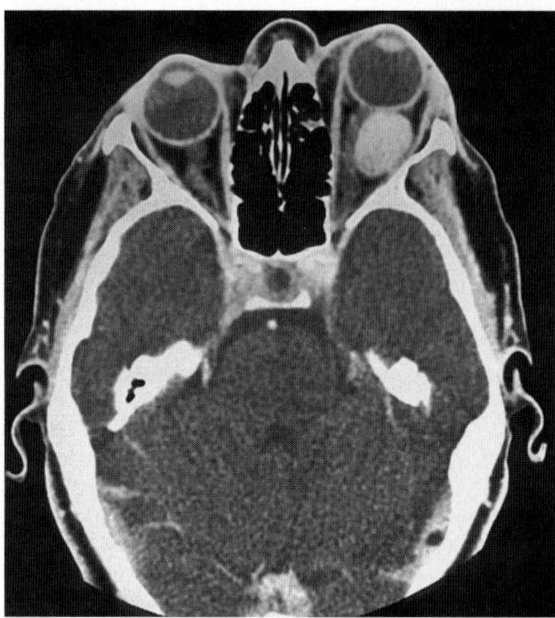

Figure 8-35

SOLITARY FIBROUS TUMOR

Axial computerized tomography (CT) shows a well-circumscribed, dense, homogeneous, oval tumor in the right orbit.

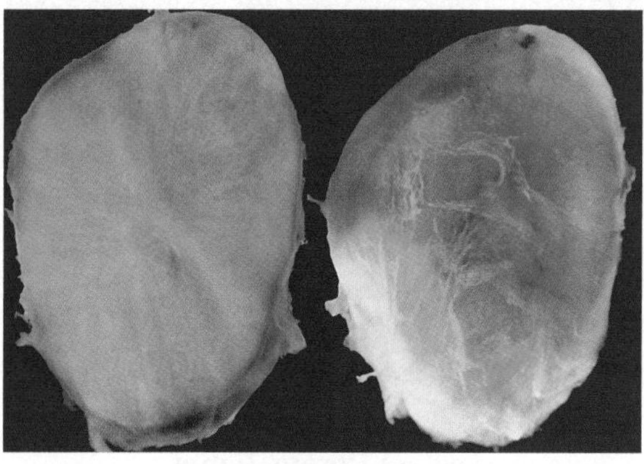

Figure 8-36

SOLITARY FIBROUS TUMOR

The tumor is well-circumscribed, yellow and tan, with white fibrous tracts.

course have been reported in other sites and occasionally in the orbit (98).

Clinical Features. SFT of the orbit affects patients between 10 and 72 years of age, with an average of 45 to 52 years (98,99). Clinically, there is painless, progressive proptosis. Lesions are located within or outside the muscle cone.

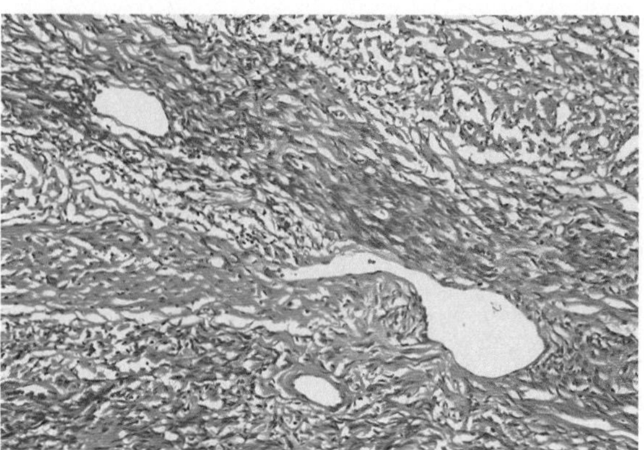

Figure 8-37

SOLITARY FIBROUS TUMOR

The tumor is composed of slender spindle-shaped cells with extracellular collagen deposits and telangiectatic vessels.

CT scans show isolated, well-circumscribed masses with contrast enhancement and foci of radiolucency (fig. 8-35) (99). MRI reveals a well-circumscribed, round mass which shows isointensity to the gray matter on T1-weighted sequences, a low signal on T2-weighted images with intralesional signal heterogeneity, and heterogeneous postcontrast enhancement.

Gross and Microscopic Findings. Grossly, SFT is a well-circumscribed or encapsulated, round to oval, rubbery mass with a white to tan cut surface that contains fibrous strands (fig. 8-36). Histologically, the tumor is composed of spindle cells with twisted nuclei organized in loosely arranged fascicles within a myxoid stroma (fig. 8-37). Bands of hyalinized, densely sclerotic collagen are invariably present between the tumor cells. Cellular pleomorphism varies from mild to moderate, with little or no mitotic activity. Branching blood vessels may resemble the staghorn configuration observed in hemangiopericytomas. The histologic features associated with malignant behavior are high cellularity, mitotic counts over 4 per 10 high-power fields, nuclear pleomorphism, and necrosis.

Immunohistochemical Findings. Lesions are strongly positive for CD34, CD99, bcl-2, and vimentin, and focally positive for desmin, but negative for smooth muscle actin, S-100-protein, CD31, pankeratin, and epithelial membrane antigen (fig. 8-38). The MIB-1 label index may be used to delineate further the tumor behavior.

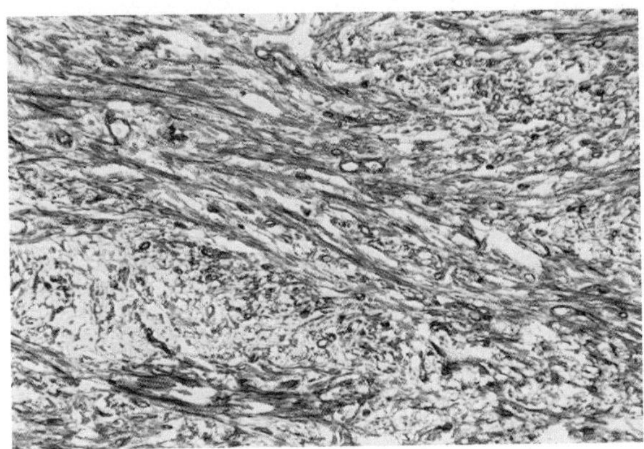

Figure 8-38

SOLITARY FIBROUS TUMOR

Most cells are positive for CD34 antibody.

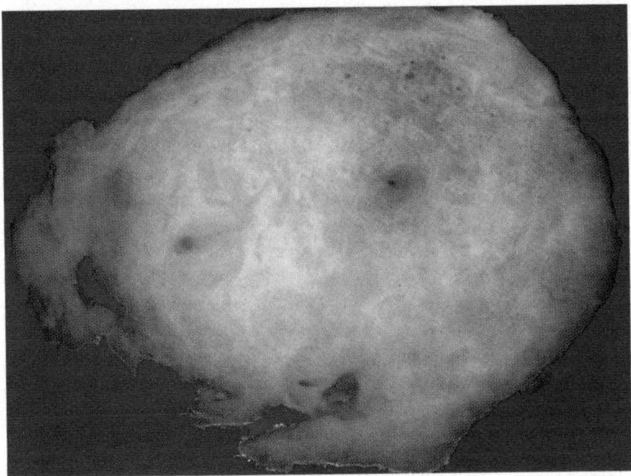

Figure 8-39

EPITHELIOID HEMANGIOMA

The irregular, solid, nodular mass contains yellowish tan nodules.

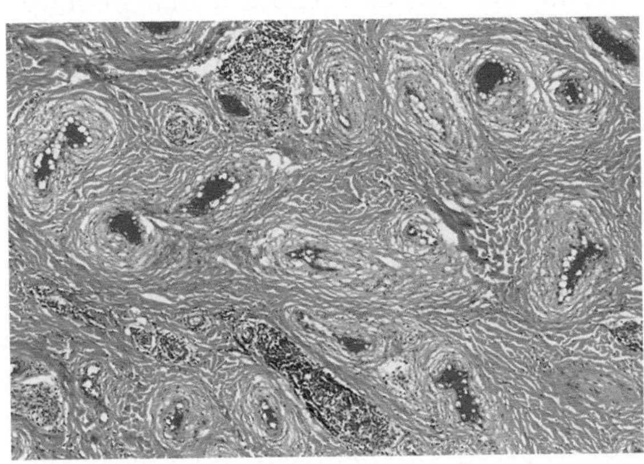

Figure 8-40

EPITHELIOID HEMANGIOMA

Low-power microscopic view shows blood vessel proliferation and lymphocytic foci.

Cytologic Findings. Typically, the tumor cells are oval to polygonal, with variable cellularity ranging from scant to moderate (95). The background contains irregular, ropy fragments of collagen and a few inflammatory cells. Most cells are dispersed singly, but loose aggregates of cells enmeshed in a collagenous matrix are usually observed. The nuclei are uniformly bland, with evenly distributed, finely granular chromatin. The cells are immunoreactive for CD34.

Differential Diagnosis. SFTs should be differentiated from hemangiopericytoma, fibrous histiocytoma, and schwannoma.

Treatment and Prognosis. Approximately 20 cases of SFT of the orbit have been reported; it appears that the orbital location is associated with benign behavior (99). Recurrences do occur, and patients should be followed closely for a long period (98). Treatment is complete surgical excision.

Epithelioid Hemangioma

Epithelioid hemangioma is an uncommon but distinctive benign vascular lesion originally described as *angiolymphoid hyperplasia with eosinophilia* (100). The affected patients are usually middle-aged women without evidence of similar lesions elsewhere. Some patients have a history of trauma or enucleation (101).

Grossly, the tumors have an irregular, nodular shape with a white-yellow cut surface (fig. 8-39). Histopathologically, there are clusters of small blood vessels with myxoid degeneration of the smooth muscle layer (fig. 8-40). Quite distinctively, the vessels are lined by swollen endothelial cells with abundant eosinophilic cytoplasm that contains conspicuous vacuoles, which gives a characteristic, plump, "epithelioid" appearance (figs. 8-41, 8-42). In addition, a variable, chronic inflammatory infiltrate that includes lymphoid aggregates and abundant eosinophils may be found in some lesions. The cells possess ultrastructural features of normal endothelium and stain for endothelial cell markers, factor VIII–related antigen, and *Ulex europaeus* agglutinin I.

Epithelioid hemangioma should be distinguished clinically and histopathologically from

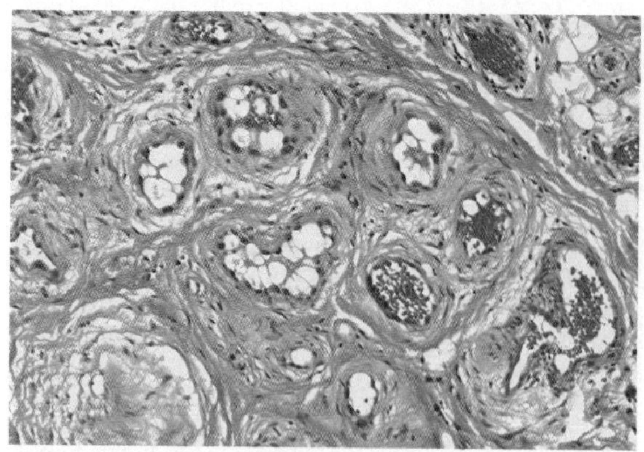

Figure 8-41

EPITHELIOID HEMANGIOMA

Proliferated blood vessels are lined by plump endothelial cells with cytoplasmic strands.

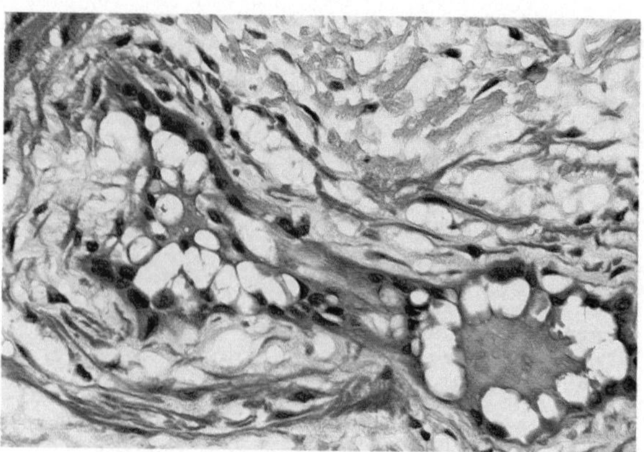

Figure 8-42

EPITHELIOID HEMANGIOMA

The Movat pentachrome stain shows the swollen endothelial cells within the lumen of the vascular spaces.

Kimura's disease, epithelioid hemangioendothelioma, epithelioid angiosarcoma, and bacillary angiomatosis (101). Confusion exists between epithelioid hemangioma (angiolymphoid hyperplasia with eosinophilia) and Kimura's disease, and many reports use both names interchangeably.

Kimura's disease, first described in 1948 by Kimura et al. (102) in Japan, is a distinctive clinical and histopathologic entity. It consists of lymphadenopathy, with or without an inflammatory mass, almost always accompanied by increased serum immunoglobulin (Ig)E and peripheral blood eosinophilia that may be associated with IgE glomerular nephropathy. These lesions occur almost exclusively in Asian males (102–104). Histopathologic examination of orbital lesions shows dense lymphoid aggregates with prominent germinal centers, including thin-walled postcapillary venules and numerous eosinophils. The vessels are lined by attenuated endothelial cells.

Complete surgical excision is the treatment of choice for epithelioid hemangioma since most lesions show only a partial response to corticosteroids, radiation, and chemotherapy. The recurrence rate after surgical excision is approximately 33 percent. In some cases the lesions regress spontaneously (101).

Arteriovenous and Venous Anomalies

Clinically, orbital vascular malformations are classified according to their hemodynamic relationships as no flow, venous flow, and arterial flow lesions (fig. 8-43) (105). Some vascular anomalies result in excision of diagnostic biopsy material (fig. 8-44). These include *orbital varix, Klippel-Trenaunay-Weber syndrome, blue rubber bleb nevus syndrome, Sturge-Weber syndrome, arteriovenous malformations (racemose hemangiomas), Wyburn-Mason syndrome, dural arteriovenous fistulas,* and *aneurysms* (106–109).

Orbital varices are usually considered to be a congenital venous malformation. Some authors believe that they are very common. Imaging studies demonstrate an enlarged ophthalmic vein, generally in the superior orbit (110). Complications such as thrombosis and spontaneous orbital hemorrhage mimic an acute orbital process. Pathologic examination of excised varices shows a single vascular space or tangles of vascular channels. Many thrombosed varices have the histologic features of benign papillary endothelial hyperplasia. Most patients with orbital varices are managed conservatively.

Intravascular Papillary Endothelial Hyperplasia

Intravascular papillary endothelial hyperplasia (IPEH) is a reactive intravascular lesion that should not be confused with angiosarcoma. In the orbit it usually occurs within a preexisting vein and rarely from a vascular malformation or an artery (111–113). Patients develop progressive proptosis over several months. CT scans show a well-circumscribed orbital lesion resembling cavernous hemangioma. Grossly, the

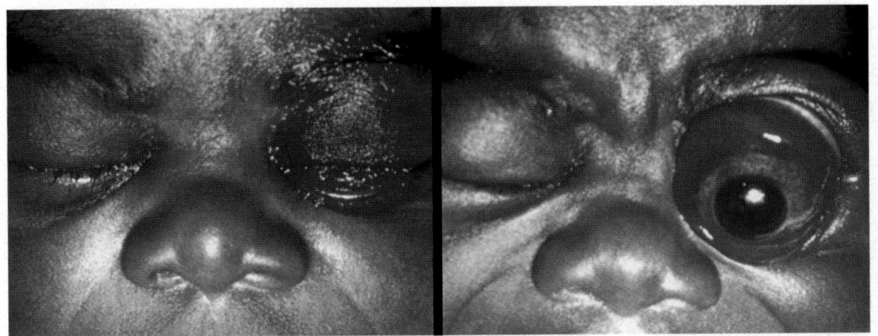

Figure 8-43

ARTERIOVENOUS MALFORMATION

The proptosis enlarges with an increase in venous pressure.

excised lesions have a dusky blue discoloration. Histopathologic examination reveals part of the wall of the preexistent vein or, rarely, artery. The lesion is composed of masses of endothelial cell proliferation with a papillary arrangement along connective tissue trabeculae. Its intravascular location is the main factor that differentiates IPEH from angiosarcoma. These lesions have a benign clinical course.

Angiosarcoma

Angiosarcoma is one of the rarest vascular tumors of the orbit (114,115). In the past, such malignant vascular tumors were termed *hemangiosarcoma, lymphangiosarcoma,* and *hemangioendothelioma*. The mean age of the patients is 11 years at diagnosis (range, 2 weeks to 66 years) (115). The orbit may also be the site of metastatic angiosarcoma. The tumors are composed of large, highly pleomorphic, hyperchromatic endothelial cells and form pseudoglandular vascular spaces that infiltrate the orbital soft tissues. A papillary pattern with multiple layers of malignant endothelial cells is characteristically present. Immunohistochemistry demonstrates staining with CD31 and CD34. The results with factor VIII–related antigen and *Ulex europaeus* agglutinin I are less specific. Adults have a rapidly fatal outcome.

PERIPHERAL NERVE SHEATH TUMORS

Primary nerve sheaths tumors of the orbit originate from sensory nerves (116–118). Most frequently, they are located in the superior and medial orbital compartments. Extension to the superior orbital fissure is seen in almost half of the cases. Primary nerve sheath tumors comprise 4 percent of all primary orbital tumors: 2 percent are plexiform neurofibromas associated with neurofibromatosis type 1; 1 percent are isolated

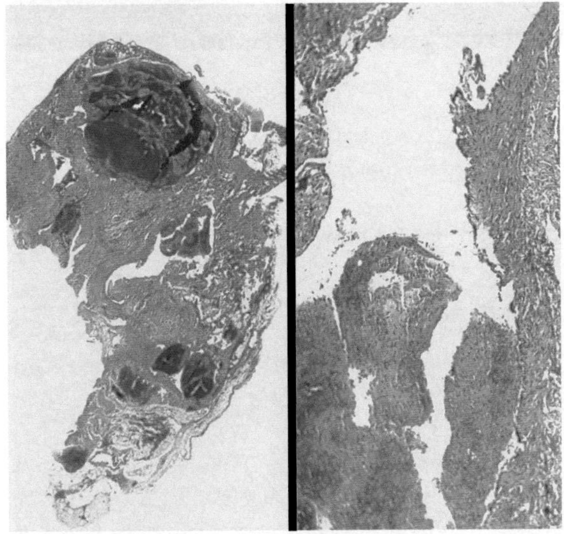

Figure 8-44

ARTERIOVENOUS MALFORMATION

Irregular vascular spaces are seen in the same lesion as depicted in figure 8-43.

neurofibromas; and 1 percent are isolated schwannomas. Postamputation neuromas of the orbit are rare and have been described following blunt or surgical trauma (119,120). Granular cell tumor is currently recognized as a benign neural tumor.

Neurofibroma

Definition. Neurofibroma is a benign tumor of the nerve sheath that may occur in the orbit as a *plexiform neurofibroma, diffuse neurofibroma,* or *isolated neurofibroma*.

General and Clinical Features. The plexiform neurofibroma is a pathognomonic feature of neurofibromatosis type 1 (von Recklinghausen's disease). The first symptoms usually

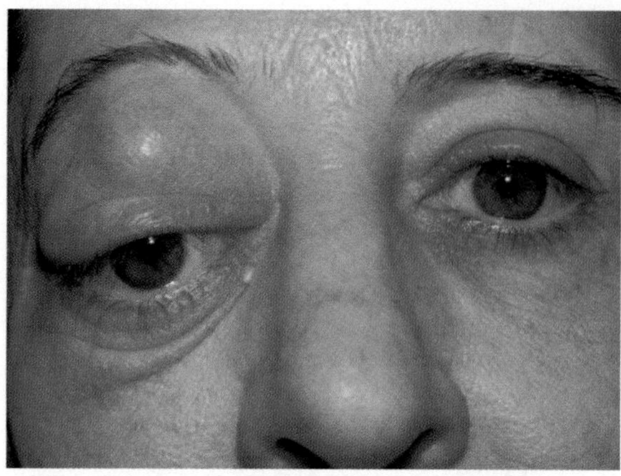

Figure 8-45

NEUROFIBROMA

Nodular tumor in the right upper eyelid.

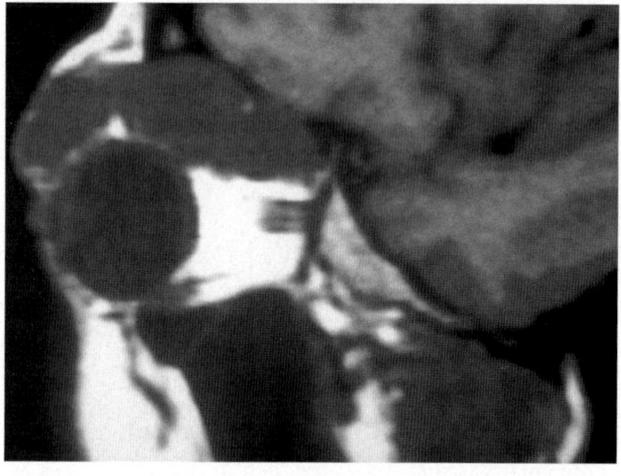

Figure 8-46

NEUROFIBROMA

MRI of the tumor seen in figure 8-45 shows an elongated mass that extends to the posterior orbit.

appear in the first decade of life. The lesions may involve the orbital structures, including the lacrimal gland. The sphenoid bone may be dysplastic and associated with pulsatile exophthalmos or enophthalmos (121). Occasionally, benign neurofibromatous nerve growths adopt an infiltrative pattern. These tumors are named diffuse neurofibromas and are less likely to be associated with neurofibromatosis. Isolated (localized or circumscribed) neurofibromas are nonencapsulated, well-circumscribed lesions, first seen in the third to fifth decades of life (fig. 8-45) (122). They may be multiple and bilateral

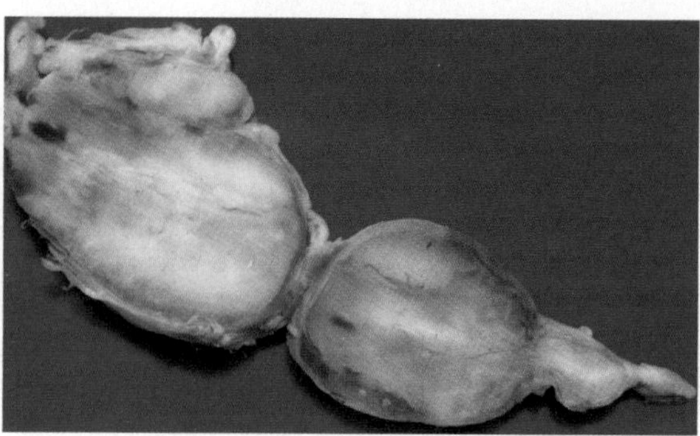

Figure 8-47

NEUROFIBROMA

Gross appearance of an isolated neurofibroma with a myxoid matrix.

but usually occur sporadically (123,124). Imaging studies, including ultrasonography and MRI, differentiate neurofibroma from other primary orbital tumors (fig. 8-46).

Gross Findings. Plexiform neurofibroma is a nonencapsulated tumor that grows in a "crabgrass" fashion to involve the orbital tissues. In contrast, isolated neurofibroma is well-circumscribed and may have a pseudocapsule. One or more peripheral nerves are usually attached to or in continuity with the lesion (fig. 8-47). Diffuse infiltrating neurofibroma involves the orbital tissues without circumscription (fig. 8-48).

Microscopic Findings. Neurofibromas are composed of wavy bundles of peripheral nerve sheath cells (fig. 8-49). The cells are represented by Schwann cells and endoneural and perineural fibroblasts. The Schwann cells may form pacinian corpuscles (fig. 8-50). Special stains (Bodian) usually demonstrate myelinated axons. Typically, the stroma is rich in hyaluronic acid and contains variable amounts of collagen.

Immunohistochemical Findings. The Schwann cells of neurofibromas are usually focally immunoreactive for S-100 protein. The perineural cells may be positive for epithelial membrane antigen.

Electron Microscopic Findings. The Schwann cells are invested by a thin continuous basement membrane. Patches of banded basement membrane (Luse bodies) may be present along the plasma membrane (125).

Treatment and Prognosis. Malignant degeneration of orbital plexiform neurofibromas can occur but is extremely rare (126,127). The result

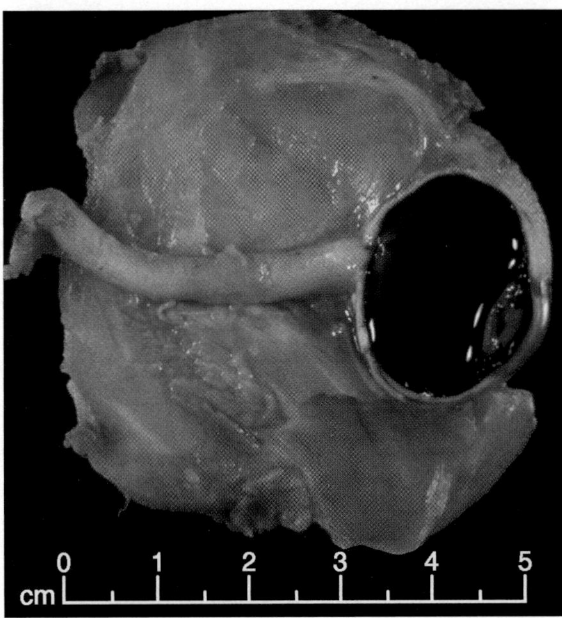

Figure 8-48

DIFFUSE INFILTRATING NEUROFIBROMA

Orbital exenteration specimen shows a diffuse, infiltrating, yellowish tumor.

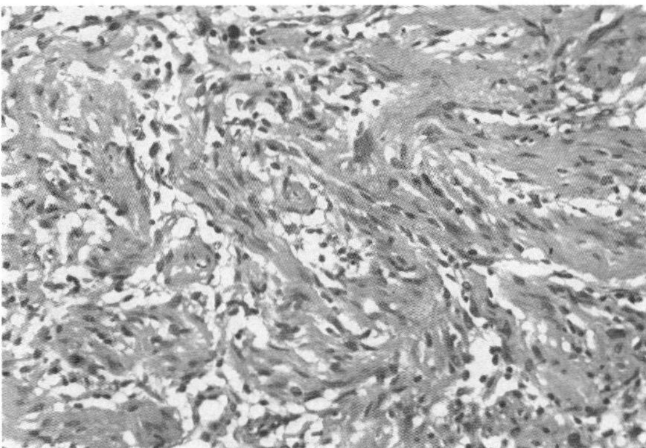

Figure 8-49

NEUROFIBROMA

Wavy bundles of peripheral nerve sheath cells are seen.

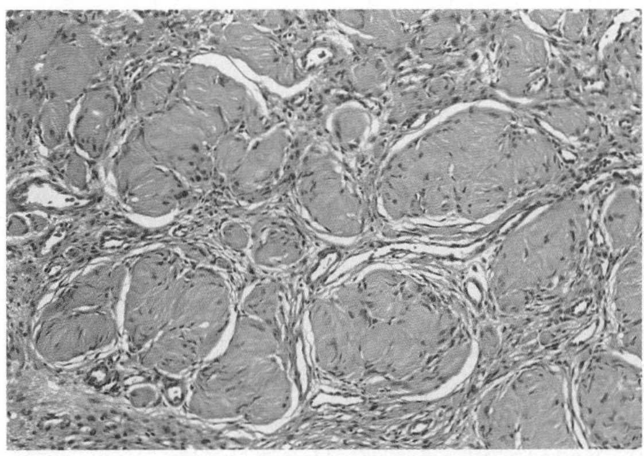

Figure 8-50

DIFFUSE INFILTRATING NEUROFIBROMA

Pacinian corpuscles from the exenteration specimen seen in figure 8-48.

of surgical excision depends upon the type of growth, either localized, plexiform, or diffuse.

Schwannoma (Neurilemoma)

Definition. *Schwannoma,* also termed *neurilemoma,* is a peripheral nerve sheath tumor composed predominately of Schwann cells. Most schwannomas are sporadic, but a few occur in patients with neurofibromatosis type 2.

General and Clinical Features. Schwannomas are similar to neurofibromas of the orbit and originate from either the supraorbital or infraorbital nerves (fig. 8-51) (128). Patients present with longstanding proptosis (129). The results of imaging studies are virtually identical to those of neurofibroma (130). T1-weighted MRI with fat suppression and gadolinium enhancement usually demonstrates a cystic mass, representing mucinous degeneration (131). The lesions usually are well vascularized.

Gross and Microscopic Findings. Schwannomas are well-circumscribed tumors that are encapsulated by the epineurium of the nerve of origin (fig. 8-52). The cut surface is white to yellow, with reddish tan areas because of hemorrhage (fig. 8-53). Classically, there is palisading of nuclei forming solid cellular areas (Antoni A pattern) (fig. 8-54) alternating with areas of loose, stellate cells suspended in a mucinous matrix (Antoni B pattern). Nuclear palisading and highly oriented, polar cytoplasmic processes (Verocay bodies) may be observed (fig. 8-55). Longstanding lesions (*ancient schwannomas*) have areas of cystic degeneration with thickening of the vessel walls, nuclear hyperchromasia, hemorrhage, and lipidized histiocytes (xanthoma cells). One case of orbital *melanotic schwannoma* has been reported (132).

Immunohistochemical Findings. The spindle-shaped cells are strongly positive for S-100 protein in all cases.

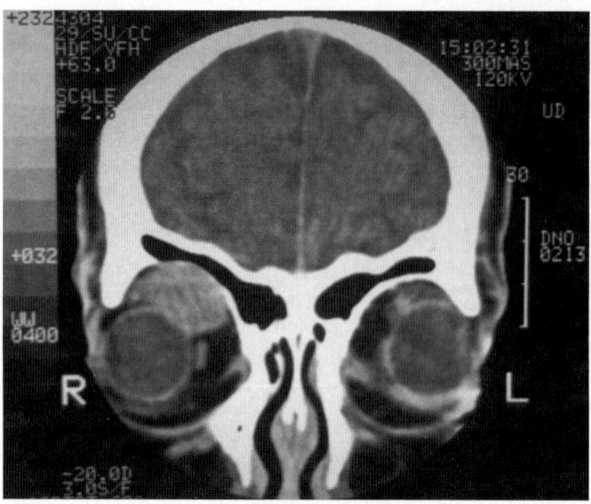

Figure 8-51

SCHWANNOMA

Coronal CT scan shows an oval, well-circumscribed mass involving the superior orbit.

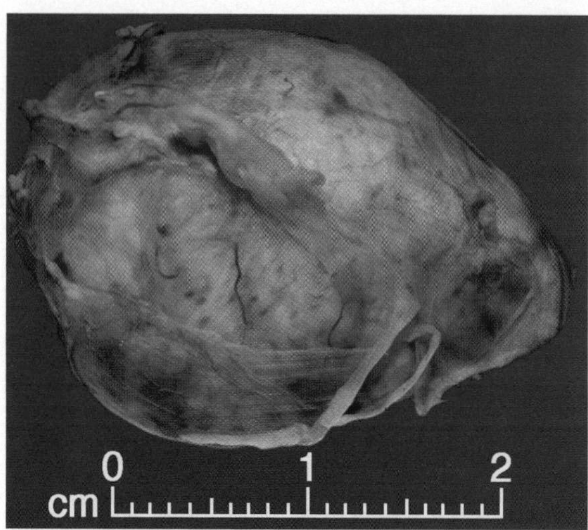

Figure 8-52

SCHWANNOMA

The mass depicted in figure 8-51 is yellowish tan and encapsulated.

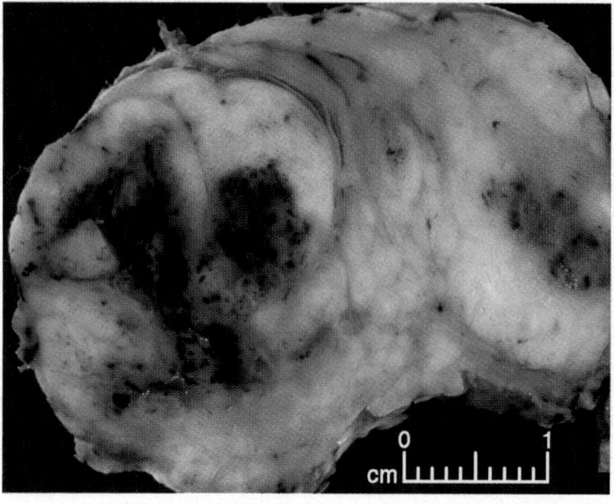

Figure 8-53

SCHWANNOMA

This recurrent orbital schwannoma has a well-circumscribed, bilobed, yellowish tan surface with multiple blood-filled cystic areas.

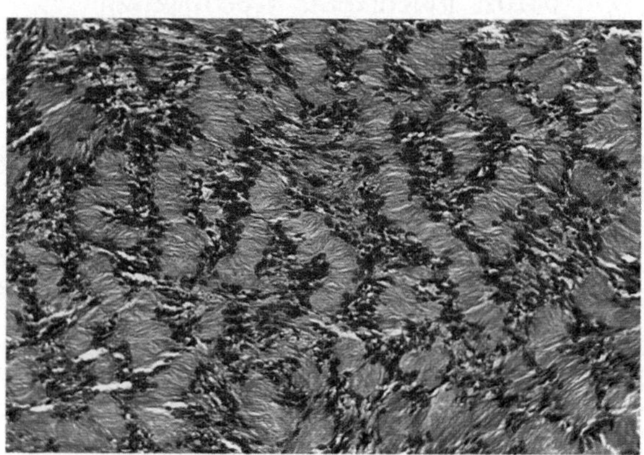

Figure 8-54

SCHWANNOMA

The typical Antoni A pattern is seen (Masson trichrome stain).

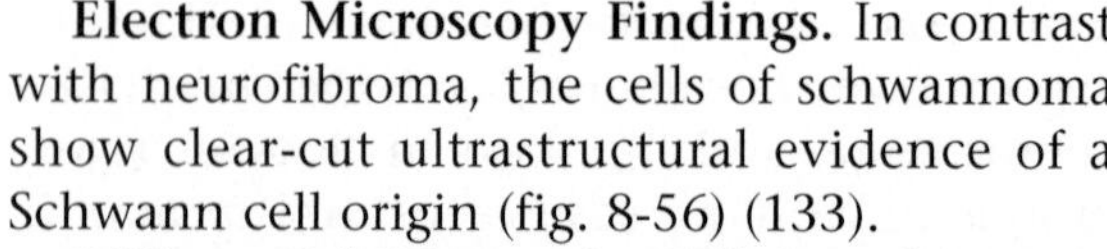

Electron Microscopy Findings. In contrast with neurofibroma, the cells of schwannoma show clear-cut ultrastructural evidence of a Schwann cell origin (fig. 8-56) (133).

Differential Diagnosis. Cellular schwannomas should be differentiated from fibroblastic or smooth muscle spindle cell tumors that show different immunohistochemical profiles and specific tissue markers. The presence of neurofilament protein helps in the distinction of neurofibroma from schwannoma.

Treatment and Prognosis. Schwannomas are surgically removed. They tend to recur if incompletely excised (134). Although rare, malignant transformation of an orbital schwannoma has been reported (135,136).

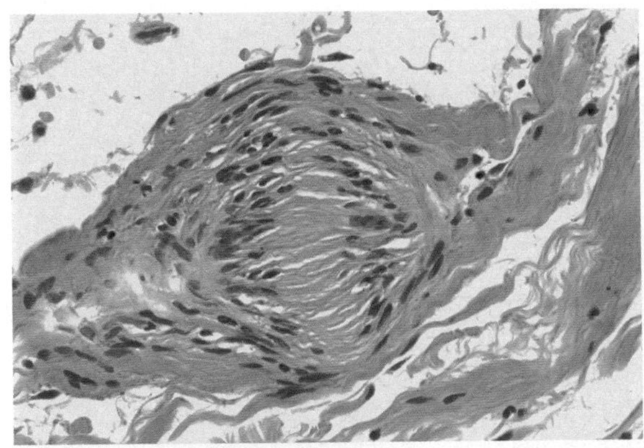

Figure 8-55

SCHWANNOMA

Verocay body in an orbital schwannoma with a fusiform appearance.

Granular Cell Tumor

Granular cell tumor is a neoplasm of peripheral nerve sheath origin that is usually benign. It has been reported in the orbital soft tissues, particularly involving extraocular muscles in about half of the cases (137–140). Microscopic examination reveals a nonencapsulated mass with invasive borders. It is composed of lobules and cords of polyhedral and spindle cells with eosinophilic, granular cytoplasm. The cytoplasmic inclusions are PAS positive and diastase resistant, and contain lipid. Electron microscopy shows the presence of basement membrane and numerous autophagosomes, with lipid and membranous inclusions within the cytoplasm (138). The cells are immunoreactive for S-100 protein, CD68, and leu-7. Treatment is wide local excision, but lesions may recur (140).

Malignant Peripheral Nerve Sheath Tumor

Definition. *Malignant peripheral nerve sheath tumor* (MPNST) has been variously designated *neurofibrosarcoma, perineural fibrosarcoma, malignant schwannoma,* and *neurogenic sarcoma.* The term MPNST acknowledges the tumor's origin not only from Schwann cells, but also from perineural cells and endoneural or epineural fibroblasts (141).

General Features. Although MPNST of soft tissue may arise from preexisting neurofibromas, the orbital lesions also originate in a preexisting schwannoma (142). A history of neurofibromatosis type 1 is present in 2 to 29 percent of patients (141).

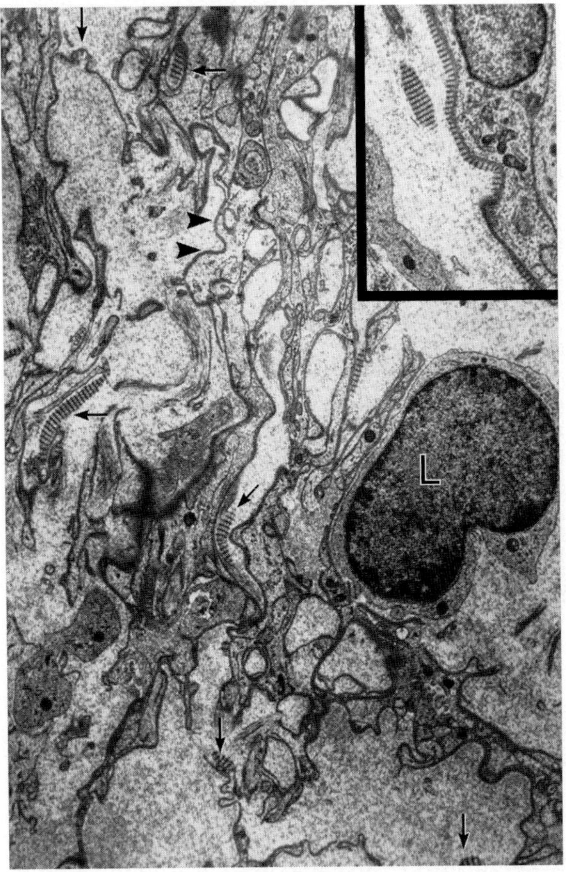

Figure 8-56

SCHWANNOMA

Electron microscopy shows cell processes. Patches of banded basement membrane (Luse bodies) are observed along the plasmalemmae.

Clinical Features. Patient age varies from 4 days to 75 years (142–145). There is a history of rapid tumor growth associated with pain and hyperesthesia in the distribution of the involved nerves. Most lesions develop in the superomedial aspect of the orbit from the supraorbital branch of the trigeminal nerve; on palpation they frequently feel cystic (fig. 8-57) (144).

Gross and Microscopic Findings. Tumors that originate from preexisting peripheral nerve tumors may appear encapsulated and circumscribed by the epineurium (fig. 8-58). Microscopically, dense fascicles of spindle cells alternate with less cellular areas. Many lesions are biphasic, featuring asymmetric tapered spindle cells with

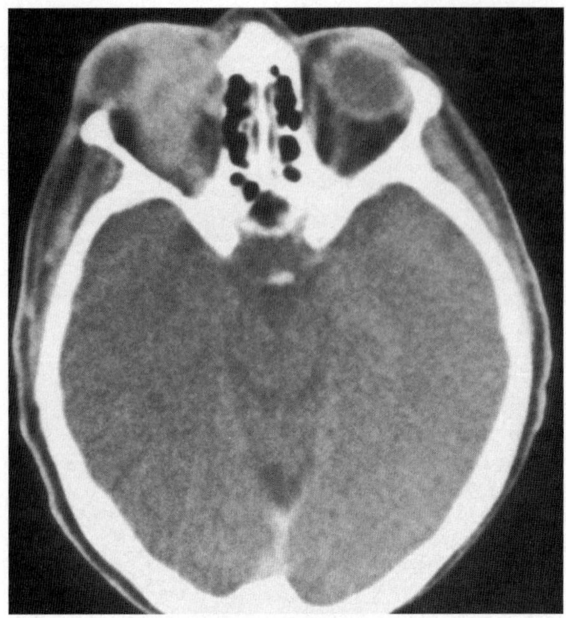

Figure 8-57

MALIGNANT PERIPHERAL NERVE SHEATH TUMOR

CT scan shows a recurrent orbital tumor with ill-defined margins.

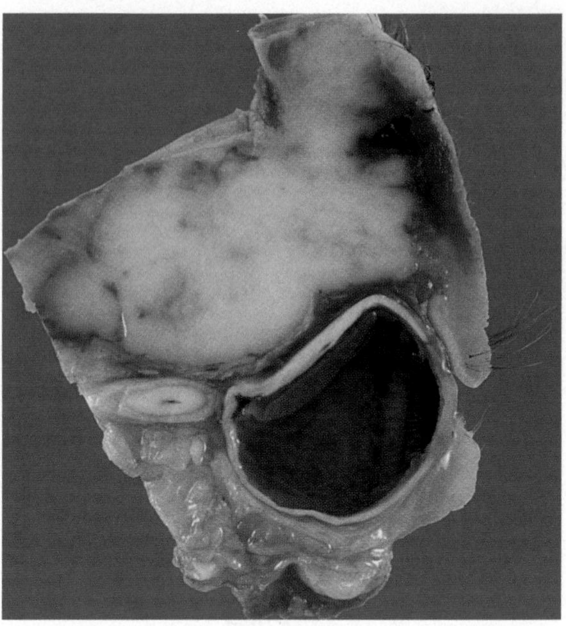

Figure 8-58

MALIGNANT PERIPHERAL NERVE SHEATH TUMOR

The exenteration specimen, a rubbery, yellowish mass with infiltrating margins, is located supranasally. The attached calotte is free of tumor. (Figs. 8-58–8-60 are from the same patient.)

buckled, wavy nuclei, as well as an epithelioid cell component (fig. 8-59). The mitotically active spindle cells frequently exhibit abundant eosinophilic cytoplasm and oval, vesicular nuclei. Necrosis may be seen in the spindle cell areas; the neoplastic cells tend to palisade around foci of necrosis. Areas resembling fibrosarcoma or chondrosarcoma have been described in excised MPNSTs of the orbit.

Immunohistochemical Findings. S-100 protein is positive in 50 to 90 percent of MPNSTs, often in differentiated spindle cell areas (fig. 8-60). Heterologous elements may show focal positivity for cytokeratin, muscle-specific actin, and neuron-specific enolase.

Electron Microscopic Findings. The spindle cells have numerous cytoplasmic processes that interdigitate with those of other cells and occasionally form junctional complexes. Noncontinuous basement membrane and long-spacing collagen are also found.

Differential Diagnosis. MPNSTs may be confused with other orbital tumors observed in children or adults, including fibrous histiocytoma, leiomyosarcoma, and fibrosarcoma.

Treatment and Prognosis. The best management for MPNST of the orbit is radical surgery, including exenteration. After incomplete excision the tumors tend to recur within a few months (146). Recurrent tumors may extend intracranially or metastasize to regional lymph nodes, mediastinum, and lungs. The survival rate is poor: more than half of the reported patients died between 1 and 5 years after surgery (144,145).

BONE TUMORS

Fibro-osseous tumors of the orbit arise from the orbital bones and adjacent paranasal sinuses (147–149). They include osteoma, fibrous dysplasia, ossifying fibroma, osteoblastoma, osteosarcoma, and giant cell tumors (148,149). This heterogeneous group of lesions constitutes approximately 2 percent of orbital tumors (149). Osteomas of the orbit may be part of Gardner's syndrome; therefore, younger patients may benefit from gastrointestinal consultation (150). Cartilaginous tumors of the orbit, either primary or secondary from surrounding structures, are rare.

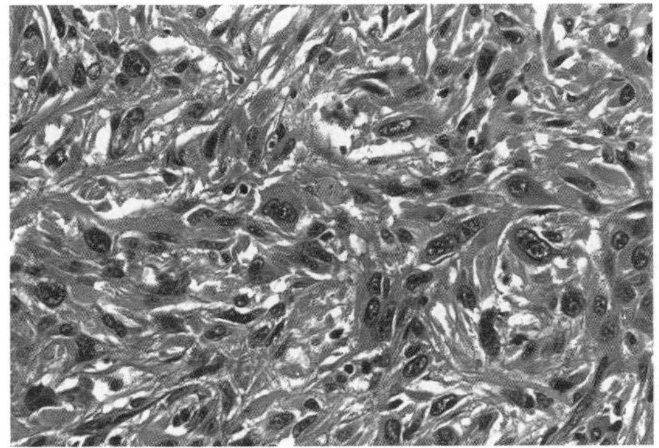

Figure 8-59

MALIGNANT PERIPHERAL NERVE SHEATH TUMOR

Plump spindle cells exhibit large pleomorphic nuclei with prominent nucleoli and abundant eosinophilic cytoplasm.

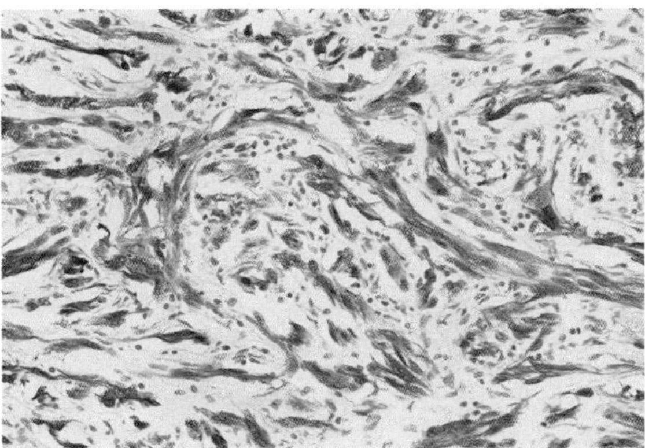

Figure 8-60

MALIGNANT PERIPHERAL NERVE SHEATH TUMOR

The tumor cells are strongly immunoreactive for S-100 protein.

Fibrous Dysplasia

Fibrous dysplasia may develop around the orbit to involve the frontal bone, the sphenoid bone, and the maxilla (151). It presents almost exclusively in children and adolescents. Most orbital lesions are isolated and not part of multifocal (polyostotic) disease. Imaging studies show a poorly demarcated, sclerotic lesion within the orbital bones that may display lytic foci and cystic areas (fig. 8-61). Pathologically, the trabeculae are composed of woven bone within a fibrous stroma without osteoblastic rimming (figs. 8-62, 8-63). The bony trabeculae assume a variety of shapes that resemble Chinese characters. The best management in symptomatic patients is wide local excision. Malignant transformation is rare.

Ossifying Fibroma

Ossifying fibroma is differentiated from fibrous dysplasia by its more aggressive behavior, which is not restricted to younger individuals (Table 8-5; fig. 8-64). It may recur after incomplete excision. Ossifying fibroma originates from any of the orbital bones but frequently involves the frontal bone and the sphenoethmoidal region (152). CT scans show a delimited lesion with sclerotic margins that contains a less radiodense center with foci of calcification (fig. 8-65). MRI demonstrates an isodense lesion on T1- and a hypointense lesion on T2-weighted images, which enhance significantly after gadolinium injection.

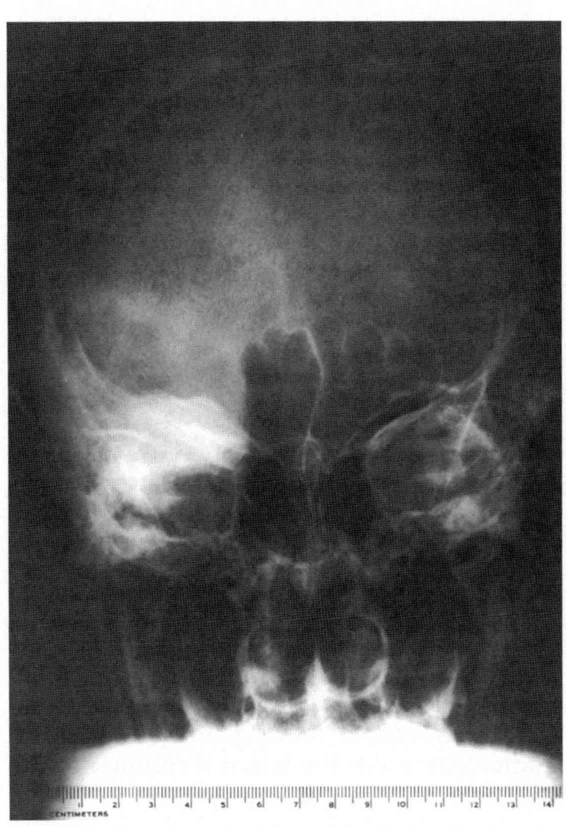

Figure 8-61

FIBROUS DYSPLASIA

Plain X ray delineates an osteoblastic lesion of the orbital bones. The edges have a linear frayed appearance.

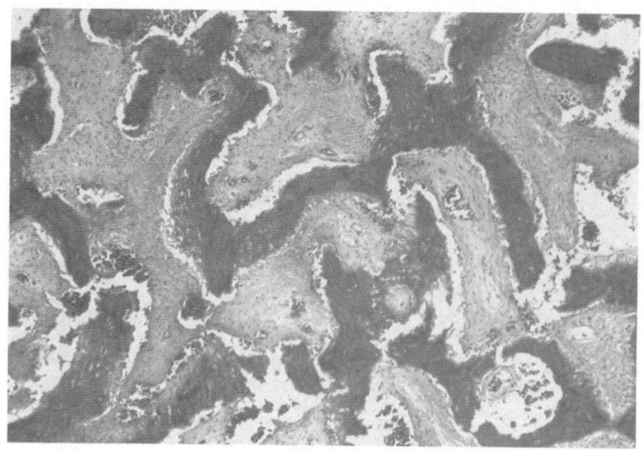

Figure 8-62

FIBROUS DYSPLASIA

The lesion shows the "Chinese characters" of the bony trabeculae which are devoided of osteoblastic rimming. (Figs. 8-62 and 8-63 are from the same patient.)

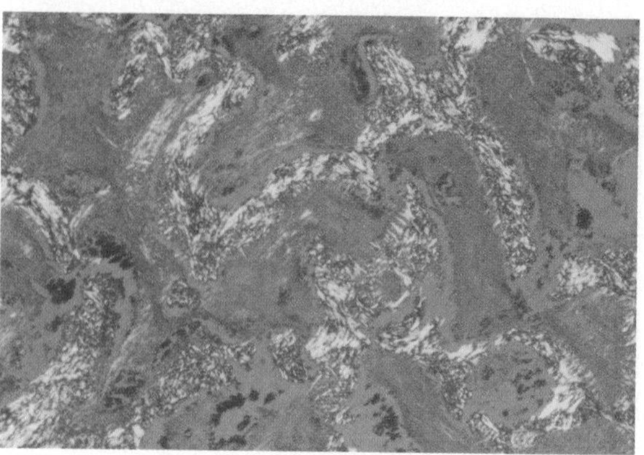

Figure 8-63

FIBROUS DYSPLASIA

The woven, birefringent, immature pattern of the bony trabeculae is seen.

Table 8-5

COMPARATIVE FEATURES OF FIBROUS DYSPLASIA AND OSSIFYING FIBROMA OF THE ORBIT

Characteristics	Fibrous Dysplasia	Ossifying Fibroma
Age at onset	More common 1st decade	2nd and 3rd decades
Sex	No sex predilection	Females more common
Rate of growth	May be progressive	Slow growing
Site	Cranial and long bones	Cranial bones (mandible)
Bone involvement	Monostotic or polyostotic	Monostotic
X ray	Ill-defined borders	Well-circumscribed
CT scan	Poorly demarcated	Well-demarcated
MRI	Central enhancement	Peripheral enhancement
Type of bone	Woven, no osteoblastic rimming	Lamellar, osteoblastic rimming
Polarized light	Random birefringence	Parallel lines birefringence

Microscopically, the lesion is composed of a highly vascularized, fibrous stroma in which spicules of lamellar bone are surrounded by osteoblasts (fig. 8-66). The bone spicules may adopt a round "psammomatous" type of configuration, which may be confused with meningioma or the cementicles of a cementifying fibroma. Wide local excision is the preferred method of treatment (153).

Osteosarcoma

Osteogenic sarcoma, also termed *osteosarcoma*, most commonly develops from the paranasal sinuses and extends secondarily into the orbit. It is seen in young children as an isolated lesion arising "de novo," arising from fibrous dysplasia, or in survivors of retinoblastoma who have had or have not had previous orbital radiation (fig. 8-67) (154,155). The

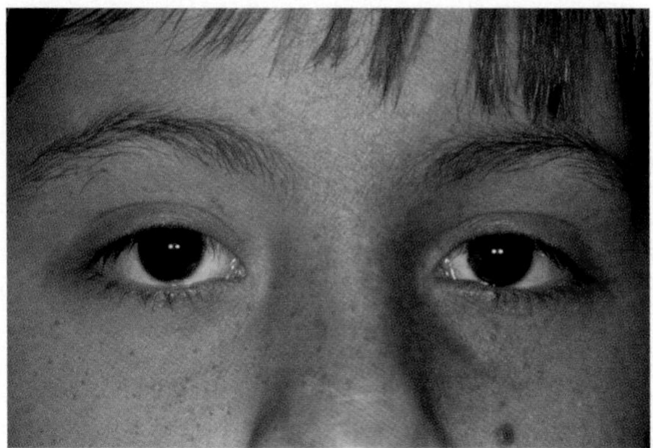

Figure 8-64

PSAMMOMATOID OSSIFYING FIBROMA

Lesion of the right orbit. (Figs. 8-64–8-66 are from the same patient.)

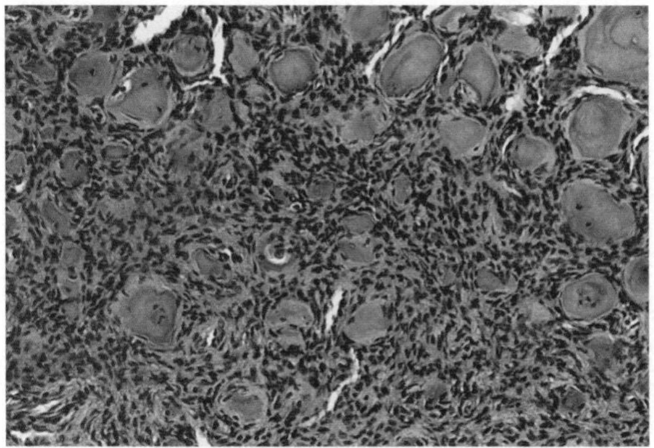

Figure 8-66

PSAMMOMATOID OSSIFYING FIBROMA

Dense spindle cells surround the irregular bony structures resembling psammoma bodies.

histopathologic findings do not differ from those of osteogenic sarcoma in other locations (fig. 8-68). The prognosis of patients with craniofacial osteosarcoma is guarded and treatment requires radical local excision with preoperative and postoperative chemotherapy and radiotherapy.

A clinical subtype, *parosteal osteosarcoma,* is an uncommon tumor that usually affects long bones; it is extremely rare in the orbit (156). It is a low-grade sarcoma that tends to recur locally after excision but has a favorable prognosis. Primary osteosarcoma should be differentiated from metastatic osteosarcoma (157).

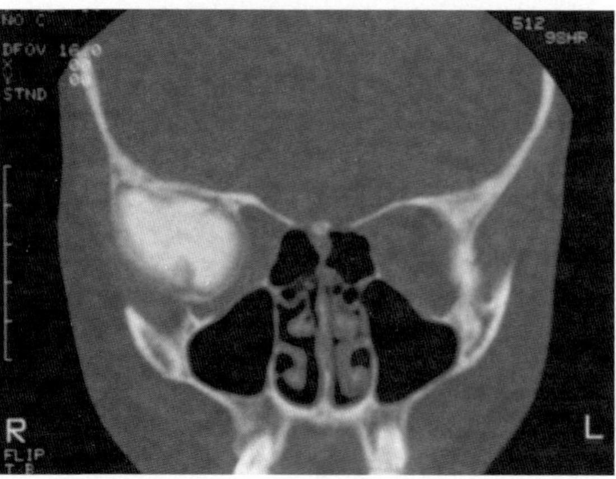

Figure 8-65

PSAMMOMATOID OSSIFYING FIBROMA

A dense, sclerotic, bony mass is surrounded by a thin lucent layer.

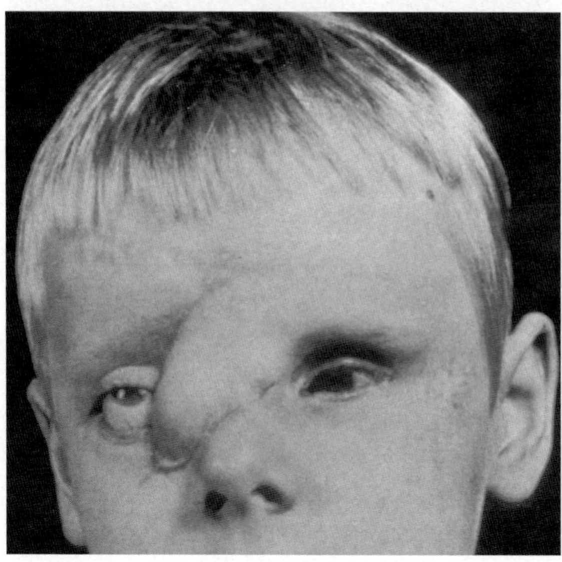

Figure 8-67

OSTEOSARCOMA POSTRADIATION

Tumor on the bridge of the nose of a child with bilateral retinoblastoma.

Mesenchymal Chondrosarcoma

Mesenchymal chondrosarcoma is a malignant tumor that develops within bone or soft tissues (*extraskeletal mesenchymal chondrosarcoma*) of the orbit in young adults (158). Microscopically, the stroma of the lesion is composed of mesenchymal areas resembling hemangiopericytoma

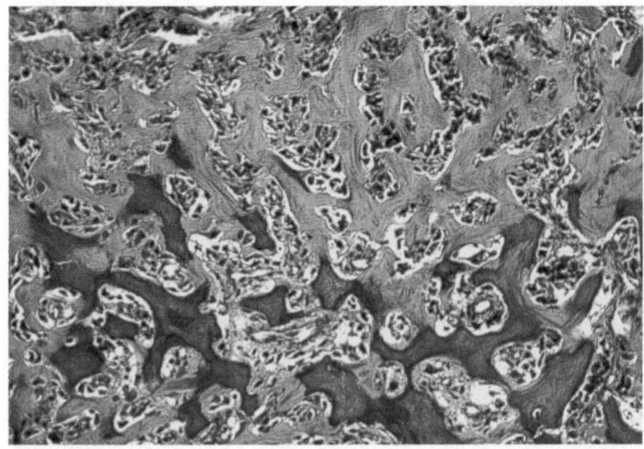

Figure 8-68

OSTEOSARCOMA POSTRADIATION

The malignant cells are forming osteoid and bony trabeculae.

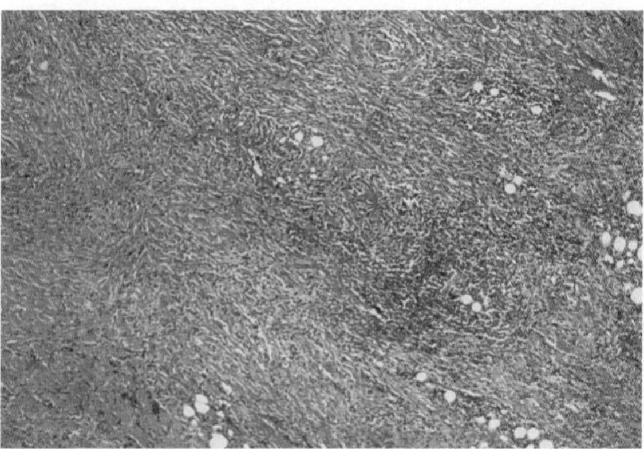

Figure 8-70

IDIOPATHIC INFLAMMATORY PSEUDOTUMOR

Areas of dense sclerotic collagen are intermixed with lymphocytes and mononuclear cells.

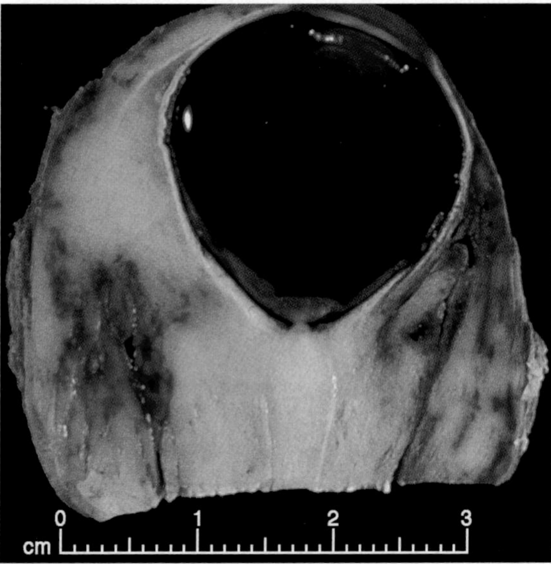

Figure 8-69

IDIOPATHIC INFLAMMATORY PSEUDOTUMOR

Orbital exenteration specimen from the files of the Armed Forces Institute of Pathology (AFIP) shows a diffuse yellowish tan orbital mass. The eye is free of tumor.

with islands of cartilage. The metastatic potential is inherent in the hemangiopericytomatous stromal component and can become apparent after long follow-up.

LYMPHOID TUMORS

Because the lacrimal gland and orbit are normally devoid of substantial lymphoid aggregates or fully formed lymph nodes, the occurrence of lymphatic tissue within these sites is always pathologic (159). Lymphoid lesions represent 8 percent of orbital tumors in the general population and 28 percent in older adults (160). Proliferative lymphoid lesions, either reactive or neoplastic, should be differentiated from inflammatory pseudotumor of the orbit, a proteiform clinicopathologic entity characterized histopathologically by polymorphic cellularity from different cell lineages (figs. 8-69, 8-70) (161).

The diagnosis and classification of lymphoid proliferations are the most difficult and challenging problems encountered by the pathologist dealing with adnexal-ocular specimens. These lesions include reactive lymphoid hyperplasia and malignant lymphoma. A gray zone exists that has received names such as atypical lymphoid hyperplasia and indeterminate lymphoid lesions, which reflects the uncertainly of microscopic diagnosis (162). Modern immunophenotypic and molecular techniques have established a more precise characterization of many of these lesions (163,164). Dissemination of the disease only occurs in monoclonal lesions that are considered lymphomas (164–167). Hodgkin's disease and plasma cell myeloma are now recognized as lymphoid neoplasms. Orbital involvement in Hodgkin's disease is extremely rare and usually is secondary to localized involvement in other anatomic regions (neck, mediastinum, etc) and rarely from disseminated disease (168–171). The orbit may be affected in patients with post-transplantation proliferative disorders (172).

Reactive Lymphoid Hyperplasia

General Features. *Reactive lymphoid hyperplasia* (RLH) represents approximately 16 percent of all lymphoproliferative lesions of the orbit (162).

Clinical Features. Clinical and radiologic criteria cannot be used to determine the benign or malignant nature of orbital lymphoid proliferations in a reliable or reproducible form (173). Although the mean age of patients with RLH is slightly less than that of patients with lymphoma, the difference is not clinically significant.

Gross and Microscopic Findings. Surgical samples show a gray-white solid mass that may have fine vascularization. Microscopically, there is dense infiltration of small dark lymphocytes with scanty fibrous stroma. There is usually an admixed cell population consisting of plasma cells and histiocytes, as well as focal capillary proliferation with plump endothelial cells. Most lesions show reactive lymphoid follicles of varying size surrounded by a mantle of mature lymphocytes. Mitotic activity is restricted to the follicular centers where tingible body macrophages are observed.

Immunohistochemical Findings. The lesions are composed of a mixture of T and B lymphocytes, with the T-cell infiltrate varying between 42 and 65 percent (174,175). The B-cell component is polyclonal regarding kappa and lambda light chains. The proliferative cell population, as demonstrated with MIB-1 staining, is restricted to the germinal centers.

Treatment and Prognosis. Treatment includes corticosteroids and low-dose radiotherapy (162). Most cases remain localized or resolve. Molecular genetic analysis of RLH of the orbit has detected clonal immunoglobulin gene rearrangements suggestive of early neoplastic transformation (175). Consequently, clinical follow-up is recommended in all cases.

Lymphoma

General Features. *Lymphomas* of the ocular adnexa (eyelid, conjunctiva, orbit, and lacrimal gland) represent approximately 8 percent of all extranodal lymphomas (176). Although simultaneous involvement of the conjunctiva and orbit occur, and recent series suggest that the degree of malignancy does not differ between them, for the purpose of clarity only orbital lesions are discussed here.

Malignant lymphoma is the most common orbital tumor in the older adult population (160). More than 50 percent of orbital lymphomas represent primary disease at the time of diagnosis (164,177). In one study of patients with systemic lymphoma, 5.3 percent had adnexal ocular involvement (176). The orbital involvement was found either at time of presentation or as late as 53 months after primary diagnosis (164).

Clinical Features. Although patients with orbital lymphoma are generally older adults (median age, 62 years), children and young adults can be affected as well (164,177). Orbital lymphoma occurs in females slightly more often than males. The main signs and symptoms include proptosis and upper lid ptosis (164). Motility disturbances suggest extraocular muscle involvement. The superior orbit is more commonly affected, with involvement of the superior rectus muscle and the levator palpebrae superioris. There may be a salmon-colored patch on the bulbar conjunctiva or superior fornix. In one series of lymphoproliferative lesions of the ocular adnexa, bilateral lesions as well as pain associated with bone erosion were observed only in patients with lymphoma (173).

Orbital lymphomas are seen in males aged 22 to 44 years who have human immunodeficiency virus (HIV) infection (178). For patients with *acquired immunodeficiency syndrome (AIDS)-associated lymphoma*, the diagnosis of AIDS precedes the onset of lymphoma in up to 72 percent of cases, often with an accompanying history of opportunistic infections. AIDS-associated orbital lymphomas generally exhibit a rapid onset and aggressive course. The most frequent types of AIDS-associated lymphomas are *large B- or T-cell lymphoma, Burkitt's lymphoma,* and *large cell immunoblastic lymphoma* (179–181).

Burkitt's lymphoma with ocular involvement is most common in children in equatorial Africa and New Guinea, who have the endemic form of the disease (182). The sporadic form of the disease is observed in young adults and older patients, and is present worldwide (183). In the advanced stage, local disease may invade the eye (figs. 8-71, 8-72) (184).

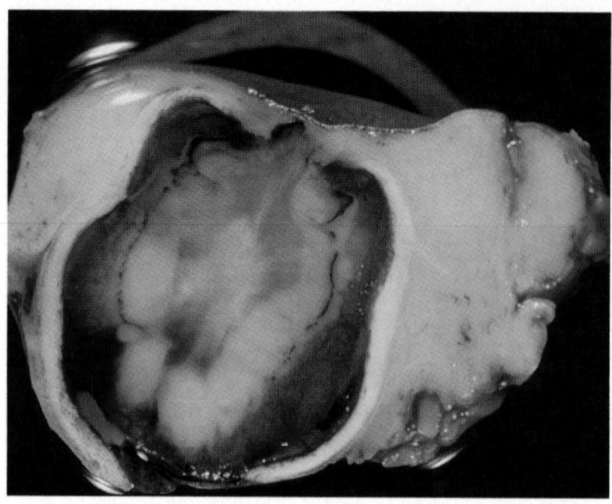

Figure 8-71

BURKITT'S LYMPHOMA

Tumor of the soft tissues of the orbit with intraocular involvement.

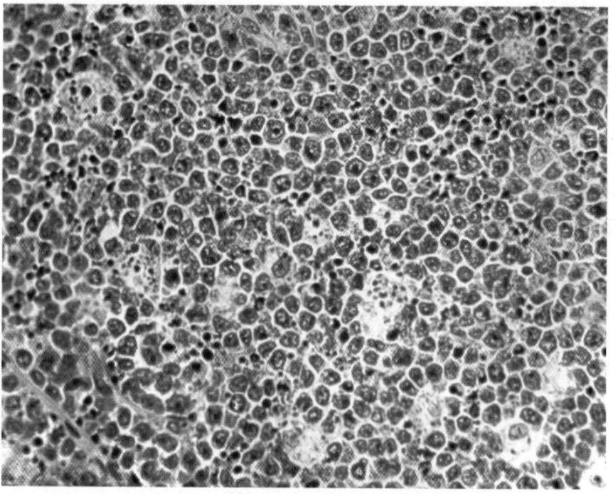

Figure 8-72

BURKITT'S LYMPHOMA

Large cell lymphoma with numerous apoptotic bodies (starry sky pattern).

Microscopic Findings. The microscopic appearance varies according to the type of lymphoma. The current Revised European-American Classification of Lymphoid Neoplasms (REAL) is based on morphology, immunophenotype, and molecular genetic features (185). The most frequent type of orbital lymphoma is *extranodal marginal zone B-cell lymphoma*, a tumor that has very similar features to the mucosa-associated lymphoid tissue lymphoma (164,177). In decreasing order of frequency, other lymphoma types include *follicular center cell lymphoma, lymphoplasmacytic lymphoma, diffuse large B-cell lymphoma*, and *B-cell chronic lymphocytic leukemia/small lymphocytic lymphoma*. The rarest variants of orbital lymphoma are *mantle cell lymphoma, B-cell precursor lymphoblastic leukemia/lymphoma, diffuse large T-cell lymphoma, mycosis fungoides/Sézary's syndrome*, and *angiocentric T-cell lymphoma* (177,186).

Cytologic Findings. Cytologic preparations of fresh specimens, "squash" technique and touch imprints, preserve the morphologic details of the tumor cells, which is especially important when evaluating lymphoid lesions (187). Additionally, multiple smears can be prepared simultaneously for ancillary studies such as immunocytochemistry. Fine-needle aspiration biopsy provides a rapid cytologic diagnosis of orbital tumors without the necessity of surgery (188).

Cytologic specimens show abundant cellularity composed of lymphoid cells with morphologic features according with the type of lymphoma. The cytologic features of the reactive lymphoid hyperplasia include a polymorphic lymphoid population intermixed with scattered tingible body macrophages.

Immunohistochemical Findings and Special Studies. A panel that includes the following antibodies is commonly used for immunophenotyping the most common lymphomas of the ocular adnexa: CD20, CD3, CD5, CD10, CD23, cyclin D1, bcl-2, Ig light chains (kappa and lambda), and Ig heavy chains (164,185). Staining with MIB-1 (Ki-67 index) and p53 may provide additional information regarding the severity of the disease. Low-grade lymphomas with MIB-1 cell counts higher than 20 percent have a more aggressive biologic behavior. P53 overexpression has proven to be of prognostic significance with regard to stage at presentation, disease course, and risk of lymphoma-related death (164).

Immunoglobulin gene rearrangement analysis is useful for the determination of B-cell origin and the presence of monoclonality or polyclonality in doubtful cases. In a large series of lymphomas studied with current techniques, 80 percent were monoclonal and 5 percent oligoclonal (167). All reactive lymphoid hyperplasias were polyclonal. In a study of five specimens considered borderline by light microscopy, four were reclassified as lymphoma based on the results of immunoglobulin polymerase chain reaction (PCR) amplification (164). The presence of cytologic atypia and Dutcher bodies is consistently associated with monoclonality (166).

Treatment and Prognosis. The risk of extraorbital spread and lymphoma-related death ranges from low to high in the following order: marginal zone B-cell lymphoma, lymphoplasmacytic lymphoma, follicular center cell lymphoma, and mantle cell lymphoma (177). According to the Ann Arbor classification of lymphoma, most low-grade malignant lymphomas of the orbit are classified as stage IE (extranodal) (189). Absence of dissemination is demonstrated in 86 to 93 percent of stage IE lymphomas of the ocular adnexa with follow-up periods ranging from 3.6 and 4.2 years. A subset of low-grade lymphomas with high MIB-1 staining, p53 positivity, and CD5-positive cells is associated with more advanced clinical stages (II and III). Stages III and IV represent a secondary manifestation of lymphoma involving the orbit and ocular adnexa. In the latter group, the tumors usually are large B-cell lymphomas and T-cell lymphomas.

Although a few patients are cured with local excisional surgery, the preferred treatment for those with orbital disease stage IE is radiotherapy; 80 percent of these patients achieve complete remission. Patients with stage II, III, or IV disease usually are evaluated by an oncologist and treated with localized radiation therapy and systemic chemotherapy. The mean time to relapse for patients with orbital marginal zone B-cell lymphoma is 6.3 years, suggesting that such patients be followed beyond 5 years (164).

Orbital Plasmacytoma

General Features. Pure plasmacytic proliferations of the orbit are rare. Two forms are well characterized: *solitary extramedullary plasmacytoma* and *plasmacytoma associated with multiple myeloma* (190). It is important to make the distinction between them, because they are significantly different regarding prognosis and treatment.

Clinical Features. Solitary plasmacytoma of the orbit occurs more frequently in male patients in the sixth to seventh decades, while multiple myeloma is seen in the seventh and eight decades (191). Both extramedullary plasmacytoma and multiple myeloma may present with painless proptosis. It is the primary manifestation of multiple myeloma in up to 75 percent of the cases with orbital involvement.

Microscopic Findings. Both proliferations are characterized by a dense monomorphous infiltrate of plasma cells with a variable degree of differentiation.

Immunohistochemical Findings. Normal and neoplastic plasma cells express mature B-cell antigens (CD38 and CD79a), and show intracytoplasmic but not surface immunoglobulin. Monoclonality is demonstrated for kappa or lambda immunoglobulin light chains (192,193).

Treatment and Prognosis. Patients with a histopathologic diagnosis of plasma cell proliferation should be studied for systemic manifestations, including radiographic skeletal survey, serum and urine protein analyses, and bone marrow examination. Patients with multiple myeloma usually have a chronic clinical course with a median survival period of 3 years. Patients with solitary plasmacytoma of the orbit require only localized radiation treatment, and have a better prognosis, with a mean survival time of 8.3 years (191).

LEUKEMIC DISORDERS

Granulocytic disorders produce the most common leukemic orbital infiltrates: *acute lymphocytic leukemia* in children and *chronic lymphocytic leukemia* in adults (194–196). When orbital disease develops, bilateral proptosis may occur (197). Because lymphoma of the orbit is rare in children, the pathologist should always include leukemia in the differential diagnosis of childhood lymphoma. Leukemic cells display more watery, vesicular nuclei than the coarse heterochromatin observed in lymphoma cells. Immunohistochemical methods should be performed to accurately identify the immunophenotype. The results of the peripheral blood cell count and bone marrow biopsy may provide additional useful clinical information.

Granulocytic Sarcoma

Granulocytic sarcoma, also known as *myeloid sarcoma,* is a soft tissue or visceral focus of infiltrating leukemic cells in the absence of peripheral

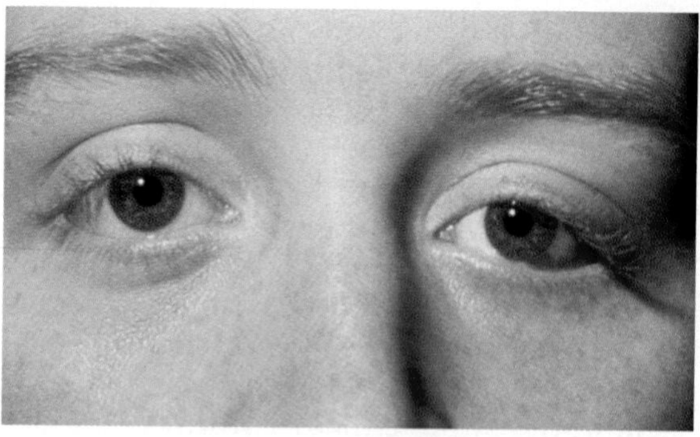

Figure 8-73

GRANULOCYTIC SARCOMA

An 18-year-old male has a growing mass involving the left lacrimal gland.

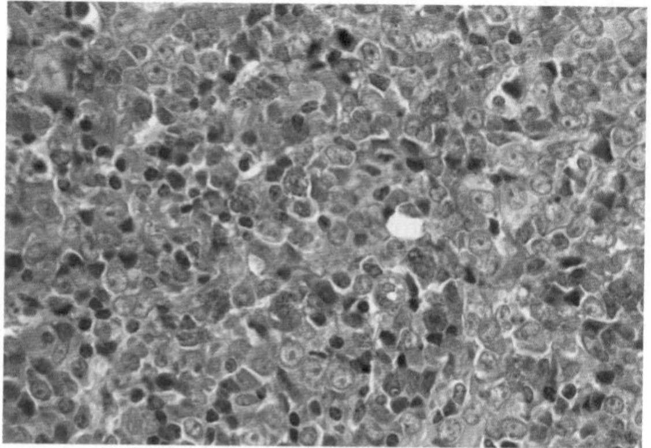

Figure 8-74

GRANULOCYTIC SARCOMA

Immature blasts are intermixed with eosinophilic myelocytes.

blood involvement (198). The name *chloroma*, used in the past, refers to the greenish hue observed clinically and grossly as a result of the presence of myeloperoxidase. Adnexal involvement is preferentially observed in young patients, whose median age at presentation is 7 years (199). Characteristic clinical features include bilateral or lateral orbital involvement and lack of osteolysis or subperiosteal infiltration (fig. 8-73). MRI studies show hypointensity in T1- and intermediate intensity in T2-weighed images.

Microscopically, evidence of granulocytic differentiation takes the form of immature myelocytes and metamyelocytes (fig. 8-74). The Leder stain for esterase or immunohistochemical

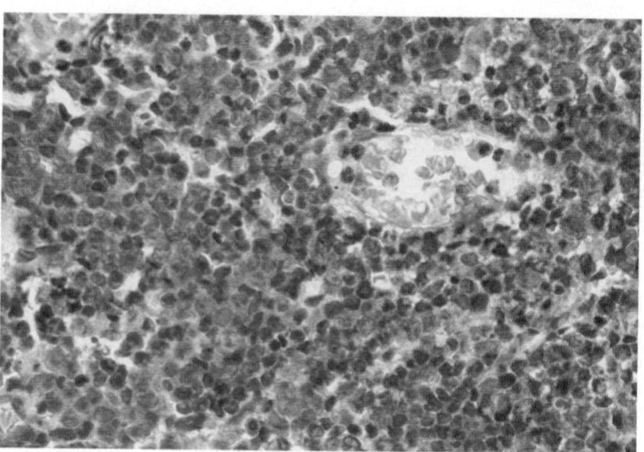

Figure 8-75

GRANULOCYTIC SARCOMA

The immature myeloid cells are positive with the Leder stain.

stains for myeloperoxidase (MPO-7), and lysozyme (muramidase) establish the diagnosis unequivocally (fig. 8-75) (200) Overt leukemia may occur within 2 to 12 months after diagnosis. Tumors with 11q23/*MML* gene rearrangements may be associated with acute monoblastic leukemia (AML M5) (201). Cure is possible if appropriate chemotherapy is promptly introduced, aborting the leukemic process before bone marrow or peripheral blood disease occurs (figs. 8-76, 8-77). If there is massive proptosis that threatens vision, localized orbital radiotherapy combined with chemotherapy may be needed.

HISTIOCYTOSIS

The Histiocyte Society redefined the classification of the histiocytosis of childhood (202). Class I includes all Langerhans cell histiocytoses, class II includes all the histiocytoses of the mononuclear phagocytes excluding Langerhans cells, and class III includes the malignant histiocytic disorders. A minor revision of this classification has recently been proposed, and the three major groups are now termed dendritic cell-related disorders, of which Langerhans cell histiocytosis is by far the most common; erythrophagocytic macrophage-related disorders; and malignant histiocytosis.

Langerhans Cell Histiocytosis

Langerhans cell histiocytosis (LCH) is a group of idiopathic disorders characterized by the proliferation of specialized bone marrow–derived

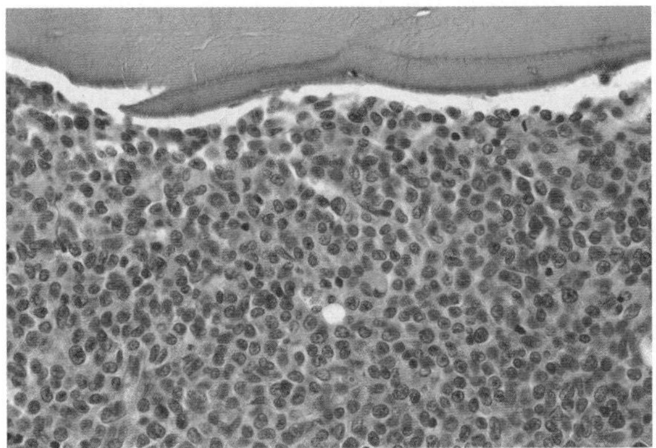

Figure 8-76

GRANULOCYTIC SARCOMA

Bone marrow from the iliac crest from the patient depicted in figure 8-73. Sheets of myeloblasts replace the marrow elements.

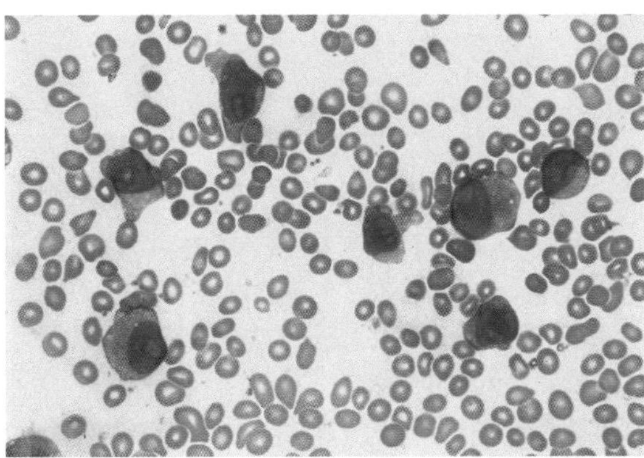

Figure 8-77

GRANULOCYTIC SARCOMA

Peripheral blood from the patient seen in figure 8-73 shows numerous myeloblasts, some with monocytoid features.

Langerhans cells and mature eosinophils. The clinical spectrum of LCH includes, on one end, an acute, fulminant, disseminated disease called Letterer-Siwe disease and, on the other end, solitary or few, indolent and chronic lesions of bone or other organs called eosinophilic granulomas. The orbit is usually involved with the unifocal, localized disease known as eosinophilic granuloma (fig. 8-78) (202,203). LCH affects mainly the supertemporal frontal bone, and a lytic lesion with sclerotic margins is demonstrated by imaging studies (fig. 8-79). Children and adolescents are usually affected, although it may be seen sporadically in adults (204).

Biopsy specimens show large cells with grooved and folded nuclei among a mixed cellular infiltrate composed of pale bilobed histiocytes, eosinophils, multinucleated giant cells, lymphocytes, and plasma cells (figs. 8-80, 8-81). Immunohistochemical staining is positive for CD1a, fascin, and S-100 protein, supporting the derivation from dendritic cells (fig. 8-82) (205,206). The two most important criteria for the demonstration of Langerhans cells are the presence of Birbeck granules, which appear as pentalaminar, rod-shaped intracellular structures when visualized by electron microscopy (fig. 8-83) (207), and the strong presence of CD1a antigen on the surface of the cells.

The management of unifocal LCH (eosinophilic granuloma) of the orbit is close observation for focal lesions (208), local injection of corticosteroids, or low-dose radiotherapy. Curettage is reserved for easily accessible lesions. Children diagnosed at preschool age should undergo complete clinical examination to rule out multisystem disease.

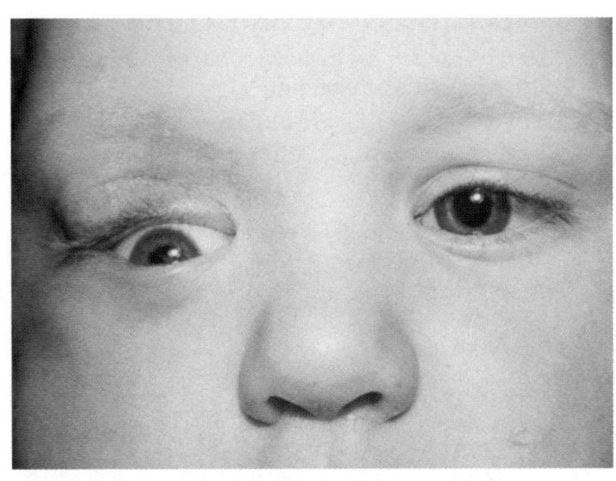

Figure 8-78

LANGERHANS CELL HISTIOCYTOSIS

A mass in the right orbital rim.

Histiocytic Disorders of Mononuclear Phagocytes

Localized or systemic histiocytic proliferations that involve the orbit include *sinus histiocytosis with massive lymphadenopathy* (209–212), *juvenile xanthogranuloma* (213), *adult orbital xanthogranuloma* (214), *necrobiotic xanthogranuloma*

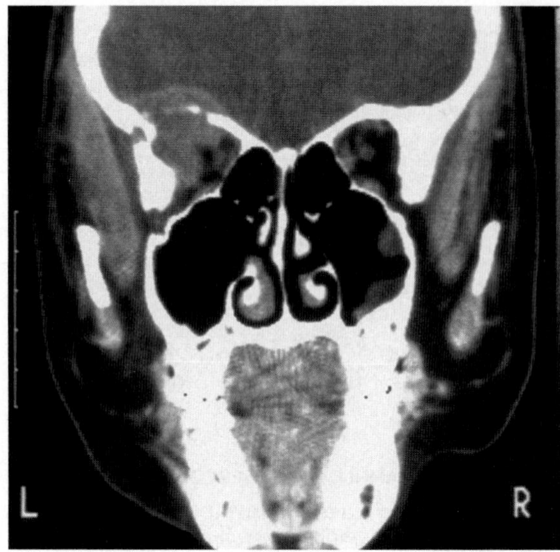

Figure 8-79

LANGERHANS CELL HISTIOCYTOSIS

CT scan of the left orbit shows a bilobed orbital mass and destruction of the orbital rim.

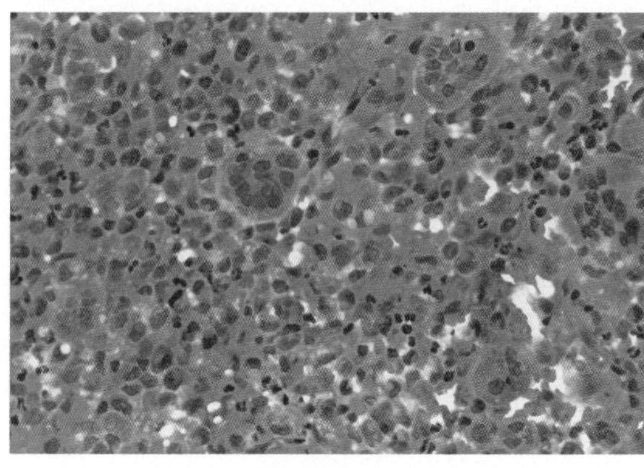

Figure 8-81

LANGERHANS CELL HISTIOCYTOSIS

Masses of acidophilic histiocytes with reniform nuclei are intermixed with scattered eosinophils and foci of hemorrhage.

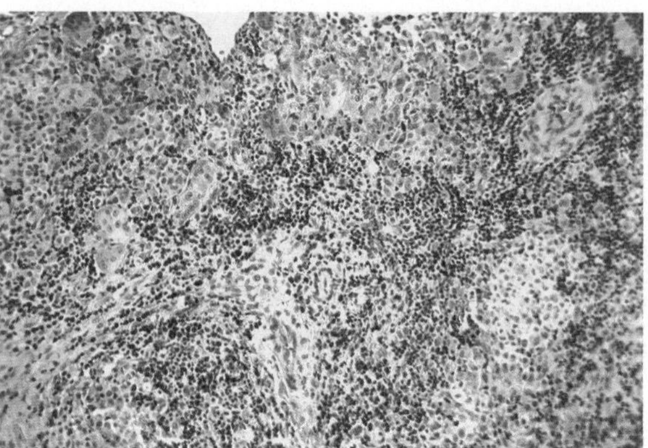

Figure 8-80

LANGERHANS CELL HISTIOCYTOSIS

The infiltrate is composed of numerous eosinophils intermixed with nodules of histiocytes with abundant eosinophilic cytoplasm.

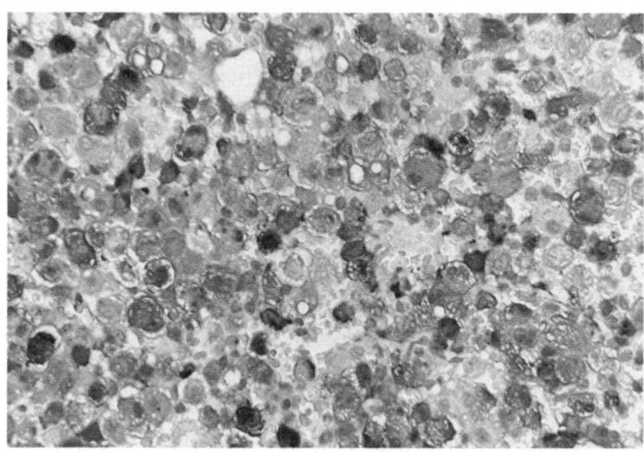

Figure 8-82

LANGERHANS CELL HISTIOCYTOSIS

The cells display strong immunoreactivity for S-100 protein.

(215–217), *Erdheim-Chester disease* (218–220), and others. Extranodal sinus histiocytosis of the orbit is mainly seen in children (209,210). Bilateral or unilateral proptosis is produced by massive collections of histiocytes intermixed with lymphocytes in the orbital tissues (fig. 8-84) (211,212). The histiocytes are positive for CD68, HAM56, and S-100 protein. The overall prognosis generally is good, without evidence of extraorbital or visceral involvement.

Xanthogranulomatous diseases have in common the presence of Touton giant cells. Necrobiotic xanthogranuloma is a severe condition associated with paraproteinemia and other hematologic abnormalities and an increased risk of hematologic and lymphoproliferative malignancies (217). Several ocular tissues including the orbit may be affected. Histopathologically, the lesions consist of necrobiotic centers surrounded by palisading granuloma and inflammatory cells, including many Touton giant cells

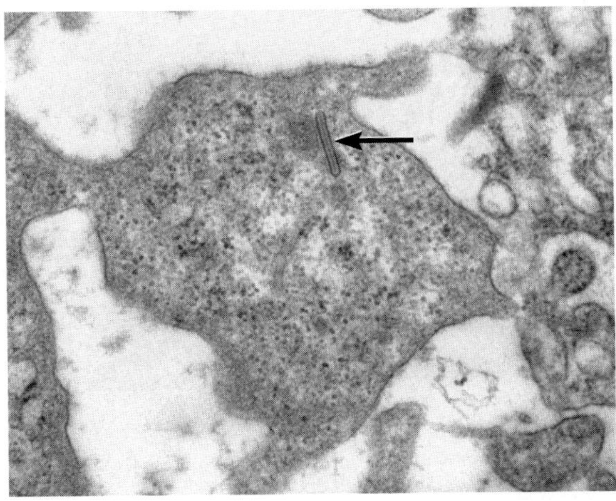

Figure 8-83

LANGERHANS CELL HISTIOCYTOSIS

Electron micrograph shows a Langerhans cell with an elongated Birbeck granule in the cytoplasm (arrow).

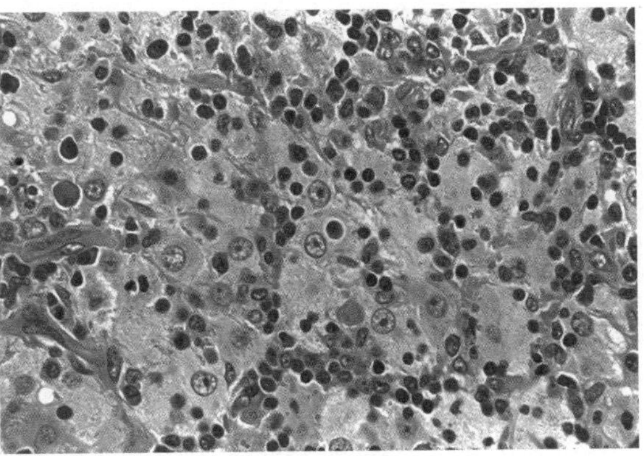

Figure 8-84

ORBITAL EXTRANODAL SINUS HISTIOCYTOSIS

The infiltrate is composed of large pale histiocytes, lymphocytes, and plasma cells with Russell bodies. The histiocytes contain engulfed lymphocytes (emperipolesis).

and xanthoma cells. A highly characteristic finding is the presence of cholesterol clefts within the foci of necrobiotic collagen. The cells are S-100 protein negative. Necrobiotic xanthogranuloma is distinguished from juvenile xanthogranuloma and Erdheim-Chester disease by the characteristic necrobiotic foci, which are not observed in the latter. Radiotherapy has been reported to be effective in a case with eyelid and orbit involvement (221). Patients with isolated orbital xanthogranulomas may present with adult-onset asthma and nasal polyps (222).

Erdheim-Chester disease is a rare idiopathic disease that consists of xanthomatous lesions in several organs and tissues (218). Patients with adnexal and orbital involvement have a poor prognosis (220). Patients present with bilateral orbital disease and xanthelasma-type lesions (219). The typical posterior orbital involvement is commonly associated with compressive optic neuropathy. Systemic findings include cardiomyopathy, renal failure, and lung disease.

MISCELLANEOUS ORBITAL TUMORS

Epithelial Cystic Choristoma

Definition. *Dermoid, epidermoid, conjunctival,* and *respiratory cysts of the orbit* are the result of small inclusions of more differentiated embryonic ectodermal tissues that become entrapped within the soft tissues, particularly involving the developing sutures of the orbital bones (223,224). *Choristomatous cysts* may also arise in the orbit from ectopic lacrimal gland (225).

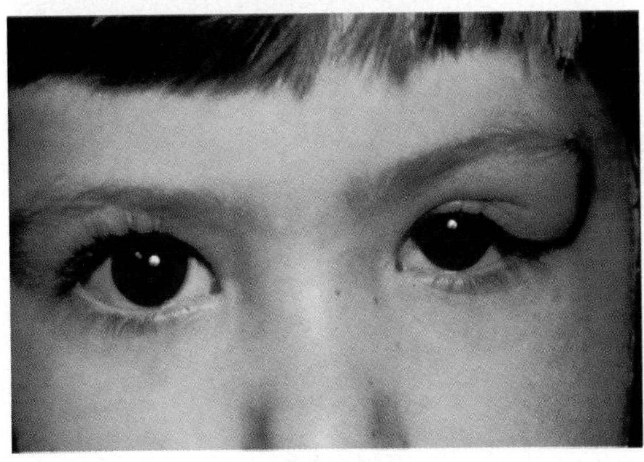

Figure 8-85

DERMOID CYST

Tumor of the outer border of the eyebrow on the left side.

General and Clinical Features. Dermoid cysts are the most common cystic lesions that have a propensity for the supertemporal or supranasal anterior quadrants of the orbit (fig. 8-85) (226). They represent 30 to 50 percent of the excised orbital tumors in children (227,228). CT scan demonstrates the bony relationship to the cystic lesion in 87 percent of the cases (fig. 8-86) (229). Dermoid cysts may undergo spontaneous or post-traumatic rupture, releasing the irritating keratinous debris of the cyst contents,

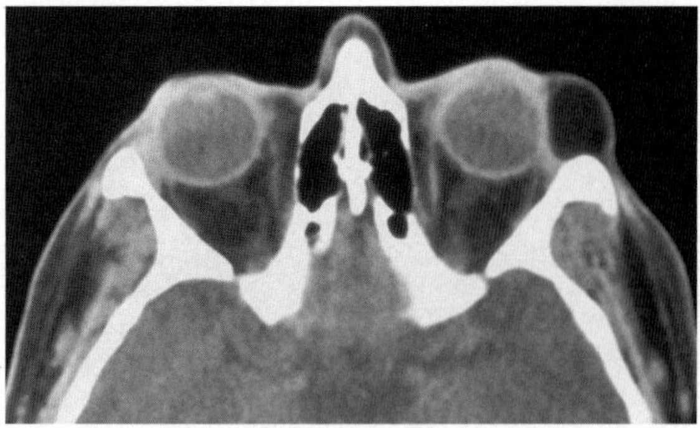

Figure 8-86

DERMOID CYST

Axial CT scan shows a well-circumscribed cystic mass of the temporal, anterior orbital rim.

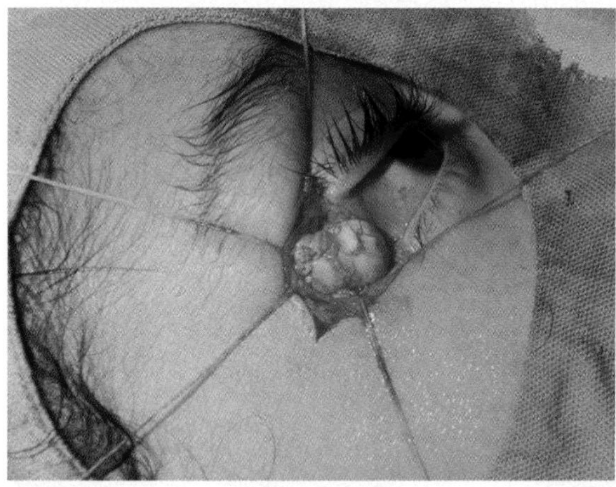

Figure 8-87

DERMOID CYST

Intraoperative appearance of a dermoid cyst shows a yellow mass.

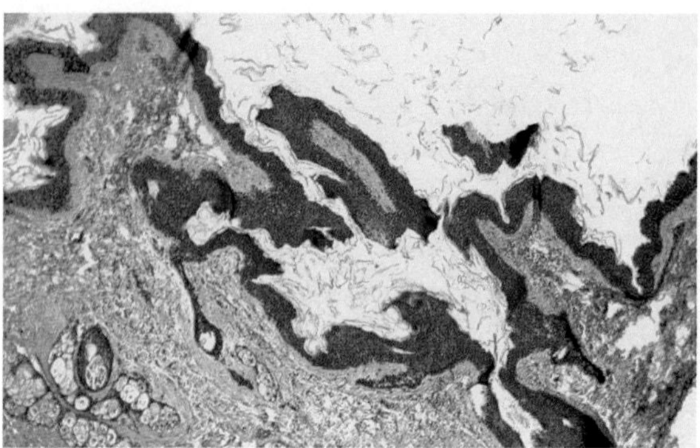

Figure 8-88

DERMOID CYST

The wall of the cyst is lined by keratinized squamous epithelium that resembles the epidermis, as well as lobules of sebaceous glands.

with subsequent inflammation (230,231). The abrupt onset of manifestations may suggest the development of a malignant tumor.

Gross and Microscopic Findings. Dermoid cysts have a thin capsule and contain a lumen with keratinous debris, hairs, and yellow lipid deposits (fig. 8-87). The lining of the cyst is composed of stratified squamous epithelium identical to that of the epidermis (fig. 8-88). Pilosebaceous units are identified in the cyst walls. When cysts rupture, the lining is partly replaced by a lipogranulomatous inflammatory response that extends into the adjacent orbital tissues. Rarely, the cyst is lined by a double layer of cuboidal epithelium resembling conjunctiva (dermoid cysts of conjunctival origin), or ciliated cells (intraorbital cyst lined by respiratory epithelium) (232,233).

Differential Diagnosis. Cholesterol granuloma (cholesteatoma) of the orbit is a well-characterized lesion that must be distinguished from a ruptured dermoid cyst (234). The former usually occur in adults and involve the supertemporal quadrant of the orbit. Imaging studies disclose a well-outlined solid lesion within the diploe of the bone. Histopathologically, the lesion is composed of cholesterol clefts surrounded by mononucleated and multinucleated giant cells. No evidence of an epithelial lining is present.

Mucoceles are expansile lesions of the paranasal sinuses that extend into the orbit; they likely are the result of chronic sinusitis (235). Frontal and ethmoidal mucoceles are the most common types. Mucoceles generally develop in older patients. The walls of a mucocele contain thinned bone fragments, chronic inflammatory cells, and ciliated, respiratory-type epithelium. In cases of chronic inflammation, the epithelium may display squamous metaplasia.

Treatment and Prognosis. The management of orbital dermoid cysts is local surgical excision. Dermoid cysts have almost no capacity for malignant transformation. Invasive squamous cell carcinomas arising from choristomatous orbital cysts have been reported in adult patients (236,237).

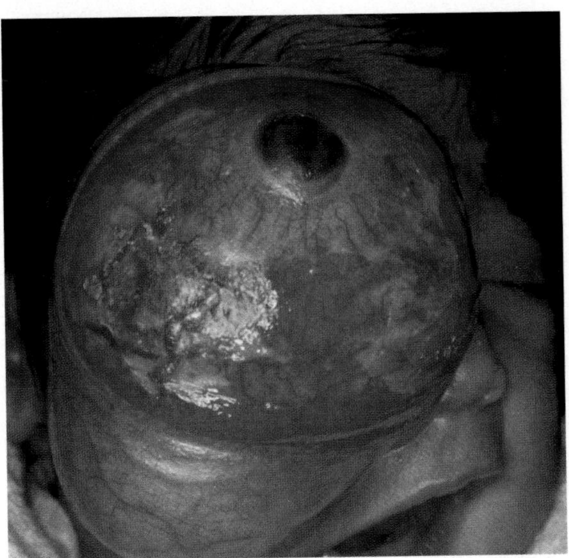

Figure 8-89

TERATOMA

A large orbital teratoma in a child exposes the globe.

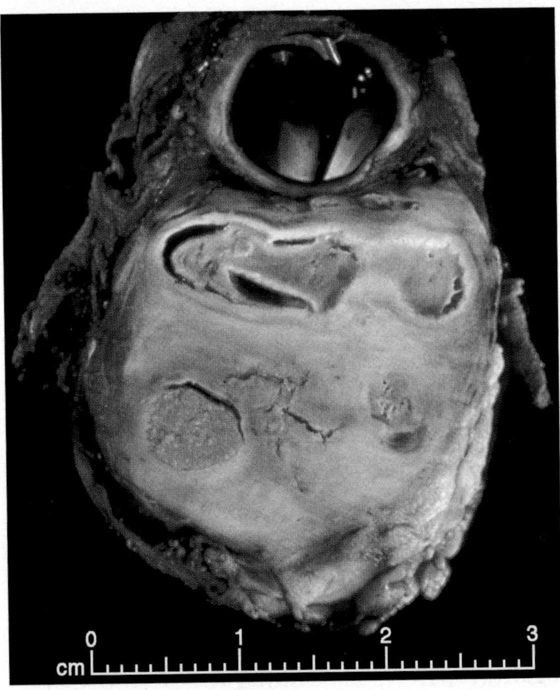

Figure 8-90

TERATOMA

An eye and attached orbital tumor with multiple large cystic spaces.

Teratoma

Teratomas are rare germ cell tumors. In the orbit, they arise from misdirected or ectopic germ cells (238–241). They comprise approximately 1 percent of orbital tumors in childhood. The congenital orbital tumor may be large at the time of birth (fig. 8-89) (241). Pathologic examination discloses a circumscribed but not encapsulated, often multicystic lesion that contains tissue from all germ layers (figs. 8-90, 8-91). The preferred treatment is local excision with preservation of the eye if possible. Malignant transformation is extremely rare (242,243).

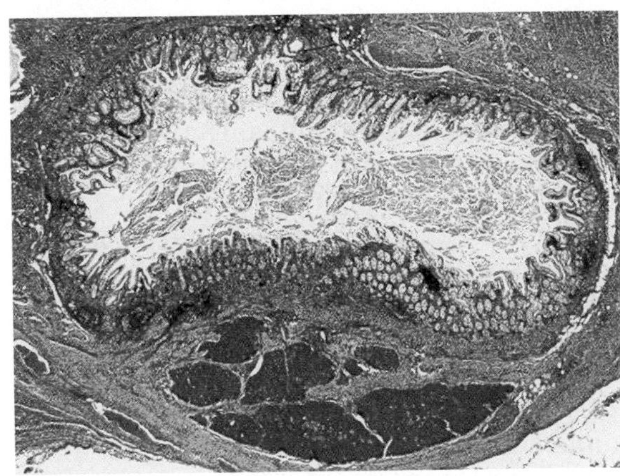

Figure 8-91

TERATOMA

The cavity is lined by multilayered epithelium of the intestinal tract and lobules of pancreatic tissue (bottom).

Endodermal Sinus Tumor

Endodermal sinus tumor (yolk sac tumor) arises from midline extragonadal sites including intracranial and orbital locations. This malignant tumor is composed of primitive germ cells. The five reported orbital cases were seen in infants, median age 13 months (244). The rapid clinical growth may simulate a rhabdomyosarcoma. Histologically, the tumor is composed of cuboidal embryonal cells arranged around blood vessels. The perithelial accumulation of cells resembles embryonic renal glomeruli (Schiller-Duval bodies). There is considerable atypia and mitotic activity. Immunohistochemistry is positive for alpha-fetoprotein in all cases. Although the prognosis of patients with endodermal sinus tumor is poor, the orbital lesions behave better than extranodal germ cell tumors.

Pigmented Retinal Choristoma

The rare *pigmented retinal choristoma*, also called *melanotic progonoma, retinal anlage tumor,* or *pigmented neuroectodermal tumor of infancy*, often develops in the maxilla in young children and may secondarily invade the orbit (245, 246). Microscopically, the tumor has an adenomatous appearance composed of tubules and cords of pigmented cells having large melanosomes. Zimmerman (247) recognized that the melanosomes resemble those present in the retinal pigment epithelium and recommended the term pigmented retinal choristoma.

Ewing's Family of Tumors

The Ewing's family of tumors includes *Ewing's tumor of bone, extraosseous Ewing's tumor, primitive neuroectodermal tumors* (*peripheral neuroepithelioma*), and *Askin's tumor* (248). About 95 percent of cases have a t(11;22) or t(21;22) translocation (249). The resulting fusion of the *EWS* gene and *FLI-1* gene results in a chimeric protein that can be used for immunohistochemical analyses (FLI-1) and molecular diagnosis (250,251). Primitive neuroectodermal tumors (PNETs) are malignant tumors of adolescents and young adults. Involvement of the orbit is extremely rare (252–256). These tumors should be differentiated mainly from rhabdomyosarcoma, neuroblastoma, lymphoma, and orbital invasion from retinoblastoma. The overall prognosis for patients with Ewing's sarcoma is better than that for patients with PNET.

Orbital Ewing's tumors are usually seen in children and adolescents (range, 2 to 61 years), either as metastases from distant sites, secondary from a primary tumor affecting the mandible, or, rarely, primary (extraosseous Ewing's tumor) (257,258). The individual cells of classic Ewing's tumor contain round to oval nuclei with fine, dispersed chromatin without nucleoli. The cytoplasm varies in amount but generally is clear and contains glycogen, which can be highlighted with the PAS stain, with and without diastase pretreatment. The cells are positive with CD99 (MIC2 gene product, O-13) and vimentin antibodies (259). Treatment is chemotherapy, with or without radiotherapy. Approximately 50 percent of patients with orbital involvement develop metastatic disease (260).

Primary Orbital Carcinoid and Paraganglioma

Primary orbital carcinoid is extremely rare (261,262). Most frequently, orbital carcinoid is a metastasis from the gastrointestinal tract or lung (263). Microscopically, the tumors exhibit a mixture of basaloid, trabecular, tubular, and rosette-like patterns. Two types of cells are present: one type has clear cytoplasm and a round nucleus with fine, stippled chromatin; the other type has eosinophilic cytoplasm and a small, hyperchromatic nucleus. The cells demonstrate both argentophilic and argyrophilic granules. Immunohistochemical studies show reactivity for chromogranin A, synaptophysin, and serotonin, among other neuropeptides (263).

Orbital paraganglioma, also called *chemodectoma* or *glomus body tumor*, originates from the ciliary ganglion (264,265). Histologically, the cells are arranged in spherical aggregates separated by capillaries. There are two type of cells: sustentacular cells disclosing a dark, basophilic nucleus and scanty cytoplasm, and neurosecretory cells. Immunohistochemistry demonstrates the expression of synaptophysin, chromogranin, and neurofilament among other neural markers. S-100 protein is expressed at the periphery of the cell groups. Although most of the reported orbital lesions were benign, the management should be complete local excision to prevent recurrences.

Primary Melanoma

Malignant melanoma of the orbit occurs in the following settings: 1) primary, frequently associated with a blue nevus, congenital melanosis oculi or nevus of Ota (266,267); 2) secondary from direct extension from a uveal, conjunctival, eyelid, or paranasal sinus melanoma; and 3) metastatic from nonocular melanomas or from contralateral uveal melanomas (268). Primary malignant melanomas represent less that 1 percent of the tumors of the orbit (fig. 8-92). Tellado et al. (269) reported 21 of 24 cases among 288 cases of orbital melanoma from the files of the AFIP and mentioned 31 previously reported cases up to 1996. The median age was 42 years, with a range from 15 to 84 years. Signs and symptoms included painless proptosis, blurred vision, and diplopia. Some form of congenital melanosis was present in 47 percent of the

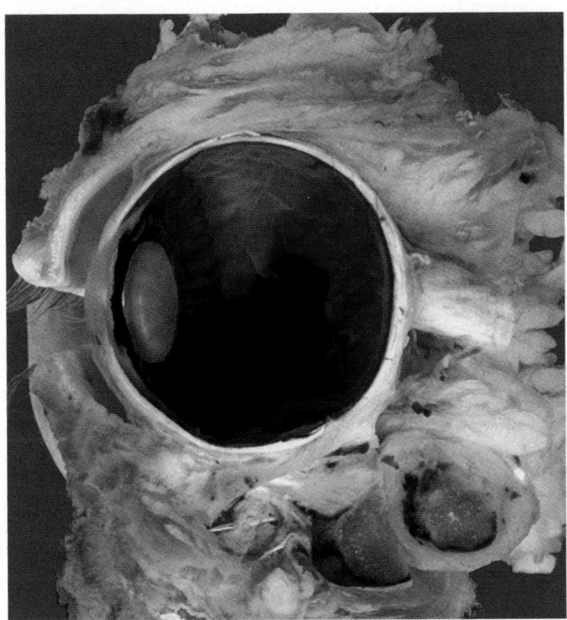

Figure 8-92

PRIMARY ORBITAL MELANOMA

A multinodular pigmented tumor is in the posterior orbit inferiorly.

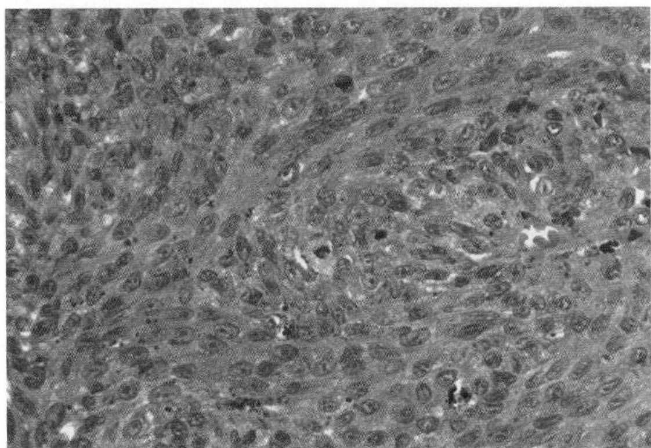

Figure 8-93

PRIMARY ORBITAL MELANOMA

The tumor depicted in figure 8-92 was composed of variably pigmented, plump, spindle-shaped cells with ovoid nuclei and prominent nucleoli.

patients. Histologically, the tumors were of spindle or mixed cell types (fig. 8-93); evidence of an associated blue nevus was observed in 90 percent of the 21 cases studied. Eight patients died of metastatic disease.

Alveolar Soft Part Sarcoma

Alveolar soft part sarcoma is a malignant tumor of unknown origin. In contrast to other body locations the orbital lesions have an indolent course with few recurrences (270). The average age at presentation is 23 years, range 11 months to 69 years. Grossly, the tumors are usually well circumscribed, rubbery, and pink, tan, or reddish brown. Microscopically, the tumor cells are arranged in a pseudoalveolar or organoid pattern. The cells are polyhedral with distinct, abundant, granular cytoplasm. PAS stain highlights the presence of diastase-resistant, crystalline rhomboid or rod-like structures. The cells may occasionally express S-100 protein, muscle-specific actin, MyoD1, and desmin. The differential diagnosis includes metastatic renal cell carcinoma, paraganglioma, and granular cell tumor. Complete surgical excision is the recommended treatment in most cases. Only 2 of 15 patients with sufficient follow-up developed metastases.

SECONDARY TUMORS

Direct invasion of the orbit by lesions located in the surrounding structures or in the periorbital adnexal ocular tissues accounts for about 11 to 24 percent of orbital tumors. In decreasing order of frequency, the most common sources of tumors invading the orbit are paranasal sinuses (271), eyelid skin and conjunctiva (272–274), eyeball (275,276), and cranial cavity.

The vast majority of secondary malignant tumors of the orbit are either squamous cell carcinomas of the paranasal sinuses or carcinomas from the skin and conjunctiva. Basal cell carcinoma, squamous cell carcinoma, and sebaceous carcinoma of the eyelid may invade the orbit, particularly in neglected cases. Intraocular retinoblastoma and medulloepithelioma in children, and uveal malignant melanoma and carcinoma of the nonpigmented ciliary epithelium in adults, may invade the orbit. Extraocular extension carries a poor prognosis (276).

From the intracranial cavity, meningiomas are the most frequent invasive tumors. Meningiomas usually develop from the greater wing of the sphenoid and are associated with hyperostosis, lid edema, and proptosis. Other tumors extending into the orbit from the nose or oropharynx are inverted papilloma, nasopharyngeal lymphoepithelial carcinoma, esthesioneuroblastoma, nasopharyngeal angiofibroma, and ameloblastoma (277–279). Secondary orbital tumors are the most frequent cause of orbital exenteration (280).

METASTATIC TUMORS

Definition. Metastatic disease of the orbit refers to malignant orbital tumors from distant organs or the contralateral eye or orbit. Excluded are hematopoietic diseases and systemic lymphoma, and any direct extension from the eye, intracranial cavity and brain, paranasal sinuses, nasopharynx, and mandible.

General Features. Metastatic tumors constitute approximately 3 percent of all orbital diseases and 10 percent of orbital neoplasms in most series (281–283). The prevalence of ocular and orbital metastases in patients with cancer varies from 0.7 percent to 12.0 percent, depending on whether the analysis was clinical or was performed in autopsy series (284,285). The frequencies of the site of origin parallel the general incidence of the tumors (286). Breast in women, lung and prostate in men, and cutaneous melanoma are the most frequent primary sites (287–289); however, metastases from a large variety of tumors have been reported to occur in the orbit. According to different series, 47 to 91 percent of orbital metastases were accompanied by metastases in other sites (290). The mean interval between the diagnosis of the primary tumor and the first orbital symptoms has been as long as 60 months, breast carcinoma and thyroid carcinoma being the longest. In more recent series, approximately 20 percent of metastatic tumors presented first as orbital masses and in 10 percent the primary site could not be demonstrated (281).

Clinical Features. The age of patients with metastatic orbital disease correlates with the prevalence of malignant tumors in each age group. Patients with metastases have a relatively rapid onset of symptoms, including motility disturbances, proptosis, mass, ptosis, eyelid swelling, and pain. Enophthalmos may occur in tumors with a prominent scirrhous stromal reaction. Metastases that involve bone or grow rapidly may present with ecchymosis (fig. 8-94) (291). Bilateral orbital involvement is observed in approximately 7 percent of the cases. Breast carcinoma and malignant melanoma have a strong tendency to metastasize to extraocular muscles, while prostate and thyroid carcinomas have a predilection for bone. CT scans and MRI studies show the location and extent of the disease (fig. 8-95) (292).

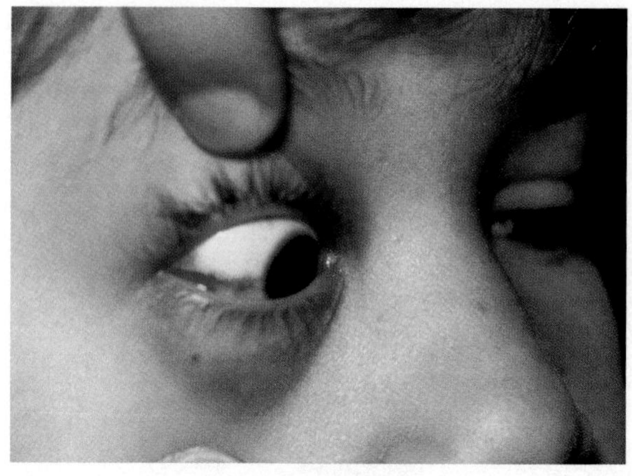

Figure 8-94

NEUROBLASTOMA

Young girl with bluish discoloration of the inferior right eyelid and conjunctival hemorrhage.

Microscopic Findings. Orbital metastases may adopt an infiltrative, nodular, or mixed growth pattern. In general, the neoplastic cells retain the characteristics of the primary tumor. Metastatic carcinomas, mainly from breast, may have an infiltrative pattern with a histiocytic or monocytic appearance (293). In these cases, the finding of intracytoplasmic lumens, mucosecretion, and positive keratin stain by immunohistochemistry may resolve the diagnosis. Metastatic neuroblastoma in children should be differentiated from extraocular extension of a retinoblastoma or lymphoma (fig. 8-96). Several types of sarcoma may disseminate into the orbit (294).

Cytologic Findings. One of the main indications for fine-needle aspiration biopsy of the orbit is presumed metastatic disease (295). In adequately obtained specimens immunostaining for surface antigens and hormonal receptors can be performed. The results of fine-needle aspiration biopsy can be misleading or the aspirate insufficient in tumors associated with inflammation or with abundant stromal (scirrhous) reaction. In tumors such as malignant melanoma and renal carcinoma, the slides

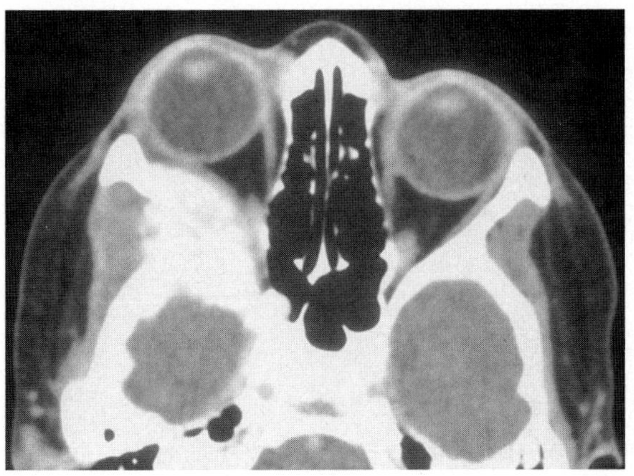

Figure 8-95

NEUROBLASTOMA

Axial CT scan shows a mass in the orbital bones and proptosis.

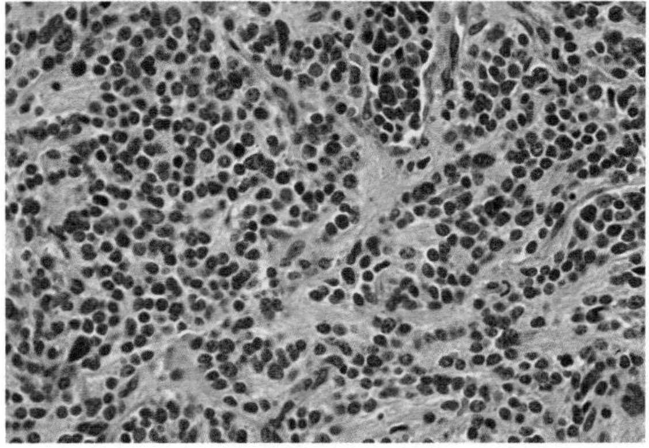

Figure 8-96

NEUROBLASTOMA

Histopathologic specimen of primary neuroblastoma.

may have a very bloody background due to tumor vascularity, which makes identification of isolated neoplastic cells difficult.

Immunohistochemical Findings. A large panel of monoclonal antibodies have been developed for the specific tissue diagnosis of tumors (296). The antibodies routinely used are those related to the primary tumors that most frequently disseminate to the orbit.

Treatment and Prognosis. Survival and treatment of patients with orbital metastases depend on the type of primary tumor and the results of the general physical examination. Palliative radiation therapy is indicated for the treatment of localized orbital metastatic disease (297). Surgery may be used for the treatment of isolated, easily accessible, circumscribed metastases, or as a decompressive procedure for bulky tumors. The overall mean survival period after the diagnosis of metastatic disease to the orbit is approximately 15 months, range 3 to 96 months (283).

STAGING AND GRADING OF SARCOMAS OF THE ORBIT

The clinical classification of orbital sarcomas (Table 8-6) is based on symptoms and signs relating to visual loss, degree of proptosis or displacement, papilledema, and optic atrophy. Diagnostic tests include radiographs of the orbit, CT, MRI, and angiography. This system is recommended by the Task Force for Staging of Cancer of the Eye of the American Joint Committee on Cancer (298).

It should be noted that the grading system and stages for rhabdomyosarcoma are mentioned separately in accord with the recommendation of the Intergroup Rhabdomyosarcoma Study Group, Soft Tissue Sarcoma Committee of the Children Oncology Group (see Tables 8-3, 8-4).

Table 8-6

CLINICAL CLASSIFICATION OF ORBITAL SARCOMAS

T-Primary Tumor

TX Primary tumor cannot be assessed
T0 No evidence of primary tumor
T1 Tumor 15 mm or less in greatest dimension
T2 Tumor more than 15 mm in greatest dimension
T3 Tumor of any size with diffuse invasion of orbital tissues and/or bony walls
T4 Tumor invades beyond the orbit to adjacent sinuses and/or cranium

N-Regional Lymph Nodes (submandibular, parotid [preauricular] and cervical)

NX Regional lymph nodes cannot be assessed
N0 No regional lymph node metastasis
N1 Regional lymph node metastasis

M-Distant Metastasis

MX Distant metastasis cannot be assessed
M0 No distant metastasis
M1 Distant metastasis

Histologic Type

Sarcomas of the orbit include a broad spectrum of soft tissue tumors and sarcomas of bone

G-Microscopic Grading

GX Grade cannot be assessed
G1 Well differentiated
G2 Moderately differentiated
G3 Poorly differentiated
G4 Undifferentiated

Stage Grouping

Stage	Primary Tumor	Grade	Regional Lymph Node	Distant Metastasis
IA	T1	G1 or G2	No	No
IB	T2	G1 or G2	No	No
IIA	T3	G1 or G2	No	No
IIB	T1	G3 or G4	No	No
IIC	T2	G3 or G4	No	No
III	T4	G3 or G4	No	No
IV	Any T	Any G	Any N	M1

REFERENCES

Classification and Frequency

1. Weiss SW, Goldblum JR. Enzinger and Weiss's soft tissue tumors, 4th ed. St. Louis: Mosby Inc; 2001.
2. Campbell RJ, Sobin LH. Histological typing of tumours of the eye and its adnexa. Berlin Heildelberg: Springer Verlag; 1998:26–30.
3. Kennedy RE. An evaluation of 820 orbital cases. Trans Am Ophthalmol Soc 1984;82:134–57.
4. Gunalp I, Gunduz K. Biopsy-proven orbital lesions in Turkey. A survey of 1092 cases over 30 years. Orbit 1994;13:67–79.
5. Iliff WJ, Green WR. Orbital tumors in children. In: Jakobiec FA, ed. Ocular and adnexal tumors. Birmingham, AL: Aesculapius; 1978:669–84.
6. Bullock JD, Goldberg SH, Rakes SM. Orbital tumors in children. Ophthal Plast Recons Surg 1989;5:13–6.
7. Kodsi SR, Shetlar DJ, Campbell RJ, Garrity JA, Bartley BB. A review of 340 orbital tumors in children during a 60-year period. Am J Ophthalmol 1994;117:177–82.
8. Demirci H, Shields CL, Shields JA, Honavar SG, Mercado GJ, Tovilla JC. Orbital tumors in the older adult population. Ophthalmology 2002; 109:243–8.
9. Margo CE, Mulla ZD. Malignant tumors of the orbit. Analysis of the Florida Center Registry. Ophthalmology 1998;105:185–90.

9a. Kempson RL, Fletcher CD, Evans HL, Hendrickson MR, Sibley RK. Tumors of the soft tissues. Atlas of Tumor Pathology, 3rd Series, Fascicle 30. Washington, DC: Armed Forces Institute of Pathology; 2001.

9b. Unni KK, Inwards CY, Bridge, JA, Kindblom L, Wold, LE. Tumors of the bones and joints. AFIP Atlas of Tumor Pathology, 4th Series, Fascicle 2. Silver Spring, MD: American Registry of Pathology; 2005.

9c. Warnke RA, Weiss LM, Chan JK, Cleary ML, Dorfman RF. Tumors of the lymph nodes and spleen. Atlas of Tumor Pathology, 3rd Series, Fascicle 14. Washington, DC: Armed Forces Institute of Pathology; 1995.

Fibromatosis

10. MacKenzie DH. The Differential diagnosis of fibroblastic disorders. Oxford: Blackwell; 1970.
11. Maillard AA, Kountakis SE. Pediatric sino-orbital desmoid fibromatosis. Ann Otol Rhinol Laryngol 1996;105:463–6.
12. Fornelli A, Salvi F, Mascalchi M, Marchetti C, Foschini MP. Orbital (desmoid type) fibromatosis. Orbit 1999;18:203–10.
13. Campbell RJ, Garrity JA. Juvenile fibromatosis of the orbit: a case report with review of the literature. Br J Ophthalmol 1991;75:313–6.
14. Duffy MT, Harris M, Hornblass A. Infantile myofibromatosis of orbital bone. A case report with computed tomography, magnetic resonance imaging, and histologic findings. Ophthalmology 1997;104:1471–4.
15. Hidayat AA, Font RL. Juvenile fibromatosis of the periorbital region and eyelid. A clinicopathologic study of six cases. Arch Ophthalmol 1980;98:280–5.

Nodular Fasciitis

16. Bernstein KE, Lattes R. Nodular (pseudosarcomatous) fasciitis, a nonrecurrent lesion: clinicopathologic study of 134 cases. Cancer 1982;49: 1668–78.
17. Font RL, Zimmerman LE. Nodular fasciitis of the eye and adnexa. A report of ten cases. Arch Ophthalmol 1966;75:475–81.
18. Sakamoto T, Ishibashi T, Ohnishi Y, Inomata H. Immunohistological and electron microscopical study of nodular fasciitis of the orbit. Br J Ophthalmol 1991;75:636–8.
19. Shields JA, Shields CL, Christian C, Eagle RC Jr. Orbital nodular fasciitis simulating a dermoid cyst in an 8-month-old child. Case report and review of the literature. Ophthal Plast Reconstr Surg 2001;17:144–8.

Fibroma

20. Mortada A. Fibroma of the orbit. Br J Ophthalmol 1971;55:350–2.
21. Case T, LaPiana F. Benign fibrous tumor of the orbit. Am J Ophthalmol 1975;7:813–5.

Fibrous Histiocytoma

22. Jakobiec FA, Howard GM, Jones IS, Tannenbaum M. Fibrous histiocytomas of the orbit. Am J Ophthalmol 1974;77:333–45.
23. Font RL, Hidayat AA. Fibrous histiocytoma of the orbit. A clinicopathologic study of 150 cases. Hum Pathol 1982;13:199–209.
24. Dalley RW. Fibrous histiocytoma and fibrous tissue tumors of the orbit. Radiol Clin North Am 1999;37:185–94.

Fibrosarcoma

25. Eifrig DE, Foos RY. Fibrosarcoma of the orbit. Am J Ophthalmol 1969;67:244–8.
26. Jakobiec FA, Tannenbaum M. The ultrastructure of orbital fibrosarcoma. Am J Ophthalmol 1974;77:899–917.
27. Weiner JM, Hidayat AA. Juvenile fibrosarcoma of the orbit and eyelid. A study of five cases. Arch Ophthalmol 1983;101:253–9.

Lipomatous Tumors

28. Johnson BL, Linn JG Jr. Spindle cell lipoma of the orbit. Arch Ophthalmol 1979;97:133–4.
29. Bartley GB, Yeatts RP, Garrity JA, Farrow GM, Campbell RJ. Spindle cell lipoma of the orbit. Am J Ophthalmol 1985;100:605–9.
30. Daniel CS, Beaconsfield M, Rose GE, Luthert PJ, Heathcote JG, Clark BJ. Pleomorphic lipoma of the orbit: a case series and review of literature. Ophthalmology 2003;110:101–5.
31. Brown HH, Kersten RC, Kulwin DR. Lipomatous hamartoma of the orbit. Arch Ophthalmol 1991; 109:240–3.
32. Jakobiec FA, Rini F, Char D, et al. Primary liposarcoma of the orbit. Problems in the diagnosis and management of five cases. Ophthalmology 1989;96:180–91.
33. Cai YC, McMenamin ME, Rose G, Sandy CJ, Cree IA, Fletcher CD. Primary liposarcoma of the orbit: a clinicopathologic study of seven cases. Ann Diagn Pathol 2001;5:255–66.
34. McNab AA, Moseley I. Primary orbital liposarcoma: clinical and computed tomographic features. Br J Ophthalmol 1990;74:437–9.
35. Weiss SW, Goldblum JR. Enzinger and Weiss's soft tissue tumors, Fourth ed. St. Louis: Mosby Inc; 2001:685–6.
36. Cockerham KP, Kennerdell JS, Celin SE, Fechter HP. Liposarcoma of the orbit: a management challenge. Ophthal Plast Reconstr Surg 1998;14:370–4.

Smooth Muscle Tumors

37. Jakobiec FA, Howard GM, Rosen M, Wolff M. Leiomyoma and leiomyosarcoma of the orbit. Am J Ophthalmol 1975;80:1028–42.
38. Jakobiec FA, Jones IS, Tannenbaum M. Leiomyoma. An unusual tumor of the orbit. Br J Ophthalmol 1973;57:825–31.
39. Kulkarni V, Rajshekhar V, Chandi SM. Orbital apex leiomyoma with intracranial extension. Surg Neurol 2000;54:327–30.
40. Henderson JW, Harrison EG Jr. Vascular leiomyoma of the orbit: report of a case. Trans Am Acad Ophthalmol Otolaryngol 1970;74:970.
41. Meekins BB, Dutton Proia AD. Primary orbital leiomyosarcoma. A case report and review of the literature. Arch Ophthalmol 1988;106:82–6.
42. Font RL, Jurco S 3rd, Brechner RJ. Postradiation leiomyosarcoma of the orbit complicating bilateral retinoblastoma. Arch Ophthalmol 1983; 101:1557–61.
43. Folberg R, Cleasby G, Flanagan JA, Spencer WH, Zimmerman LE. Orbital leiomyosarcoma after radiation therapy for bilateral retinoblastoma. Arch Ophthalmol 1983;101:1562–5.
44. Minkovitz JB, Dickersin GR, Dallow RL, Albert DM. Leiomyosarcoma metastatic to the orbit. Arch Ophthalmol 1990;108:1525–6.
45. Kaltreider SA, Destro M, Lemke BN. Leiomyosarcoma of the orbit. A case report and review of the literature. Ophthal Plast Reconstr Surg 1987;3:35–41.

Rhabdomyosarcoma

46. Horn RC, Enterline HT. Rhabdomyosarcoma: a clinicopathologic study and classification of 39 cases. Cancer 1958;11:181.
47. Porterfield JF, Zimmerman LE. Rhabdomyosarcoma of the orbit: a clinicopathologic study of 55 cases. Virchows Arch Pathol Anat Physiol Klin Med 1962;335:329–44.
48. Ashton N, Morgan G. Embryonal sarcoma and embryonal rhabdomyosarcoma of the orbit. J Clin Pathol 1965;18:699–714.
49. Jones IS, Reese AB, Kraut J. Orbital rhabdomyosarcoma. An analysis of 62 cases. Am J Ophthalmol 1966;61:721–36.
50. Kirk RC, Zimmerman LE. Rhabdomyosarcoma of the orbit in a survivor of rhabdomyosarcoma of the kidney. Arch Ophthalmol 1969;81:559–64.
51. Knowles DM, Jakobiec FA, Potter GD, Jones IS. Ophthalmic striated muscle neoplasms. Surv Ophthalmol 1976;21:219–61.
52. Shields JA, Bakewell B, Augsburger JJ, Donoso LA, Bernardino V. Space-occupying orbital masses in children. A review of 250 consecutive biopsies. Ophthalmology 1986;93:379–84.
53. Porterfield JF. Orbital tumors in children: a report on 214 cases. Ophthalmol Clin 1962;2: 319–35.
54. Shields CL, Shields JA, Honavar SG, Demirci H. Clinical spectrum of primary ophthalmic rhabdomyosarcoma. Ophthalmology 2001;108: 2284–92.
55. Mullaney PB, Nabi NU, Thorner P, Buncic R. Ophthalmic involvement as a presenting feature of nonorbital childhood parameningeal embryonal rhabdomyosarcoma. Ophthalmology 2001;108:179–82.

56. Wang NP, Marx J, McNutt MA, Rutledge JC, Gown AM. Expression of myogenic regulatory proteins (myogenin and MyoD1) in small blue round cell tumors in childhood. Am J Pathol 1995;147:1799–810.
57. Polack FM, Kanai A, Hood CI. Light and electron microscopic studies of orbital rhabdomyosarcoma. Am J Ophthalmol 1971;71:75–83.
58. Wharam M, Beltangady M, Hays D, et al. Localized orbital rhabdomyosarcoma. An interim report of the Intergroup Rhabdomyosarcoma Study Committee. Ophthalmology 1987;94:251–4.
59. Mannor GE, Rose GE, Plowman PN, Kingston J, Wright JE, Vardy SJ. Multidisciplinary management of refractory orbital rhabdomyosarcoma. Ophthalmology 1997;104:1198–201.
60. Raney RB, Anderson JR, Kollath J, et al. Late effects of therapy in 94 patients with localized rhabdomyosarcoma of the orbit: report from the Intergroup Rhabdomyosarcoma Study (IRS)-III, 1984-1991. Med Pediatr Oncol 2000;34:413–20.
61. Crist WM, Garnsey L, Beltangady MS, et al. Prognosis in children with rhabdomyosarcoma: a report of the intergroup rhabdomyosarcoma studies I and II. Intergroup Rhabdomyosarcoma Committee. J Clin Oncol 1990;8:443–52.
62. Crist W, Gehan EA, Ragab AH, et al. The Third Intergroup Rhabdomyosarcoma Study. J Clin Oncol 1995;13:610–30.
63. Lawrence W Jr, Gehan EA, Hays DM, Beltangady M, Maurer HM. Prognostic significance of staging factors of the UICC staging system in childhood rhabdomyosarcoma: a report from the Intergroup Rhabdomyosarcoma Study (IRS-II). J Clin Oncol 1987;5:46–54.
64. Lawrence W Jr, Anderson JR, Gehan EA, Maurer H. Pretreatment TNM staging of childhood rhabdomyosarcoma: a report of the Intergroup Rhabdomyosarcoma Study Group. Children's Cancer Study Group. Pediatric Oncology Group. Cancer 1997;80:1165–70.

Miscelaneous Skeletal Muscle Tumors

65. Knowles DM 2nd, Jakobiec FA. Rhabdomyoma of the orbit. Am J Ophthalmol 1975;80:1011–8.
66. Rootman J, Damji KF, Dimmick JE. Malignant rhabdoid tumor of the orbit. Ophthalmology 1989;96:1650–4.
67. Gunduz K, Shields JA, Eagle RC Jr, Shields CL, De Potter P, Klombers L. Malignant rhabdoid tumor of the orbit. Arch Ophthalmol 1998;116:243–6.

Capillary Hemangioma

68. Gunalp I, Gunduz K.Vascular tumors of the orbit. Doc Ophthalmol 1995;89:337–45.
69. Haik BG, Jakobiec FA, Ellsworth RM, Jones IS. Capillary hemangioma of the lids and orbit: an analysis of the clinical features and therapeutic results in 101 cases. Ophthalmology 1979;86:760–89.
70. Haik BG, Karcioglu ZA, Gordon RA, Pechous BP. Capillary hemangioma (infantile periocular hemangioma). Surv Ophthalmol 1994;38:399–426.
71. Aldave AJ, Shields CL, Shields JA. Surgical excision of selected amblyogenic periorbital capillary hemangiomas. Ophthalmic Surg Lasers 1999;30:754–7.
72. Kushner BJ. Intralesional corticosteroid injection for infantile adnexal hemangioma. Am J Ophthalmol 1982;93:496–506.
73. Hastings MM, Milot J, Barsoum-Homsy M, Hershon L, Dubois J, Leclerc JM. Recombinant interferon alfa-2b in the treatment of vision-threatening capillary hemangiomas in childhood. JAAPOS 1997;1:226–30.

Cavernous Hemangioma

74. Harris GJ, Jakobiec FA. Cavernous hemangioma of the orbit. A clinicopathologic analysis of sixty-six cases. In: Jakobiec FA, ed. Ocular and adnexal tumors. Birmingham, AL: Aesculapius Publishing Co; 1978:741–81.
75. McNab AA, Wright JE. Cavernous hemangiomas of the orbit. Aust N Z J Ophthalmol 1989;17:337–45.
76. Sklar EL, Quencer RM, Byrne SF, Sklar VE. Correlative study of the computed tomographic, ultrasonographic, and pathologic characteristics of cavernous versus capillary hemangiomas of the orbit. J Clin Neuroophthalmol 1986;6:14–21.
77. Iwamoto T, Jakobiec FA. Ultrastructural comparison of capillary and cavernous hemangioma of the orbit. Arch Ophthalmol 1979;97:1144–53.
78. Jakobiec FA, Font RL. Orbital infections. In: Spencer WH, ed. Ophthalmic pathology. An atlas and textbook, 3rd ed. Philadelphia: WB Saunders; 1985;2459–812.

Lymphangioma

79. Jones IS. Lymphangioma of the ocular adnexa: an analysis of 62 cases. Trans Am Ophthalmol Soc 1959;57:602–65.
80. Iliff WJ, Green WR. Orbital lymphangiomas. Ophthalmology 1979;86:914–29.
81. Wright JE, Sullivan TJ, Garner A, Wulc AE, Moseley IF. Orbital venous anomalies. Ophthalmology. 1997;104:905–13.
82. Rootman J, Hay E, Graeb D, Miller R. Orbit-adnexal lymphangiomas. A spectrum of hemodynamically isolated vascular hamartomas. Ophthalmology 1986;93:1558–70.

83. Katz SE, Rootman J, Vangveeravong S, Graeb D. Combined venous lymphatic malformations of the orbit (so-called lymphangiomas). Association with noncontiguous intracranial vascular anomalies. Ophthalmology 1998;105:176–84.
84. Bond JB, Haik BG, Taveras JL, et al. Magnetic resonance imaging of orbital lymphangioma with and without gadolinium contrast enhancement. Ophthalmology 1992;99:1318–24.
85. Selva D, Strianese D, Bonavolonta G, Rootman J. Orbital venous-lymphatic malformations (lymphangiomas) mimicking cavernous hemangiomas. Am J Ophthalmol 2001;131:364–70.
86. Harris GJ, Sakol PJ, Bonavolonta G, De Conciliis C. An analysis of thirty cases of orbital lymphangioma. Pathophysiologic considerations and management reccomendations. Ophthalmology 1990;97:1583–92.

Hemangiopericytoma

87. Fletcher CD. Haemangiopericytoma, a dying breed? Reappraison of an "entity" and its variant: a hypothesis. Curr Diagn Pathol 1994;1:19–23.
88. Croxatto JO, Font RL. Hemangiopericytoma of the orbit: a clinicopathologic study of 30 cases. Hum Pathol 1982;13:210–8.
89. Boniuk M, Messmer EP, Font RL. Hemangiopericytoma of the meninges of the optic nerve. A clinicopathologic report including electron microscopic observations. Ophthalmology 1985;92:1780–7.
90. Kikuchi K, Kowada M, Sageshima M. Orbital hemangiopericytoma: CT, MR, and angiographic findings. Comput Med Imaging Graph 1994;18:217–22.
91. Setzkorn RK, Lee D, Iliff NT, Green WR. Hemangiopericytoma of the orbit treated with conservative surgery and radiotherapy. Arch Ophthalmol 1987;105:1103–5.
92. Carew JF, Singh B, Kraus DH. Hemangiopericytoma of the head and neck. Laryngoscope 1999;109:1409–11.

Solitary Fibrous Tumor

93. Klemperer P, Rabin CB. Primary neoplasm of the pleura: a report of five cases. Arch Pathol 1931;11:385–412.
94. Weiss SW, Goldblum JR. Enzinger and Weiss's soft tissue tumors, 4th ed. St. Louis: Mosby Inc; 2001:1021–31.
95. Ing EB, Kennerdell JS, Olson PR, Ogino S, Rothfus WE. Solitary fibrous tumor of the orbit. Ophthal Plast Reconstr Surg 1998;14:57–61.
96. Carrera M, Prat J, Quintana M. Malignant solitary fibrous tumour of the orbit: report of a case with 8 years follow-up. Eye 2001;15(Pt 1):102–4.
97. Fenton S, Moriarty P, Kennedy S. Solitary fibrous tumor of the orbit. Eye 2001;15:124–6.
98. Polito E, Tosi M, Toti P, Schurfeld K, Caporossi A. Orbital solitary fibrous tumor with aggressive behavior. Three cases and review of the literature. Graefes Arch Clin Exp Ophthalmol 2002;240:570–4.
99. Gigantelli JW, Kincaid MC, Soparkar CN, et al. Orbital solitary fibrous tumor: radiographic and histopathologic correlations. Ophthal Plastic Reconstr Surg 2001;17:207–14.

Epthelioid Hemangioma

100. Wells GC, Whimster IW. Subcutaneous angiolymphoid hyperplasia with eosinophilia. Br J Dermatol 1969;81:1–14.
101. McEachren TM, Brownstein S, Jordan DR, Montpetit VA, Font RL. Epithelioid hemangioma of the orbit. Ophthalmology 2000;107: 806–10.
102. Kimura T, Yoshimura S, Ishikawa E. On the unusual granulation combined with hyperplastic changes of lymphatic tissues. Trans Soc Pathol Jpn 1948;37:179–80.
103. Hidayat AA. Cameron JD, Font RL, Zimmerman LE. Angiolymphoid hyperplasia with eosinophilia (Kimura's disease) of the orbit and ocular adnexa. Am J Ophthalmol 1983;96:176–89.
104. Buggage RR, Spraul CW, Wojno TH, Grossniklaus HE. Kimura disease of the orbit and ocular adnexa. Surv Ophthalmol 1999;44:79–91.

Venous Anomalies and Malformations

105. Harris GJ. Orbital vascular malformations: a consensus statement on terminology and its clinical implications. Orbital Society. Am J Ophthalmol 1999;127:453–5.
106. Rathbun J, Hoyt WF, Beard C. Surgical management of orbitofrontal varix in Klippel-Trenaunay-Weber syndrome. Am J Ophthalmol 1970;70:109–12.
107. Rennie IG, Shortland JR, Mahood JM, Browne BH. Periodic exophthalmos associated with the blue rubber bleb naevus syndrome: a case report. Br J Ophthalmol 1982;66:594–9.
108. Chang EL, Rubin PA. Bilateral multifocal hemangiomas of the orbit in the blue rubber bleb nevus syndrome. Ophthalmology 2002;109: 537–41.
109. Hofeldt AJ, Zaret CR, Jakobiec FA, Behrens MM, Jones IS. Orbitofacial angiomatosis. Arch Ophthalmol 1979;97:484–8.
110. Bullock JD, Goldberg SH, Connelly PJ. Orbital varix thrombosis. Ophthalmology 1990;97:251–6.

Intravascular Papillary Endothelial Hyperplasia

111. Weber FL, Babel J. Intravascular papillary hyperplasia of the orbit. Br J Ophthalmol 1981;65: 18–22.
112. Font RL, Wheeler TM, Boniuk M. Intravascular papillary endothelial hyperplasia of the orbit and ocular adnexa. A report of five cases. Arch Ophthalmol 1983;101:1731–6.
113. Werner MS, Hornblass A, Reifler DM, Dresner SC, Harrison W. Intravascular papillary endothelial hyperplasia: collection of four cases and a review of the literature. Ophthal Plast Reconstr Surg 1997;13:48–56.

Angiosarcoma

114. Messmer EP, Font RL, McCrary JA 3rd, Murphy D. Epithelioid angiosarcoma of the orbit presenting as Tolosa-Hunt syndrome. A clinicopathologic case report with review of the literature. Ophthalmology 1983;90:1414–21.
115. Hufnagel T, Ma L, Kuo TT. Orbital angiosarcoma with subconjunctival presentation. Report of a case and literature review. Ophthamology 1987;94:72–7.

Peripheral Nerve Sheath Tumors

116. Coleman DJ, Jack RL, Franzen LA. High resolution B-scan ultrasonography of the orbit. IV. Neurogenic tumors of the orbit. Arch Ophthalmol 1972;88:380–4.
117. Lyons CJ, McNab AA, Garner A, Wright JE. Orbital malignant peripheral nerve sheath tumours. Br J Ophthalmol 1989;73:731–8.
118. Rose GE, Wright JE. Isolated peripheral nerve sheath tumours of the orbit. Eye 1991;5(Pt 6):668–73.
119. Messmer EP, Camara J, Boniuk M, Font RL. Amputation neuroma of the orbit. Report of two cases and review of the literature. Ophthalmology 1984;91:1420–3.
120. Okubo K, Asai T, Sera Y, Okada S. A case of amputation neuroma presenting [with] proptosis. Ophthalmologica 1987;194:5–8.

Neurofibroma

121. Harkens K, Dolan KD. Correlative imaging of sphenoid dysplasia accompanying neurofibromatosis. Ann Otol Rhinol Laryngol 1990;99: 137–41.
122. Krohel GB, Rosenberg PN, Wright JE, Smith RS. Localized orbital neurofibromas. Am J Ophthalmol 1985;100:458–64.
123. Shields JA, Shields CL, Lieb WE, Eagle RC. Multiple orbital neurofibromas unassociated with von Recklinghausen's disease. Arch Ophthalmol 1990;108:80–3.
124. Meyer DR, Wobig JL. Bilateral localized orbital neurofibromas. Ophthalmology 1992;99:1313–7.
125. Erlandson RA, Woodruff JM. Peripheral nerve sheath tumors: an electron microscopic study of 43 cases. Cancer 1982;49:273–87.
126. Lyons CJ, McNab AA, Garner A, Wright JE. Orbital malignant peripheral nerve sheath tumours. Br J Ophthalmol 1989;73:731–8.
127. Jakobiec FA, Font RL, Zimmerman LE. Malignant peripheral nerve sheath tumors of the orbit: a clinicopathologic study of eight cases. Trans Am Ophthalmol Soc 1985;83:332–66.

Schwannoma

128. Mohan H, Sen DK. Orbital neurilemmoma. Presenting as retrobulbar neuritis. Br J Ophthalmol 1970;54:206–7.
129. Rootman J, Goldberg C, Robertson W. Primary orbital schwannomas. Br J Ophthalmol 1982;66:194–204.
130. Dervin JE, Beaconsfield M, Wright JE, Moseley IF. CT findings in orbital tumors of nerve sheath origin. Clin Radiol 1989;40:475–9.
131. Carroll GS, Haik BG, Fleming JC, Weiss RA, Mafee MF. Peripheral nerve tumors of the orbit. Radiol Clin North Am 1999;37:195–202.
132. Jensen OA, Bretlau P. Melanotic schwannoma of the orbit. Immunohistochemical and ultrastructural study of a case and survey of the literature. APMIS 1990;98:713–23.
133. Nishida S. Fine structural studies of a neurilemoma in the orbit. Folia Ophthalmol Jpn 1977;28:438–47.
134. Chisholm IA, Polyzoidis K. Recurrence of benign orbital neurilemmoma (schwannoma) after 22 years. Can J Ophthalmol 1982;17:271–3.
135. Schatz H. Benign orbital neurilemmoma. Sarcomatous transformation in von Recklinghausen's disease. Arch Ophthalmol 1971;86: 268–73.
136. Nieuwenhuis I, Witschel H. [Benign and malignant schwannoma of the orbit—clinical picture and histopathologic diagnosis.] Fortschr Ophthalmol 1988;85:782–5. (German.)

Granular Cell Tumor

137. Morgan G. Granular cell myoblastoma of the orbit. Report of a case. Arch Ophthalmol 1976;94:2135–42.
138. Goldstein BG, Font RL, Alper MG. Granular cell tumor of the orbit: a case report including electron microscopic observation. Ann Ophthalmol 1982;14:231–2, 236–8.
139. Karcioglu ZA, Hemphill GL, Wool BM. Granular cell tumor of the orbit: case report and review of the literature. Ophthalmic Surg 1983; 14:125–9.

140. Jaeger MJ, Green WR, Miller NR, Harris GJ. Granular cell tumor of the orbit and ocular adnexae. Surv Ophthalmol 1987;31:417–23.

Malignant Peripheral Nerve Sheath Tumors

141. Wanebo JE, Malik JM, VandenBerg SR, Wanebo HJ, Driesen N, Persing JA. Malignant peripheral nerve sheath tumors. A clinicopathologic study of 28 cases. Cancer 1993;71:1247–53.
142. Grinberg MA, Levy NS. Malignant neurilemoma of the supraorbital nerve. Am J Ophthalmol 1974;78:489–92.
143. Mortada A. Solitary orbital malignant neurilemmoma. Br J Ophthalmol 1968;52:188–90.
144. Jakobiec FA, Font RL, Zimmerman LE. Malignant periperal nerve sheath tumors of the orbit: a clinicopathologic study of eight cases. Trans Am Ophthalmol Soc 1985;83:332–66.
145. Briscoe D, Mahmood S, O'Donovan DG, Bonshek RE, Leatherbarrow B, Eyden BP. Malignant peripheral nerve sheath tumor in the orbit of a child with acute proptosis. Arch Ophthalmol 2002;120:653–5
146. Dutton JJ, Tawfik HA, DeBacker CM, Lipham WJ, Gayre GS, Klintworth GK. Multiple recurrences in malignant peripheral nerve sheath tumor of the orbit: a case report and a review of the literature. Ophthal Plast Reconstr Surg 2001;17:293–9.

Bone Tumors

147. Blodi FC. Pathology of orbital bones. The XXXII Edward Jackson Memorial Lecture. Am J Ophthalmol 1976;81:1–26.
148. Spencer WH, ed. Ophthalmic pathology: an atlas and textbook, 4th ed. Philadelphia: Saunders; 1996.
149. Selva D, White VA, O'Connell JX, Rootman J. Primary bone tumors of the orbit. Surv Ophthalmol 2004;49:328–42.
150. Whitson WE, Orcutt JC, Walkinshaw MD. Orbital osteoma in Gardner's syndrome. Am J Ophthalmol 1986;101:236–41.
151. Moore AT, Buncic JR, Munro IR. Fibrous dysplasia of the orbit in childhood. Clinical fetaures and management. Ophthalmology 1985;92:12–20.
152. Margo CE, Ragsdale BD, Perman KI, Zimmerman LE, Sweet DE. Psammomatoid (juvenile) ossifying fibroma of the orbit. Ophthalmology 1985;92:150–9.
153. Hartstein ME, Grove AS Jr, Woog JJ, Shore JW, Joseph MP. The multidisciplinary management of psammomatoid ossifying fibroma of the orbit. Ophthalmology 1998;105:591–5.
154. Abramson DH, Ellsworth RM, Zimmerman LE. Nonocular cancer in retinoblastoma survivors. Trans Am Acad Ophthalmol Otolaryngol Am Acad Ophthalmol Otolaryngol 1976;81:454–7.
155. Roarty JD, McLean IW, Zimmerman LE. Incidence of second neoplasms in patients with bilateral retinoblastoma. Ophthalmology 1988;95:1583–7.
156. Parmar DN, Luthert PJ, Cree IA, Reid RP, Rose GE. Two unusual osteogenic orbital tumors: presumed parosteal osteosarcomas of the orbit. Ophthalmology 2001;108:1452–6.
157. Misra A, Misra S, Chaturvedi A, Srivastava PK. Osteosarcoma with metastasis to orbit. Br J Ophthalmol 2001;85:1387–8.
158. Shinaver CN, Mafee MF, Choi KH. MRI of mesenchymal chondrosarcoma of the orbit: case report and review of the literature. Neuroradiology 1997;39:296–301.

Lymphoid Tumors

159. Jakobiec FA, Knowles DM. An overview of ocular adnexal lymphoid tumors. Trans Am Ophthalmol Soc 1989;87:420–44.
160. Demirci H, Shields CL, Shields JA, Honavar SG, Mercado GJ, Tovilla JC. Orbital tumors in the older adult population. Ophthalmology 2002;109:243–8.
161. Knowles DM, Jakobiec FA, McNally L, Burke JS. Lymphoid hyperplasia and malignant lymphoma occurring in the ocular adnexa (orbit, conjunctiva, and eyelids): a prospective multiparametric analysis of 108 cases during 1977 to 1987. Hum Pathol 1990;21:959–73.
162. Jakobiec FA, McLean I, Font RL. Clinicopathologic characteristics of orbital lymphoid hyperplasia. Ophthalmology 1979;86:948–66.
163. Medeiros LJ, Harris NL. Lymphoid infiltrates of the orbit and conjunctiva. A morphologic and immunophenotypic study of 99 cases. Am J Surg Pathol 1989;13:459–71.
164. Coupland SE, Krause L, Delecluse HJ, et al. Lymphoproliferative lesions of the ocular adnexa. Analysis of 112 cases. Ophthalmology 1998;105:1430–41.
165. Jenkins C, Rose GE, Bunce C, et al. Histological features of ocular adnexal lymphoma (REAL classification) and their association with patient morbidity and survival. Br J Ophthalmol 2000; 84:907–13.
166. Knowles DM 2nd, Jakobiec FA. Ocular adnexal lymphoid neoplasms: clinical, histopathologic, electron microscopic, and immunologic characteristics. Hum Pathol 1982;13:148–62.

167. Jakobiec FA, Neri A, Knowles DM 2nd. Genotypic monoclonality in immunophenotypically polyclonal orbital lymphoid tumors. A model of tumor progression in the lymphoid system. The 1986 Wendell Hughes lecture. Ophthalmology 1987;94:980–94.
168. Sen DK, Mohan H, Chatterjee PK. Hodgkin's disease in the orbit. Int Surg 1971;55:183–6.
169. Fratkin JD, Shammas HF, Miller SD. Disseminated Hodgkin's disease with bilateral orbital involvement. Arch Ophthalmol 1978;96:102–4.
170. Patel S, Rootman J. Nodular sclerosing Hodgkin's disease of the orbit. Ophthalmology 1983;90:1433–6.
171. Park KL, Goins KM. Hodgkin's lymphoma of the orbit associated with acquired immunodeficiency syndrome. Am J Ophthalmol 1993;116:111–2.
172. Pomeranz HD, McEvoy LT, Lueder GT. Orbital tumor in a child with posttransplantation lymphoproliferative disorder. Arch Ophthalmol 1996;114:1422–3.
173. Westacott S, Garner A, Moseley IF, Wright JE. Orbital lymphoma versus reactive lymphoid hyperplasia: an analysis of the use of computed tomography in differential diagnosis. Br J Ophthalmol 1991;75:722–5.
174. Knowles DM 2nd, Jakobiec FA. Quantitative determination of T cells in ocular lymphoid infiltrates. An indirect method for distinguishing between pseudolymphomas and malignant lymphomas. Arch Ophthalmol 1981;99:309–16.
175. Garner A, Rahi AH, Wright JE. Lymphoproliferative disorders of the orbit: an immunological approach to diagnosis and pathogenesis. Br J Ophthalmol 1983;67:561–9.
176. Bairey O, Kremer I, Rakowsky E, Hadar H, Shaklai M. Orbital and adnexal involvement in systemic non-Hodgkin's lymphoma. Cancer 1994;73:2395–9.
177. Medeiros LJ, Harmon DC, Linggood RM, Harris NL. Immunohistologic features predict clinical behavior of orbital and conjunctival lymphoid infiltrates. Blood 1989;74:2121–9.
178. Reifler DM, Warzynski MJ, Blount WR, Graham DM, Mills KA. Orbital lymphoma associated with acquired immune deficiency syndrome (AIDS). Surv Ophthalmol 1994;38:371–80.
179. Font RL, Laucirica R, Patrinely JR. Immunoblastic B-cell malignant lymphoma involving the orbit and maxillary sinus in a patient with acquired immune deficiency syndrome. Ophthalmology 1993;100:966–70.
180. Antle CM, White VA, Horsman DE, Rootman J. Large cell orbital lymphoma in a patient with acquired immunodeficiency syndrome: case report and review. Ophthalmology 1990;97:1494–8.
181. Brooks HL Jr, Downing J, McClure JA, Engel HM. Orbital Burkitt's lymphoma in a homosexual man with acquired immune deficiency. Arch Ophthalmol 1984;102:1533–7.
182. Ziegler JL. Burkitt's lymphoma. N Engl J Med 1981;305:735–45.
183. Sandy CJ, Rose GE, Clark BJ, Plowman PN. Sporadic Burkitt's lymphoma presenting as solely orbital disease in a 78-year-old. Eye 2001;15(Pt 1):113–5.
184. Payne T, Karp LA, Zimmerman LE. Intraocular involvement in Burkitt's lymphoma. Arch Ophthalmol 1971;85:295–8.
185. Harris NL, Jaffe ES, Stein H, et al. A revised European-American classification of lymphoid neoplasms: a proposal from the International Lymphoma Study Group. Blood 1994;84:1361–92.
186. Lauer SA, Fischer J, Jones J, Gartner S, Dutcher J, Hoxie JA. Orbital T-cell lymphoma in human T-cell leukemia virus-I infection. Ophthalmology 1988;95:110–5.
187. Laucirica R, Font RL. Cytologic evaluation of lymphoproliferative lesions of the orbit/ocular adnexa: an analysis of 46 cases. Diagn Cytopathol 1996;15:241–5.
188. Nassar DL, Raab SS, Silverman JF, Kennerdell JS, Sturgis CD. Fine-needle aspiration for the diagnosis of orbital hematolymphoid lesions. Diagn Cytopathol 2000;23:314–7.
189. Carbone PP, Kaplan HS, Musshoff K, Smithers DW, Tubiana M. Report of the Committee on Hodgkin's Disease Staging Classification. Cancer Res 1971;31:1860–1.

Orbital Plasmacytoma

190. Rodman HI, Font RL. Orbital involvement in multiple myeloma. Review of the literature and report of three cases. Arch Ophthalmol 1972;87:30–5.
191. De Smet MD, Rootman J. Orbital manifestation of plasmacytic lymphoproliferations. Ophthalmology 1987;94:995–1003.
192. Knowles DM 2nd, Halper JA, Trokel S, Jakobiec FA. Immunofluorescent and immunoperoxidase characteristics of IgDlambda myeloma involving the orbit. Am J Ophthalmol 1978;85:485–94.
193. Khalil MK, Huang S, Viloria J, Duguid WP. Extramedullary plasmacytoma of the orbit: case report with results of immunocytochemical studies. Can J Ophthalmol 1981;16:39–42.

Leukemic Disorders

194. Kincaid MC, Green WR. Ocular and orbital involvement in leukemia. Surv Ophthalmol 1983;27:211–32.
195. Rubinfeld RS, Gootenberg JE, Chavis RM, Zimmerman LE. Early onset acute orbital involvement in childhood acute lymphoblastic leukemia. Ophthalmology 1988;95:116–20.
196. Hatton MP, Rubin PA. Chronic lymphocytic leukemia of the orbit. Arch Ophthalmol 2002;120:990–1.
197. Jha BK, Lamba PA. Proptosis as a manifestation of acute myeloid leukemia. Br J Ophthalmol 1971;55:844–7.
198. Davis JL, Parke DW 2nd, Font RL. Granulocytic sarcoma of the orbit. A clinicopathologic study. Ophthalmology 1985;92:1758–62.
199. Zimmerman LE, Font RL. Ophthalmologic manifestations of granulocytic sarcoma (myeloid sarcoma or chloroma). The third Pan American Association of Ophthalmology and American Journal of Ophthalmology Lecture. Am J Ophthalmol 1975;80:975–90.
200. Shome DK, Gupta NK, Prajapi NC, Raju GM, Choudhury P, Dubey AP. Orbital granulocytic sarcomas (myeloid sarcomas) in acute nonlymphocytic leukemia. Cancer 1992;70:2298–301.
201. Johansson B, Fioretos T, Kullendorff CM, et al. Granulocytic sarcomas in body cavities in childhood acute myeloid leukemias with 11q23/MLL rearrangements. Genes Chromosomes Cancer 2000;27:136–42.

Langerhans Cell Histiocytosis

202. Malone M. The histiocytoses of childhood. Histopathology 1991;19:105–19.
203. Feldman RB, Moore DM, Hood CI, Hiles DA, Romano PE. Solitary eosinophilic granuloma of the lateral orbital wall. Am J Ophthalmol 1985;100:318–23.
204. Kramer TR, Noecker RJ, Miller JM, Clark LC. Langerhans cell histiocytosis with orbital involvement. Am J Ophthalmol 1997;124:814–24.
205. Tazi A, Bonay M, Grandsaigne M, Battesti JP, Hance AJ, Soler P. Surface phenotype of Langerhans cells and lymphocytes in granulomatous lesions from patients with pulmonary histiocytosis X. Am Rev Respir Dis 1993;147(Pt 1):1531–6.
206. Pinkus GS, Lones MA, Matsumura F, Yamashiro S, Said JW, Pinkus JL. Langerhans cell histiocytosis immunohistochemical expression of fascin, a dendritic cell marker. Am J Clin Pathol 2002;118:335–43.
207. Birbeck MS, Breathnach AS, Everall JD. An electron microscope study of basal melanocytes and high-level clear cells (Langerhans cells) in vitiligo. J Invest Dermatol 1961;37:51–64.
208. Smith JH, Fulton L, O'Brien JM. Spontaneous regression of orbital Langerhans cell granulomatosis in a three-year-old girl. Am J Ophthalmol 1999;128:119–21.

Histiocytic Disorders of Mononuclear Phagocytes

209. Friendly DS, Font RL, Rao NA. Orbital involvement in 'sinus' histiocytosis. A report of four cases. Arch Ophthalmol 1977;95:2006–11.
210. Foucar E, Rosai J, Dorfman RF. The ophthalmologic manifestations of sinus histiocytosis with massive lymphadenopathy. Am J Ophthalmol 1979;87:354–67.
211. Zimmerman LE, Hidayat AA, Grantham RL, et al. Atypical cases of sinus histiocytosis (Rosai-Dorfman disease) with ophthalmological manifestations. Trans Am Ophthalmol Soc 1988;86: 113–35.
212. Marion JR, Geisinger KR. Sinus histiocytosis with massive lymphadenopathy: bilateral orbital involvement spanning 17 years. Ann Ophthalmol 1989;21:55–8.
213. Zimmerman LE. Ocular lesions of juvenile xanthogranuloma. Nevoxanthoendothelioma. Am J Ophthalmol 1965;60:1011–35.
214. Nasr AM, Johnson T, Hidayat A. Adult onset primary bilateral orbital xanthogranuloma: clinical, diagnostic, and histopathologic correlations. Orbit 1991;10:13–22.
215. Robertson DM, Winkelmann RK. Ophthalmic features of necrobiotic xanthogranuloma with paraproteinaemia. Am J Ophthalmol 1984; 97:173–83.
216. Bullock JD, Bartley GB, Campbell RJ, Yanes B, Connelly PJ, Funkhouser JW. Necrobiotic xanthogranuloma with paraproteinemia. Case report and a pathogenic theory. Trans Am Ophthalmol Soc 1986;84:342–54.
217. Ugurlu S, Bartley GB, Gibson LE. Necrobiotic xanthogranuloma: long-term outcome of ocular and systemic involvement. Am J Ophthalmol 2000;129:651–7.
218. Alper MG, Zimmerman LE, Piana FG. Orbital manifestations of Erdheim-Chester disease. Trans Am Ophthalmol Soc 1983;81:64–85.
219. Shields JA, Karcioglu ZA, Shields CL, Eagle RC, Wong S. Orbital and eyelid involvement with Erdheim-Chester disease. A report of two cases. Arch Ophthalmol 1991;109:850–4
220. Sheidow TG, Nicolle DA, Heathcote JG. Erdheim-Chester disease: two cases of orbital involvement. Eye 2000;14(Pt 4):606–12
221. Char DH, LeBoit PE, Ljung BM, Wara W. Radiation therapy for ocular necrobiotic xanthogranuloma. Arch Ophthalmol 1987;105:174–5.

222. Jakobiec FA, Mills MD, Hidayat AA, et al. Periocular xanthogranulomas associated with severe adult-onset asthma. Trans Am Ophthalmol Soc 1993;91:99–129.

Dermoid

223. Jakobiec FA, Bonanno PA, Sigelman J. Conjunctival adnexal cysts and dermoids. Arch Ophthalmol 1978;96:1040–9.
224. Newton C, Dutton JJ, Klintworth GK. A respiratory epithelial choristomatous cyst of the orbit. Ophthalmology 1985;92:1754–7.
225. Rush A, Leone CR Jr. Ectopic lacrimal gland cyst of the orbit. Am J Ophthalmol 1981;92:198–201.
226. Sherman RP, Rootman J, Lapointe JS. Orbital dermoids: clinical presentation and management. Br J Ophthalmol 1984;68:642–52.
227. Gotzamanis A, Desphieux JL, Pluot M, Ducasse A. [Dermoid cysts. Epidemiology, clinical and anatomo-pathologic aspects, therapeutic management.] J Fr Ophtalmol 1999;22:549–53. (French.)
228. Shields JA, Kaden IH, Eagle RC Jr, Shields CL. Orbital dermoid cysts: clinicopathologic correlations, classification, and management. The 1997 Josephine E. Schueler Lecture. Ophthal Plast Reconstr Surg 1997;13:265–76.
229. Chawda SJ, Moseley IF. Computed tomography of orbital dermoids: a 20-year review. Clin Radiol 1999;54:821–5.
230. Abou-Rayyah Y, Rose GE, Konrad H, Chawla SJ, Moseley IF. Clinical, radiological and pathological examination of periocular dermoid cysts: evidence of inflammation from an early age. Eye 2002;16:507–12.
231. Colombo F, Holbach LM, Naumann GO. Chronic inflammation in dermoid cysts: a clinicopathologic study of 115 patients. Orbit 2000;19:97–107.
232. Boynton JR, Searl SS, Ferry AP, Kaltreider SA, Rodenhouse TG. Primary nonkeratinized epithelial ('conjunctival') orbital cysts. Arch Ophthalmol 1992;110:1238–42.
233. Mee JJ, McNab AA, McKelvie P. Respiratory epithelial orbital cysts. Clin Experiment Ophthalmol 2002;30:356–60.
234. Parke DW 2nd, Font RL, Boniuk M, McCrary JA 3rd. 'Cholesteatoma' of the orbit. Arch Ophthalmol 1982;100:612–6.
235. Iliff CE. Mucoceles in the orbit. Arch Ophthalmol 1973;89:392–5.
236. Wright J, Morgan G. Squamous cell carcinoma developing in an orbital cyst. Arch Ophthalmol 1977;95:635–7.
237. Holds JB, Anderson RL, Mamalis N, Kincaid MC, Font RL. Invasive squamous cell carcinoma arising from asymptomatic choristomatous cyst of the orbit. Two cases and a review of the literature. Ophthalmology 1993;100:1244–52.

Teratoma

238. Hoyt WF, Joe S. Congenital teratoid cyst of the orbit. A case report and review of the literature. Arch Ophthalmol 1962;68:196–201.
239. Levin ML, Leone CR Jr, Kincaid MC. Congenital orbital teratomas. Am J Ophthalmol 1986;102:476–81.
240. Weiss AH, Greenwald MJ, Margo CE, Myers W. Primary and secondary orbital teratomas. J Pediatr Ophthalmol Strabismus 1989;26:44–9.
241. Kivela T, Tarkkanen A. Orbital germ cell tumors revisited: a clinicopathological approach to classification. Surv Ophthalmol 1994;38:541–54.
242. Garden JW, McManis JC. Congenital orbital-intracranial teratoma with subsequent malignancy: case report. Br J Ophthalmol 1986;70:110–3.
243. Wilson DJ, Dailey RA, Wobig JL, Dimmig JW. Neuroblastoma within a congenital orbital teratoma. Arch Ophthalmol 2002;120:213–5.

Endodermal Sinus Tumor

244. Margo CE, Folberg R, Zimmerman LE, Sesterhenn IA. Endodermal sinus tumor [yolk sac tumor] of the orbit. Ophthalmology 1983;90:1426–32.

Pigmented Retinal Choristoma

245. Lurie H. Congenital melanocarcinoma, melanotic adamantinoma, retinal anlage tumor, progonoma, and pigmented epulis of infancy. Summary and review of the literature and report of the first case in an adult. Cancer 1961;14:1090–108.
246. Lamping KA, Albert DM, Lack E, Dickersin GR, Chapman PH, Walton DS. Melanotic neuroectodermal tumor of infancy (retinal anlage tumor). Ophthalmology 1985;92:143–9.
247. Lamping KA, Albert DM, Lack E, Dickersin GR, Chapman PH, Walton DS. Melanotic neuroectodermal tumor of infancy (retinal anlage tumor). Ophthalmology 1985;92:143–9.

Ewing's Family of Tumors (Ewing's Sarcoma, Primitive Neuroectodermal Tumor)

248. Delattre O, Zucman J, Melot T, et al. The Ewing family of tumors—a subgroup of small-round-cell tumors defined by specific chimeric transcripts. N Engl J Med 1994;331:294–9.
249. Denny CT. Gene rearrangements in Ewing's sarcoma. Cancer Invest 1996;14:83–8.

250. Meier VS, Kuhne T, Jundt G, Gudat F. Molecular diagnosis of Ewing tumors: improved detection of EWS-FLI-1 and EWS-ERG chimeric transcripts and rapid determination of exon combinations. Diagn Mol Pathol 1998;7:29–35.
251. Jimenez RE, Folpe AL, Lapham RL, et al. Primary Ewing's sarcoma/primitive neuroectodermal tumor of the kidney: a clinicopathologic and immunohistochemical analysis of 11 cases. Am J Surg Pathol 2002;26:320–7.
252. Howard GM. Neuroepithelioma of the orbit. Am J Ophthalmol 1965;59:934–7.
253. Wilson WB, Roloff J, Wilson HL. Primary peripheral neuroepithelioma of the orbit with intracranial extension. Cancer 1988;62:2595–601.
254. Arora R, Sarkar C, Betharia SM. Primary orbital primitive neuroectodermal tumor with immunohistochemical and electron microscopy confirmation. Orbit 1993;12:7.
255. Singh AD, Husson M, Shields CL, De Potter P, Shields JA. Primitive neuroectodermal tumor of the orbit. Arch Ophthalmol 1994;112:217–21.
256. Alyahya GA, Heegaard S, Fledelius HC, Rechnitzer C, Prause JU. Primitive neuroectodermal tumor of the orbit in a 5-year-old girl with microphthalmia. Graefes Arch Clin Exp Ophthalmol 2000;238:801–6.
257. Dutton JJ, Rose JG Jr, DeBacker CM, Gayre G. Orbital Ewing's sarcoma of the orbit. Ophthal Plast Reconstr Surg 2000;16:292–300.
258. Wilson DJ, Dailey RA, Griffeth MT, Newton CJ. Primary Ewing sarcoma of the orbit. Ophthal Plast Reconstr Surg 2001;17:300–3.
259. Ambros IM, Ambros PF, Strehl S, Kovar H, Gadner H, Salzer-Kuntschik M. MIC2 is a specific marker for Ewing's sarcoma and peripheral primitive neuroectodermal tumors. Evidence for a common histogenesis of Ewing's sarcoma and peripheral primitive neuroectodermal tumors from MIC2. Cancer 1991;67:1886–93.
260. Hyun CB, Lee YR, Bemiller TA. Metastatic peripheral primitive neuroectodermal tumor (PNET) masquerading as liver abscess: a case report of liver metastasis in orbital PNET. J Clin Gastroenterol 2002;35:93–7.

Primary Orbital Carcinoid and Paraganglioma

261. Riddle PJ, Font RL, Zimmerman LE. Carcinoid tumors of the eye and orbit: a clinicopathologic study of 15 cases with histochemical and electron microscopic observations. Hum Pathol 1982;13:459–69.
262. Zimmerman LE, Stangl R, Riddle PJ. Primary carcinoid tumor of the orbit. A clinicopathologic study with histochemical and electron microscopic observations. Arch Ophthalmol 1983;101:1395–8.
263. Shetlar DJ, Font RL, Ordonez N, el-Naggar A, Boniuk M. A clinicopathologic study of three carcinoid tumors metastatic to the orbit. Immunohistochemical, ultrastructural, and DNA flow cytometric studies. Ophthalmology 1990;97:257–64.
264. Archer KF, Hurwitz JJ, Balogh JM, Fernandes BJ. Orbital nonchromaffin paraganglioma. A case report and review of the literature. Ophthalmology 1989;96:1659–66.
265. Ahmed A, Dodge OG, Kirk RS. Chemodectoma of the orbit. J Clin Pathol 1969;22:584–8.

Primary Melanoma of the Orbit

266. Jakobiec FA, Ellsworth R, Tennenbaum M. Primary orbital melanoma. Am J Ophthalmol 1974;78:24–39.
267. Dutton JJ, Anderson RL, Schelper RL, Purcell JJ, Tse DT. Orbital malignant melanoma and oculodermal melanocytosis: report of two cases and review of the literature. Ophthalmology 1984;91:497–507.
268. Font RL, Naumann G, Zimmerman LE. Primary malignant melanoma of the skin metastatic to the eye and orbit. Report of ten cases and review of the literature. Am J Ophthalmol 1967;63:738–54
269. Tellada M, Specht CS, McLean IW, Grossniklaus HE, Zimmerman LE. Primary orbital melanomas. Ophthalmology 1996;103:929–32.

Alveolar Soft Part Sarcoma

270. Font RL, Jurco S 3rd, Zimmerman LE. Alveolar soft-part sarcoma of the orbit: a clinicopathologic analysis of seventeen cases and a review of the literature. Hum Pathol 1982;13:569–79.

Secondary Tumors

271. Johnson LN, Krohel GB, Yeon EB, Parnes SM. Sinus tumors invading the orbit. Ophthalmology 1984;91:209–17.
272. Amoaku WM, Bagegni A, Logan WC, Archer DB. Orbital infiltration by eyelid skin carcinoma. Int Ophthalmol 1990;14:285–94.
273. Howard GR, Nerad JA, Carter KD, Whitaker DC. Clinical characteristics associated with orbital invasion of cutaneous basal cell and squamous cell tumors of the eyelid. Am J Ophthalmol 1992;113:123–33.
274. Johnson TE, Tabbara KF, Weatherhead RG, Kersten RC, Rice C, Nasr AM. Secondary squamous cell carcinoma of the orbit. Arch Ophthalmol 1997;115:75–8.
275. Rootman J, Ellsworth RM, Hofbauer J, Kitchen D. Orbital extension of retinoblastoma: a clinicopathological study. Can J Ophthalmol 1978;13:72–80.

276. Affeldt JC, Minckler DS, Azen SP, Yeh L. Prognosis in uveal melanoma with extrascleral extension. Arch Ophthalmol 1980;98:1975–9.
277. Rakes SM, Yeatts RP, Campbell RJ. Ophthalmic manifestations of esthesioneuroblastoma. Ophthalmology 1985;92:1749–53.
278. Bonovolonta G, Villari G, de Rosa G, Sammartino A. Ocular complications of juvenile angiofibroma. Ophthalmologica 1980;181:334–9.
279. Weiss JS, Bressler SB, Jacobs EF Jr, Shapiro J, Weber A, Albert DM. Maxillary ameloblastoma with orbital invasion. A clinicopathologic study. Ophthalmology 1985;92:710–3.
280. Levin PS, Dutton JJ. A 20-year series of orbital exenteration. Am J Ophthalmol 1991;112:496–501.

Metastatic Tumors

281. Goldberg RA, Rootman J, Cline RA. Tumors metastatic to the orbit: a changing picture. Surv Ophthalmol 1990;35:1–24.
282. Font RL, Ferry AP. Carcinoma metastatic to the eye and orbit. III. A clinicopathologic study of 28 cases metastatic to the orbit. Cancer 1976;38:1326–35.
283. Shields JA, Shields CL, Brotman HK, Carvalho C, Perez N, Eagle RC Jr. Cancer metastatic to the orbit: the 2000 Robert M. Curts Lecture. Ophthal Plast Reconstr Surg 2001;17:346–54.
284. Albert DM, Rubenstein RA, Scheie HG. Tumor metastasis to the eye. I. Incidence in 213 adult patients with generalized malignancy. Am J Ophthalmol 1967;63:723–6.
285. Bloch RS, Gartner S. The incidence of ocular metastatic carcinoma. Arch Ophthalmol 1971;85:673–5.
286. Amemiya T, Hayashida H, Dake Y. Metastatic orbital tumors in Japan: a review of the literature. Ophthalmic Epidemiol 2002;9:35–47.
287. Font RL, Ferry AP. Carcinoma metastatic to the eye and orbit: III. A clinicopathologic study of 28 cases metastatic to the orbit. Cancer 1976;38:1326–35.
288. Carriere VM, Karcioglu ZA, Apple DJ, Insler MS. A case of prostate carcinoma with bilateral orbital metastases and review of the literature. Ophthalmology 1982;89:402–6.
289. Orcutt JC, Char DH. Melanoma metastatic to the orbit. Ophthalmology 1988;95:1033–7.
290. Tijl J, Koornneef L, Eijpe A, Thomas L, Gonzalez DG, Veenhof C. Metastatic tumors to the orbit—management and prognosis. Graefes Arch Clin Exp Ophthalmol 1992;230:527–30.
291. Musarella MA, Chan HS, DeBoer G, Gallie BL. Ocular involvement in neuroblastoma: prognostic implications. Ophthalmology 1984;91:936–40.
292. Patrinely JR, Osborn AG, Anderson RL, Whiting AS. Computed tomographic features of nonthyroid extraocular muscle enlargement. Ophthalmology 1989;96:1038–47.
293. Hood CI, Font RL, Zimmerman LE. Metastatic mammary carcinoma in the eyelid with histiocytoid appearance. Cancer 1973;31:793–800.
294. Das DK, Das J, Kumar D, Bhatt NC, Banot K, Natarajan R. Leiomyosarcoma of the orbit: diagnosis of its recurrence by fine-needle aspiration cytology. Diagn Cytopathol 1992;8:609–13.
295. Dresner SC, Kennerdell JS, Dekker A. Fine needle aspiration biopsy of metastatic orbital tumors. Surv Ophthalmol 1983;27:397–8.
296. Winkler CF, Goodman GK, Eiferman R, Yam LT. Orbital metastasis from prostatic carcinoma. Identification by an immunoperoxidase technique. Arch Ophthalmol 1981;99:1406–8.
297. Glassburn JR, Klionsky M, Brady LW. Radiation therapy for metastatic disease involving the orbit. Am J Clin Oncol 1984;7:145–8.

Staging and Grading

298. American Joint Committee on Cancer. AJCC cancer staging manual, 5th ed. Philadelphia: Lippincott-Raven; 1997.

9 PATHOLOGIC EXAMINATION OF OCULAR SPECIMENS

The following is a set of guidelines for the handling, processing, gross examination, microscopic sampling, and reporting of surgical specimens from the ocular and adnexal tissues. Because of the text restrictions for in-depth coverage of the technical aspects of processing the eye, as well as to references on special techniques regarding staining, immunohistochemistry, electron microscopy, and molecular biology techniques especially adapted to ocular specimens.

THE GLOBE

Enucleation

Enucleation is the surgical procedure in which the globe and a portion of the optic nerve are removed from the orbit.

Fixation. The enucleated globe, obtained surgically or at autopsy, should be fixed promptly in 10 percent neutral-buffered formalin using a volume 20 times that of the eye (300 ml) to fix the ocular tissues properly (1). Generally, the globe must not be opened or punctured in any way and the fixative should never be injected into the vitreous body. Fixation is usually completed in 24 to 48 hours.

Before examination, the eye is washed in running tap water for 5 to 15 minutes and, preferably, placed in 60 to 70 percent ethanol for 1 to 2 hours. The purpose of immersion in alcohol is twofold: to render the eye more firm for cutting and to restore the red color of blood vessels.

Gross Examination. The orientation of the globe is determined by identification of extraocular muscle insertions, optic nerve, and other landmarks as illustrated in figure 9-1. The terms temporal and nasal are used in place of lateral and medial with reference to ocular anatomy. From the position and direction of the superior and inferior oblique muscle attachments, the specimen can be readily identified as a left or right globe and oriented properly. As seen in figure 9-1, the insertion of the superior oblique muscle, which is tendinous, corresponds roughly to the superior part of the eye, and its free end points towards the anterior nasal

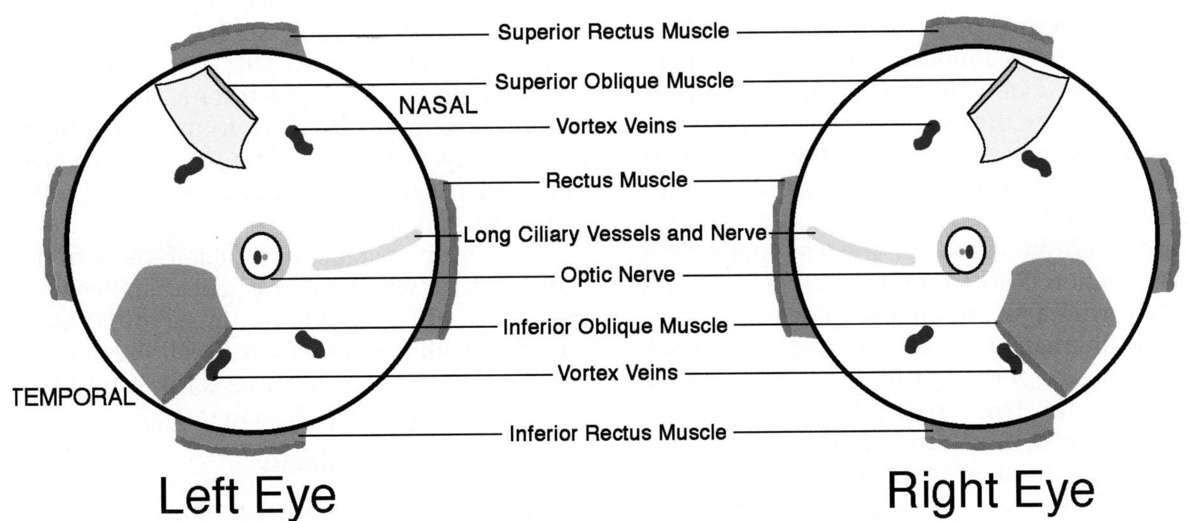

Figure 9-1

LANDMARKS FOR PROPER IDENTIFICATION OF LEFT AND RIGHT EYES

side where it is inserted in the trochlea. From the posterior view, the inferior oblique muscle has a fleshy muscular insertion temporally over the region of the macula, with its fibers running inferiorly. The optic nerve is surrounded on both sides by the short posterior ciliary arteries. Nasally, the bare sclera permits the visualization of the long posterior ciliary artery and nerve. Four or more vortex veins are seen piercing through the sclera in the four quadrants beyond the equator. The front view shows the cornea with an oblong appearance: the horizontal axis slightly longer (approximately +1 mm) than the vertical axis.

The measurements of the eye are described, the size recorded in millimeters (anteroposterior x horizontal x vertical). The length and diameter of the optic nerve are measured and a cross section of the optic nerve is obtained. Transillumination of the eye, together with data provided by the ophthalmic surgeon, permits the localization of the intraocular tumor. The normal eye transmits light well except in the ciliary body/iris region and at the site of the optic nerve and scleral insertions of the extraocular muscles. The shadow produced by the tumor is outlined on the sclera with a marking pencil. Samples from the vortex veins at the episcleral level are obtained, labeled, and submitted in separated cassettes for embedding.

The eye is usually opened with a razor blade from back to front. The plane of section should begin adjacent to the optic nerve and end about 1 mm inside the limbus through the peripheral cornea. The meridian plane of section (horizontal, vertical, or oblique) is dependent on where the tumor is located, so that the optic nerve, the larger cut area of the tumor, and the pupil are included in the same section (fig. 9-2). The central section is known as the pupil-optic nerve (PO) section (7 to 8 mm in thickness), and the other two fragments are the calottes.

An alternative to the conventional form is to cut the eye at the equator in a frontal or coronal plane (2). This is particularly useful for correlation of clinical funduscopic features and pathologic findings, and visualization of ciliary body tumors. The appearance of the internal structures are described with particular reference to the largest diameter, shape and height, and approximate volume of the tumor; degree of pigmentation, necrosis, and calcification; and the presence of rupture of Bruch membrane, or invasion of the retina, vitreous body, choroid and, particularly, the sclera. The distance of the tumor to the limbus anteriorly and to the optic disc posteriorly is also recorded.

In eyes removed for retinoblastoma, a sample of fresh tumor tissue may be required for genetic studies. Once the laterality has been determined, the location of the tumor is identified by transillumination. Before opening the eye, a sample from the distal line of surgical excision of the optic nerve is obtained and placed in a separate cassette for processing. Then a small window through the sclera overlying the tumor is opened to obtain a small sample of tumor. Retinoblastoma is a friable tumor; therefore, all maneuvers should be performed gently to minimize the artifactitious seeding of tumor cells on the sclera and surface of the optic nerve.

Embedding and cutting of globes may require special processing techniques. At least three different levels of the tumor are cut, one of them passing through the optic disc.

Excision

An excision of a small segment of the iris is known as an iridectomy. It may include the whole lesion or a sample of a larger lesion that extends to or from the ciliary body. Localized tumors of the ciliary body are removed, in general, by resecting the segment of the ciliary body containing the tumor; such a procedure is known as a cyclectomy. This procedure is usually extended to include the iris (iridocyclectomy), sclera (sclerocyclectomy), peripheral choroid (cyclochoroidectomy), and so on, when the ciliary body tumor extends to involve these adjacent structures.

Iridectomy specimens, similar to those of the conjunctiva (see below), are better handled with a piece of filter paper to minimize infolding of the tissue samples. Due to the small size of some specimens, the excised tissue is inked for identification of the surgical margins.

Biopsy

Direct biopsy of choroidal tumors may be performed with either a vitreous cutter using standard vitrectomy techniques or incisional microsurgical techniques from the vitreous side

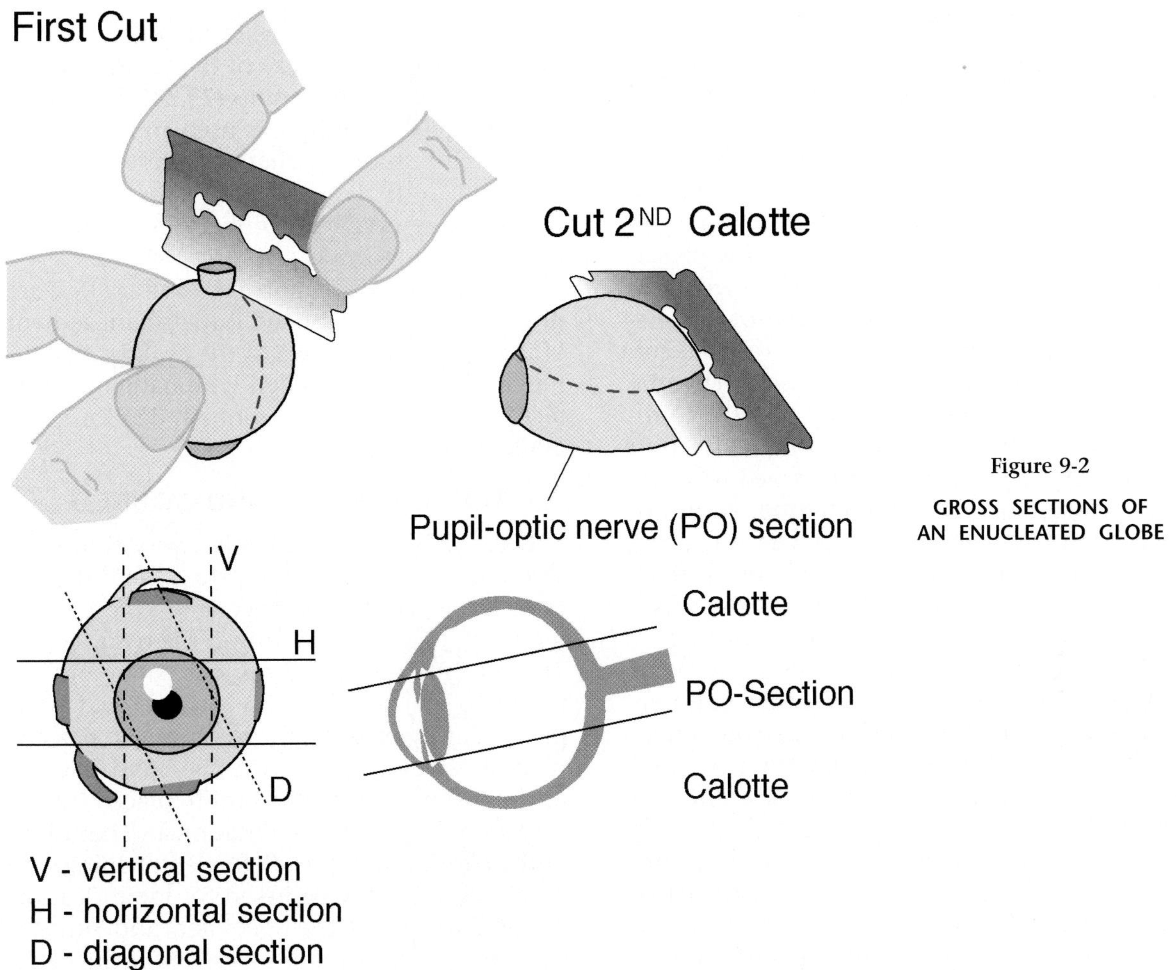

Figure 9-2

GROSS SECTIONS OF AN ENUCLEATED GLOBE

(2). Due to the size, processing of small biopsy samples should be handled with care by using special techniques (4–6).

Fine-Needle Aspiration Biopsy

Fine-needle aspiration biopsy (FNAB) of intraocular tumors of the anterior and posterior segments is indicated when an accurate diagnosis may affect management (7–12). This procedure should not be used in eyes suspected of harboring a retinoblastoma (13–15).

FNAB of the iris is performed with a tuberculin syringe and an sterile 26- to 30-gauge needle (16,17). The needle is inserted through the peripheral cornea and applied to the surface of the anterior chamber mass with the bevel down at 45° to 90°. Approximately 0.2 to 0.3 mL of fluid is obtained by gentle aspiration. Two or more slides for cytologic studies and immunohistochemistry can usually be obtained using the cytospin technique. For ciliary body tumors, the needle is inserted through the cornea and directed parallel to the visual axis towards the tumor without crossing the pupil, and outside the periphery of the lens (17). Posterior segment tumors are approached through the pars plana from the opposite site of the tumor (17,18). A small volume of culture media or transport fluid (RPMI) is aspirated before preparing the cytologic slides. Small fragments of tissue may be processed for conventional light microscopic examination (6).

All available material should be carefully examined as diagnostic cells may be few and irregularly distributed throughout the prepared slides (18). In addition to the microscopic description and conclusion, all reports must include a record of the number of slides examined.

Cytologic Samples

Vitreous specimens in cases of neoplasia are obtained to establish or rule out the presence of a primary vitreoretinal lymphoma. Surgical techniques include vitreous biopsy, vitrectomy, and chorioretinal biopsy. For vitreous biopsy, 0.5 to 1.0 mL of undiluted vitreous fluid is obtained by aspiration or vitrectomy. The preservation of cells is a critical step. The specimens should be either sent immediately for processing or preserved in the refrigerator (4°C) in culture medium (RPMI) until processing. The material received in the vitrectomy cassette is processed using the thin prep technique, fixed in 95 percent ethyl alcohol, and stained with the Papanicolaou or Diff-Quick method. Additionally, a cell block is obtained by centrifugation for 10 minutes at 2000 rpm. The cell block, fixed in 10 percent buffered formalin or Bouin's fixative, is embedded in paraffin for sectioning.

Aspiration of a drop of aqueous humor with a 30-gauge needle attached to a tuberculin syringe is useful in cases of leukemia or other neoplastic lesions that may simulate a pseudohypopyon or appear as cells in the anterior chamber (19,20). Smears from undiluted samples or cytospin preparations may be examined with conventional cytologic stains (Papanicolaou, Diff-Quick method), hematoxylin and eosin, as well as immunohistochemistry for diagnostic confirmation.

THE EYELIDS

Tumors of the eyelid are either biopsied or completely excised on the initial surgical approach. Cytologic evaluation of lid tumors is also possible (21,22). The handling, examination, and reporting of eyelid biopsies are similar to those of the skin elsewhere. Excision of eyelid tumors are full-thickness wedge resections that include the free margin of the eyelid, the internal conjunctival surface, and the outer skin surface. Proper orientation and embedding are required to identify the nasal and temporal surgical margins.

Sebaceous gland carcinoma of the eyelid may resemble other inflammatory and neoplastic lesions clinically. For this reason, it is convenient to save in 10 percent neutral-buffered formalin solution a representative sample of the lesion for frozen section evaluation and oil red-O staining for lipid. Frozen section evaluation of surgical margins in eyelid tumors is used to minimize the critical size of the excised tissue, preserving functional results (23,24). The Mohs' microsurgical technique is used and the surgical margins studied either after embedding or by using fresh tissue (25,26). This technique should be reserved for primary eyelid tumors that have a high risk of recurrence.

Lymph node dissection and examination are not routinely used in the initial management of malignant neoplasms of the eyelid and conjunctiva. Recently, guided lymphangiographic techniques have been recommended for high-grade tumors (27).

THE CONJUNCTIVA AND CARUNCLE

Because the conjunctiva is a very thin foldable tissue, it is convenient to adhere the excised tissue to a firm surface, like a piece of filter paper, to prevent curling of the tissue edges. The specimen is placed on lens paper and exposed to air for 15 to 30 seconds and then placed gently into a vial containing 10 percent neutral-buffered formalin. A free-hand diagram of the lesion or a marker suture placed by the surgeon is helpful for orientation and handling of the surgical margins. Before embedding, the whole sample may be inked for identification of the surfaces of the specimen and surgical margins. Surgical margins are either reported as noninfiltrated, infiltrated, or cannot be assessed with certainty, explaining the reason why not (28).

Multiples small biopsies of the conjunctiva are required for the staging of primary acquired melanosis and the management of melanoma of the conjunctiva arising from primary acquired melanosis. Map biopsies are particularly important in determining the extent of the disease, since clinically involved conjunctiva may appear normal (29). Each biopsy should be placed in a separate container and properly labeled. Any suspicious area on the conjunctiva and lid margins should be biopsied, and one or two biopsy samples obtained from each conjunctival quadrant, tarsal conjunctiva, fornices, and inner canthal structures (caruncle and plica semilunaris).

Proper handling of unfixed tissue from lymphoid lesions of the conjunctiva requires preservation in RPMI to perform flow cytometry for immunophenotyping and cytogenetic analysis.

THE ORBIT AND OPTIC NERVE

Most specimens from the orbit are either biopsy specimens or excised soft tissue tumors. In some instances, frozen sections are required for soft tissue tumors of the orbit. When the clinical diagnosis is uncertain and a lymphoid tumor cannot be ruled out, intraoperative examination of cytologic specimens prepared by the touch or the squash technique may provide a rapid diagnosis for further evaluation and management of the specimen.

The main indication for FNAB of the orbit is for lesions suspected to be metastatic (30–33). In addition, FNAB may be sufficient to confirm the diagnosis in patients with a previous history of systemic lymphoma (34). Because of the low morbidity and complications of FNAB of the orbit, this technique is also used as a primary diagnostic procedure in some solid and infiltrating, nonvascular orbital tumors.

Orbital exenteration is a procedure involving, in most cases, total removal of the orbital contents and the partial or total removal of the eyelids and conjunctiva. A variant technique, named eyelid-sparing exenteration, is used for malignant orbital tumors that do not involve the eyelid or conjunctiva.

Ocular tissues from exenteration specimens should be properly inked in order to provide information about the adequacy of the surgical margins. Orientation of the surgical specimen is generally facilitated by identification of suture markers made by the surgeon. The review of computerized tomography (CT) scans and magnetic resonance imaging (MRI) studies of the orbit at the time of grossing of the specimen is helpful to determine the precise location of the tumor. Gross examination includes measurement in the three dimensions. Usually, a vertical section, including the upper and lower eyelids and the globe, is processed together with additional samples from the surgical margins as well as a section of the posterior plane including the optic nerve (corresponding to the apex of the orbit).

THE LACRIMAL GLAND AND SAC

Pleomorphic adenoma of the lacrimal gland usually is removed in toto with an intact pseudocapsule, without a previous incisional biopsy to prevent recurrences. A diagnostic incisional biopsy specimen is considered in cases in which the clinical findings and imaging studies are suggestive of an infiltrative malignant epithelial tumor. The use of frozen section evaluation in the diagnosis of epithelial lacrimal gland tumors is limited, because very few surgeons are willing to perform extensive surgery on the basis of a frozen section diagnosis. The use of FNAB in the diagnosis of presumably malignant tumors of the lacrimal gland has increased during the last years (35). FNAB may be used for screening of presumed lymphoid tumors; however, a biopsy is required in order to determine whether the lesion is inflammation, reactive lymphoid hyperplasia, or malignant lymphoma (36).

Most excised lesions of the lacrimal sac represent chronic dacryocystitis. In the case of tumors, multiple step samples of the specimen are obtained and embedded for microscopic examination.

REFERENCES

1. Torczynski E. Preparation of ocular specimens for histopathologic examination. Ophthalmology 1981;88:1367–71.
2. Folberg R, Verdick R, Weingeist TA, Montague PR. The gross examination of eyes removed for choroidal and ciliary body melanomas. Ophthalmology 1986;93:1643–7.
3. Bechrakis NE, Foerster MH, Bornfeld N. Biopsy in indeterminate intraocular tumors. Ophthalmology 2002;109:235–42.
4. Engel H, de la Cruz ZC, Jimenez-Abalahin LD, Green WR, Michels RG. Cytopreparatory techniques for eye fluid specimens obtained by vitrectomy. Acta Cytol 1982;26:551–60.
5. Chess J, Sebag J, Tolentino FL, et al. Pathologic processing of vitrectomy specimens. A comparison of pathologic findings with celloidin bag and cytocentrifugation preparation of 102 vitrectomy specimens. Ophthalmology 1983;90:1560–4.
6. LoRusso FJ, Font RL. Use of agar in ophthalmic pathology: a technique to improve the handling and diagnosis of temporal artery biopsies, subfoveal membranes, lens capsules, and other ocular tissues. Ophthalmology 1999;106:2106–8.
7. Augsburger JJ, Shields JA. Fine needle aspiration biopsy of solid intraocular tumors: indications, instrumentation and techniques. Ophthalmic Surg 1984;15:34–40.
8. Davey CC, Deery AR. Through the eye, a needle: intraocular fine needle aspiration biopsy. Trans Ophthalmol Soc U K 1986;105(Pt 1):78–83.
9. Augsburger JJ. Fine needle aspiration biopsy of suspected metastatic cancers to the posterior uvea. Trans Am Ophthalmol Soc 1988;86:499–560.
10. Char DH, Miller TR, Crawford JB. Cytopathologic diagnosis of benign lesions simulating choroidal melanomas. Am J Ophthalmol 1991;112:70–5.
11. Char DH, Miller T. Accuracy of presumed uveal melanoma diagnosis before alternative therapy. Br J Ophthalmol 1995;79:692–6.
12. El-Harazi SM, Kellaway J, Font RL. Melanocytoma of the ciliary body diagnosed by fine-needle aspiration biopsy. Diagn Cytopathol 2000;22:394–7.
13. Glasgow BJ, Brown HH, Zargoza AM, Foos RY. Quantitation of tumor seeding from fine needle aspiration of ocular melanomas. Am J Ophthalmol 1988;105:538–46.
14. Karcioglu ZA. Fine needle aspiration biopsy (FNAB) for retinoblastoma. Retina 2002;22:707–10.
15. O'Hara BJ, Ehya H, Shields JA, Augsburger JJ, Shields CL, Eagle RC Jr. Fine needle aspiration biopsy in pediatric ophthalmic tumors and pseudotumors. Acta Cytol 1993;37:125–30.
16. Grossniklaus HE. Fine-needle aspiration biopsy of the iris. Arch Ophthalmol 1992;110:969–76.
17. Shields JA, Shields CL, Ehya H, Eagle RC Jr, De Potter P. Fine-needle aspiration biopsy of suspected intraocular tumors. The 1992 Urwick Lecture. Ophthalmology 1993;100:1677–84.
18. Cohen VM, Dinakaran S, Parsons MA, Rennie IG. Transvitreal fine needle aspiration biopsy: the influence of intraocular lesion size on diagnostic biopsy result. Eye 2001;15(Pt 2):143–7.
19. Novakovic P, Kellie SJ, Taylor D. Childhood leukemia: relapse in the anterior segment of the eye. Br J Ophthalmol 1989;73:354–9.
20. O'Keefe JS, Sippy BD, Martin DF, Holden JT, Grossniklaus HE. Anterior chamber infiltrates associated with systemic lymphoma: report of two cases and review of the literature. Ophthalmology 2002;109:253–7.
21. Jakobiec FA, Chattock A. Aspiration cytodiagnosis of lid tumors. Arch Ophthalmol 1979;97:1907–10.
22. Arora R, Rewari R, Betheria SM. Fine needle aspiration cytology of eyelid tumors. Acta Cytol 1990;34:227–32.
23. Margo CE, Waltz K. Basal cell carcinoma of the eyelid and periocular skin. Surv Ophthalmol 1993;38:169–92.
24. Reifler DM, Hornblass A. Squamous cell carcinoma of the eyelid. Surv Ophthalmol 1986;30: 349–65.
25. Mohs FE. Chemosurgical treatment of cancer of the eyelid. A microscopically controlled method of excision. Arch Ophthalmol 1948;39: 43–59.
26. Leshin B, Yeatts P, Anscher M, Montano G, Dutton JJ. Management of periocular basal cell carcinoma. Mohs' micrographic surgery versus radiotherapy. Surv Ophthalmol 1993;38:193–212.
27. Amato M, Esmaeli B, Ahmadi MA, et al. Feasibility of preoperative lymphoscintigraphy for identification of sentinel lymph nodes in patients with conjunctival and periocular skin malignancies. Ophthal Plast Reconstr Surg 2003; 19:102–6.

28. Buus DR, Tse DT, Folberg R, Buuns DR. Microscopically controlled excision of conjunctival squamous cell carcinoma. Am J Ophthalmol 1994;117:97–102.
29. Margo CE, Grossniklaus HE. Intraepithelial sebaceous neoplasia without underlying invasive carcinoma. Surv Ophthalmol 1995;39:293–301.
30. Kennerdell JS, Dekker A, Johnson BL, Dubois PJ. Fine-needle aspiration biopsy. Its use in orbital tumors. Arch Ophthalmol 1979;97:1315–7.
31. Midena E, Segato T, Piermarocchi S, Boccato P. Fine needle aspiration biopsy in ophthalmology. Surv Ophthalmol 1985;29:410–22.
32. Zajdela A, de Maublanc MA, Schlienger P, Haye C. Cytologic diagnosis of orbital and periorbital palpable tumors using fine-needle sampling without aspiration. Diagn Cytopathol 1986;2:17–20.
33. Watts P, Sullivan S, Davies S, Rao N, Stock D. Electromyography and computed tomography scan-guided fine needle aspiration biopsy of discrete extraocular muscle metastases. J AAPOS 2001;5:333–5.
34. Nassar DL, Raab SS, Silverman JF, Kennerdell JS, Sturgis CD. Fine-needle aspiration for the diagnosis of orbital hematolymphoid lesions. Diagn Cytopathol 2000;23:314–7.
35. Sturgis CD, Silverman JF, Kennerdell JS, Raab SS. Fine-needle aspiration for the diagnosis of primary epithelial tumors of the lacrimal gland and ocular adnexa. Diagn Cytopathol 2001;24:86–9.
36. Jeffrey PB, Cartwright D, Atwater SK, Char DH, Miller TR. Lacrimal gland lymphoma: a cytomorphologic and immunophenotypic study. Diagn Cytopathol 1995;12:215–22.

Index*

*Numbers in boldface indicate table and figure pages.

C

D

E

F

K

L

M

N

O

P

R

V

W

X

Y

Z